CONDITIONS IN OCCUPATIONAL THERAPY

EFFECT ON
OCCUPATIONAL
PERFORMANCE

FIFTH EDITION

CONDITIONS IN OCCUPATIONAL THERAPY

EFFECT ON OCCUPATIONAL PERFORMANCE

BEN J. ATCHISON, PhD, OTR/L, FAOTA

Professor and Chair
Department of Occupational Therapy
Western Michigan University
Kalamazoo, Michigan

DIANE POWERS DIRETTE, PhD, OTL, FAOTA

Professor
Department of Occupational Therapy
Western Michigan University
Kalamazoo, Michigan

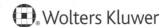

Philadelphia • Baltimore • New York • London
Buenos Aires • Hong Kong • Sydney • Tokyo

Acquisitions Editor: Michael Nobel
Product Manager: Linda G. Francis
Marketing Manager: Shauna Kelley
Production Project Manager: David Saltzberg
Design Coordinator: Holly McLaughlin
Art Director: Jennifer Clements
Manufacturing Coordinator: Margie Orzech
Production Service: SPi Global

5th Edition

Library of Congress Cataloging-in-Publication Data
  Names: Atchison, Ben, editor. | Dirette, Diane Powers, editor.
  Title: Conditions in occupational therapy: effect on occupational performance / [edited by] Ben J. Atchison,
  Diane Powers Dirette.
  Description: Fifth edition. | Philadelphia : Wolters Kluwer, [2017] | Includes bibliographical references and index.
  Identifiers: LCCN 2016018266 | ISBN 9781496332219
  Subjects: | MESH: Occupational Therapy | Case Reports
  Classification: LCC RM735 | NLM WB 555 | DDC 615.8/515—dc23 LC record available at https://lccn.loc.gov/2016018266

To my wife, Marcia, my best friend

—*Ben J. Atchison*

To the Mexican Monday Crew; Claire, Madeleine, Jayce, Jordan, and Dave. Thank you for the love, laughter, and support that make Mondays the best day of the week!

—*Diane Powers Dirette*

Contributors

Ben J. Atchison, PhD, OTR/L, FAOTA
Professor and Chair
Department of Occupational Therapy
Western Michigan University
Kalamazoo, Michigan

Shirley Blanchard, PhD, OTR/L, ABDA, FAOTA, FHDR
Associate Professor
Department of Occupational Therapy
Creighton University
Omaha, Nebraska

Ann Chapleau, DHS, OTRL
Associate Professor
Department of Occupational Therapy
Western Michigan University
Kalamazoo, Michigan

Gerry E. Conti, PhD, OTRL, FAOTA
Assistant Professor
Occupational Therapy Program
Wayne State University
Detroit, Michigan

Joan Ziegler Delahunt, OTD, MS, OTR/L
Rockhurst University
Kansas City, Missouri

Diane Powers Dirette, PhD, OTL, FAOTA
Professor
Department of Occupational Therapy
Western Michigan University
Kalamazoo, Michigan

Rosanne DiZazzo-Miller, PhD, DrOT, OTRL, CDP
Assistant Professor Occupational Therapy Program
Wayne State University
Detroit, Michigan

Kathryn Ellsworth, MA, CCC-SLP
Speech-Language Pathologist
St. Paul, Minnesota

Joanne Phillips Estes, PhD, OTR/L
Assistant Professor
Department of Occupational Therapy
Xavier University
Cincinnati, Ohio

Jennifer L. Forgach, MS, OTR/L
Forgach-Smith
Team Rehabilitation
Bingham Farms, Michigan

Joyce Fraker, MS, OTR/L
Occupational Therapist
Physical Medicine and Rehabilitation Service
VA Ann Arbor Healthcare System
Ann Arbor, Michigan

Cynthia A. Grapczynski, EdD, OTR, FAOTA
Professor and Chair
Occupational Science and Therapy Department
Grand Valley State University
Allendale, Michigan

Jennifer Harrison, PhD, MSW
Faculty Specialist II
School of Social Work
Western Michigan University
Kalamazoo, Michigan

Nancy Hock, OTR/L, CHT
Faculty Specialist II and Site Coordinator
Department of Occupational Therapy
Western Michigan University
Grand Rapids, Michigan

Heather Javaherian-Dysinger, OTD, OTR/L
Associate Professor and MOT Program Director
Department of Occupational Therapy
Loma Linda University
Loma Linda, California

Reese Martin, MS, OTR/L
Instructor
Department of Occupational Therapy
Western Michigan University
Kalamazoo, Michigan

Laura V. Miller, MS, OTR/L, CDI, CDRS
Private Practitioner, Occupational Therapy
Certified Driver Rehabilitation Specialist, Driver's
Rehabilitation Center of Michigan
Livonia, Michigan

Brandon G. Morkut, MS, OTR/L
Adjunct Faculty
Department of Occupational Therapy
Western Michigan University
Kalamazoo, Michigan

Timothy M. Mullen, PhD, OTR/L, CHT
Director of Clinical Operations
Orthopedic Physicians of Alaska
Anchorage, Alaska

Shelley Mulligan, PhD, OTR/L, FAOTA
Associate Professor
Department of Occupational Therapy
University of New Hampshire
Durham, New Hampshire

Linda M. Olson, PhD, OTRL
Chair and Assistant Professor
Department of Occupational Therapy
College of Health Sciences
Rush University
Chicago, Illinois

Rebecca Ozelie, DHS, OTR/L, BCPR
Assistant Professor and Academic Fieldwork
Coordinator
Department of Occupational Therapy
Rush University
Chicago, Illinois

Sharon L. Pavlovich, MAM, COTA/L
Assistant Professor
Department of Occupational Therapy
Loma Linda University
Loma Linda, California

Emily Raphael-Greenfield, EdD, OTRL, FAOTA
Assistant Professor
Programs in Occupational Therapy
Columbia University Medical Center
New York, New York

Mylene Schriner, PhD, OTR/L
Chair and Associate Professor of Occupational
Therapy Education
Rockhurst University
Kansas City, Missouri

Michelle A. Suarez, PhD, OTR/L
Associate Professor
Department of Occupational Therapy
Western Michigan University
Kalamazoo, Michigan

Suzänne Fleming Taylor, PhD, MBA/HCM, OTR/L
Cancer Rehabilitation, Clinician IV
Adjunct Instructor, Department of Occupational
Therapy
Virginia Commonwealth University Medical Center
Richmond, Virginia

Michael J. Urban, MS, OTR/L, MBA, CEAS, CWCS
Department of Veterans Affairs
Healthcare System of Connecticut
West Haven, Connecticut

Christine K. Urish, PhD, OTR/L, BCMH, FAOTA
Professor
Department of Occupational Therapy
St. Ambrose University
Davenport, Iowa

Amy Wagenfeld, PhD, OTR/L, SCEM, FAOTA
Assistant Professor
Department of Occupational Therapy
Western Michigan University
Kalamazoo, Michigan

Andrea L. Washington, BS, OTR/L
Clinical Occupational Therapy Specialist
Inpatient Rehabilitation
Children's Hospital of Michigan
Detroit, Michigan

Mary Steichen Yamamoto, MS, OTL
Occupational Therapist
Private Practice
Ann Arbor, Michigan

Jayne Yatczak, PhD, OTRL
Assistant Professor and Director, Occupational
Therapy Program
Eastern Michigan University
Ypsilanti, Michigan

Preface

In this fifth edition of *Conditions in Occupational Therapy: Effect on Occupational Performance*, we continue with the approach used in previous editions which includes common conditions seen by occupational therapists as published in the executive summary of the most recent practice analysis published by the National Board for Certification of Occupational Therapists (NBCOT, 2012). The book is designed to facilitate the teaching and learning of conditions from an occupational therapy perspective. We honor Dr. Ruth Hansen, Professor Emeritus, Eastern Michigan University, for her significant contributions as the founding coeditor of this textbook in which she created the design for analysis of conditions using an "occupational therapy way of thinking." Dr. Hansen's original idea continues to hold forth in Chapter 1, *Thinking Like an OT*, which begins with an overview and relevance of the philosophy and values of occupational therapy in relation to understanding a given condition and its impact on occupational performance.

In this new edition, we organized the conditions into units including pediatric, mental, and physical conditions. Each chapter is consistent in its structure to include an opening case, definition and descriptions, incidence and prevalence, signs and symptoms, course and prognosis, medical/surgical management, and impact on occupational performance, followed by two case illustrations. We continue to incorporate the language of the *Occupational Therapy Practice Framework*, third edition (OTPF) where relevant, as this is the most current "language of the profession."

Following a national review of faculty who have used the fourth edition of our textbook and their helpful input, new content has been included. We are pleased to announce new chapters in this edition. These include Obsessive Compulsive and Related Disorders, Somatic Symptoms and Related Disorders, Feeding and Eating Disorders, Sensory Processing Disorders, Substance Related and Addictive Disorders, Personality Disorders, Cancer, and Obesity. Where relevant, chapters have included updates published in the *Diagnostic and Statistical Manual of Mental Disorders*, fifth edition (American Psychiatric Association, 2013). As always, each chapter has incorporated the most recent information available. The notion that occupational therapists treat diagnoses is on ongoing point of discussion and debate. As emphasized in Chapter 1, we are mindful of the importance of "person first" philosophy that a person is more than a sum of his or her diagnosis. Simultaneously, it is essential that occupational therapists understand the distinct client factors of a given condition that impact a person's ability to regain function necessary to resume occupational roles.

Each chapter in this edition provides the authors' interpretation of the effects of the condition on occupational performance and is not necessarily all inclusive. Our goal is that the information will motivate occupational therapy students to expand their knowledge and understanding of the given condition. We expect that each chapter is a starting point for discussion and analysis of the condition which then will lead to the development of effective intervention planning.

Ben J. Atchison
Diane Powers Dirette

American Psychiatric Association. (2013). *Diagnostic and statistical manual of mental disorders* (5th ed.). Washington, DC: Author.

National Board for Certification of Occupational Therapists. (2012). *Practice analysis of the occupational therapist registered: Executive summary*. Gaithersburg, MD: Author.

To review key terms and their definitions, visit http://thePoint.lww.com/Atchison5e, and use the access code on the inside front cover of this book. Resources for instructors include a test generator, PowerPoint presentations, and an image bank.

Contents

1

Thinking Like an OT

Diane Powers Dirette and Ben J. Atchison

KEY TERMS

Altruism
Client factors
Context and
    environment
Core values
Equality
Evidence-based practice
Freedom
Justice
Occupations
Performance patterns
Performance skills
Personalized medicine
Person-first language
Philosophical
    assumptions
Practice Framework
Prudence
Truth

It is more important to know what kind of person has the disease than what kind of disease the person has.

—Sir William Osler (Address at Johns Hopkins University, February 1905)

Lindsey is finishing her course work in occupational therapy and is now beginning her first level II fieldwork experience. Throughout her education, she has learned the importance of evidence-based practice to guide her treatment decisions. Her challenge now is to develop her clinical reasoning skills to merge the science she has learned with the art of practice. To achieve this, she must understand the person's diagnosis, analyze the person's unique set of problems based on the person's individual characteristics, and determine the impact on occupational performance. The first step of this process is the referrals she receives. Each referral gives her some basic information about the person including the person's diagnosis. Her job is to decide what to do next.

How does a student learn to correlate general information about a diagnosis with the needs of a particular person and to identify the problems that require occupational therapy intervention? How does a staff therapist set priorities for problems and decide which require immediate attention? How much problem identification can be done before the therapist actually sees the patient? How does a supervisor know when a student or therapist is doing a "good job" of screening referrals and anticipating the dysfunction that the patient might be experiencing? These are precursors to the actual intervention process and are essential to effective and efficient clinical reasoning (Benamy, 1996).

The clinical reasoning procedure used by each health care professional is somewhat different. The information that is the main focus of intervention for a speech therapist will differ from that of a psychologist or a nurse. The basic tenet of the occupational therapy profession is that practitioners gather and use information to help people function in their daily activities. Such data gathering and analysis provide the therapist with the foundation for a treatment plan through a prioritized list of anticipated problems or dysfunctions for an individual.

To comprehend the unique aspects of occupational therapy requires an understanding of the core values, philosophical assumptions, and domain of concern of the profession, as well as the language that is used to communicate information clearly and precisely.

CORE VALUES OF OCCUPATIONAL THERAPY

The core values of occupational therapy are set forth in the document "Core Values and Attitudes of Occupational Therapy Practice" (Kanny, 1993). Seven have been identified: altruism, dignity, equality, freedom, justice, truth, and prudence.

1. *Altruism* is the unselfish concern for the welfare of others. This concept is reflected in actions and attitudes of commitment, caring, dedication, responsiveness, and understanding.
2. *Dignity* emphasizes the importance of valuing the inherent worth and uniqueness of each person. This value is demonstrated by an attitude of empathy and respect for self and others.
3. *Equality* requires that all individuals be perceived as having the same fundamental human rights and opportunities. This value is demonstrated by an attitude of fairness and impartiality.
4. *Freedom* allows the individual to exercise choice and to demonstrate independence, initiative, and self-direction.
5. *Justice* places value on the upholding of such moral and legal principles as fairness, equity, truthfulness, and objectivity.
6. *Truth* requires that we be faithful to facts and reality. Truthfulness or veracity is demonstrated by being accountable, honest, forthright, accurate, and authentic in our attitudes and actions.
7. *Prudence* is the ability to govern and discipline oneself through the use of reason. To be prudent is to value judiciousness, discretion, vigilance, moderation, care, and circumspection in the management of one's affairs, to temper extremes, make judgments, and respond on the basis of intelligent reflection and rational thought (Kanny, 1993).

These values are the foundation of the belief system that occupational therapists (OTs) use as a moral guide when making clinical decisions.

PHILOSOPHICAL ASSUMPTIONS

The philosophical assumptions of the profession guide OTs in providing client-centered therapy that meets the needs of the client and society. These assumptions express our basic beliefs about the client and the context in which the client functions (Mosey, 1996). These assumptions are as follows:

- Each individual has a right to a meaningful existence: the right to live in surroundings that are safe, supportive, comfortable, and over which he or she has some control; to make decisions for himself or herself; to be productive; to experience pleasure and joy; and to love and be loved.
- Each individual is influenced by the biological and social nature of the species.
- Each individual can only be understood within the context of his or her family, friends, community, and membership in various cultural groups.
- Each individual has the need to participate in a variety of social roles and to have periodic relief from participation.
- Each individual has the right to seek his or her potential through personal choice, within the context of accepted social constraints.
- Each individual is able to reach his or her potential through purposeful interaction with the human and nonhuman environment.
- Occupational therapy is concerned with promoting functional interdependence through interactions directed toward facilitating participation in major social roles (occupational performance) and development of biological, cognitive, psychological, and social components (client factors) fundamental to such roles.
- The extent to which intervention is focused on the context, on the areas of occupational performance, or on the client factors depends on the needs of the particular individual at any given time.

PERSONALIZED MEDICINE

The core values and philosophical assumption of the profession of OT lead practitioners of OT to a focus on personalized medicine. According to Burke, Trinidad, and Press (2014), "personalized medicine is best understood as a comprehensive process to determine the best health care options for a particular patient, deriving from a partnership between patient and clinician. This approach offers the opportunity to weigh personal values and preferences as well as clinical findings" (p. 196). In addition, Topol (2014) defines personalized medicine as the tailoring of medical treatments to the individual characteristics of each patient with a focus on the individual as the source of medical data and as the driver of health care.

The core values, especially dignity, equality, and freedom, are the profession's moral guide to personalized medicine. They guide us to value differences, to treat people equally despite those differences, and to allow individuals to make their own choices based on differing perspectives and preferences.

The philosophical assumptions summarize the OT profession's basic beliefs about focusing on the rights and preferences of individuals relative to their biological and social environments. In addition, the philosophical assumptions help guide practitioners to form a partnership with each individual to determine the focus of the intervention. Each of these concepts form a practice in which personalized medicine is an essential element.

Whereas the primary purpose of this book is to describe the potential impact of a condition on occupational performance, the descriptions should not be considered prescriptive or exhaustive. It is necessary to understand common facts of these conditions, including etiology, basic pathogenesis, commonly observed signs and symptoms, and precautions. However, it is equally important to recognize that the effects of a condition on occupational well-being will also be dependent on contextual factors such as age, developmental stage, health status, and the physical, social, and cultural environment (Dunn, Brown, & McGuigan, 1994). Rather than viewing an individual as a diagnostic entity, as a condition, or as the sum of biological cells, the treatment must be personalized.

LANGUAGE

Although many language systems and mechanisms are available, we will discuss language from two perspectives. First is a philosophical discussion of using person-first language. Second is the use of the *Occupational Therapy Practice Framework: Domain and Process, Third Edition* (AOTA, 2014) that presents the professional language and the occupational therapy domain of concern.

■ Person-First Language

In many cases, the literature and the media, both popular and professional, describe a person with a given condition as the condition—the arthritic, the C.P. kid, the schizophrenic, the alcoholic, the burn victim, the mentally disabled. All of these terms label people as members of a large group rather than as a unique individual. The use of person-first language requires that the person be identified first and the disease used as a secondary descriptor. For example, a woman, who is a physicist, is active in her church and has arthritis; the fourth grade boy, who is a good speller, loves baseball and has cerebral palsy. The condition does not and should not be the primary identity of any person.

Consider the following: a father is introducing his son to his coworkers. Which of the following is the best introduction?

"Hey, everyone, this is my disabled son, John."

"Hey, everyone, this is my son, John, who is disabled and loves soccer and video games."

"Hey, everyone, this is my son, John. He loves soccer and video games."

Of course, the third statement is the best choice. Yet it is common when describing a person who has a disability to emphasize the disability first. The consequence is a labeling process. "Although such shorthand language is commonplace in clinics and medical records, it negates the individuality of the person. Each of us is a person, with a variety of traits that can be used to describe aspects of our personality, behavior, and function. To use a disease or condition as the adjective preceding the identifying noun negates the multiple dimensions that make the person a unique individual" (Hansen, 1998).

THE OCCUPATIONAL THERAPY PRACTICE FRAMEWORK

The official language for the profession of occupational therapy was revised in 2014 and presented in a document titled the *Occupational Therapy Practice Framework: Domain and Process, Third Edition* (AOTA, 2014). The Practice Framework outlines the language and constructs that describe the occupational therapy profession's domain of concern. The domain defines the area of human activity to which the occupational therapy process is applied. The process facilitates engagement in occupation to support participation in life. The specific aspects of the domain are outlined in the language of the Practice Framework.

The Framework is organized into five aspects— occupations, client factors, performance skills, performance patterns, and context and environment. **Occupations** are various kinds of life activities in which individuals, groups, or populations engage. Occupations include activities of daily living, instrumental activities of daily living, rest and sleep, education, work, and play, leisure, and social participation. **Client factors** are values, beliefs, and spirituality, the body functions, and the body structures that reside within the person. These client factors influence the person's participation on occupations. **Performance skills** are observable elements of action that have an implicit functional purpose. These skills are separated into the categories of motor skills, process skills, and social interaction skills. **Performance patterns** are the habits, routines, roles, and rituals used by the person in the process of engaging in occupations or activities. These patterns may enhance or hinder occupational performance. **Context and environment** refers to a variety of interrelated conditions that are within and surrounding the person. Those conditions include cultural, personal, temporal, and virtual contexts. Environments are the physical and social conditions that surround the person (Table 1.1).

Each of these aspects has a relationship and influence on the others. The outcome is, of course, the ability to function and engage in occupations. Although at a given time you may focus on an occupation or client factors, the ultimate concern is whether the individual is able to function in daily life. For example, a therapist may evaluate a person's attention span, but not in isolation. Attention span is evaluated within the realm of the performance patterns and context of the person— the attention span required to work on an assembly line, to drive a car, to learn a card game, or to conduct a business meeting.

Once a therapist knows the diagnosis and age of the person, he or she can use this Practice Framework to examine systematically the deficits that occur in the client factors, as well as how these particular deficits can and do alter the person's ability to complete functional activities relevant to occupations. In other instances, the therapist may focus primarily on the occupation or the context, without paying much attention to the underlying client factors that influence the occupational performance. Definitions of all terms are provided in the Glossary at the back of the book.

TABLE **1.1** Occupational Therapy Practice Domains				
Occupations	**Client Factors**	**Performance Skills**	**Performance Patterns**	**Context and Environment**
Activities of daily living	Values, beliefs, and spirituality	Motor skills	Habits	Cultural
Instrumental activities of daily living	Body functions	Process skills	Routines	Personal
Rest and sleep	Body structures	Social interaction skills	Roles	Temporal
Education			Rituals	Virtual
Work				Physical
Play and leisure				Social
Social participation				

EVIDENCE-BASED PRACTICE

There has been a call to action in the health professions to practice health care based on evidence of the effectiveness of each treatment approach (Gutman, 2010). High levels of evidence are based on studies that compare groups of people, usually with similar conditions. Evidence, especially high levels of evidence, on which to base one's practice, however, might be limited (Dirette, Rozich, & Viau, 2009). First, it is limited by an insufficient number of resources to support specific treatment approaches for specific conditions. Second, it might be limited by the fact that groups of people with "average" results do not always represent the unique situation of the person with whom the therapist is working.

Therefore, while we support the idea of evidence-based practice in general, there is clearly a need for therapists to develop clinical reasoning skills that will not only help them decide which evidence to use with people who have particular conditions but also help them decide what to do with the unique individual with whom they are working. Understanding the condition with which the individual presents is often the first step in the clinical reasoning process. This textbook provides information about common conditions seen by OTs and provides the first steps in the clinical reasoning process by providing ideas about the potential impact on occupational performance.

FRAMEWORK OF THIS TEXTBOOK

As an instructional tool, this book provides an opportunity to examine each condition closely. The reader is urged to use the information as a springboard for further study of the conditions included here and the many other conditions that OTs encounter in practice. The analysis of the impact on occupational performance for a particular condition is dynamic, and the identification of the most important areas of dysfunction and, therefore, treatment will vary from practitioner to practitioner. In addition, factors such as secondary health problems, age, gender, family background, and culture contribute greatly to the development of a unique occupational performance profile for each individual served.

The occupational performance approach to the identification of dysfunction described in this book can be used to examine the effects of any condition on a person's daily life. This process will enable the therapist to identify and set a priority for problems in occupational performance, which, in turn, will serve as the foundation for creating an effective intervention plan.

REFERENCES

American Occupational Therapy Association. (2014). Occupational therapy practice framework: Domain and process, 3rd edition. *American Journal of Occupational Therapy, 68*(Suppl. 1), S1–S51. Retrieved from http://dx.doi.org/10.5014/ajot.2014.682006

Benamy, B. C. (1996). *Developing clinical reasoning skills*. San Antonio, TX: Therapy Skill Builders.

Burke, W., Trinidad, S. B., & Press, N. A. (2014). Essential elements of personalized medicine. *Urologic Oncology: Seminars and Original Investigations, 32*, 193–197. Retrieved from http://dx.doi.org/10.1016/j.urolonc.2013.09.002

Dirette, D., Rozich, A., & Viau, S. (2009). Is there enough evidence for evidence-based practice in occupational therapy? *American Journal of Occupational Therapy, 63*, 782–786. Retrieved from http://dx.doi.org/10.5014/ajot.63.6.782

Dunn, W., Brown, C., & McGuigan, A. (1994). Ecology of human performance: A framework for considering the effect of context. *American Journal of Occupational Therapy, 48*(7), 595–607.

Gutman, S. A. (2010). From the desk of the editor: AJOT publication priorities. *American Journal of Occupational Therapy, 64*, 679–681. Retrieved from http://dx.doi.org/10.5014/ajot.2010.064501

Hansen, R. A. (1998). Ethical implications. In J. Hinojosa & P. Kramer (Eds.), *Evaluation: Obtaining and interpreting data*. Bethesda, MD: AOTA.

Kanny, E. (1993). Core values and attitudes of occupational therapy practice. *American Journal of Occupational Therapy, 47*, 1085–1086.

Mosey, A. C. (1996). *Applied scientific inquiry in the health professions: An epistemological orientation* (2nd ed.). Bethesda, MD: American Occupational Therapy Association.

Topol, E. J. (2014). Individualized medicine from pre-womb to tomb. *Cell, 157*, 241–253. Retrieved from http://dx.doi.org/10.1016/j.cell.2014.02.012

Pediatric Conditions

The Pediatric Conditions Unit includes the most common conditions that children have who are treated by occupational therapists as determined by the National Board of Certification in Occupational Therapy. These chapters focus on conditions that are typically diagnosed in childhood, but many of them affect people throughout their lifespan. Each chapter provides information about the etiology, incidence and prevalence, signs and symptoms, course and prognosis, diagnosis, medical/surgical management, and impact on occupational performance of these conditions. Case illustrations are used to provide examples of lives affected by the condition. The conditions included in this unit are the following:

Chapter 2: Cerebral Palsy
Chapter 3: Autism Spectrum Disorders
Chapter 4: Intellectual Disability
Chapter 5: Muscular Dystrophy
Chapter 6: Attention Deficit Disorder/ADHD
Chapter 7: Sensory Processing Disorder

2

Cerebral Palsy

Mary Steichen Yamamoto

A couple who had been trying to conceive a child for several years were thrilled when a family friend asked if they would be interested in adopting a baby girl that had just been born to a young unmarried woman in her church. The baby was born 6 weeks early and her weight was 4 lb, but she appeared to be healthy. After initiating the paperwork for a private adoption, they brought the baby home and named her Jill. By the time of Jill's 6-month well-baby visit, her parents had become concerned. She appeared to be a bright baby who smiled and cooed and enjoyed reaching for and playing with toys, but her legs seemed stiff and she was not yet rolling over. They spoke with their family doctor about their concerns, but he assured them that Jill was developing normally and they had nothing to be concerned about. By the time of Jill's 9-month well-baby visit, her parents' concerns were only growing. Jill was still not sitting up and had not yet learned to roll over or crawl. Her doctor decided to refer Jill to the county early intervention program for a developmental assessment. Jill was assessed by the early intervention team consisting of an occupational therapist, physical therapist, and speech and language pathologist. The occupational therapist noted some mildly increased tone and incoordination in her upper extremities and a 2- to 3-month delay in fine motor and self-help skills. The physical therapist noted that Jill had hypertonicity and retained primitive reflexes in her lower extremities, which was causing significant delay in the acquisition of gross motor skills. The speech and language therapist found Jill's cognitive, language, and social skills to be at age level. The team suggested to the parents that they have a pediatric neurologist assess Jill, as she was demonstrating some of the signs and symptoms of cerebral palsy. Both the occupational and physical therapist recommended that therapy services begin as soon as possible. An IFSP (Individualized Family Service Plan) was developed at a subsequent meeting, and Jill began receiving weekly physical and occupational therapy services.

Jill's parents took her to a pediatric neurologist who diagnosed her with spastic diplegia, a type of cerebral palsy. Her parents were initially overwhelmed and devastated by the diagnosis. The next year was very difficult as they grieved the loss of so many dreams that they had for Jill and faced so much uncertainty about her future. They waded through an array of possible therapy approaches and medical and surgical interventions that were recommended trying to decide which would be right for Jill and their family. They struggled to find time to work on home exercises that had been prescribed for Jill. The strain became so great that they even separated for a period but eventually reconciled. By the time Jill turned 3 years old, she was walking with a walker and able to sit in a chair independently, although she needed assistance with changing positions. She was feeding herself but not yet dressing herself. They enrolled her in a preschool special education classroom where she received therapy services. By kindergarten, Jill was in a regular education classroom with a paraeducator for safety and support. Jill was a happy child, who had many friends and did well academically. Jill most likely will continue to need some type of additional support in order to be an independent adult, but all involved were optimistic about her future.

DESCRIPTION AND DEFINITION

Sigmund Freud, in his monograph entitled "Infantile Cerebral Paralysis," points out that a well-known painting by Spanish painter Jusepe Ribera (1588–1656), which depicts a child with infantile hemiplegia, proves that cerebral paralysis existed long before medical investigators began paying attention to it in the mid-1800s (Freud, 1968). Freud's work as a neurologist is not generally well known, and at the time that his monograph was published in 1897, he was already deep into his work in the area of psychotherapy. However, he was recognized at the time as the prominent authority on the paralyses of children. Today, cerebral paralysis is known as cerebral palsy.

Cerebral palsy is not one specific condition but rather a grouping of clinical syndromes that affect movement, muscle tone, and coordination as a result of an injury or lesion of the immature brain. It is not considered a disease, but is classified as a developmental disability since it occurs early in life and interferes with the development of motor and sometimes cognitive skills. Historically, cerebral palsy has been classified as and is still sometimes diagnostically referred to as a static encephalopathy (Brooke, 2010). This is now considered inaccurate due to recognition of the fact that the neurological manifestations of cerebral palsy often change or progress over time. Static encephalopathy is permanent and unchanging damage to the brain and includes other developmental problems such as fetal alcohol syndrome, cognitive impairments, and learning disabilities. Many individuals with cerebral palsy perform well academically and vocationally without any signs of cognitive dysfunction associated with the term encephalopathy (Johnson, 2004).

A child is considered to have cerebral palsy if all of the following characteristics apply:

The injury or insult occurs when the brain is still developing. It can occur anytime during the prenatal, perinatal, or postnatal periods. There is some disagreement about the upper age limit for a diagnosis of cerebral palsy during the postnatal period. An upper age limit ranging from 2 to 8 years of age is applied to postneonatally acquired brain injury (Smithers-Sheedy et al., 2009).

1. It is not progressive. Once the initial insult to the brain has occurred, there is no further worsening of the child's condition or further damage to the central nervous system. However, the characteristics of the disabilities affecting an individual often change over time.
2. It always involves a disorder in sensorimotor development that is manifested by abnormal muscle tone and stereotypical patterns of movement. The severity of the impairment ranges from mild to severe.
3. The sensorimotor disorder originates specifically in the brain. The muscles

themselves and the nerves connecting them with the spinal cord are normal. Although some cardiac or orthopedic problems can result in similar postural and movement abnormalities, they are not classified as cerebral palsy.

4. It is a lifelong disability. Some premature babies demonstrate temporary posture and movement abnormalities that look similar to patterns seen in cerebral palsy but resolve typically by 1 year of age. For children with cerebral palsy, these difficulties persist.

ETIOLOGY

Historically, birth asphyxia was considered the major cause of cerebral palsy. When the British surgeon William Little first identified cerebral palsy in 1860, he suggested that a major cause was a lack of oxygen during the birth process (Little, 1862). In 1897, Sigmund Freud disagreed, suggesting that the disorder might have roots earlier in life. Freud wrote, "Difficult birth, in certain cases is merely a symptom of deeper effects that influence the development of the fetus" (Freud, 1968). Although Freud made these observations in the late 1800s, it was not until the 1980s that research supported his views (Freeman & Nelson, 1988; Illingsworth, 1985). Only a small percentage of cases of cerebral palsy are a result of birth complications. The majority of children (70% to 80%) who are diagnosed with cerebral palsy have congenital cerebral palsy, that is, the injury to the brain occurred prior to their birth (Johnson, 2004).

There are a large number of risk factors that can result in cerebral palsy, and the interplay between these factors is often complex, making it difficult to identify the specific cause (Blickstein, 2003). The presence of risk factors does not always result in a subsequent diagnosis of cerebral palsy. The presence of one risk factor may not result in cerebral palsy unless it is present to an overwhelming degree. Current thought is that often two or more risk factors may interact in such a way as to overwhelm natural defenses, resulting in damage to the developing brain. The strongest risk factors are prematurity and low birth weight (Lawson & Badawi, 2003). During the postpartum period, premature and low birth weight infants are at greater risk for developing complications, especially in the circulatory and pulmonary systems.

These complications can lead to brain hypoxia and result in cerebral palsy.

Additional risk factors include intrauterine exposure to infection and disorders of coagulation (National Institute of Neurological Disorders and Stroke, 2015). Maternal infection is a critical risk factor for cerebral palsy, both during prenatal development and at the time of delivery. The infection does not necessarily produce signs of illness in the mother, which can make it difficult to detect. In a study conducted in the mid-1990s, it was determined that mothers with infections at the time of birth had a higher risk of having a child with cerebral palsy (Grether & Nelson, 1997). Table 2.1 lists specific risk factors related to both congenital and acquired types of cerebral palsy.

There are four types of injuries to the brain that often result in cerebral palsy (National Institute of Neurological Disorders and Stroke, 2015):

1. Periventricular leukomalacia (PVL) involves damage to the white matter in the brain adjacent to the lateral ventricles due to ischemia, or restriction in blood supply to the brain tissue. Necrosis occurs resulting in empty areas or cysts that fill up with fluid. This is most often associated with premature birth before 32 weeks of gestation. Sixty to one hundred percent of premature infants with PVL later show signs of cerebral palsy (Zach, 2010).

2. Hypoxic-ischemic encephalopathy (HIE), commonly known as perinatal asphyxia, occurs when there is a loss of oxygen resulting in damage to brain tissue. It most often occurs in the full-term infant in the perinatal period and can be caused by many factors related to birth and delivery as well as fetal stroke.

3. Intraventricular hemorrhage (IVH) involved bleeding into the brain's ventricular system. This most often occurs in infants born more than 10 weeks prematurely due to the blood vessels in the brain not being fully developed at this gestational period. It is rarely present at birth, but develops during the first several days of life. There are four types or grades of IVF based upon the amount of bleeding that occurs. Grades 1 and 2 involve a smaller amount of bleeding and typically do not result in any long-term developmental

TABLE 2.1   Cerebral Palsy: Contributing Risk Factors and Causes

Preconception (Parental Background)

Biological aging (parent or parents older than 35)

Biological immaturity (very young parent or parents)

Environmental toxins

Genetic background and genetic disorders

Malnutrition

Metabolic disorders

Radiation damage

First Trimester of Pregnancy

Endocrine: thyroid function, progesterone insufficiency

Nutrition: malnutrition, vitamin deficiencies, amino acid intolerance

Toxins: alcohol, drugs, poisons, smoking

Maternal disease: thyrotoxicosis, genetic disorders

Second Trimester of Pregnancy

Infection: cytomegalovirus, rubella, toxoplasma, HIV, syphilis, chickenpox, subclinical uterine infections

Placental pathology: vascular occlusion, fetal malnutrition, chronic hypoxia, growth factor deficiencies

Third Trimester of Pregnancy

Prematurity and low birth weight

Blood factors: Rh incompatibility, jaundice

Cytokines: neurological tissue destruction

Inflammation

Hypoxia: placental insufficiency, perinatal hypoxia

Infection: listeria, meningitis, streptococcus group B, septicemia, chorioamnionitis

Intrapartum Events

Premature placental separation

Uterine rupture

Acute maternal hypotension

Prolapsed umbilical cord

Ruptured vasa previa

Tightened true knot of the umbilical cord

Perinatal Period and Infancy

Endocrine: hypoglycemia, hypothyroidism

Hypoxia: perinatal hypoxia, respiratory distress syndrome

Infection: meningitis, encephalitis

Multiple births: death of a twin or triplet

Stroke: hemorrhagic or embolic stroke

Trauma: abuse, accidents

Adapted from UCP Research and Educational Foundation. Factsheet: Cerebral Palsy: Contributing Factors and Causes. September, 1995.

problems. Grades 3 and 4 involve more severe bleeding. **Hydrocephalus** can occur when blood presses on or leaks into the brain tissue resulting in blood clots blocking the flow of cerebral spinal fluid. Grades 3 and 4 bleeds are most often associated with cerebral palsy.

4. Cerebral dysgenesis is a brain malformation. It differs from the other three causes of cerebral palsy that are due to lesions or brain injuries. With cerebral dysgenesis, the brain did not grow properly or fully develop. The first 20 weeks of gestation are most critical for brain development, and factors such as maternal infections or trauma can result in a brain malformation. The severity of brain malformations can vary greatly with a more severe type resulting in cerebral palsy.

In a small percentage of children with cerebral palsy, the condition was acquired after birth. Causes in the postnatal and early childhood periods include cerebrovascular accidents (CVA's; infections such as meningitis or encephalitis; poisoning; trauma such as near-drowning and strangulation; child abuse; and illnesses such as endocrine disorders; Grether & Nelson, 1997; Marmer, 1997). Closed-head injury that occurs during this period is now classified as traumatic brain injury, even though the resulting impairments are very similar to cerebral palsy.

INCIDENCE AND PREVALENCE

Cerebral palsy is the most common motor disability in childhood (Jones, Morgan, Shelton, & Thorogood, 2007). The Autism and Developmental Disabilities Monitoring Network has been monitoring the incidence of cerebral palsy in children in four areas of the United States. Estimates of the incidence of cerebral palsy in the United States range from 3.1 to 3.6 per 1,000 live births (Christensen et al., 2014). They also found that it was significantly more common among boys than among girls at a ratio of 1.4:1. It is also more common among black children than among white or Hispanic children. There was a 70% increase in prevalence in middle- and low-income areas as compared with upper class areas (Centers for Disease Control and Prevention, 2004; Cerebral Palsy International Research Foundation, 2009).

The United Cerebral Palsy Association estimated as of 2012 that 764,000 children and adults in the United States show one or more symptoms of cerebral palsy. They estimated that each year, 10,000 infants and 1,200 to 1,500 preschool-aged children are diagnosed with cerebral palsy (United Cerebral Palsy Research and Education Foundation Factsheet, 2012).

There has been considerable advancement in obstetric and neonatal care during the past three to four decades. Many hoped these advancements would reduce the incidence of cerebral palsy. Unfortunately, the rate has remained relatively stable over this period. This is probably a result of increased survival rates of very low birth weight and premature infants. Another factor may be the use of fertility treatments by older women that have resulted in an increase in the number of multiple births. Multiple births tend to result in infants who are smaller and premature and are at greater risk for health problems. On the average, they are half the weight of other babies at birth and arrive 7 weeks earlier. There is a 400% increase in the probability of cerebral palsy in twin births than in a single birth (United Cerebral Palsy Research and Educational Foundation, 1997).

SIGNS AND SYMPTOMS

The early signs and symptoms common to all types of cerebral palsy are abnormal muscle tone, reflex and postural abnormalities, delayed motor development, and atypical motor performance.

■ Tone Abnormalities

Tone abnormalities include **hypertonicity**, **hypotonicity**, and fluctuating tone. Fluctuating tone shifts in varying degrees from hypotonic to hypertonic. Muscle tone can be characterized as the degree of resistance when a muscle is stretched. For instance, when there is hypotonicity and the elbow is passively extended, there will be little to no resistance to the movement and hypermobility in the elbow joint. With hypertonicity, there will be increased resistance, and it may be difficult to pull the elbow into full extension if the tone is strong. Most infants with cerebral palsy initially demonstrate hypotonia. Later, the infant may develop hypertonicity and fluctuating tone or continue to demonstrate hypotonia, depending on the type of cerebral palsy.

■ Reflex Abnormalities

With hypertonicity, reflex abnormalities such as **hyperreflexia**, **clonus**, overflow, enhanced **stretch reflex**, and other signs of upper motor neuron lesions are present. Retained primitive infantile reflexes and a delay in the acquisition of righting and equilibrium reactions occur in conjunction with all types of abnormal tone. When hypotonia is present, there may be areflexia or an absence of **primitive reflexes**. These reflexes should be present during the first several months of life, and it is of concern when they are not.

■ Atypical Posture

The presence of primitive reflexes and muscle tone abnormalities causes the child to have atypical positions at rest and to demonstrate stereotypical and uncontrollable postural changes during movement. For instance, in an infant lying supine with hypertonicity in the lower extremities, the hips are typically internally rotated and adducted and the ankles plantar flexed. This posture is caused by a combination of hypertonicity in the affected muscles and the presence of the crossed extension reflex (Fig. 2.1). In contrast, when an infant with hypotonicity in the lower extremities is lying supine, the hips are typically abducted, flexed, and externally rotated because of low muscle tone, weakness in the affected muscles, and the influence of gravity.

■ Delayed Motor Development

Cerebral palsy is always accompanied by a delay in the attainment of motor milestones. One of the signs that often alerts the pediatrician to the problem is a delay in the child's ability to sit independently or to crawl. While cerebral palsy is often present at birth, it is often not recognized until the child fails to achieve these early motor milestones.

■ Atypical Motor Performance

The way in which a child moves when performing skilled motor acts is also affected. Depending on the type of cerebral palsy, the child may demonstrate a variety of motor abnormalities such as asymmetrical hand use, unusual crawling method or gait, uncoordinated reach, or difficulty sucking, chewing, and swallowing.

TYPES OF CEREBRAL PALSY

Types of cerebral palsy are classified neurophysiologically into three major types: spastic, athetoid, and ataxia. Each results from damage in different parts of the brain (Fig. 2.2).

1. Spastic is characterized by hypertonicity. Deep tendon reflexes are present in affected limbs, and motor control is affected by the hypertonicity. This type is the most common and accounts for approximately 80% of people with cerebral palsy (Centers for Disease Control and Prevention, 2015). The spasticity is a result of upper motor neuron

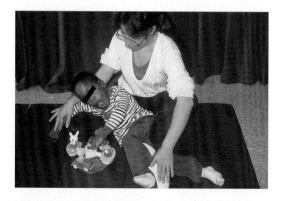

Figure 2.1 Child with spasticity in upper and lower extremities. Note hip adduction and scissoring in his legs, internal rotation at shoulders, fisted hand position, and overflow movements in his mouth. (From Hatfield, N. T. (2013). *Introductory maternity and pediatric nursing.* Philadelphia, PA: Lippincott Williams & Wilkins.)

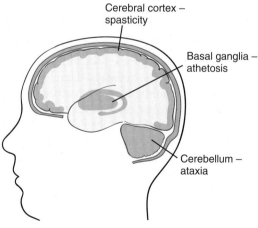

Figure 2.2 Cerebral palsy. Shown are the major parts of the brain involved in each of the three major types of cerebral palsy: spastic, athetoid, and ataxic. (From Wilkins, E. M. (2012). *Clinical practice of the dental hygienist* (11th ed.). Philadelphia, PA: Wolters Kluwer Health.)

involvement (Porter & Kaplan, 2009). Within this category, types are further subdivided anatomically according to the parts of the body that are affected.

2. **Athetoid** also known as **dyskinetic** type is characterized by involuntary and uncontrolled movements. These movements are typically slow and writhing. This type is much less common and results from basal ganglia involvement (Porter & Kaplan, 2009).

3. **Ataxia** is characterized by unsteadiness and difficulties with balance, particularly when ambulating. It is the least common type of cerebral palsy and results from involvement of the cerebellum or its pathways (Porter & Kaplan, 2009).

It is common for there to be mixed forms where two of the types occur together as a result of diffuse brain damage. The most common is spastic with athetoid. Persons with this type have signs of athetosis, and postural tone that fluctuates from hypertonicity to hypotonia. Athetoid combined with ataxia is less common (Porter & Kaplan, 2009).

■ Spastic

Spastic cerebral palsy is characterized by hypertonicity, retained primitive reflexes in affected areas of the body, and slow, restricted movement. The impact on motor function can range from a mild impairment that does not interfere with functional skills, such as not having isolated finger movement, to a severe impairment, where there is an inability to reach and grasp. **Contractures**, where there is permanent shortening of a muscle or joint and deformities, are common (Fig. 2.3). Spastic cerebral palsy is categorized anatomically according to the area of the body that is affected. Spastic hemiplegia, spastic diplegia, and spastic quadriplegia are the most common types. Spastic triplegia has similar features to spastic quadriplegia with three limbs involved. Typically, it is both lower extremities and one upper extremity. There are often mild coordination difficulties in the non-involved upper extremity. Monoplegia, where one limb is affected, is rare and, when it does occur, is typically mild (Molnar & Alexander, 1998).

Spastic Hemiplegia

Spastic hemiplegia involves one entire side of the body, including the head, neck, and trunk. Usually, the upper extremity is most affected.

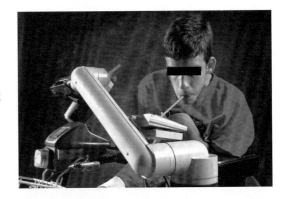

Figure 2.3 Due to spasticity and limited controlled movement and range of motion in upper extremities and hands, this person is using a mouth stick to activate a computer. Note wrist flexion contracture. (From Carter, P. J. (2011). *Lippincott textbook for nursing assistants.* Philadelphia, PA: Lippincott Williams & Wilkins.)

Early signs include asymmetrical hand use during the first year or dragging one side of the body when crawling or walking. The child learns to walk later than is typical, and when walking, the child typically hyperextends the knee, and the ankle is in **equinovarus** or **equinovalgus** position on the involved side. The child often lacks righting and equilibrium reactions on the involved side and will avoid bearing weight on this side. The shoulder is held in adduction, internal rotation; the elbow is flexed; the forearm is pronated; the wrist is flexed and ulnar deviated; the thumb is adducted, and the fingers are flexed (Fig. 2.4). Spasticity increases during physical activities and emotional excitement. Arm and hand use is limited on the involved side, depending on the severity. The child may use more primitive patterns of grasping and lacks precise and coordinated movement. In more severe cases, the child may totally neglect the involved side or use it only as an assist during bilateral activities.

Spastic Diplegia

Spastic diplegia involves both lower extremities, with mild incoordination, tremors, or less severe spasticity in the upper extremities. It is most often attributed to premature birth and low birth weight and is, therefore, on the rise as more infants born prematurely survive as a result of medical advances. The ability to sit independently can be delayed up to 3 years of age or older because of inadequate hip flexion and extensor and

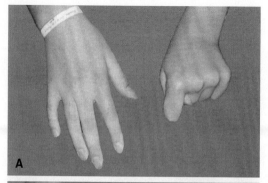

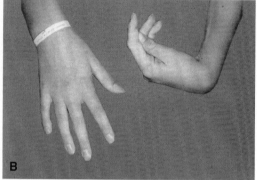

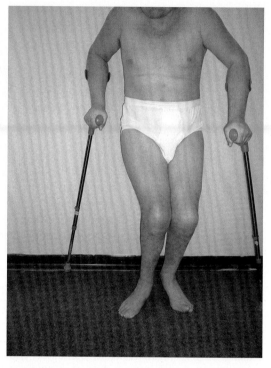

Figure 2.4 Abnormal hand position due to spasticity. Note thumb adduction and flexion in **(A)**. When wrist is flexed, thumb is released and tone reduced but still not in a position for a functional grasp. **(B)** (From Salter, R. B. (1998). *Textbook of disorders and injuries of the musculoskeletal system.* Philadelphia, PA: Lippincott Williams & Wilkins.)

Figure 2.5 Atypical posture and structural deformities seen in spastic diplegia. Note crouched posture due to abnormal muscle tone and strength: hip flexion and internal rotation, knee flexion, and equinovalgus positioning of the feet. (From Liebenson, C. (2014). *Functional training handbook.* Philadelphia, PA: Wolters Kluwer Health.)

adductor hypertonicity in the legs (Bobath, 1980). Frequently, the child will rely on the arms for support. The young child will move forward on the floor by pulling along with flexed arms while the legs are stiffly extended. Getting up to a creeping position is difficult because of spasticity in the lower extremities. Similarly, standing posture and gait are affected to varying degrees, depending on severity. Because of a lack of lower extremity equilibrium reactions, excessive trunk and upper extremity compensatory movements are used when walking. Lumbar **lordosis**, hip flexion and internal rotation (scissoring), plantar flexion of the ankles, and difficulty shifting weight when walking are common (Fig. 2.5). Many of these problems result in contractures and deformities, including dorsal spine **kyphosis**, lumbar spine lordosis, hip subluxation or dislocation, flexor deformities of hips and knees, and equinovarus or equinovalgus deformity of the feet (Bobath, 1980). Approximately 80% to 90% of children

with diplegia will walk independently, some requiring assistive devices such as crutches or a walker to do so (Sola & Grant, 1995). Walking will be slower and more labored with a crouched gait sometimes developing.

Spastic Quadriplegia

With spastic **quadriplegia**, the entire body is involved. The arms typically demonstrate spasticity in the flexor muscles, with spasticity in the extensor muscles in the lower extremities. Because of the influence of the tonic labyrinthine reflex (TLR), shoulder retraction and neck hyperextension are common, particularly in the supine position. This results in difficulty with transitional movements such as rolling or coming up to sitting. In the prone position, there is increased flexor tone, also a result of TLR influence, causing difficulty with head raising and bearing weight on the arms. Independent sitting and standing are difficult for the child because of hypertonicity,

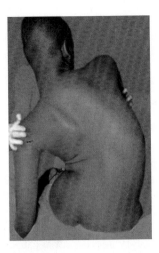

Figure 2.6 Severe scoliosis with pelvic obliquity in person with spastic quadriplegia. Scoliosis with this severity can compromise respiratory function. (From Flynn, J. M., & Wiesel, S. W. (2010). *Operative techniques in pediatric orthopaedics.* Philadelphia, PA: Lippincott Williams & Wilkins.)

the presence of primitive reflex involvement, and a lack of righting and equilibrium reactions. Only a small percentage of children with quadriplegia are able to walk independently (Sola & Grant, 1995). Oral musculature is usually affected, with resulting dysarthria, eating difficulties, and drooling (Molnar & Alexander, 1998). Individuals are susceptible to contractures and deformities, particularly hip dislocation and **scoliosis**, and must be closely monitored (Fig. 2.6).

◼ Athetosis

Athetosis is the most common type of dyskinesia or dystonia, characterized by slow, writhing involuntary movements of the face and extremities or the proximal parts of the limbs and trunk. Abrupt, jerky distal movements (choreiform) may also appear. The movements increase with emotional tension and are not present during sleep. Head and trunk control is often affected, as is the oral musculature, resulting in drooling, **dysarthria**, and eating difficulties. Whereas spasticity is characterized by hypertonicity in the affected muscle groups and restricted movement, fluctuating tone and excessive movement characterize athetosis. Contractures are rare, but hypermobility may be present because of fluctuating hypotonicity.

◼ Ataxia

Ataxia is characterized by a wide-based, staggering, and unsteady gait. Children with ataxia often walk quickly to compensate for their lack of stability and control. Controlled movements are clumsy. Intention tremors may be present. The ability to perform refined movements such as handwriting is affected. Hypotonicity is often present (Low, 2010).

ASSOCIATED DISORDERS

In addition to the motor impairments, there are a number of disorders and difficulties associated with cerebral palsy that can significantly affect functional abilities. In some cases, associated disorders can have a more significant impact on function than the motoric aspects of cerebral palsy.

◼ Cognitive Impairment

Of all the associated disorders with cerebral palsy, cognitive impairment has the most significant impact upon functional outcomes. Estimates of the incidence of cognitive or intellectual impairment with cerebral palsy range from 30% to 50% (Molnar & Alexander, 1998). In about one-third of these instances, the cognitive impairment is mild. The most significant impairments most often occur with mixed types and severe spastic quadriplegia. Athetoid–type cerebral palsy has the least occurrence of cognitive impairment. Many children with spastic hemiplegia and diplegia have average intelligence (Molnar & Alexander, 1998; Porter & Kaplan, 2009).

◼ Seizure Disorder

Reports of the incidence of seizures in people with cerebral palsy range from 25% to 60% (Porter & Kaplan, 2009). The incidence varies across the diagnostic categories. It is most common in spastic hemiplegia and quadriplegia and rare with spastic diplegia and athetosis (Centers for Disease Control and Prevention, 2004; Johnson, 2004; Molnar & Alexander, 1998; Porter & Kaplan, 2009). A population-based study published in 2003 found that the frequency of epilepsy in children with cerebral palsy was 38%. Partial seizures were the most common type, and children with cognitive impairments had a higher frequency of a seizure disorder (Carlsson, Hagberg, & Olsson, 2003).

■ Visual and Hearing Impairments

Visual and hearing impairments occur at a higher rate with cerebral palsy than in the general population. Common visual defects include **strabismus**, **nystagmus**, and difficulties with visual fixation and tracking (Molnar & Alexander, 1998). Some other visual defects are known to occur related to specific types of cerebral palsy. **Homonymous hemianopsia** can occur in children with spastic hemiplegia, paralysis of upward gaze in children with athetosis, and nystagmus and lack of depth perception can occur with ataxia (Dufresne, Dagenais, Shevell, & REPACQ Consortium, 2014). Hearing impairments most often include sensorineural hearing loss, due to congenital nervous system infections (Johnson, 2004). Conductive hearing losses, caused by persistent fluid in the ears and middle ear infections, occur when there is severe motor involvement in children who spend a lot of time in a prone or supine position (Blackman, 1997).

■ Oral Motor

If the oral musculature is affected, the individual with cerebral palsy may have significant difficulty with speaking and eating. Dysarthria, if it is severe, may affect functional communication resulting in the need for alternative forms of communication. Eating difficulties can result in increased risk of aspiration, limited amount of foods consumed, and difficulty with chewing and swallowing. Drooling is a significant problem in about 10% of the cases of cerebral palsy (Stanley & Blair, 1994). It can be due to many factors including oral motor muscular control, impaired oral sensation, inefficient and infrequent swallowing, poor lip closure, decreased jaw control, and poor head control.

Dental problems occur frequently in individuals with cerebral palsy. Motor problems and oral sensitivity can make tooth brushing more difficult. The combination of enamel dysplasia, mouth breathing, and poor hygiene leads to increased tooth decay and periodontal diseases (Molnar & Alexander, 1998).

■ Gastrointestinal

Gastrointestinal difficulties occur frequently in cerebral palsy. **Gastroesophageal reflux** can create much discomfort and can result in refusal to eat or difficulty transitioning to solid foods. It requires medical intervention such as medication or in more serious cases surgery. Constipation is common due to decreased mobility and exercise as well as inadequate intake of water or unusual diets due to difficulties with oral motor control (Molnar & Alexander, 1998).

■ Pulmonary

Individuals with more severe motor impairments such as spastic quadriplegia often develop scoliosis or other spinal deformities that can impact respiration. The respiratory muscles themselves may be affected, which results in poor respiration. These individuals are prone to frequent upper respiratory infections that can significantly impact their health. When difficulty chewing and swallowing is associated with poor breathing and inadequate or decreased ability to cough, this can result in increased aspiration pneumonia. A barium swallow study can be conducted to rule out aspiration as a cause of frequent pneumonia. In cases where there is aspiration, a gastric feeding tube may need to be inserted. Premature infants who had **bronchopulmonary dysplasia** also have compromised pulmonary systems (Molnar & Alexander, 1998).

DIAGNOSIS

No definitive test will diagnose cerebral palsy. Several factors must be considered. Physical evidence includes a history of delayed achievement of motor milestones; however, delayed motor development can occur with a host of other developmental disabilities and genetic syndromes. The quality of movement is the factor that helps provide a differential diagnosis. The findings of atypical or stereotypical movement patterns, the presence of infantile reflexes, and abnormal muscle tone all point toward a diagnosis of cerebral palsy. However, other causes must be ruled out, such as progressive neurological disorders, mucopolysaccharidosis, muscular dystrophy, or a spinal cord tumor. Many of these disorders can be ruled out by laboratory tests, although some must be differentiated by clinical or pathological criteria. A magnetic resonance imaging (MRI) or computed tomography (CT) scan may provide evidence of hydrocephalus, help determine the location and extent of structural lesions, and help to rule out other conditions. However, these scans are not definitive as far as making a diagnosis of cerebral palsy and are not predictive as far as the child's functioning (Miller & Bachrach, 2006). The yield of finding an abnormal CT scan in a child with cerebral palsy is 77% and for an MRI it is about 89% (Ashwal et al., 2004). An electroencephalogram (EEG) should not be used to determine the cause of cerebral palsy but should be obtained if there is an indication that the child may be having seizures. Because of the high occurrence of associated conditions, children with cerebral palsy should be screened for cognitive, visual, and hearing impairments, as well as speech and language disorders.

Cerebral palsy often is not evident during the first few months of life and is rarely diagnosed that early. Most cases, however, are detected by 12 months, and nearly all can be diagnosed by 18 months (Miller & Bachrach, 2006). In some cases, early postural and tonal abnormalities in premature infants can resemble cerebral palsy, but the signs are transient with normal subsequent development.

COURSE AND PROGNOSIS

The course of cerebral palsy varies depending on type, severity, and the presence of associated problems. With mild motor involvement, the child will continue to make motor gains and compensate for motor difficulties. With more severe forms, little progress may be made in attaining developmental milestones and performing functional tasks. As the child grows older, secondary problems such as contractures and deformities will become more common, especially with spasticity. Adults with cerebral palsy experience musculoskeletal difficulties and loss of function at an earlier age than do their nondisabled peers. One study found that 75% of individuals with cerebral palsy had stopped walking by age 25 due to fatigue and walking insufficiency (Murphy, Molnar, & Lankasky, 1995). Another study of young adults found clinical evidence of arthritis in 27% of the subjects with cerebral palsy as compared to 4% in the general population (Cathels & Reddihough, 1993).

The survival rate for adults with cerebral palsy is good but lower than that of the general population. A study in Great Britain found that there was an 86% survival rate at age 50 for adults with cerebral palsy compared to 96% for the general population. After age 50, the relative risk of death was only slightly higher in women with cerebral palsy as compared to the general population. The risk for men with cerebral palsy was the same as the general population. Adults with cerebral palsy were more likely to die of respiratory disease than the general population but less likely to die from an accident or injury (Hemming, Hutton, & Pharoah, 2006).

MEDICAL/SURGICAL MANAGEMENT

Because of the complexity and diversity of difficulties affecting the individual with cerebral palsy, medical management requires a team approach using the skills of many professionals. Depending on the type of cerebral palsy and the presence of associated problems, team members typically include an occupational therapist, physical therapist, speech pathologist, educational psychologist, nurse, and social worker. The emphasis of intervention is on helping the child gain as much motor control as possible, positioning the child to minimize the effects of abnormal muscle tone, instructing the parents and caregivers on handling techniques and ways to accomplish various activities of daily living, recommending adaptive equipment and assistive technology to increase the child's ability to perform desired activities, providing methods to improve feeding and speech if difficulties are present, and helping parents manage behavioral concerns and family stresses.

The primary physician treats the usual childhood disorders and helps with prevention of many health problems. Physicians with various medical specialties may also be involved. These include a neurologist to assess neurological status and help control seizures, if present; an orthopedist to prescribe orthotic devices and any necessary surgeries; and an ophthalmologist to assess and treat any visual difficulties.

Medical management includes both surgical and nonsurgical approaches, with much of the focus on techniques to decrease spasticity. Oral medications such as diazepam (Valium), dantrolene (Dantrium), and baclofen have been used to reduce spasticity in severe cases with mixed results (Johnson, 2004). Intrathecal baclofen infusion (ITB) administered through a pump implanted in the abdominal wall to the spinal cord fluid has shown to be more effective than oral medications in reducing severe spasticity and dystonia in cerebral palsy (Albright, 1996). There is however the potential for serious side effects, and the long-term consequences are not yet known (Stempien & Tsai, 2000). Another treatment more widely used in recent years is the injection of botulinum toxin (Botox) into muscles. Spasticity is reduced for a period of 3 to 6 months after injection. Botox is injected into specific muscles, which, in addition to reducing tone, increases range of motion and reduces deformities as well as provides an opportunity to work on muscle strengthening. Minimal side effects have been reported; however, its long-term effectiveness on function has not been demonstrated (Steinbok, 2006).

Orthotics and splinting are used to improve function and prevent contractures and deformities. Upper extremity resting or night splints are used to maintain range of motion. Soft splints, dynamic splints, and those allowing movement of the fingers and thumb are used during waking hours and functional activities to reduce tone and promote more typical patterns of movement. Ankle-foot orthosis (AFO) and variants are often used to control spastic equinus, promote alignment of the hind foot, and control midfoot and excessive knee extension when standing (Molnar & Alexander, 1998) (Fig. 2.7). Inhibitory and progressive casting has gained acceptance as an alternative to bracing in recent years. A molded footplate is constructed that inhibits the primitive reflexes, thus reducing spasticity. The footplate is surrounded by a snug, bivalve below the knee cast. Inhibitory and progressive casting also is used with the upper extremities.

Surgical approaches are used to improve the function and appearance of affected areas of the body and to prevent or correct deformities. Common surgical procedures include tendon lengthening to increase range of motion and tendon transfers to decrease spastic muscle imbalances. These procedures, commonly used on the lower extremities, are performed more selectively in the upper extremities (Steinbok, 2006). Selective dorsal rhizotomy (SDR) is a neurosurgical technique that is used to reduce spasticity and improve function in carefully selected individuals (Berman, Vaughan, & Peacock, 1990; The Cleveland Clinic, 2015; Feger, Lunsford, Sauer, Novicoff, & Abel, 2015; Kinghorn, 1992; Peacock & Staudt, 1991). The procedure involves dividing the lumbosacral posterior nerve root into four to seven rootlets. Each rootlet is stimulated electrically. The dorsal rootlets causing spasticity are cut,

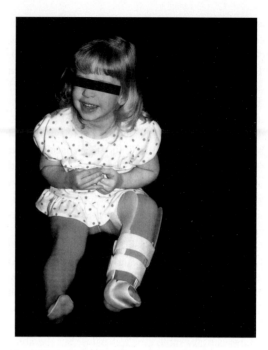

Figure 2.7 Child wearing knee-ankle-foot orthosis (KAFO). (From Hatfield, N. T. (2013). *Introductory maternity and pediatric nursing.* Philadelphia, PA: Lippincott Williams & Wilkins.)

leaving the normal rootlets intact. This approach is highly successful for individuals who meet the selection criteria (Berman et al., 1990; Kinghorn, 1992). The most likely candidates are children with diplegia or severe quadriplegia (Berman et al., 1990; Kinghorn, 1992; Peacock & Staudt, 1991). For children with diplegia, the goal is to improve gait and leg function. For children with spastic quadriplegia who have very limited movement, the goal is to increase their independence by allowing them to sit for longer periods of time enabling them to use a wheelchair or potty chair as well as making daily care easier for their caregivers by reducing spasticity, which makes dressing and other daily living tasks more manageable. An essential part of this treatment approach includes intensive postsurgical physical and occupational therapy for a period of several weeks.

IMPACT ON OCCUPATIONAL PERFORMANCE

Virtually all of the body function categories can be affected in the individual that has cerebral palsy. Which of the categories are affected depends on the type of cerebral palsy, the severity of the condition, and the presence of associated disorders. Milder forms of cerebral palsy may have limited impact upon occupational performance. Some individuals will require physical assistance, additional training, or assistive technology to participate fully in occupational performance areas, while individuals with severe forms of cerebral palsy will be limited in their performance of all areas of occupation. The body function category that is always affected in individuals with cerebral palsy is neuromusculoskeletal and movement-related function. If spasticity is present, it affects joint mobility and results in limited active or passive range of motion or both. Joint stability is affected in all types of cerebral palsy. With spastic type, uneven muscle pull affects stability and joint cocontraction; fluctuating movement and tone affects stability in athetoid type; and ataxic type is characterized by a lack of joint stability. Underlying the tone abnormalities is decreased muscle power. Tone abnormalities affect muscle endurance. It requires much more effort to complete motor tasks with both hypotonia and hypertonia, and endurance is often diminished. Endurance is also decreased if respiratory muscles are affected. In movement functions, primitive motor reflexes such as the stretch reflex, asymmetrical tonic neck reflex (ATNR), or grasp reflex are retained in the child with spasticity and continue to influence movement throughout life. Individuals with all types of cerebral palsy have impaired involuntary movement reactions such as decreased righting and equilibrium reactions. Involuntary movements impact individuals with athetoid cerebral palsy. Some individuals with ataxia have intention tremors. Gait patterns are affected in all types of cerebral palsy; however, in milder cases, they may have little effect on occupational performance.

All sensory functions can be affected. All types of cerebral palsy have associated visual difficulties such as strabismus, visual tracking and fixation difficulties, or hearing impairments. Some individuals with cerebral palsy demonstrate sensory processing difficulties with either hypersensitivity to sensory input or their ability to discriminate sensory input.

Mental functions, both global and specific, can be affected, particularly if there is an associated learning disability, attention deficit hyperactive disorder, or cognitive impairment. Voice and speech functions can be affected if the oral motor and respiratory muscles have tonal abnormalities. Functions of the cardiovascular and respiratory system can be affected in a variety of ways, such as associated spinal deformities that can compromise respiration or decreased physical endurance or stamina as a result of the amount of effort that it takes to move. The digestive system can be affected by a number of different medical and physical factors such as reflux and feeding difficulties. Urinary functions are impacted by decreased control of muscles used in urination and in some cases cognitive factors.

It is important for the occupational therapist to be aware of all the client factors that can be affected in individuals with cerebral palsy but to not make any assumptions based upon the type of cerebral palsy and known associated disorders but to directly assess each factor and its impact on occupational performance. Each individual is unique and will have their own set of strengths and challenges.

CASE STUDY 1

A.K. is a 2-year-old girl who lives with her parents and older brother. She was born at 37 weeks of gestation at a birth weight of 5 lb 10 oz. Pregnancy and birth were unremarkable. She was healthy at birth, but by her well-baby visit at 9 months of age, she was not yet rolling, crawling, or sitting independently. Her pediatrician referred her to a pediatric neurologist who diagnosed her with spastic diplegia at 11 months of age. The neurologist referred her to a physical medicine and rehabilitation (PM&R) physician at the local children's hospital as well as the local school district for early intervention services. The PM&R physician signed a referral for her to the orthotics department to fit her with AFO's (ankle-foot orthosis) to help her with standing and walking. He has also recommended botulinum toxin (Botox) injections and selective posterior rhizotomy for consideration as future treatments. Through the early intervention program, she received a multidisciplinary team assessment, which included physical, occupational, and speech and language assessments. Delays were noted in gross motor, fine motor, and self-help skills. Speech and language, social, and cognitive skills were all determined to be at age level. Weekly occupational and physical therapy home-based services were recommended.

Affected performance skills are in the motor area, which includes posture, mobility, coordination, and strength/effort. She demonstrates spasticity in all lower extremities and her trunk. Her movement patterns reflect significant spasticity in her legs. Her joint range of motion is significantly limited in her hamstrings and hip adductors with mild limitations in her heel cords bilaterally. A.K. can sit independently; however, it is difficult for her to sit on the floor with her legs extended in front of her as a result of hamstring and hip adductor tightness. She requires assistance moving in and out of sitting. In prone, she can push up to hands and knees and can crawl for short distances. She bears weight on her legs in supported standing with knees in a slightly flexed position, hips adducted, and feet plantar flexed

and pronated. She has begun ambulating with a walker for short distances.

In her upper extremities, there is mildly increased muscle tone bilaterally as well as some incoordination. A.K. grasps pegs and small blocks and releases objects into a container. She can place a peg in a pegboard but is not yet able to stack objects or complete a shape sorter. Areas of occupation that are affected include activities of daily living (ADLs) and play. Because she is only 2 years old, instrumental activities of daily living, student, work, and leisure areas of occupational are not yet relevant areas for her. In ADLs, because of her age, she would not yet be expected to be independent. Given this, A.K.'s affected activities of daily living include bathing, dressing, feeding, and functional mobility. A.K. needs assistance with dressing skills such as undressing and removing shoes and socks. She is independent in feeding with some adaptations. She requires assistance with maintaining a stable sitting position in the bathtub and requires assistance getting in and out of the bath tub. She needs assistance with functional mobility, such as getting in and out of chairs and moving from one place to another.

Exploratory play* skills are affected by A.K.'s difficulty with moving about her environment to obtain toys she wants to play with. Participation is affected by the need for a stable position in which to free up her upper extremities to manipulate toys. She uses a bench with a pelvis stabilizer and tray for refined fine motor tasks.

CASE STUDY 2

L.N. is a 54-year-old woman with cerebral palsy, spastic quadriplegic type. She has lived alone in an apartment complex for the elderly and disabled for the past 15 years. She supports herself on supplemental security income (SSI) and disability payments from the state. A personal care attendant provided by the Department of Social Services comes in each morning and evening to assist her with activities of daily living, such as meal preparation, bathing, and dressing. L.N. has never been employed but has done volunteer work. She writes articles for a newsletter on her computer and has worked in her church's Sunday school. She has no family support but has many friends. She enjoys learning and taking classes through continuing education.

Spasticity, fluctuating tone, and retained primitive reflexes severely restrict L.N.'s purposeful movement. She has limited range of motion in her left upper extremity and both lower extremities. When reaching with the left arm, she cannot bring it to shoulder height or behind her back. She has a gross grasp in her right upper extremity and can grasp a joystick to operate her electric wheelchair. She cannot write or perform other activities requiring fine motor dexterity. Her left upper extremity is used as an assist for bilateral activities, with no grasping ability present. She can maintain an upright position in sitting, but her weight is shifted to the left (with resulting scoliosis). She can bring her head to an upright position, but neck flexion increases with activities requiring effort. Oral motor muscles are affected, resulting in severe dysarthria, drooling, and difficulty eating. Endurance is a problem, and L.N. becomes easily fatigued.

Communication/interaction skills are also affected. Articulation and modulation when speaking are affected by L.N.'s oral motor control. Limited dexterity and restrictions in movement limit her ability to use gestures and to orient her body in relation to others when engaged in social interactions.

All areas of occupation are affected. In activities of daily living, L.N. needs assistance with bathing, personal hygiene and grooming, toilet hygiene, and dressing. She brushes her teeth and performs light hygiene, such as washing her face, independently. She can transfer herself between her wheelchair and her bed. She needs assistance transferring to the shower seat she uses for bathing. She can transfer on and off the toilet in her apartment with grab bars and the toilet seat at the proper height and position, although it takes her a while to do this. In eating, L.N. can feed herself with adaptations if the food is set up for her, but the process is slow and messy. She drinks from a straw. She takes her own medications if they are set out for her.

In instrumental activities of daily living, L.N. needs assistance in clothing care, cleaning her apartment, household maintenance, and meal preparation. She can use a handheld portable vacuum cleaner for small cleanups. She has a cat that she cares for. She shops independently but needs assistance getting money out of her wallet at the cash register. All areas of activities of daily living are affected except socialization. L.N. uses a computer for written communication. She uses a speaker phone for telephone communication. If she falls or is in danger at home, she has an emergency alert system that she can activate. Because her speech is difficult to understand, she has an augmented output device for communication but uses it infrequently. She uses a motorized wheelchair for mobility. In the community, L.N. uses public transportation with no difficulty. She has some difficulty transferring herself to and from the toilet when using public restrooms, which sometimes results in incontinence.

In work activities, L.N. has never been employed but has worked as a volunteer for the past several years in the religious education program at her church. She enjoys the interaction with the children who are in the classes.

In leisure activities, L.N. has varied interests. She is an avid reader and enjoys computer games. Social activities include getting together with friends frequently and going out into the community, either alone or with friends. L.N. participates in church retreats as well as community-based trips through an independent living center.

RECOMMENDED LEARNING RESOURCES

Bowers, E. (2008). *Finnie's handling the young child with cerebral palsy at home* (4th ed.). Waltham, MA: Butterworth-Heinemann.
This book was written with the aim of helping parents assist their child with cerebral palsy achieve most comfortable independence in all activities and assists professionals new to the field in understanding, supporting, and encouraging young children with cerebral palsy and their families.

Levitt, S. (2003). *Treatment of cerebral palsy and motor delay* (4th ed.). Oxford, UK: Blackwell Science LTP.
This book was written for occupational and physical therapists working with children with cerebral palsy. Good discussion of treatment approaches, principles of treatment, and description of procedures.

Miller, F., & Bachrach, S. (2006). *Cerebral palsy: A complete guide for caregivers* (2nd ed.). Baltimore, MD: John Hopkins University Press.
Written by a team of experts, the book is organized into three parts: explanation of the condition, practical advice regarding caregiving, and an extensive encyclopedia of medical terms, procedures, and devices related to cerebral palsy.

Morris, S., & Klein, M. (2000). *Pre-feeding skills* (2nd ed.). Tucson, AZ: Psychological Corp.
Excellent reference for oral-motor and feeding therapy for children. Very thorough and good overall approach to feeding issues including those occurring in children with cerebral palsy.

United Cerebral Palsy National Office
1660 L Street, NW Suite 700
Washington, DC 20036

Tel: (202) 776-0406; toll free: (800) 872-5827
ucp.org
Leading source of information on cerebral palsy
and national advocacy group.

**Children's Hemiplegia and Stroke Association
(CHASA)**
4101 West Green Oaks Blvd.
Suite 305-149
Arlington, TX 76016
Tel: (817) 492-4325
www.chasa.org

**A comprehensive, practical resource related to
children with hemiplegia–type cerebral palsy.**

**National Institute of Neurological Disorders
and Stroke (NINDS). Cerebral Palsy
Information Page.**
Retrieved from www.ninds.nih.gov/disorders/
cerebral_palsy.htm. Lists resources including
organizations, publications, links, and general
information about cerebral palsy.

REFERENCES

Albright, A. (1996). Intrathecal baclofen in cerebral palsy movement disorders. *Journal of Child Neurology, 11,* S29.

Ashwal, S., Russman, B. S., Blasco, P. A., Miller, G., Sandler, A., Shevell, M., & Stevenson, R. (2004). Practice parameter: Diagnostic assessment of the child with cerebral palsy. *Neurology, 62,* 851–863. Retrieved from http://dx.doi.org/10.1212/01. WNL.0000117981.35364.1B, doi: 10.1212/01. WNL.0000117981.35364.1B#_blank

Berman, B., Vaughan, C. L., & Peacock, W. J. (1990). The effect of rhizotomy on movement in patients with cerebral palsy. *American Journal of Occupational Therapy, 44,* 6. Retrieved from http://dx.doi.org/10.5014/ajot.44.6.511, doi: 10.5014/ajot.44.6.511#_blank

Blackman, J. (1997). *Medical aspects of developmental disabilities in children birth to three* (3rd ed.). Iowa City, IA: The University of Iowa.

Blickstein, A. (2003). Cerebral palsy: A look at etiology and new task force conclusions. *OBG Management, 15,* 5.

Bobath, K. (1980). *Neurological basis for the treatment of cerebral palsy.* Philadelphia, PA: JB Lippincott.

Brooke, H. (2010). *Cerebral palsy as a cause of static encephalopathy in infants.* Retrieved from http:// www.associatedcontent.com/article/2688287/cerebral_palsy_as_a_cause_of_static.html?cat=5

Carlsson, M., Hagberg, G., & Olsson, I. (2003). Clinical and etiological aspects of epilepsy in children with cerebral palsy. *Developmental Medicine & Child Neurology, 45*(6), 371–376. Retrieved from http://dx.doi.org/10.1111/j.1469-8749.2003. tb00415.x, doi: 10.1111/j.1469-8749.2003. tb00415.x#_blank

Cathels, B., & Reddihough, D. (1993). The health care of young adults with cerebral palsy. *The Medical Journal of Australia, 159*(7), 444–446.

Centers for Disease Control and Prevention. (August 4, 2004). *Metropolitan Atlanta Developmental Disabilities Surveillance Program (MADDSP).* Retrieved from http://www.cdc.gov/ncbddd/developmentaldisabilities/MADDSP.html

Centers for Disease Control and Prevention. (2015). *Facts about cerebral palsy.* Retrieved from http:// www.cdc.gov/ncbddd/cp/facts.html

Cerebral Palsy International Research Foundation. (2009). *Racial disparities in the prevalence of cerebral palsy.* Retrieved from http://cpirf.org/stories/478

Christensen, D., Van Naarden Braun, K., Doernberg, N., Maenner, M., Ameson, C., Durkin, M., Ameson, C., … Yeargin-Allsopp, M. (2014). Prevalence of cerebral palsy, co-occurring autism spectrum disorders, and motor functioning-Autism and Developmental Disabilities Monitoring Network. *Developmental Medicine and Child Neurology, 2014, 56*(1), 59–65. Retrieved from http://dx.doi.org/10.1111/dmcn.12268

Cusick, B. (1990). *Progressive casting and splinting for lower extremity deformities in children with neuromuscular dysfunction.* Tucson, AZ: Therapy Skill Builders.

Dufresne, D., Dagenais, L., Shevell, M. I., & REPACQ Consortium. (2014). Spectrum of visual disorders in a population-based cerebral palsy cohort. *Pediatric Neurology, 50*(4), 324–328. Retrieved from http://dx.doi.org/10.1016/j. pediatrneurol.2013.11.022

Feger, M. A., Lunsford, C. D., Sauer, L. D., Novicoff, W., & Abel, M. F. (2015). Comparative effects of multilevel muscle tendon surgery, osteotomies, and dorsal rhizotomy on functional and gait outcome measures for children with cerebral palsy. *American Journal of Physical Medicine and Rehabilitation, 7*(5), 485–493. Retrieved from http://dx.doi.org/10.1016/j.pmrj.2014.11.002

Freeman, J., & Nelson, K. (1988). Intrapartum asphyxia and cerebral palsy. *Pediatrics, 82,* 240–249.

Freud, S. (1968). *Infantile cerebral paralysis.* Coral Gables, FL: University of Miami Press.

Grether, J. K., & Nelson, K. B. (1997). Maternal infection and cerebral palsy in infants of normal birth weight. *Journal of the American Medical Association*, 278(3), 207–211. Retrieved from http://dx.doi.org/10.1001/jama.1997.03550030047032, doi: 10.1001/jama.1997.03550030047032#_blank

Hemming, K., Hutton, J., & Pharoah, P. (2006). Long-term survival for a cohort of adults with cerebral palsy. *Developmental Medicine and Child Neurology*, 48(2), 90–95. Retrieved from http://dx.doi.org/10.1017/S0012162206000211, doi: 10.1017/S0012162206000211#_blank

Illingsworth, R. S. (1985). A pediatrician asks—why is it called a birth injury? *British Journal of Med Obstetrics and Gynecology*, 92(2), 122–130. Retrieved from http://dx.doi.org/10.1111/j.1471-0528.1985.tb01063.x, doi: 10.1111/j.1471-0528.1985.tb01063.x#_blank

Johnson, M. (2004). Encephalopathies. In R. Behrman, R. Kliegman, & H. Jenson (Eds.), *Nelson's textbook of pediatrics* (17th ed.). Philadelphia, PA: Saunders.

Jones, M., Morgan, E., Shelton, J. E., & Thorogood, C. (2007). Cerebral palsy: Introduction and diagnosis (part 1). *Journal of Pediatric Health Care*, 21(3), 146–152. Retrieved from http://dx.doi.org/10.1016/j.pedhc.2006.06.007, doi: 10.1016/j.pedhc.2006.06.007#_blank

Kinghorn, J. (1992). Upper extremity functional changes following selective posterior rhizotomy in children with cerebral palsy. *American Journal of Occupational Therapy*, 46, 502–507. Retrieved from http://dx.doi.org/10.5014/ajot.46.6.502, doi: 10.5014/ajot.46.6.502#_blank

Lawson, R. D., & Badawi, N. (2003). Etiology of cerebral palsy. *Hand Clinics*, 19(4), 547–556. Retrieved from http://dx.doi.org/10.1016/S0749-0712(03)00040-4, doi: 10.1016/S0749-0712(03)00040-4#_blank

Little, W. J. (1862). On the influence of abnormal parturition, difficult labor, premature birth and physical condition of the child, especially in relation to deformities. *Transactions of the Obstetrical Society of London*, 3, 243–344. Retrieved from http://www.neonatology.org/classics/little.html

Low, J. (2010). *Ataxic cerebral palsy*. Retrieved from www.disabled-world.com/health/neurology/cerebral-palsy/ataxic.php

Marmer, L. (1997). *ACDC tracks disability in kids ages 3 to 10. Advance for Occupational Therapists.* King of Prussia, PA: Merion Publications, Inc.

Miller, F., & Bachrach, S. (2006). *Cerebral palsy: A complete guide for caregiving.* Baltimore, MD: John Hopkins Press.

Molnar, G., & Alexander, M. (Eds.). (1998). *Pediatric rehabilitation* (3rd ed.). University of California Davis, CA: Hanley & Belfus.

Murphy, K. P., Molnar, G. E., & Lankasky, K. (1995). Medical and functional status of adults with cerebral palsy. *Developmental Medicine and Child Neurology*, 37(12), 1075–1084. Retrieved from http://dx.doi.org/10.1111/j.1469-8749.1995.tb11968.x, doi: 10.1111/j.1469-8749.1995.tb11968.x#_blank

National Institute of Neurological Disorders and Stroke. (2015). *Cerebral palsy: Hope through research*. Retrieved from http://www.ninds.nih.gov/disorders/cerebral_palsy/cerebral_palsy.htm

Peacock, W. J., & Staudt, L. A. (1991). Functional outcomes following selective posterior rhizotomy in children with cerebral palsy. *Journal of Neurosurgery*, 74(3), 380–385. Retrieved from http://dx.doi.org/10.3171/jns.1991.74.3.0380, doi: 10.3171/jns.1991.74.3.0380#_blank

Porter, R., & Kaplan, M. (Eds.). (2009). *The Merck manual online*. Rahway, NJ: Merc Sharp & Dohme Corp. Retrieved from http://www.merck.com/mmpe/sec19/ch283/ch283b.html

Sola, D. A., & Grant, A. D. (1995). Prognosis for ambulation in cerebral palsy. *Developmental Medicine and Child Neurology*, 37(11), 1020–1026. Retrieved from http://dx.doi.org/10.1111/j.1469-8749.1995.tb11959.x, doi: 10.1111/j.1469-8749.1995.tb11959.x#_blank

Smithers-Sheedy, H., McIntyre, S., Watson, L., Yeargin-Allsop, M., Blair, E., & Cans, C. (2009). Report of the international survey of cerebral palsy registers and surveillance systems. *Cerebral Palsy Institute*. Retrieved from http://www.cpresearch.org.au/pdfs/Report-of-the-international-survey-of-cerebral-palsy-registers-and-surveillance-systems-2009.pdf

Stanley, F., & Blair, E. (1994). Cerebral palsy. In Press, I. B. (Ed.), *The epidemiology of childhood disorders*. New York, NY: Oxford University Press.

Steinbok, P. (2006). Selection of treatment modalities in children with spastic cerebral palsy: Management options. *Neurosurgery Focus*, 21(2). Retrieved from http://www.medscape.com/viewarticle/550745_2

Stempien, L., & Tsai, T. (2000). Intrathecal baclofen pump use for spasticity: A clinical survey. *American Journal of Physical Medicine and Rehabilitation*, 6, 536–541. Retrieved from http://dx.doi.org/10.1097/00002060-200011000-00010, doi: 10.1097/00002060-200011000-00010#_blank

The Cleveland Clinic Health Information Center. (2015). *Selective dorsal rhizotomy*. Retrieved from http://my.clevelandclinic.org/services/selective_dorsal_rhizotomy/ns_overview.aspx

United Cerebral Palsy Research and Educational Foundation. (1997). *Multiple births and developmental brain damage.* Retrieved from http://cpirf.org/stories/364

United Cerebral Palsy Research and Education Foundation Factsheet. (2012). *Cerebral palsy facts and figures.* Retrieved from http://www.ucp.org/wp-content/uploads/2013/02/cp-fact-sheet.pdf

Zach, T. (2010). *Pediatric Periventricular leukomalacia.* Retrieved from http://emedicine.medscape.com/article/975728-overview

CHAPTER

3

Autism Spectrum Disorders

Michelle A. Suarez and Kathryn Ellsworth

Rachel was a beautiful firstborn daughter, and during her first year of life, she appeared to be a typically developing child. She responded to people and objects in her environment with interest and enjoyment. Though slightly delayed in learning to walk, she mastered this skill between 14 to 16 months of age. In contrast, many of her language skills developed strongly during her first year. Rachel was exposed to two different languages in her home and learned several vocabulary words in each language by the time she was 14 months old.

When Rachel was approximately 14 months old, her parents noticed a startling change in her behavior. Eye contact became rare, and she no longer turned in response when her mother called her name. As a result of this decreased responsiveness, her parents worried she was losing her hearing. However, an audiologic test indicated normal hearing abilities. Dressing this little girl became a challenge. Suddenly, she did not easily tolerate the sensation of clothes against her skin. She became intensely distressed when her mother tried to brush her hair or clip her nails. The vocabulary of approximately 30 words that she had previously developed was replaced by silence or babbling. Upon reflection, her mother realized Rachel had never used specific communicative gestures such as waving to greet others or pointing. Engaging Rachel in daily activities became increasingly difficult for she appeared frustrated, unable to express her needs and wants, and unable to leave familiar, preferred activities without becoming highly agitated. During these episodes of tantrums, Rachel would hit herself or bang her head repeatedly against a wall while crying. Her mother described that overall, "she no longer seemed happy." When Rachel was 2 years and 6 months old, her parents brought their concerns to the attention of early intervention specialists. As a result, Rachel began receiving occupational therapy, speech-language therapy, and special education services. During her preschool class, these specialists observed the same concerning characteristics her parents had described. Additionally, they noted she did not appear interested in the other children in her preschool class. Transitioning from room to room consistently distressed her, causing "meltdowns" during which she flung herself on the floor and cried inconsolably. She used only a few real words or echoed words of others but did not appear to understand what they meant. Many times, the classroom environment seemed to provide her with far too much sensory input. As a result, she would close her eyes or seek out places away from others. Yet Rachel still showed moments of attachment and joy, such as a strong, loving connection toward her parents and grandparents. Additionally, she smiled, laughed, and shared eye contact during specific activities, such as swinging, playing peekaboo, or singing.

Despite these moments of engagement, the changes and gaps in her development caused her parents and therapists to seek further neurodevelopmental testing. Rachel was therefore assessed by a team of specialists including a developmental pediatrician, a psychologist, a speech and language pathologist, and an occupational therapist who confirmed the suspicions of her family and therapists: Rachel presented with autism spectrum disorder.

DESCRIPTION AND DEFINITIONS

Autism spectrum disorder (ASD) is characterized by impairments in social interaction and social communication and by the presence of restricted and repetitive behaviors (American Psychiatric Association, 2013b). Individuals with this developmental disorder often have difficulty with things like participating in conversation or may misread nonverbal social cues from others. This can make it difficult to make friends and interact with peers. In addition, people who have ASD can have unusual responses to sensory information (e.g., tactile, auditory, visual stimulus) or be highly sensitive to changes in their environment or overly dependent on routines.

The *Diagnostic and Statistical Manual of Mental Disorders*, by the American Psychiatric Association, provides differential diagnosis criteria for autism. In 2013, the *Diagnostic and Statistical Manual of Mental Disorders, Fifth Edition (DSM-5)* was published and provided major changes to the way individuals with autism are diagnosed. In the earlier manual, the *Diagnostic and Statistical Manual of Mental Disorders, Fourth Edition (DSM-IV)*, individuals could be diagnosed with one of five main disorders under the autism spectrum umbrella. These disorders included autistic disorder, Asperger's disorder (also known as Asperger's syndrome), pervasive developmental disorder not otherwise specified (PDD-NOS),

childhood disintegrative disorder, and Rett's disorder (American Psychiatric Association, 2000).

In a major departure from the presence of multiple categories of autism, the DSM-5 provides for one universal ASD diagnosis. The rational for this change was the inconsistent and inaccurate use of the DSM-IV criteria (American Psychiatric Association, 2013a, DSM-5 ASD Fact Sheet). Researchers found that across clinics and professionals, there were few reliability data to support this continued separation of five separate disorders. In the DSM-5, anyone with a DSM-IV diagnosis should still meet the criteria for ASD. In addition, the DSM-5 provides new specifiers to more accurately describe the variants and severity of ASD, theoretically making it of more practical use for defining a treatment plan for an individual based on their specific presentation of this condition. For example, an individual who was previously diagnosed with Asperger's disorder (a previous variant of autism where intelligence is normal, language skills are intact, but social skills are impaired) might now be diagnosed with ASD *with or without* intellectual impairment or *with or without* language impairment.

Children with ASD share the following diagnostic characteristics (American Psychiatric Association, 2013b):

1. Impairment in social communication and social interaction that occurs over several contexts
2. Restricted, **repetitive** behavior, interests, and/ or activities

A child with ASD is deviant from, as well as delayed in, typical patterns of development. Some children evidence problems from birth, such as appearing aloof and making far less eye contact than other infants. In other cases, the characteristics of autism noticeably emerge between 12 to 36 months of age. Recognition of symptoms at this age is often due to one of two reasons. During the 12- to 36-month period, there is typically an explosion of language skills. Children with ASD may have been developing more slowly overall, and then this language burst fails to occur. Alternatively, 12- to 36-month-old children with ASD may lose language skills that they had demonstrated during earlier months in their development (Strock, 2004).

ASD is considered a "lifelong" disability, and there is no cure. However, intervention to improve skills, particularly in challenging areas that significant limit participation in meaningful occupation, can have a positive and powerful impact on quality of life for individuals with this disorder.

ETIOLOGY

Though researchers believe that certain factors (e.g., genetics) are more likely than others to cause ASD, no one etiologic factor has clearly emerged. Therefore, ASD is diagnosed based on observed behaviors using diagnostic criteria. Autism was first described in literature in 1943 by Dr. Leo Kanner (Kanner, 1943), and his initial hypotheses was that autism was caused by "cold" or unresponsive parents (Bettelheim, 1967). This hypothesis has been proven false and summarily rejected. Rather, autism is a neurologic disability (Lord & McGee, 2001) that likely originates in utero due to errors in genes causing abnormalities in brain structure and function (Autism Society of America, 2004).

■ Abnormalities in Brain Structure/ Function

Children with ASD develop, process, and react differently to their world than typically developing children. This diversion from normal development may be due to the possibility that children with autism begin life with brains that are physically different from those of typically developing children. Additionally, the way in which life experiences are mapped onto the brain is altered as a

result of these physical differences (Siegel, 2003). The precise distinctions are not yet entirely clear, since autism is not caused by a single obvious lesion in the brain. In fact, studies have indicated subtle differences in several areas of the brain with researchers unsure which area, or combination of areas, results in the manifestation of autism (United Kingdom Medical Research Council, 2001).

Through the study of postmortem brain tissue and imaging studies such as positron emission tomography (PET) scan and magnetic resonance imaging (MRI), consistencies have emerged in the research of brain abnormalities.

1. The brain is made up of about 100 billion **neurons**, or single cells, that interconnect and communicate information among the various brain regions and from other areas of the body. The behaviors of autism may result from abnormalities in the neural networking between the multiple areas of the brain, rather than in one area, as the brain processes complex information (Piven, Saliba, Bailey, & Arndt, 1997).

2. Though children with autism are born with normal head circumferences, increased brain volume and head circumference become evident in children with autism when they are 3 to 4 years old (United Kingdom Medical Research Council, 2001).

3. There is a growing body of research that suggests that dysfunction of the cerebellum is a likely contributor to autism. This area of the brain has been traditionally known for its role in the coordination of movement. But the **cerebellum**, which sits over the brainstem, may also play a role in sensory discrimination, attention, emotions, mental imagery, problem solving, and some aspects of language processing; the speed, consistency, and appropriateness of mental and cognitive processes; and visual-spatial orientation, spatial orientation, and visuomotor function (Bauman, 2004; Kemper & Bauman, 1998). Neurons in the cerebellum known as **Purkinje cells** form a layer near the surface of the cerebellum and convey signals away from the cerebellum. In autistic individuals, an important deviation consistently noted is a decrease in the Purkinje cell number.

4. In the brainstem, the neurons in the inferior olive of individuals with autism also showed deviations depending on age. Cells were initially larger than normal but typical in appearance in young children; in adulthood, these cells were unusually small and pale (Kemper & Bauman, 1998; United Kingdom Medical Research Council, 2001).

5. **Inferior olives** are connected to Purkinje cells by climbing fibers, and this bond from the inferior olive to the Purkinje cell is made at 28 to 30 weeks of gestation. Once this union occurs, if a Purkinje cell dies, then the inferior olive will also deplete. As previously noted, Purkinje cells are reduced in number in children with autism, but the cells of the inferior olive are normal in quantity. The implication is that damage to the Purkinje cells in children with ASD would have likely occurred in utero before the bond was established, prior to 30 weeks of gestation (Bauman, 2004; Kemper & Bauman, 1998).

6. Imaging studies have indicated reduced activation of the frontal lobe in individuals diagnosed with autism (United Kingdom Medical Research Council, 2001). Additionally, some areas of the frontal lobe appear markedly larger in children with autism compared with typically developing children (Carper & Courchesne, 2005). The frontal lobe's function is voluntary control of the body's movements. Specific regions of this lobe are also responsible for social behavior, spontaneous production of language, initiation of motor activity, processing sensory stimuli, and then planning reaction as a result of the input, abstract thinking, problem solving, and judgment (Kemper & Bauman, 1998). How the abnormalities affect the frontal lobe's ability to conduct these roles remains unclear, though many symptoms of autism appear related to problems in frontal lobe functioning (Fig. 3.1).

7. Within the **limbic system**, a network of structures that regulates emotion, structures known as the **amygdala** and **hippocampus**, appear abnormal in the brains of individuals with ASD.

"Memories, the desire to produce language, feelings, and the emotional coloring of thought are all mediated by the limbic system. Anatomical systems necessary for cognitive

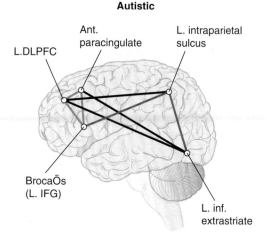

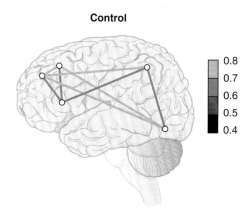

Figure 3.1 Autism: Connectivity in the brain. The behaviors of autism may result from reduced connectivity among the different regions of the brain. This figure illustrates reliably lower functional connectivity for autism participants between pairs of key areas during sentence comprehension tasks. **Darker end** of scale denotes lower connectivity (slide courtesy of Marcel Just, Carnegie Mellon University).

functions, such as language, spatial concepts, understanding of meaning in life, and so forth are all intimately linked to the limbic system" (Helm-Estabrooks & Albert, 2003, p. 15).

Since the functioning of these abilities is impacted in individuals with autism, it has been a logical step to focus research in this area. Thus far, anomalies include decreased size of the neurons that make up the structures of the limbic system, with a higher number of these neuronal cells packed into their respective spaces (Kemper & Bauman, 1998) (Fig. 3.2).

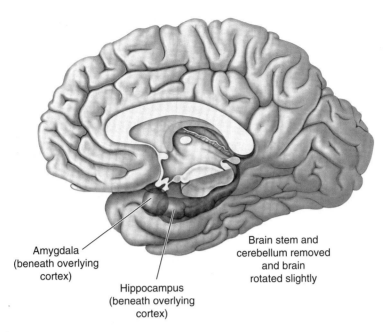

Amygdala
(beneath overlying
cortex)

Brain stem and
cerebellum removed
and brain
rotated slightly

Hippocampus
(beneath overlying
cortex)

Figure 3.2 Cerebral cortex. Left lateral view of the brain, including the four lobes of the cerebrum and the cerebellum. (From Bickley, L. S., & Szilagyi, P. (2003). *Bates' guide to physical examination and history taking* (8th ed.). Philadelphia, PA: Lippincott Williams & Wilkins.)

Scientists are persistently closing in on the differences in the brain structure and function of this population. In the meantime, the question arises: What has happened in a child's system to cause these deviations in the brain to occur?

Parents of children with ASD, upon hearing their child's diagnosis, typically search for reasons why this condition occurred in their child. The professionals who work with these parents must act as guides to discuss the most recent and accurate information in the autism field. Parents are likely to question professionals about many of the factors that will be discussed in the following sections. It is important to share with parents those theories that are likely and those that seem implausible based on current research.

■ Genetics

The differences in the neurobiology of children with autism are most likely accounted for by genetics. **Genes** are composed of DNA and, through heredity, determine the particular characteristics that distinguish one human from another. Genes are encoded instructions—the brain's written guidelines for function. If any abnormalities lie in a brain's genes, the brain deviates from a course of typical development (Siegel, 2003). No single gene has been found to cause ASD; therefore, current research is focused on finding a combination of genes that may be responsible for an individual's susceptibility to autism (United Kingdom Medical Research Council, 2001; Veenstra-VanDerWeele, Cook, & Lombroso, 2003).

Support for Genetic Etiology

- In sibling studies, where one monozygotic (identical) twin was diagnosed with autism, the other was also diagnosed somewhere on the spectrum in 90% to 95% of cases. For dizygotic (fraternal) twins, both children received an ASD diagnosis in only 10% of cases studied. These statistics imply that shared genetic codes significantly increase the likelihood of autism occurrence (Rapin & Katzman, 1998; Veenstra-VanDerWeele et al., 2003).

- In the general population, an individual has a 0.2% chance of having autism (Veenstra-VanDerWeele et al., 2003). Siblings of children with autism, however, are at a higher risk for presenting somewhere on the autism spectrum. For parents, the probability of having a second child with autism is 3% to 7% if the first child is male and has autism. If the first child is female with autism, the likelihood of a second child with autism increases to approximately 7% to 14% (Rapin & Katzman, 1998). A higher rate of speech-language disorders has also been found among these families (Rutter, Silberg, O'Connor, & Simonoff, 1999), suggesting that these siblings received some, but not all, of the genes responsible for autism (Siegel, 2003).

- Relatives of these children more commonly displayed traits of autism (e.g., anxiety, aloofness) than did relatives of other children. The presence of these traits in family members may be genetically linked to the manifestation of autism (Jick & Kaye, 2003).
- Additional weight is given to the genetic link since a disproportionately higher number of males are diagnosed with autism, with three to four males diagnosed for every one female (Rapin & Katzman, 1998).

Because specific genes have not yet been identified as the cause of autism, current research is exploring other factors as possible etiologies or covariables. Researchers are also considering that autism may be caused by a different combination of variables for each child on the spectrum.

■ Environmental Factors

Environmental factors are external influences that may cause damage to people's systems if they are overexposed or exposed during a period of critical development. The United Kingdom Medical Research Council (2001) reviewed the following environmental risk factors as possible causes of autism: prenatal or postnatal exposure to viruses, infections, drugs/alcohol, endocrine factors, and carbon monoxide. However, these factors are thus far not significantly linked to ASDs. In terms of obstetric complications, most mothers reported entirely normal prenatal or perinatal experiences. Researchers have paid particular attention to the measles-mumps-rubella (MMR) vaccination (which protects against those diseases) in recent years, with some researchers speculating that the mercury in this vaccination is responsible for causing changes in a person's system that lead to the symptoms of autism. When further investigated, a valid association between the MMR vaccine and autism was not found. Though exposure to mercury may lead to impairments that look similar to those found in autism, children with autism have not consistently evidenced elevated levels

of mercury in their systems. In contrast, children with behavioral and/or developmental difficulties were discovered to have a higher level of lead in their systems, though it is unclear if exposure to lead results in autism (United Kingdom Medical Research Council, 2001).

■ Physiologic Abnormalities

Children with autism need to be closely monitored for additional medical concerns, since many of these children are not able to clearly express a medical problem. For those children who are nonverbal, acting out with inappropriate behaviors may be their only form of expressing discomfort. If a child demonstrates sudden aggressive, severe, or unusual behaviors, or awakens frequently from sleep, then medical attention by an experienced physician is necessary (Horvath, Papadimitriou, Rabsztyn, Drachenburg, & Tildon, 1999).

One medical condition a child with autism may experience is a **gastrointestinal (GI) disorder**, which is a disorder of the digestive tract. Unusually high rates of GI disorders in children with autism have been documented in recent years, including GI reflux, gastritis, persistent gas, diarrhea, and constipation (Horvath et al., 1999; Levy, Mandell, Merhar, Ittenbach, & Pinto-Martin, 2003, p. 418; McQueen & Heck, 2002). These problems should be treated by a gastroenterologist, a physician who specializes in GI disorders. A common, though unproven, theory hypothesizes that children with autism experience abnormal digestion of **gluten**, a mixture of proteins that may be found in wheat and other products (e.g., some snack foods or delicatessen meats), and **casein**, a protein found in cow's milk. This theory suggests that children with autism lack an enzyme that efficiently digests these substances; as a result, opioid or morphine-like substances accumulate and may be the reason these children socially withdraw or engage in repetitive behaviors (Levy & Hyman, 2003; McCandless, 2003).

It has been widely debated that children with autism have increased vulnerability to immune system disorders. While this idea has gathered interest, similar to theories of food allergies, there is a current lack of research to prove or disprove this factor.

■ Combination of Factors

It is plausible that the interaction of gene susceptibility and environmental factors gives rise to autism. In other words, an individual may be genetically at risk for this disorder, but in order for characteristics to appear, an individual would also need to be exposed to a yet-to-be-identified environmental factor (United Kingdom Medical Research Council, 2001).

INCIDENCE AND PREVALENCE

ASD impacts approximately 1% of the world's population (CDC, 2014), and in the United States, 3.5 million Americans live with this disability (Ostrow, 2014). For reasons that are not entirely clear, the prevalence of autism has been rising steadily and increased by 119.4% from the year 2000, where 1 in 150 were diagnosed with autism, to the year 2010 where 1 in 68 children were diagnosed (CDC, 2014). This makes autism the fastest growing developmental disability. Though this increase has raised speculation of a possible "epidemic," the rise in prevalence likely results from better identification and availability of services, along with changes in diagnostic criteria that allow more children to fit the diagnosis of autism (Fombonne, 1999; Jick & Kaye, 2003; Rapin, 2002).

The likelihood of an autism diagnosis can vary by community and by demographic characteristics (CDC, 2014). For example, only 1 in 175 children were diagnosed in some areas of Alabama whereas 1 in 45 were diagnosed in New Jersey. In addition, white children are much more likely to be given an autism diagnosis than black or Hispanic children. This may be a reflection of availability of services in rural versus urban areas and availability of resources to some underserved populations. Finally, boys are just about five times more likely to be identified with ASD than girls. This difference may be due to differences in the biological structures of the male and female brain. The concept of autism being caused by "extreme maleness" has been explored (Baron-Cohen, Knickmeyer, & Belmonte, 2005). This theory relates to the population generality that the male brain is more geared toward "systemizing" and the female brain generally more geared toward empathizing. Overall, prevalence information can be useful to inform policy and education of health care professionals so that all children on the spectrum have access to services that can impact quality of life.

Incidence, or the measure of new cases per year, is best studied in disorders that have a clear onset. Because the age of onset in autism is usually unclear, accurate incident rates are difficult to measure. Estimates range from 2.1 to 8.3 per 10,000 for all children diagnosed with an ASD (United Kingdom Medical Research Council, 2001).

SIGNS AND SYMPTOMS

Children with ASD all have difficulty with social communication and interaction as well as restricted and repetitive behaviors. However, the severity and functional presentation of these symptoms vary widely from one individual to the next. In addition, these core behavior deficits do not encompass the entire picture for these complex human beings. Motor abnormalities, **sensory processing disorders**, feeding disorders, and co-occurring medical disorders (e.g., seizures, sleep disturbances, GI problems) are only some of the additional concerns that arise in this population. Every child with autism displays a separate matrix of strengths and challenges with individual differences resulting from personality and experiences (United Kingdom Medical Research Council, 2001). Core symptoms, described below, are drawn from the DSM-5 diagnostic criteria for ASD (American Psychiatric Association, 2013b).

■ Core Symptoms

The first of the core symptoms, difficulty in social interaction, includes limited use of eye contact, facial expressions, and social gestures (e.g., pointing, shrugging, reaching arms up to be lifted). Additionally, children on the autism spectrum are usually challenged to accurately interpret the body language and facial expressions of other people. A child with ASD may not seek out others to share enjoyment, share interest in the same objects with peers, or look for approval or reassurance from parents. Moreover, individuals experience challenges in developing friendships with same-age peers. These obstacles range from showing a lack of interest in others to desiring friends but having difficulty understanding how to relate appropriately to peers.

Problems with interaction may be partially due to the fact that children with autism are hypothesized to have limitations in **theory of mind,** which is the ability to understand another person's thoughts, feelings, or intentions. It is how an individual "reads" someone's thoughts, understands another person's perspective on an issue, and predicts another's feelings (Leslie & Frith, 1987). Without this ability, a person is not able to predict or understand the actions of others. Other social disturbances that manifest in children with autism include a preference for playing alone, limited or repetitive play routines, and limited or absent pretend play skills (National Research Council, 2001; Rapin, 1991).

Social communication and language impairments in the autism population include delays in language development as well as abnormalities in language use. Typically, developing children progress through several communication milestones in their first few years (Strock, 2004). During a child's first year of life, a toddler gazes at others with interest, begins babbling, and reacts to sounds and voices. By 12 months, gestures and first words emerge and the child shows recognition of his or her name and some words and phrases. By 2 years of age, the child has built a substantial vocabulary and combines words into two- to three-word phrases. However, children with autism frequently show delays in learning to speak, with some children unable to use words until their school-age years (Strock, 2004). In severe cases of autism, spoken language may not be acquired at all. A child's ability to respond to voices or comprehend verbal language (**auditory processing**) may also be impacted. Many parents report that their child with autism does not respond when spoken to or called by name. Social impairments further affect these children's communication because they may not be motivated to communicate with others, are typically challenged to use or understand social cues such as intonation and facial expressions to interpret meaning, and have difficulty maintaining the "give and take" of conversations (e.g., a child may discuss only his or her topic of interest without allowing others to take a turn).

The language of verbal children often appears even more peculiar because of the presence of echolalia, pronoun reversal, and out-of-context words. **Echolalia** is speech in which the child echoes back what he or she has previously heard. Though all young children use echolalia as they are learning language, children with autism retain this characteristic and often apply it in abnormal ways. It results from poor auditory processing

while auditory memory remains intact (Siegel, 1996). Echolalia may be immediate, meaning that it occurs just after another speaker's utterance, or delayed, occurring significantly after hearing a speaker (e.g., reciting an entire children's book from memory an hour or day later). Though it may appear unusual in conversation, children with autism frequently use this inappropriate device in meaningful ways (e.g., reciting lines from his favorite movie as a self-calming strategy when he feels anxious). Because children with autism often fail to understand language, pronouns (e.g., "you" and "me") are also often used incorrectly. Other times, these individuals may use language in a context that seems out of place; for instance, saying "ball" when actually requesting juice.

The second core feature of autism is in the area of **restrictive and repetitive behaviors.** Individuals with ASD may exhibit an abnormal or intense preoccupation with routines or patterns. For instance, a child may line up blocks or toy cars for hours without playing with others or using these toys in pretend play. Additionally, the child may scream or cry in reaction to someone joining the child's play or moving the lined-up toys. Obsessions with specific topics are common, such as showing an unusual interest in elevators or numbers and letters (Strock, 2004). Additional common characteristics include rigidity in daily routines; abnormal, stereotyped behaviors such as repetitive hand-flapping or body rocking; and unusual, nonfunctional preoccupation with parts of an object (e.g., spinning the wheels of a toy car without showing interest in any other type of play with this toy) (American Psychiatric Association, 2013a; Strock, 2004).

All children diagnosed with ASD demonstrate some combination of these social, social language, and behavioral symptoms. However, the range of severity and functional presentation of these symptoms is vast. The DSM-5 provides additional specifiers to more accurately capture the impact of these symptoms on individual functioning that is useful for treatment planning and research purposes. First, the presence or absence of intellectual disability, language disorder, associated medical condition, and/or catatonia is captured. Then, severity level for the two core symptoms is captured on a three-point scale from mild to severe. Examples of function within this hierarchy, adapted from the DSM 5, are included in Table 3.1.

The DSM-5 provides for one umbrella diagnosis of ASD and offers new categorical descriptors

TABLE 3.1   Levels of Severity within the Autism Spectrum

Level 1: Mild to Moderate on Autism Spectrum	Level 2: Severe to Moderate on Autism Spectrum	Level 3: Very Severe on Autism Spectrum
Has use of sentence level language but often has difficulty using language functionally without support	May have some use of language but verbal and nonverbal communication is limited	Often does not have verbal language and/or use of language is very limited and atypical
May have less interest in social engagement than typically developing peers or is sometimes described as odd or atypical	Difficulty with meaningful engagement with others and attempts are often viewed as odd or unusual	Does not seek engagement with others except occasionally to get needs met
Attempts to make friends may fail when social cues are missed	May attempt conversation around a restricted interest like trains, numbers, or electricity and unable to shift to a topic of mutual interest	When attempting to communicate a need, does so with unusual and often ineffectual attempts
		Frequently ignores or does not respond to even very direct attempts from others to engage socially
Is most comfortable in a well-worn routine	Insistence on sameness and inflexibility is noticeable to others outside of the child's immediate social circle.	Extreme inflexibility and resistance to change. May have self-injurious behavior with changes in routine
This child benefits from intervention to engage in meaningful occupations at a greater depth and to improve the richness of social relationships.	This child requires substantial intervention to engage in meaningful occupations.	Even with intervention, this child's autism very significantly interferes with participation in meaningful occupations.

to pinpoint the specific presentation of this disorder for an individual. Since the degree of functional impairment varies widely for individuals with autism, this has the potential to allow for more individualized treatment. However, the move from having five diagnostic categories (i.e., Asperger's syndrome, pervasive developmental disability not otherwise specified, childhood disintegrative disorder, Rett's syndrome, and autism disorder) is not without controversy. Detractors are concerned that diagnosis may be more restricted and that people being newly diagnosed with autism may not fit the new criteria and may not have access to services and support previously provided (Kulage, Smaldone, & Cohn, 2014). The impact of this major change will be followed for years to come, and the evaluation of

the usefulness of this new diagnostic structure will be determined by the successful identification of children in need of services to mediate the functional limitations that are often caused by symptoms of autism.

■ Co-occurring Conditions

The core symptoms of autism cause many challenges to engagement in everyday life for individuals with ASD and the people who love and support them. These challenges can be compounded by co-occurring conditions that are commonly found in individuals ASD. Sensory processing disorder and possibly related fine and gross motor deficits, **food selectivity**, sleep disturbances, and GI issues can create additional stressors that profoundly influence the quality of life in this population.

Sensory Processing Disorder

Hypo- and hyperreactivity to sensory information and/or unusual preoccupation with the sensory aspects of the environment are included in the diagnostic criteria in the DSM-5 under restricted and repetitive behaviors. However, many children with autism have sensory processing problems that go beyond hypo- and hyperreactivity. Also, beginning with the pioneering work of the prominent occupational therapist Jean Ayres, sensory processing disorders are of special interest to occupational therapists and are therefore covered separately here.

In the 1970s, Jean Ayres, an occupation therapist with training in neuroscience and education, developed the theory of sensory integration to explain learning differences in children who struggled with interpreting sensation from their bodies and the environment (Ayres, 1994). Today, estimates of atypical sensory processing in children with ASD range as high as 95% (Baranek, David, Poe, Stone, & Watson, 2006). Sensory processing disorders are organized into several subtypes that manifest in difficulty modulating sensory experiences in order to maintain a calm alert state (i.e., under- or hyporesponsivity [SUR], over- or hyperresponsivity [SOR], sensory seeking [SS], or craving [SC]), difficulty with motor skills (i.e., dyspraxia and postural instability), and difficulty with discrimination of the quality of sensory stimulus (Miller, 2014). The severity and type of sensory processing problems in children with ASD contribute substantially to success in daily functioning. Table 3.2 contains the sensory processing disorder subtypes with behavioral examples and the connection between the subtype and children with ASD.

Fine and Gross Motor Impairment

As described in the table above, children with autism have motor impairments that may be related to their ability to use sensation to plan, guide, and execute movement. Fine and gross motor impairments include problems in skilled movement, hand-eye coordination, speed, praxis and imitation, posture, and balance (Dawson & Watling, 2000). A particularly debilitating abnormality in individuals with autism includes deficits in motor imitation skills despite intact perceptual and motor capacities, which are most apparent in younger groups of children (Williams, Whiten, & Singh, 2004). Furthermore, these children perform poorly on tasks of executing a sequence of movements,

such as a sequence of hand or facial actions in imitation (Hughes, 1996). Reduced stride lengths, increased stance times, increased hip flexion at toe-off, reduced knee extension at initial ground contact, abnormal heel strikes, and decreased knee extension and ankle dorsiflexion at ground contact were noted in an earlier study of children with autism (Vilensky, Damasio, & Maurer, 1981).

In addition, a disproportionate number of children with autism display ambiguous hand preference (~40%) long past the age that dominant hand preference typically develops. A person who is ambidextrous will usually choose one hand for a specific task (e.g., left hand for writing, right hand for throwing a football). An **ambiguous hand preference**, however, refers to switching hands within the same activity (Hauck & Dewey, 2001). When this behavior persists into the school-age years, it may indicate abnormal functioning of the brain.

Food Selectivity

Children with ASD often have an extremely self-restricted diets and disruptive behaviors during mealtime (Schreck, Williams, & Smith, 2004). These children may refuse to eat more than 5 to 10 very specific foods. For example, a child with ASD might insist on eating a specific brand and shape of macaroni and cheese at every meal. They may insist that food be arranged on the plate a particular way with foods not touching other foods. They may refuse to eat any foods from a particular food group and have meltdowns and/or gag or vomit when encouraged to eat a nonpreferred food. It is common for children with autism and **food selectivity** to refuse to eat any fruits and vegetables (Suarez & Crinion, 2015). This behavior causes worry and stress for caregivers and can make mealtime unpleasant for the entire family (Suarez, Atchison, & Lagerwey, 2014). Also, depending on the degree of food refusal, **food selectivity** can threaten health and development due to lack of consumption of essential nutrients (Bandini et al., 2010).

Sleep Disturbance

Poor quality sleep is common in the ASD population and up to approximately 70% have some form of sleep disturbance (Souders et al., 2009). Children with autism may resist going to bed and require extensive time to fall asleep (Liu, Hubbard, Fabes, & Adam, 2006). They may have long periods of awakenings, awaken many times during the night, or wake-up very early in

TABLE 3.2   **Sensory Processing Disorder in Children with ASD**

Sensory Processing Disorder Subtype (Miller, 2014)	Behavioral Example	Implications Specific to ASD
Sensory Modulation Disorder		
SOR Sometimes called "sensory defensiveness." Behavioral response to stimuli that is more intense and longer lasting than expected	Distress with bathing and grooming Difficulty tolerating crowded places Meltdowns with unexpected noises	Strong correlation with symptoms of anxiety in children with ASD (Lane, Reynolds, & Dumenci, 2012) Linked to decreased participation in activities outside the home for children with ASD (Little, Ausderau, Sideris, & Garanek, 2015)
SUR Take longer to respond to stimuli or do not notice sensory information that is obvious to others	Does not respond to injuries Often unaware of what is going on in the environment. Leaves food on face or clothing twisted on body	Most common pattern of SMD in children with ASD (Ben-Sasson et al., 2009) Is one early predictor of joint attention and social communication skills in young children with ASD (Baranek et al., 2013; Watson, Baranek, Roberts, David, & Perryman, 2010)
SC Insatiable craving for sensory stimuli that interferes with functioning	Touches everything Is always moving Puts nonfood items in mouth	Has been associated with academic underachievement due to difficulty with sustained attention (Ashburner, Ziviani, & Rodger, 2008)
Sensory-Based Motor Disorder		
Dyspraxia Difficulty with motor planning (praxis)	Is delayed in the development of motor skills including learning to walk and/or learning to ride a bike Struggles with multistep activities, like getting dressed or making a sandwich Novel motor activities are especially difficult.	Motor coordination deficits are pervasive and some hypothesize that this may be an underlying feature of autism (Fournier, Hass, Naik, Lodha, & Cauraugh, 2010; MacNeil & Mostofsky, 2012; Roley et al., 2015) Have substantial dysfunction in praxis skills when compared to typically developing individuals (MacNeil & Mostofsky, 2012) Somatopraxis (ability to organize own body action using tactile and proprioceptive information) deficits are associated with social participation, possibly due to difficulty with imitation (Roley et al., 2015).
Postural disorder and/or poor postural strength and stability	Tires easily Has decreased balance and requires support during static motor tasks	Development of postural stability is delayed and can fail to mature to adult levels in children with ASD (Minshew, Sung, Jones, & Furman, 2004).

(continued)

TABLE 3.2 *Continued*		
Sensory Processing Disorder Subtype (Miller, 2014)	**Behavioral Example**	**Implications Specific to ASD**
Sensory Discrimination Disorder Difficulty discriminating between the qualities of distinct sensory stimulus can occur in one of more of the senses.	Difficulty with stereognosis Struggles to tell the difference between a "b" and a "d" Cannot distinguish between speech sounds	Contradictory evidence (Dickinson & Milne, 2014) for both enhanced sensory discrimination (Bertone, Mottron, Jelenic, & Faubert, 2005; Bonnel et al., 2003) and reduced tactile discrimination (Puts, Woodka, Tommerdahl, Mostofsky, & Edden, 2014)

the morning. Causes for sleep disturbance are unknown but may be related to abnormalities in the areas of the brainstem that regulate sleep and in melatonin levels (Malow et al., 2012). Children with ASD who are poor sleepers have more difficulty with daytime disruptive behavior than children who sleep well (Malow et al., 2006; Wang et al., 2015). In addition, sleep disturbance in children with ASD has implications for the sleep quality of the entire family. This can lead to additional stress on a family already struggling with core symptoms of autism.

COURSE AND PROGNOSIS

Since the symptom variability within the autism spectrum differs widely between individuals, the course and prognosis depend on the individual's presentation. Many children with autism can have significant functional improvement with treatment. However, most individuals tracked longitudinally retain characteristics of the diagnosis throughout the span (Lord & McGee, 2001). Several prognostic indicators can partially predict functional outcomes for individuals with this disorder.

■ Intellectual Disability

Some children with autism also have decreased mental capacity limiting their ability to plan, problem solve, think abstractly, and/or comprehend complex ideas (The Arc, n.d.). Intellectual abilities are measured with assessments that provide an intelligence quotient (IQ) and scores below 75 indicate significant impairment in

thinking skills. The prevalence of intellectual disability in children with ASD is likely in the 15% to 20% range (Fernell, Eriksson, & Gillberg, 2013) with estimates ranging as high as 68% (Yeargin-Allsopp et al., 2003). IQ is the number one predictor of later adaptive functioning in children with autism (Fernell et al., 2013). For example, the previous DSM (IV) included a diagnosis of Asperger's, which was characterized by social and behavioral challenges *without* presentation of cognitive deficits. Longitudinal studies suggest that prognosis is better for the Asperger's disorder with more individuals able to function independently in employment and self-sufficient living (American Psychiatric Association, 2000).

■ Language

A child's language level is also a strong predictor of functioning over the course of the lifespan. A child's ability to spontaneously, meaningfully, and consistently combine words into phrases or sentences before 5 years of age is a good prognostic indicator of cognitive, language, adaptive, and academic achievement measures (Lord and McGee, National Research Council, 2001). It is important to observe that the child is able to spontaneously construct sentences rather than echo others' utterances (echolalia) or use memorized chunks of language to communicate. In addition, a child's use of joint attention has been found to be a predictor of language outcome. **Joint attention** is the ability to use eye contact and gestures in order to share experiences with others. Children who fail to use early gestural joint attention (e.g., failing to point at an object and to turn to his mother to determine if his mother shares his interest) seem to struggle in the development of meaningful language. In Lord and McGee's review of autism research (2001), findings implied that early joint attention, symbolic play, and receptive language were strong predictors of a child's future outcomes. Another study in this review examined severity of repetitive, stereotyped behaviors and social symptoms and found that the severity later predicted adaptive functioning.

Motor Skills

Early success in hand-eye coordination may predict vocational abilities later in life. Fine motor skills also predicted later leisure pursuits (Lord & McGee, 2001). Children with autism who displayed a definite hand preference performed significantly better on motor, language, and cognitive tasks (Hauck & Dewey, 2001). The ability to imitate body movements has been linked to expressive language development, and imitation of actions with objects predicted later levels of play abilities (Lord & McGee, 2001). The more established behavioral challenges become without intervention, the more these problems persist and worsen.

SURGICAL/MEDICAL MANAGEMENT

Diagnosis

Autism is now diagnosed at a younger age than ever before because characteristics of autism have become more defined and better recognized. Researchers have employed at least two research methods to identify early indicators of ASD (Boyd, Odom, Humphreys, & Sam, 2010). Retrospective studies, using home videos of children later diagnosed with autism, and prospective studies of the younger siblings of children with autism (due to the genetic likelihood of siblings both having autism) have been used to develop an understanding of early behavioral warning signs. Key indicators include delay or disorder in social behaviors like smiling socially or response to one's name. Coordination of verbal and non-verbal communication (e.g., verbalization with a point or eye gaze, showing objects to others) is often difficult or absent in very young children that are eventually diagnosed with autism. Finally, atypical play, including spinning objects or preoccupations with parts of objects, can be an early indicator. Receiving a diagnosis at an early age is optimal because the sooner the disorder is recognized, the more likely the child can make dramatic reductions in symptoms and gains in learning (Lord & McGee, 2001; Strock, 2004). In addition, parents are able to receive valuable support and education from professionals and other family members.

A child is usually referred for an assessment because those who interact closely with him (e.g., family members, pediatrician, teachers) may observe warning signs either specific to autism or to a development delay in one or more areas. When these concerns become apparent, the child is initially screened, usually by primary care providers or early child care professionals, to look for the "red flags" that may indicate autistic behaviors. Published screening instruments for children with autism include

- The Checklist for Autism in Toddlers (CHAT) (Baron-Cohen, Allen, & Gillberg, 1992)
- The Autism Screening Questionnaire (ASQ) (Berument, Rutter, Lord, Pickles, & Bailey, 1999)
- The Screening Tool for Autism in Two-Year-Olds (Stone, Coonrod, & Ousley, 2000)
- Australian Scale for Asperger's Syndrome (Garnett & Attwood, 1998)
- Pervasive Developmental Disorders Screening Test, Stage 1 (PDDST-I) (Siegel, 1998a)
- The Modified Checklist for Autism in Toddlers (M-CHAT) (Robins et al., 2001).

If the child does not pass the screening, this indicates that enough warning signs of autism are present to warrant a thorough assessment for autism. Since each child on the ASD displays a unique matrix of strengths and weaknesses, no two children on the autism spectrum will look the same. Therefore, critical to an accurate diagnosis is an assessment with clinicians who are experienced in identifying the characteristics of autism. Additionally, a thorough diagnosis with a team of professionals can gather insight into each child's skills across several areas of development, which, in turn, helps with intervention planning. An autism evaluation team frequently consists of a developmental pediatrician, a psychologist, a speech and language pathologist, and often an occupational therapist. The following elements should be included in every sensitive, comprehensive evaluation of a child with autism:

1. *History*: Though autism is not known to result from complications during pregnancy, it is important to discuss any unusual pre- or perinatal events to rule out other disorders. Because of autism's genetic implications, it is important to determine if other family members have been diagnosed with autism, psychiatric concerns, or developmental disorders. The history portion should also include questioning about autism-specific behaviors in the areas of social, language, behavioral, play, cognitive, and sensory processing abilities (Rapin, 1997).

2. *Medical history*: During this portion of the assessment, parents report when their child's developmental milestones were reached (e.g., what age their child said his or her first word, learned to walk), if regression of developmental skills occurred at any point, or if any other medical problems are occurring (e.g., psychiatric, sleeping, or eating problems) (Filipek et al., 1999).

3. *Physical/neurological examination*: Other illnesses such as fragile X syndrome, tuberous sclerosis, or congenital rubella need to be ruled out, since these disorders may look similar to autism (Rapin, 1997). The physician also checks for other medical illnesses (e.g., GI disorders, ear infections), measures head circumference, gives a general physical examination, examines mental status, verifies that cranial nerves function normally, and performs a motor examination (Filipek et al., 1999).

4. *Parent interviewing*: Many diagnostic tools are available to gain parents' insight into their child's autism-specific behaviors. A clinician should also ask parents about their overall impression of their child, since more general questions may reveal further insight beyond the scope of these tools (Filipek et al., 1999; Lord and McGee, National Research Council, 2001).

5. Parent Interview Tools:
   - *The Autism Diagnostic Interview*: Revised (Lord, Rutter, & LeCouteur, 1994)
   - Functional Emotional Assessment Scale (FEAS) (Greenspan, DeGangi, & Wieder, 1999)
   - The Gilliam Autism Rating Scale (GARS) (Gilliam, 1995)
   - The Pervasive Developmental Disorders Screening Test, Stage 2 (PDDST-II) (Siegel, 1998b)

6. Tests in language development. Examples of tools include the following:
   - Preschool Language Scales (PLS) (Zimmerman, Steiner, & Pond, 2011)
   - Clinical Evaluation of Language Fundamentals (CELF) (Wiig, Semel, & Second, 2013)

7. Tests in cognitive development:
   - Mullen Scales of Early Learning (MSEL) (Mullen, 1995).
   - Wechsler Intelligence Scale for Children (WISC) (Wechsler, 2003)
   - Bayley Scales of Infant and Toddler Development, Third Edition (Bayley-III) (Bayley, 2005).

8. Tests in other developmental areas including sensory processing, motor, and adaptive skills.
   - Sensory Profile 2 (Dunn, 2014)
   - Peabody Developmental Motor Scales, Second Edition (PDMS-2) (Folio & Fewell, 2000)
   - Quick Neurological Screening Test 3 (QNST-3) (Mutti et al.)
   - Vineland Adaptive Behavior Scales (Sparrow, Cicchetti, & Balla, 2006)

9. Formal and informal observation of the child interacting with others. This is considered one of the most valuable pieces of the evaluation process, since it typically reveals the qualitative impairments of the child (such as lack of eye contact, limited initiation of interaction, or difficulty transitioning between tasks). A diagnostic instrument should be used that examines autistic behaviors while the clinician observes the child's interests and interactions with others. The Autism Diagnostic Observation Schedule (ADOS) (Lord & Rutter, 2000) is considered a gold standard instrument for this purpose.

10. *Audiological testing*: An audiologic evaluation is necessary to rule out hearing disorders. Children with autism are often unresponsive to verbal auditory stimuli, and it is important to determine that this behavior is not caused by a hearing impairment. If hearing loss co-occurs with autism, language comprehension may be further impacted than with a diagnosis of autism alone (Filipek et al., 1999).

11. *Other testing*: Certain tests may prove beneficial to specific circumstances.

For instance, an electroencephalograph (EEG) may be needed if the child is suspected of having seizures (Filipek et al., 1999). Some children are assessed through university studies, and MRIs are typically included in these autism assessments (Bauman, 2004; Filipek et al., 1999). Genetics testing may be appropriate for parents who are considering having another child (Filipek et al., 1999). Some parents are also concerned about heavy metal contamination and wish to pursue a lead screening for their child.

■ Medical/Surgical Treatment

Overall, treatment for autism does not heavily rely on medical intervention, and surgical interventions are not practiced for this disorder. Intensive early intervention is most effective in reducing problem behaviors while increasing language, social, sensory, motor, and cognitive skills (Lord and McGee, National Research Council, 2001; Rapin, 1997; Rogers, 1996). A variety of approaches are available, ranging from highly structured to naturalistic. Because no two children with autism present with the same set of symptoms, no one treatment plan is successful for all children with autism. Effective intervention must account for the child's individual strengths and challenges and must consider functional skills to be generalized across a variety of settings in the child's life. Substantial literature supports early intervention for children 0 to 3 years as the most beneficial time to connect new pathways for more appropriate functioning and behavior, though an individual may continue to make substantial gains following this period of development (Lord and McGee, National Research Council, 2001; Rapin, 1997; Rogers, 1996). Because it is beyond the scope of this book to discuss these approaches, this chapter focuses on current knowledge of medical interventions meant to accompany intervention techniques.

Pharmacologic Therapies

Use of medication does not cure the core social, language, and repetitive behavioral deficits of autism because "in most cases, the brain has undergone atypical cellular development dating from the earliest embryonic stages" (Rapin, 2002, p. 303). Research in this area is presently limited or inconclusive. In addition, many parents and clinicians are cautious because use of pharmacotherapy with children presents the risk of harmful side effects. Lindsay and Aman (2003) reviewed existing literature on pharmacologic intervention and found that when certain medications are used appropriately, behavioral dysregulations such as hyperactivity, irritability, anxiety, and perseveration may be reduced. For instance, risperidone, an atypical antipsychotic agent, shows promising results in emerging research for reducing tantrums, irritability, aggression, and self-injurious and repetitive behaviors (Gordon, 2002; Lindsay & Aman, 2003; Pediatric Psychopharmacology Autism Network, 2002). Because autism is likely a genetic disorder determined before the child is born, pharmacologic treatments could probably not "undo" this disorder. Therefore, these treatments are not investigated to replace educational services but rather to supplement them. For those children who respond successfully to medication, behavioral and educational intervention may be even more beneficial since they do not struggle as greatly with challenging behaviors.

Medical Conditions

Medical intervention is necessary for any co-occurring medical conditions, such as seizures or GI disorders. Children with autism need to be monitored closely for behaviors that may reflect a medical condition and should receive a complete medical workup and treatment through a physician who specializes in the child's medical condition.

Complementary and Alternative Medicine

Complementary and alternative medicine has gained popularity in the past decade as a supplementary treatment to educational services. **Complementary and alternative medicine** is defined as "a broad domain of healing resources that encompasses all health systems modalities and practices and their accompanying theories and beliefs, other than those intrinsic to the politically dominant health system" (Levy et al., 2003, p. 418). Those who support complementary and alternative medicine believe the methods target underlying medical difficulties, such as GI and sleep disorders, which are not addressed through educational intervention. The goal of many of the complementary and alternative medicine treatments is to aid in the associated problems of autism, rather than claim to cure the disorder. Statistics reveal that 30% to 50% of children with autism in the United States are using complementary and alternative medicine; however, approximately 9% are using potentially harmful treatments, and 11% are using multiple complementary and alternative medicine treatments (Levy et al., 2003). Several studies are currently underway to examine the effectiveness and the risks of these treatments since many parents have reported a decrease in associated problems (e.g., GI problems) and an increase in developmental skills. Table 3.3 summarizes the potentially harmful side effects of these methods. The following sections describe commonly used complementary and alternative medicine treatments.

Supplements

The use of vitamins and minerals to address ASD concerns purports that because children with autism experience GI inflammation and intestinal disorders, their ability to absorb nutrients is thereby reduced. As a result, development that relies on nutrients such as vitamins A, B1, B3, B5, biotin, selenium, zinc, and magnesium is altered. Frequently used supplements include vitamin C, cod liver oil (for vitamins A and D), and the combination of vitamin B6 with magnesium (Autism Society of America, 2004).

Gluten-Free, Casein-Free Diet

Parents and professionals who support the theory that gluten and casein negatively impact a child's

---

TABLE 3.3   Potential Side Effects of Complementary and Alternative Medicine

Proposed Mechanisms	Example	Potential Adverse Side Effects
Neurotransmitter production or release	DMG	No reported side effects (excessive doses)
	B6/magnesium	B6: peripheral neuropathy; Mg: arrhythmia
	Vitamin C	Renal stones
	Omega 3	No reports of side effects from excessive administration
	Fatty acids	
	Secretin	Unknown impact of long-term administration of secretin
Change in gastrointestinal function	Gluten-free/casein-free diet	If nutritional state not monitored by clinicians, at risk for inadequate calcium, vitamin D, protein intake
	Secretin	
	Pepcid	Unknown impact of long-term administration
	Antibiotics	Hepatotoxicity in high doses
		Superinfection or antibiotic resistance with long-term use, implications for population at large with resistance
Putative immune mechanism or modulators	Antifungal agents	Possible superinfections or resistance with long-term use
	Intravenous immunoglobulin	Aseptic meningitis, renal failure, or infection
	Vitamin A/cod liver oil	Hypervitaminosis A or pseudotumor cerebri
Agents that might remove toxins	Chelation—DMSA, DMPA	Renal and hepatotoxicity of oral agents
	Other detox agents or protocols	Possible magnesium intoxication from Epsom salts ingestion

Levy, S. E., & Hyman, S. L. (2003). Use of complementary and alternative medicine for children with autistic spectrum disorders is increasing. *Pediatric Annals, 32*(10), 685–691. http://dx.doi.org/10.3928/0090-4481-20031001-10. Reprinted with permission.

development recommend a diet that completely eliminates these products (McCandless, 2003). Parent reports of improvement have been inconsistent, as some parents claim to see significant improvements in their child's behavior and/or developmental skills (e.g., improved eye contact), while others report that no change occurs by implementing this diet. Data is currently limited and inconclusive. One review of five available articles researching the effectiveness of gluten- and casein-free diets for behavioral symptom management found no positive effect from this diet (Hurwitz, 2013).

Other Common Complementary and Alternative Medicine Treatments for Autism

- *Secretin*: The human body naturally produces secretin, which is a hormone produced in the small intestine that stimulates secretion by the pancreas and liver. The use of extra secretin through injections became a popular complementary and alternative medicine treatment before it was scientifically analyzed, and studies now show few changes for children with ASDs who have used the extra hormone injection (Levy & Hyman, 2003).
- *Chelation*: Because mercury poisoning produces symptoms similar to those seen in autism, mercury and other heavy metals have been suggested as causes of autism. Though research has not found a link between mercury and autism, those who believe their children have experienced metal poisoning may choose chelation, a process to remove toxins from a child's system (Levy & Hyman, 2003).
- *Antibiotic treatment*: Immune system dysfunctions and antibiotic treatments have been targeted as possible causes of autism, and those who believe in these theories use further antibiotic treatment to alter the course of the symptoms in autism (Levy & Hyman, 2003).
- *Antifungal treatment*: Yeast overgrowth in the colon is hypothesized to cause many medical disorders, including autism, with a low-sugar diet and the use of probiotic agents (which encourage helpful intestinal bacteria) used as treatments (Levy & Hyman, 2003).

The effectiveness of complementary and alternative medicine stands largely unproven and highly controversial, though attempts are underway for further studies since many parents report positive results by using these methods. Complementary and alternative medicine treatments are intended to supplement educational services rather than to replace them. Clinicians are currently encouraged to use an empathetic stance with families providing complementary and alternative medicine to their children, though no alternative method should be administered without the guidance of an experienced physician.

IMPACT ON OCCUPATIONAL PERFORMANCE

The presence or absence of intellectual and language impairments, the severity of the autism symptoms, and the influence of coexisting sensory, psychiatric, and motor deficits all have significant implications on the degree of functional impairment present in an individual with an ASD diagnosis. For example, ADLs like dressing and eating can be difficult if the individual is over-responsive to the sensations of clothing or food and/or has difficulty with maintaining the necessary postural stability to support motor planning of these tasks. IADLs like shopping or driving are difficult and even dangerous if the individual does not have adequate focused attention and emotional regulation to make in the moment safe decisions. Participation in the educational system can be hampered by difficulty with memory functions for learning and socialization skills to develop healthy relationships with peers. Play and leisure activities are sometimes limited by restricted and repetitive behaviors, making participation outside of the home stressful. Finally, individuals with autism often have difficulty obtaining and maintaining employment due to the complex nature of these tasks and the constellation of symptoms that make professional behaviors challenging. In summary, ASD is a pervasive, lifelong disability that can impact every area of occupational performance. However, intervention can facilitate functional changes to significantly improve the quality of life of the individual with autism and their family.

Global Impairment

Autism is considered a global impairment, meaning that it does not reflect damage as a result of one specific lesion in the brain. Since autism likely affects several regions of the brain, this global impact means that autism impairs multiple areas of a child's development. As a result, all areas of occupation are often impacted by this disorder.

■ Specific Mental Functions

Each individual with autism presents with different areas of strengths and weaknesses; therefore, individuals with an ASD diagnosis show various combinations of concerns in their mental skills. Concerns in this area can range from very severe, where the individual will need constant support and supervision throughout the lifespan, to very mild, where the individual can achieve complete financial and interpersonal independence. However, despite the great variability in symptom presentation, several areas of mental function are commonly impaired to a greater or lesser extent depending on the level of ASD severity.

Children with autism often have difficulty regulating their own emotions and often experience features of or possibly comorbid psychiatric disorders (Leyfer et al., 2006). The most common issue is specific phobia. Children with autism may experience phobias of typically innocuous things like crowds, bridges, or loud noises. In addition, attention deficits are nearly universal in this population. Unique patterns of attention include distractibility, disorganization, intense preoccupation for preferred, self-initiated activities for unusual lengths of time, and lack of boredom for repeating same action or play schema (Rapin, 1991). Features of obsessive-compulsive disorder are also often present in many children with autism. They may need to perform a routine a certain way, like walking through the same side of a double door to get to the lunchroom at school, or not be able to move on until a task is completed, like needing to pick all of the dandelions on the playground before they can play. Finally, approximately 10% of children with autism also have symptoms of major depression with episodes of things like sadness, hopelessness, crying, and/or flat affect (Leyfer et al., 2006). Difficulty regulating emotion in this population can lead to emotional lability (e.g., swinging from laughing to crying without apparent reason), heightened anxiety with temper tantrums, and/or aggressive behaviors such as hitting and biting, self-injury (e.g., head banging, hitting self), or self-stimulatory behaviors (body rocking).

A child with autism often shows a scattered pattern of memory functions (Hill, Berthoz, & Frith, 2004). Overall, "memory performance of individuals with autism becomes increasingly impaired as the complexity of the material increases" (Minshew & Goldstein, 2001, p. 1099). Children with autism also use fewer organizational strategies, relying on stereotyped rules regardless of the task's complexity (Minshew & Goldstein, 2001). Therefore, a child with autism performs more poorly on tasks with higher complexity. Word recall is more significantly impacted than digit recall, and these children often have difficulty recalling activities in which they have recently participated (Boucher, 1981). However, certain areas of memory remain intact, particularly in the areas of visual and rote memory. **Rote memory** describes the memorization and use of previously heard chunks of language rather than the spontaneous generation of language.

In the area of perceptual functioning, individuals with ASDs perceive sensory stimuli, but often process and react abnormally to it. Integration of perceptual and sensorimotor information allows individuals to respond appropriately with physical and emotional responses. In autism, this integration does not occur in the same efficient way; therefore, this population of individuals has difficulty responding with typical emotional and behavioral responses to the sensory stimuli around them. Between 30% and 100% of individuals with autism demonstrate deviant sensory-perceptual abilities (Dawson & Watling, 2000).

As mentioned above, cognitive impairments or intellectual disabilities are common in, though not universal to, the autism population. Individuals with cognitive deficits typically demonstrate scattered skills; in other words, they may present with strong skills in some areas with significant concerns in other areas. These children often have difficulty sequencing a series of items, imitating the actions and words of others meaningfully, generalizing concepts across a variety of situations, demonstrating **theory of mind**, and playing with toys appropriately and symbolically (Lord and McGee, National Research Council, 2001). In her 1991 literature review of autistic features, Rapin described that children with autism tend to have better visual-spatial skills than auditory verbal skills on IQ tests. Children in this population may show above-average skills in very specific areas, such as calculating numbers, completing puzzles, or demonstrating rote verbal memory, while demonstrating overall cognitive impairment. Some children with autism are able to read at a young age with minimal instruction, but they have little or no understanding of what they read. This unusual occurrence is known as **hyperlexia** (Rapin, 1991).

Studies examining higher level cognitive functions have revealed that executive functioning skills such as forward planning, cognitive flexibility, and the use of assistive strategies (e.g., creating a mnemonic such as a rhyme to assist in remembering information) in learning are impacted for those who have autism (Gordon, 2002).

As previously described, children with autism typically show language delay. Deviations from typical language are noted across all diagnostic categories. Children on the autism spectrum typically have limitations in using language in appropriate contexts and for social purposes. Some children may be highly verbal and articulate though literal, echolalic, and repetitive; other children may remain nonverbal or use very little speech (Rapin, 1997). Additionally, comprehension of language is affected and exacerbated by a decreased motivation to use language for interacting with others. Often, these children are challenged to understand what topics interest others and have difficulty interpreting nonverbal language such as gestures and facial expressions, as well as abstract language such as jokes or idioms. For those who are verbal, intonation of their voices may sound unnatural as a result of a singsong or monotone pattern. Speaking at unusually loud volumes is another unusual characteristic of children with autism. Though the words may be clear, content may be memorized chunks of language or may focus on topics that are not relevant to a conversation partner. Echolalia is also common for verbal children (Rapin, 1991). Some children do not master fluent speech and their sounds in words are difficult to understand. Decoding the sounds that they hear may be severely compromised; therefore, these children may not understand what they hear and, in turn, are unable to produce the sound accurately (Rapin, 1997).

■ Sensory Functions and Pain

"The experience of being human is imbedded in the sensory events of everyday life. When we observe how people live their lives, we discover they characterize their experiences from a sensory point of view" (Dunn, 2001, p. 608). As described above, sensory processing is particularly challenging in individuals with autism and additional information is included here. If a child's sensory system does not interpret stimuli in a typical way, it is easy to understand why this individual may react to the world differently. Sensory processing problems should be addressed through early intervention to reduce these abnormal behaviors (Lord and McGee, National Research Council, 2001; Dunn, 2001).

Visual perception is usually an area of relative strength and may be used to compensate for challenging areas. For instance, the integration of vestibular, visual, and somatosensory afferent systems is needed to maintain upright postural stability. Molloy, Dietrich, and Bhattacharya (2003) measured the postural stability in children with autism and found that these children relied on visual cues to help them maintain stability. When these visual cues were omitted, children had difficulty maintaining their upright balance and reducing their sway. One area of visual processing that is consistently impaired is integrating details of a figure into a whole (Deruelle, Rondan, Gepner, & Tardit, 2004). For instance, if given a line drawing of a house made up of geometric shapes, these children focus on the shapes rather than seeing the image of a house.

■ Functions Related to the Digestive System

Children with autism may be at a higher risk for experiencing GI problems such as reflux or gastritis, with persistent gas, diarrhea, and constipation also frequently reported (Horvath et al., 1999; Levy et al., 2003; McQueen & Heck, 2002). Additionally, hypotheses exist regarding functioning of the digestive system, such as increased intestinal permeability that allows absorption of morphine-like compounds from gluten and casein. The buildup of these substances theoretically results in the social withdrawal and stereotypical behaviors seen in autism, but as previously described, this theory has not been proven (Levy & Hyman, 2003).

■ Urinary and Reproductive Functions

In children with autism, the urinary tract is usually typical in its structure and function. However, for those children with cognitive and sensory impairments, toilet training is often complicated. Children with autism often learn to toilet train at a later age than typically developing children; evidence problems such as fear, pain, confusion, frustration, and constipation when learning to train; urinate or defecate in inappropriate places; and experience difficulty when a change of routine occurs or when entering an unfamiliar bathroom (Ruble & Dalrymple, 1993).

Because individuals with autism have difficulty interacting, inappropriate sexual behavior is also a concern. Close relationships with others are challenging for these individuals; therefore, few person-oriented behaviors are noted. Additionally, discouraging inappropriate sexual behaviors may be difficult. The most frequently reported inappropriate sexual behaviors include public masturbation or public touching of one's own private parts (Ruble & Dalrymple, 1993; Van Bourgondien, Reichle, & Palmer, 1997).

■ Brain Structure

The most significant abnormalities in a child's body structure include the anomalies of the brain that are currently under investigation. Likely caused by genetic abnormalities, these deviations in the brains of individuals with autism are not yet clearly defined, nor is it clear precisely how the differences cause the characteristics of autism. Studies have found consistent abnormalities in the cerebellum, frontal lobes, brainstem, and limbic system (Bauman & Kemper, 1996). Research is also examining potential deviations in the way different regions of the brain communicate (Piven et al., 1997).

CASE STUDY 1

At 1 year of age, Jacob was brought to an early intervention clinic because of delays in motor and cognitive skills. An initial evaluation conducted by an occupational therapist, educator, and speech-language pathologist confirmed these concerns. In the area of gross motor skills, Jacob was delayed in learning to walk and demonstrated moderate hypotonia in his trunk. Fine motor concerns included tactile defensiveness of wet or sticky substances and delays in grasping and manipulating objects appropriately. Cognitively, Jacob showed little interest in playing with toys or imitating the words and actions of others. Language impairments were not yet observed since Jacob frequently vocalized, babbled, and expressed his feelings through behaviors such as smiling or crying. At this young age, ASD was not initially suspected. Jacob was clearly a delightful little boy who showed a strong attachment to his parents and was interested in watching children and other adults in his environment.

Jacob was placed in a playgroup at the clinic where his occupational therapist and educator worked directly with him, while a speech-language pathologist monitored his language. As time passed, further concerns became evident. His language skills failed to further develop; as a result, first words did not emerge. Nor was he using gestures to indicate what he wanted. At the age of fourteen months, he evidenced limitations in language comprehension and speech production, and his use of eye contact decreased. As the months progressed, he showed frustration more frequently through crying, banging his head, throwing himself on the ground, and arching his back to pull away from a person trying to hold him.

His feeding skills were limited since he was not able to bring his hand to his mouth, and he demonstrated extreme sensitivities to many tastes and textures. He did not show an interest in other self-help skills such as learning to bathe or dress himself. While other children his age learned to imitate motor movements in songs, Jacob seemed to content to only listen to the songs. He did not demonstrate typical play skills for his age such as exploring how toys worked, taking toys in or out of a container, or taking turns with others. However, musical or flashing toys captured his attention for long periods of time. While he was engrossed with these toys, he evidenced unusual, repetitive behaviors such as rocking his body back and forth.

Through early intervention by his therapists and parents, Jacob's gross motor skills improved during the following months and he successfully learned to walk at 18 months. He delighted in walking through his home, through the early intervention center, and outside. His eye contact improved, becoming more spontaneous and consistent. His repertoire of sounds increased and he vocalized to take a turn in songs or games; in addition, he began signing "more" to request something desirable to happen again. He learned to play with toys in a more functional manner, including stacking rings and blocks and taking toys in and out of containers. Yet other skills continued to be challenging. When he was left to play on his own, he repetitively turned the pages of books or walked aimlessly around a room. He showed hypersensitivities to touching or mouthing certain textures, limited motor or imitation skills, difficulty understanding others, a lack of verbal words, and repetitive behaviors during play.

Currently, at slightly older than 2 years of age, Jacob continues to struggle in several areas of development. However, he has made steady progress in these developmental skills, and his family and team are encouraged that he will continue to make significant gains. More importantly, despite being faced with more challenges than typically developing children, Jacob is a young boy who is often able to share and express joy with others.

CASE STUDY 2

Patrick is a 38-year-old man who was diagnosed with autistic disorder at two-and-a-half years of age. His mother was first concerned he had a hearing impairment, as he did not seem to understand what people said to him, did not respond to a fire truck siren, placed his ear close to the refrigerator, and acted out with negative behaviors. Behavioral and developmental concerns persisted after testing ruled out a hearing impairment. A psychologist specializing in autism assessed Patrick's developmental skills and behaviors and diagnosed Patrick with autistic disorder.

Patrick communicated nonverbally for several years, usually by grabbing a person's hand and leading the person to an item he wanted. He had a very limited diet as a young child, eating only peanut butter, raisins, and yogurt. In time, he increased his repertoire of foods. When Patrick was three, he began attending a local school for children with autism; at the age of eight, he attended a school for children with a variety of special needs. Patrick began using words at the age of nine. He transferred to a local public high school at the age of 18, participating in the school's autism program and working in the school's kitchen to learn to work with others. He graduated high school when he was 26, receiving a diploma of completion for the school's autism program.

Following high school, Patrick moved into a condominium with two other men diagnosed with autism; he currently maintains this living situation. Patrick and his roommates receive 24-hour supervision. He also works five days per week at a therapy center that encourages functional skill building. He works alongside eight or nine other adults with autism and receives supervision in his daily tasks, which include shredding legal documents and inserting newspapers into plastic sleeves. To prevent overwhelming stimuli, the room is kept dim and without extraneous sound.

As with all individuals diagnosed with autism, Patrick shows personal strengths and unique challenges, with his own personality shining through.

Patrick has achieved several goals in activities of daily living and continues to work toward independence. He dresses himself, with the occasional need for help with fasteners. He toilets independently, though requires assistance with wiping after a bowel movement. He washes himself with verbal prompting from a supervisor and climbs in and out of the tub independently. He applies deodorant and cologne and combs his hair when directed. Once a supervisor has prepared his toothbrush, Patrick brushes his teeth for two minutes, needing occasional reminders to not swallow the toothpaste. He carries groceries into the house, takes out the trash, and wipes the table after meals.

Patrick displays unusual and stereotypical behaviors, such as rapidly bouncing or tapping a small ball on a tabletop, spinning lids, and repeatedly blowing up balloons. He eats his food very quickly and needs verbal reminders to eat at a slower pace. In the car, he often bends down to play with the hardware beneath his seat. Recently, Patrick has shown negative behaviors, such as destruction of property or soiling himself. His family and staff believe these behaviors are likely Patrick's way of showing grief from his father's death last year.

Socially, Patrick gets along well with his family, supervisors, and roommates, though he has few verbal interactions with his roommates. His family frequently brings him to community outings such as sports events; Patrick shows interest and enjoyment during these outings. He reciprocates another person's smile easily. He occasionally initiates and maintains eye contact with another person, but not with typical duration or frequency. He often responds to a speaker, but does not engage in back-and-forth conversation.

Regarding other developmental skills, Patrick currently understands more language than he uses. He follows familiar one-step directions, though sometimes needs repetition from the speaker to complete the request. He comprehends simple questions that relate to his interests and daily routines. Patrick communicates through single words and phrases. He names familiar people and objects, answers simple questions, and requests desired items and actions. He greets when prompted by another person. In the area of fine motor skills, Patrick does not demonstrate a hand preference. He writes his first name, last name, and the word "love" to sign letters and cards. Patrick shows many strengths in his gross motor skills. He enjoys playing a variety of sports, including swimming and throwing a ball back and forth with a partner. He loves to shoot basketball hoops (dribbling is more difficult for him), which

was a favorite activity he had shared with his father. He experiences some difficulty with coordination and motor planning. Cognitively, Patrick has recently learned the days of the week and loves to look at calendars. He can recite the alphabet and recognizes a few familiar written words. He does not yet tell time.

Patrick lives a very active life, filled with family, supportive staff, and opportunities to contribute to his community. His mother and professional team continuously work together to create new goals for Patrick, and he meets these challenges. He is a delightful and admirable individual.

RECOMMENDED LEARNING RESOURCES

Organizations

Autism Society of America
7910 Woodmont Ave., Suite 300
Bethesda, MD 20814-3067
www.autism-society.org/site/PageServer

Autism Speaks
http://www.autismspeaks.org
Web site includes a "100 day kit" for families whose children have recently been diagnosed with autism.

Centers for Disease Control and Prevention
http://www.cdc.gov/ncbddd/autism/index.html
Web site includes fact sheets and other helpful information for families, individuals with autism, healthcare providers, etc.

First Signs
http://www.firstsigns.org/
Web site includes valuable information on autism and an ASD video glossary

National Alliance of Autism Research
99 Wall Street, Research Park
Princeton, NJ 08540
www.naar.org

National Institute of Mental Health Office of Communications
6001 Executive Blvd
Room 8184, MSC 9663
Bethesda, MD 20892-9663
www.nimh.nih.gov/publicat/autism.cfm

Books on Autism Spectrum Disorders

Attwood, T. (1998). *Asperger's syndrome: A guide for parents and professionals.* London: Jessica Kingsley Publishers Ltd.

Greenspan, S. I., & Wieder, S. (2006). *Engaging autism: Using the floortime approach to help children relate, communicate, and think.* Cambridge, MA: Da Capo Press.

Lord, C., & McGee, J. P. (Eds.). (2001). *Educating children with autism.* Washington, DC: National Academy Press.

Ozonoff, S., Dawson, G., & McPartland, J. (2002). *A parent's guide to Asperger syndrome and high functioning autism.* New York, NY: Guilford Press.

Quill, K. A. (2000). *Do-Watch-Listen-Say: Social and communication intervention for children with autism.* Baltimore, MD: Paul H. Brookes Publishing.

Robledo, S. J., & Ham-Kucharski, D. (2005). *The autism book: Answers to your most pressing questions.* New York, NY: Penguin Group.

Siegel, B. (2003). *Helping children with autism learn: Treatment approaches for parents and professionals.* New York, NY: Oxford University Press.

Volkmar, F. R. (Ed.). (2005). *Handbook of autism and pervasive developmental disorders* (pp. 335–364). Hoboken, NJ: John Wiley & Sons, Inc.

Wing, L. (1996). *The autistic spectrum: A guide for parents and professionals.* London: Constable and Company Limited.

Books on Sensory Integration Disorder

Ayres, A. J. (1998). *Sensory integration and the child.* Los Angeles, CA: Western Psychological Services.

Kranowitz, C. S. (1998). *The out-of-sync child: Recognizing and coping with sensory integration dysfunction.* New York, NY: Perigee.

Diagnostic Guidelines Online

Filipek, P. (2006). Autism diagnostic guidelines. *Screening and Diagnosis of Autism.* Retrieved from http://www.neurology.org/cgi/reprint/55/4/468.pdf

REFERENCES

American Psychiatric Association. (2000). *Diagnostic and statistical manual of mental disorders* (4th ed.). Washington, DC: American Psychiatric Association.

American Psychiatric Association. (2013a). *DSM-5 autism spectrum disorder fact sheet.* Retrieved from http://www.dsm5.org/Documents/Autism%20Spectrum%20Disorder%20Fact%20Sheet.pdf

American Psychiatric Association. (2013b). *Diagnostic and statistical manual of mental disorders* (5th ed.). Washington, DC: American Psychiatric Association.

Ashburner, J., Ziviani, J., & Rodger, S. (2008). Sensory processing and classroom, emotional, behavioral and educational outcomes in children with autism spectrum disorder. *American Journal of Occupational Therapy, 62*, 564–573. http://dx.doi.org/10.5014/ajot.62.5.564

Autism Society of America. (2004). Bethesda, MD: Autism Society of America. Retrieved from http://www.autism-society.org, on August 4, 2015.

Ayres, J. (1994). *Sensory integration and the child.* Los Angeles, CA: WPS Publishing.

Bandini, L. G., Anderson, S. E., Curtin, C., Cermak, S., Evans, E.W., Scampini, R., et al. (2010). Food selectivity in children with autism spectrum disorders and typically developing children. *The Journal of Pediatrics, 157*(2), 259–264. http://dx.doi.org/10.1016/j.jpeds.2010.02.013

Baranek, G. T., David, F. J, Poe, M., Stone, W., & Watson, L. R. (2006). Sensory experiences questionnaire: Discriminating response patterns in young children with autism, developmental delays, and typical development. *Journal of Child Psychology and Psychiatry, 47*(6), 591–601. http://dx.doi.org/10.1111/j.1469-7610.2005.01546.x

Baranek, G. T., Watson, L. R., Boyd, B. A., Poe, M. D., David, F. J., & McGuire, L. (2013). Hyporesponsiveness to social and nonsocial sensory stimuli in children with autism, children with developmental delays, and typically developing children. *Development & Psychopathology, 25*, 307–320. http://dx.doi.org/10.1017/s0954579412001071

Baron-Cohen, S., Allen, J., & Gillberg, C. (1992). Can autism be detected at 18 months? The needle, the haystack, and the CHAT. *Br J Psychiatr, 161*, 839–843. http://dx.doi.org/10.1192/bjp.161.6.839

Baron-Cohen, S., Knickmeyer, R. C., & Belmonte, M. K. (2005). Sex differences in the brain: Implications for explaining autism. *Science, 310*(5749), 819–823. http://dx.doi.org/10.1126/science.1115455

Bauman, M. (2004, December). Innovative interventions in autism/non-verbal learning disabilities. *Conference presentation, December 3–4, 2004,* Seattle, WA.

Bauman, M. L., & Kemper, T. L. (1996). Brief report: Neuroanatomic observations of the brain in pervasive developmental disorders. *Journal of Autism and Developmental Disorders, 26*(2), 199–203. http://dx.doi.org/10.1007/BF02172012

Bayley, N. (2005). *Bayley scales of infant and toddler development* (3rd ed., Bayley III). Pearson: PsychCorp.

Ben-Sasson, A., Hen, L., Fluss, R., Cermak, S. A., Engel-Yeger, B. & Gal, E. (2009). A meta-analysis of sensory modulation symptoms in individuals with autism spectrum disorders. *Journal of Autism an dDevelopmental Disabilities, 39*, 1–11

Bertone, A., Mottron, L., Jelenic, P., & Faubert, J. (2005). Enhanced and diminished visuo-spatial information processing in autism depends on stimulus complexity. *Brain, 128*, 2430–2441. http://dx.doi.org/10.1093/brain/awh561

Berument, S. K., Rutter, M., Lord, C., Pickles, A., & Bailey, A. (1999). Autism screening questionnaire: Diagnostic validity. *Br J Psychiatr, 175*, 444–451. http://dx.doi.org/10.1192/bjp.175.5.444

Bettelheim, B. (1967). *The empty fortress: Infantile autism and the birth of the self.* New York, NY: The New York Free Press.

Bonnel, A., Mottron, L., Teretz, L., Trudel, M., Gallun, E., & Bonnel, A. M. (2003). Enhanced pitch sensitivity in individuals with autism: A signal detection analysis. *Journal of Cognitive Neuroscience, 15*(2), 226–235. http://dx.doi.org/10.1162/089892903321208169

Boucher, J. (1981). Memory for recent events in autistic children. *Journal of Autism and Developmental Disorders, 11*, 293–302. http://dx.doi.org/10.1007/BF01531512

Boyd, B. A., Odom, S. L., Humphreys, B. P., & Sam, A. M. (2010). Infants and toddlers with autism spectrum disorder: Early identification and early intervention. *Journal of Early Intervention, 32*(2), 75–98. http://dx.doi.org/10.1177/1053815110362690

Carper, R. A., & Courchesne, E. (2005). Localized enlargement of the frontal cortex in early autism. *Biological Psychiatry, 57*(2), 126–133. http://dx.doi.org/10.1016/j.biopsych.2004.11.005

Centers for Disease Control and Prevention (CDC). (2014). *10 Things to know about new autism data.* Retrieved from http://www.cdc.gov/features/dsautismdata/, on August 19, 2015.

Centers for Disease Control and Prevention (CDC). (2015). *Autism spectrum disorder data and statistics.* Retrieved from http://www.cdc.gov/ncbddd/autism/data.html, on August 19, 2015.

Dalrymple, N. J., & Ruble, L. (1992). Toilet training and behaviors of people with autism: Parent views. *Journal of Autism and Developmental Disorders, 22*(2), 265–275. http://dx.doi.org/10.1007/BF01058155

Dawson, G., & Watling, R. (2000). Interventions to facilitate auditory, visual, and motor integration in autism: A review of the evidence. *Journal of Autism and Developmental Disorders, 30*(5), 415–421. http://dx.doi.org/10.1023/A:1005547422749

Deruelle, C., Rondan, C., Gepner, B., & Tardit, C. (2004). Spatial frequency and face processing in children with autism and Asperger syndrome. *Journal of Autism and Developmental Disorders, 34*(2), 199–210. http://dx.doi.org/10.1023/B:JADD.0000022610.09668.4c

Dickinson, A., & Milne, E. (2014). Enhanced and impaired sensory discrimination in autism. *Journal of Neurophysiology, 112*(6), 1599. http://dx.doi.org/10.1152/jn.00288.2014

Dunn, W. (2001). The sensations of everyday life: Empirical, theoretical, and pragmatic considerations. *American Journal of Occupational Therapy, 55*(6), 608–620. http://dx.doi.org/10.5014/ajot.55.6.608

Dunn, W. (2014). *Sensory profile 2.* Pearson: PsychCorp.

Dunn, H. G., & MacLeod, P. M. (2001). Rett syndrome: Review of biological abnormalities. *C J Neurol Sci, 28*(1), 16–29.

Fernell, E., Eriksson, M. A., & Gillberg C. (2013). Early diagnosis of autism and impact on prognosis: A narrative review. *Clinical Epidemiology, 5*, 33–43. http://dx.doi.org/10.2147/CLEP.S41714

Filipek, P. A., Accardo, P. J., Baranek, G. T., et al. (1999). The screening and diagnosis of autistic spectrum disorders. *Journal of Autism and Developmental Disorders, 29*(6), 439–484. http://dx.doi.org/10.1023/A:1021943802493

Folio, M. R., & Fewell, R. R. (2000). *Peabody developmental motor scales, second edition (PDMS-2).* Pearson: PsychCorp.

Fombonne, E. (1999). The epidemiology of autism: A review. *Psychological Medicine, 29*, 769–786. http://dx.doi.org/10.1017/S0033291799008508

Fournier, K. A., Hass, C. J., Naik, S. K., Lodha, N., & Cauraugh, J. H. (2010). Motor coordination in autism spectrum disorders: A synthesis and meta-analysis. *Journal of Autism and Developmental Disorders, 40*(10), 1227–1240. http://dx.doi.org/10.1007/s10803-010-0981-3

Garnett, M. S., & Attwood, A. J. (1998). Australian scale for Asperger's syndrome. In: T. Attwood, (Ed.), *Asperger's syndrome: A guide for parents and professionals.* London: Jessica Kingsley.

Gillberg, C. (2010). The ESSENCE in child psychiatry: Early symptomatic syndromes eliciting neurodevelopmental clinical examinations. *Research in Developmental Disabilities, 42*(7), 1491–1497. http://dx.doi.org/10.1016/j.ridd.2010.06.002

Gilliam, G. E. (1995). *Gilliam autism rating scale.* Austin, TX: Pro-Ed.

Gordon, B. (2002). Autism and autistic spectrum disorders. In: A. K. Asbury, G. M. McKhann, W. I. McDonald, et al. (Eds.), *Diseases of the nervous system* (3rd ed., Vol. *1*, pp. 406–418). Cambridge: University Press.

Greenspan, S. I., DeGangi, G., & Wieder, S. (1999). *The functional emotional assessment scale for infancy and early childhood: A manual.* Madison, WI: International Universities Press.

Hauck, J. A., & Dewey, D. (2001). Hand preference and motor functioning in children with autism. *Journal of Autism and Developmental Disorders, 31*(3), 265–277. http://dx.doi.org/10.1023/A:1010791118978

Helm-Estabrooks, N., & Albert, M. L. (2003). *Manual of aphasia and aphasia therapy* (2nd ed.). Austin, TX: PRO-ED

Hill, E., Berthoz, S., & Frith, U. (2004). Cognitive processing of own emotions in individuals with autistic spectrum disorder and in their relatives. *Journal of Autism and Developmental Disorders, 34*(2), 229–235. http://dx.doi.org/10.1023/B:JADD.0000022613.41399.14

Horvath, K., Papadimitriou, J. C., Rabsztyn, A., Drachenburg, C., & Tildon, J. T. (1999). Gastrointestinal abnormalities in children with autistic disorder. *Journal of Pediatrics, 135*(5), 559–563. http://dx.doi.org/10.1016/S0022-3476(99)70052-1

Hughes, C. (1996). Brief report: Planning problems in autism at the level of motor control. *Journal of Autism and Developmental Disorders, 26*(1), 99–107. http://dx.doi.org/10.1007/BF02276237

Hurwitz, S. (2013). The gluten-free, casein-free diet and autism: Limited return on family investment. *Journal of Early Intervention, 35*(1), 3–19. http://dx.doi.org/10.1177/1053815113484807

Jick, H., & Kaye, J. A. (2003). Epidemiology and possible causes of autism. *Pharmacotherapy, 23*(12), 1525–1530. http://dx.doi.org/10.1592/phco.23.15.1524.31955

Kanner, L. (1943). Autistic disturbances of affective contact. *Nervous Child, 2*, 17–250.

Kemper, T. L., & Bauman, M. (1998). Neuropathology of infantile autism. *Journal of Neuropathology &*

Experimental Neurology, 57(7), 645–652. http://dx.doi.org/10.1097/00005072-199807000-00001

Kulage, K. M., Smaldone, A. M., & Cohn, E. G. (2014). How will the DSM-5 affect autism diagnosis? A systematic literature review and meta-analysis. *Journal of Autism and Developmental Disorders, 44*(8), 1918–1932. http://dx.doi.org/10.1007/s10803-014-2065-2

Lane, S. J., Reynolds, S., & Dumenci, L. (2012). Sensory overresponsivity and anxiety in typically developing children and children with autism and attention deficit hyperactivity disorder: Cause or coexistence? *American Journal of Occupational Therapy, 66*(5), 595–603. http://dx.doi.org/10.5014/ajot.2012.004523

Leslie, A. M., & Frith, U. (1987). Metarepresentation and autism: How not to lose one's marbles. *Cognition, 27*(3), 291–294. http://dx.doi.org/10.1016/S0010-0277(87)80014-8

Levy, S. E., & Hyman, S. L. (2003). Use of complementary and alternative medicine for children with autistic spectrum disorders is increasing. *Pediatric Annals, 32*(10), 685–691. http://dx.doi.org/10.3928/0090-4481-20031001-10

Levy, S. E., Mandell, D. S., Merhar, S., Ittenbach, R. F., & Pinto-Martin, J. A. (2003). Use of complementary and alternative medicine among children recently diagnosed autistic spectrum disorder. *Journal of Developmental and Behavioral Pediatrics, 24*(6), 418–423. http://dx.doi.org/10.1097/00004703-200312000-00003

Leyfer, O.T., Folstein, S.E., Bacalman, S., Davis, N.O., Dinh, E., Morgan, J., … H., Lainhart, J.E. (2006). Comorbid psychiatric disorders in children with autism: Interview development and rates of disorders. *Journal of Autism and Developmental Disorders, 36*, 849–861. DOI 10.1007/s10803-006-0123-0

Lindsay, R. L., & Aman, M. G. (2003). Pharmacologic therapies aid treatment for autism. *Pediatric Annals, 32*(10), 671–676. http://dx.doi.org/10.3928/0090-4481-20031001-08

Little, L. M., Ausderau, K., Sideris, J., & Garanek, G. T. (2015). Activity participation and sensory features among children with autism spectrum disorders. *Journal of Autism and Developmental Disorders, 45*(9), 2981–2990. http://dx.doi.org/10.1007/s10803-015-2460-3

Liu, X., Hubbard, J. A., Fabes, R. A., & Adaom, J. B. (2006). Sleep disturbances and correlates of children with autism spectrum disorders. *Child Psychiatry and Human Development, 37*, 179–191. http://dx.doi.org/10.1007/s10578-006-0028-3

Lord, C., Luyster, R. J., Gotham, K., & Guthrie, W. (2012). *Autism Diagnostic Observation Schedule, Second Edition (ADOS-2). Manual.* Torrance, CA: Western Psychological Services.

Lord, C., Rutter, M., & LeCouteur, A. (1994). Autism diagnostic interview-revised: A revised version of a diagnostic interview for caregivers of individuals with possible pervasive developmental disorders. *Journal of Autism and Developmental Disorders, 24*, 659–685. http://dx.doi.org/10.1007/BF02172145

MacNeil, L. K., & Mostofsky, S. (2012). Specificity of dyspraxia in children with autism. *Neuropsychology, 26*(2), 165–171. http://dx.doi.org/10.1037/a0026955

Malow, B. A., Adkins, K. W., McGrew, S. G., Wang, L., Goldman, S. E., Fawkes, D., & Burnette, C. (2012). Melatonin for sleep in children with autism: A controlled trial examining dose, tolerability, and outcomes. *Journal of Autism and Developmental Disorders, 42*(8), 1729–1734. http://dx.doi.org/10.1007/s10803-011-1418-3

Malow, B. S., Marzec, M. L., McGrew, S. G., Wang, L., Henderson, L. M., & Stone, W. L. (2006). Characterizing sleep in children with autism spectrum disorders: A multidimensional approach. *Sleep, 29*(12), 1563–1571.

McCandless, J. (2003). *Children with starving brains: A medical treatment guide for autism spectrum disorder* (2nd ed.). Paterson, NJ: Bramble Books.

McQueen, J. M., & Heck, A. M. (2002). Secretin for the treatment of autism. *Annals of Pharmacotherapy, 36*, 305–311. http://dx.doi.org/10.1345/aph.19113

Miller, L. J. (2014). *Sensational kids.* New York, NY: Penguin Group.

Minshew, N. J., & Goldstein, G. (2001). The pattern of intact and impaired memory functions in autism. *J Child Psychol Psychiatry, 42*(8), 1095–1101. http://dx.doi.org/10.1111/1469-7610.00808

Minshew, N. J., Sung, K., Jones, B. L., & Furman, J. M. (2004). Underdevelopment of the postural control system in autism. *Neurology, 63*, 2056–2061. http://dx.doi.org/10.1212/01.WNL.0000145771.98657.62

Molloy, C. A., Dietrich, K., & Bhattacharya, A. (2003). Postural stability in children with autism spectrum disorder. *Journal of Autism and Developmental Disorders, 33*(6), 643–652. http://dx.doi.org/10.1023/B:JADD.0000006001.00667.4c

Mullen, E. M. (1995). *Mullen scales of early learning.* Torrance, CA: Western Psychological Services.

Mutti, M., Martin, N., Sterling, H., & Spalding, N, et al. (2012). *Quick neurological screening test 3 (QNST-3).* Ann Arbor, MI: Academic Therapy Publications.

National Research Council. (2001). Educating children with autism. Committee on Educational Interventions for Children with Autism. In: C. Lord, & J. P. McGee (Eds.), *Division of behavioral and social sciences and education.* Washington, DC: National Academy Press.

Ostrow, N. (2014). Autism costs more than $2 Million over patients life. *Bloomberg Business*. Retrieved from http://www.bloomberg.com/news/articles/2014-06-09/autism-costs-more-than-2-million-over-patient-s-life, on August 19, 2015.

Panel of Definition and Description. (1995). Defining and describing complementary and alternative medicine. *Paper presented at CAM Research Methodology conference, April 7–9, Washington, DC.*

Pediatric Psychopharmacology Autism Network. (2002). Risperidone in children with autism and serious behavioral problems. *The New England Journal of Medicine, 347*(5), 314–321. http://dx.doi.org/10.1056/NEJMoa013171

Piven, J., Saliba, K., Bailey, J., & Arndt, S. (1997). An MRI study of autism: The cerebellum revisited. *Neurology, 49*(2), 546–551. http://dx.doi.org/10.1212/WNL.49.2.546

Puts, N., Woodka, E., Tommerdahl, M., Mostofsky, S., & Edden, R. (2014). Impaired tactile processing in children with autism spectrum disorders. *Journal of Neurophysiology, 111*, 1803–1822. http://dx.doi.org/10.1152/jn.00890.2013

Rapin, I. (1991). Autistic children: Diagnosis and clinical features. *Pediatrics, 87*, 751–760.

Rapin, I. (1997). Autism. *The New England Journal of Medicine, 337*, 97–104. http://dx.doi.org/10.1056/NEJM199707103370206

Rapin, I. (2002). The autistic spectrum disorders. *The New England Journal of Medicine, 347*(5), 302–303. http://dx.doi.org/10.1056/NEJMp020062

Rapin, I., & Katzman, R. (1998). Neurobiology of autism. *Annals of Neurology, 43*, 7–14. http://dx.doi.org/10.1002/ana.410430106

Robins, D. L., Fein, D., Barton, M. L., et al. (2001). The modified checklist for autism in toddlers: An initial study investigating the early detection of autism and pervasive developmental disorders. *Journal of Autism and Developmental Disorders, 21*, 131–144. http://dx.doi.org/10.1023/A:1010738829569

Rogers, S. J. (1996). Brief report: Early intervention in autism. *Journal of Autism and Developmental Disorders, 26*(2), 243–246. http://dx.doi.org/10.1007/BF02172020

Roley, S. S., Mailloux, Z., Parham, L. D., Schaaf, R. C., Lane, C. J., & Cermak, S. (2015). Sensory integration and praxis patterns in children with autism, *American Journal of Occupational Therapy, 69*, 6901220010.

Ruble, L. A., & Dalrymple, N. J. (1993). Social/sexual awareness of persons with autism: A parental perspective. *Archives of Sexual Behavior, 22*, 229–240. http://dx.doi.org/10.1007/BF01541768

Rutter, M., Silberg, J., O'Connor, T., & Simonoff, E. (1999). Genetics and child psychiatry: II Empirical research findings. *Journal of Child Psychology and Psychiatry, 40*(1), 19–55. http://dx.doi.org/10.1111/1469-7610.00423

Schreck, K. A., Williams, K., & Smith, A. F. (2004). A comparison of eating behaviors between children with and without autism. *Journal of Autism and Developmental Disorders, 34*, 4. http://dx.doi.org/10.1023/B:JADD.0000037419.78531.86

Siegel, B. (1996). *The world of the autistic child.* Oxford: Oxford University Press.

Siegel, B. (1998a). Early screening and diagnosis in autism spectrum disorders: The Pervasive Developmental Disorders Screening Test (PDDST). *Paper presented at the NIH State of the Science in Autism Screening and Diagnosis Working Conference, Bethesda, MD, June 15–17.*

Siegel, B. (1998b). *Pervasive developmental disorder screening test–II (PDDST-II).* San Antonio, TX: Harcourt. DOI:10.1177/0734282906298469

Siegel, B. (2003). *Helping children with autism to learn.* Oxford: Oxford University Press.

Souders, M. C., Mason, T. B., Valladares, O., Bucan, M., Levy, S. E., Mandell, D. S., … Pinto-Martin, J. (2009). Sleep behaviors and sleep quality in children with autism spectrum disorders. *Sleep, 32*(12), 1566–1578.

Sparrow, S., Cicchetti, D., & Balla, D. (2006). *Vineland adaptive behavior scales* (2nd ed.). Pearson: PsychCorp.

Stone, W. L., Coonrod, E. E., & Ousley, O. Y. (2000). Brief report: Screening tool for autism in two-year-olds (STAT): Development and preliminary data. *Journal of Autism and Developmental Disorders, 30*, 607–612. http://dx.doi.org/10.1023/A:1005647629002

Strock, M. (2004). *Autism spectrum disorders (Pervasive Developmental Disorders)* (p. 40) NIH Publication No. NIH-04-5511. Bethesda, MD: National Institute of Mental Health, National Institutes of Health, U.S. Department of Health and Human Services. Retrieved from http://www.nimh.nih.gov/publicat/autism.cfm

Suarez, M. A., Atchison, B. J., & Lagerwey, M. (2014). Phenomonilogical examination of the mealtime experience of children with autism and food selectivity. *American Journal of Occupational Therapy, 68*, 102. http://dx.doi.org/10.5014/ajot.2014.008748

Suarez, M. A., & Crinion, K. M. (2015). Food choices of children with autism spectrum disorders. *International Journal of School Health, 2*, 3. http://dx.doi.org/10.17795/intjsh-27502

The Arc. (n.d.). *Intellectual disability.* Retrieved from http://www.thearc.org/page.aspx?pid=2543, on August 20, 2015.

United Kingdom Medical Research Council. (2001, December). *MRC review of autism research: Epidemiology and causes.* Retrieved from http://www.mrc.ac.uk/pdf-autism-report.pdf. on July 25, 2004.

Van Bourgondien, M. E., Reichle, N. C., & Palmer, A. (1997). Sexual behavior in adults with autism. *Journal of Autism and Developmental Disorders, 27*(2), 113–125. http://dx.doi.org/10.1023/A:1025883622452

Veenstra-VanDerWeele, J., Cook, E., & Lombroso, P. J. (2003). Genetics of childhood disorders: XLVI. Autism. Part 5: Genetics of autism. *Journal of the American Academy of Child and Adolescent Psychiatry, 42*, 116–118.

Vilensky, J. A., Damasio, A. R., & Maurer, R. G. (1981). Gait disturbances in patients with autistic behavior: A preliminary study. *Archives of Neurology, 38*(10), 646–649. http://dx.doi.org/10.1001/archneur.1981.00510100074013

Wang, G., Liu, Z., Xu, G., Jiang, F., Lu, N., Baylor, A., & Owens, J. (2015). Sleep disturbances and associated factors in Chinese children with autism spectrum disorder: A retrospective and cross-sectional study. *Child Psychiatry and Human Development, 47*(2), 248–258. http://dx.doi.org/10.1007/s10578-015-0561-z

Watson, L. R., Baranek, G. T., Roberts, J. E., David, F. J., & Perryman, T. P. (2010). Behavioral and physiological responses to child-directed speech as predictors of communication outcomes in children with autism spectrum disorders. *Journal of Speech, Language, and Hearing Research, 53*(4), 1052–1064. (PMID: 20631229) http://dx.doi.org/10.1044/1092-4388(2009/09-0096

Wechsler, D. (2003). *Wechsler intelligence scale for children, fourth edition (WISC-IV)*. Pearson: PsychCorp.

Wiig, E. H., Semel, E., & Second, W. (2013). *Clinical evaluation of language fundamentals, fifth edition (CELF-5)*. Pearson: PsychCorp.

Williams, J. H. G., Whiten, A., & Singh, T. (2004). A systematic review of action imitation in autistic spectrum disorder. *Journal of Autism and Developmental Disorders, 34*(3), 285–299. http://dx.doi.org/10.1023/B:JADD.0000029551.56735.3a

Yeargin-Allsopp, M., Rice, C., Karapukar, T., Doernberg, N., Boyle, C., & Murphy, C. (2003). Prevalence of autism in US metropolitan area. *JAMA, 289*(1), 49–55. http://dx.doi.org/10.1001/jama.289.1.49

Zimmerman, I., Steiner, V., & Pond, R. (2011). *Preschool language scales, fifth edition (PLS-5)*. Pearson: PsychCorp.

CHAPTER 4

Intellectual Disability

Michelle A. Suarez and Ben J. Atchison

KEY TERMS

Cortical atrophy
Craniostenosis
Cytomegalovirus
Down syndrome
Fragile X syndrome
Hydrocephaly
Hyperphenylalaninemia
Hypoxia
PICA
Spina bifida
Tay-Sachs disease
Teratogenic
Toxemia

Jeffrey, aged 3 years, was brought to Early On at the local school district for a developmental evaluation. His parents report that his pediatrician is concerned about his language development. He smiled and interacted with examiners but was unable to express his wants and needs or follow single-step directions. An interview with his parents revealed that Jeffrey was unable to dress or undress and was not self-feeding. He was diagnosed with an intellectual disability and enrolled in early childhood special education where he is working toward language and self-care goals. His family hopes he will eventually attend mainstream kindergarten with special education support.

Michael, now 2, was diagnosed by his pediatrician shortly after his birth as having Down syndrome. He exhibits the physical characteristics such as a round face, flattened nose bridge, abnormally small head, low-set ears, short limbs, and abnormally shaped fingers. His motor development is delayed and his low muscle tone has made learning to walk difficult. Intellectual disability in children with Down syndrome is inevitable but varies in degree of severity. Michael's early intervention program provides services for Michael as well as parent support and education.

Kelly, now in second grade, is pleasant and likable. Teachers have been concerned about her inability to write letters or sound out words since kindergarten, and as the curriculum becomes more challenging, she is falling further behind. She has trouble maintaining friendships and often struggles to join peers in play. School staff conducted multidisciplinary team evaluation and diagnosed Kelly with an intellectual disability. She was placed in a special education classroom where the material is appropriate for her cognitive ability and learning pace.

DEFINITION

The term intellectual disability (ID) has evolved from the previous diagnosis of mental retardation. This terminology change reflects the shift from a view that classifies "mental retardation" as a personal trait residing solely within the individual to a holistic perspective that includes the capabilities of the person within the context of the environment. The official definition of the disability is as follows and includes three specific criteria:

"Intellectual disability is characterized by significant limitations both in intellectual functioning and in adaptive behavior as expressed in conceptual, social, and practical adaptive skills. This disability originates before age 18." (American Psychiatric Association, 2013)

■ Intellectual Functioning

The first component of this definition, intellectual functioning (or intelligence), is the general mental capability of an individual. This includes the ability to reason, plan, problem solve, think abstractly, comprehend complex ideas, and learn from experience. While it has its limitations, the accepted measure of intelligence is that which is determined by an intelligence quotient (IQ) score, which involves administration of standardized tests given by a trained professional. In the 2010 publication of the American Association on Intellectual and Developmental Disabilities (AAIDD), a "significant limitation in intellectual functioning" was defined as two standard deviations below the mean, in the context of the standard error and strengths and limitations of the specific instrument (IQ test) used in assessment (American Association on Intellectual and Developmental Disabilities, 2010). The IQ score is not a complete representation of human functioning and must be considered in the context of adaptive behavior, health, participation, and context. Therefore, clinical judgment must be used to interpret scores when considering diagnosis or service provision.

■ Adaptive Behavior

Adaptive behavior is the most related domain of concern among occupational therapists. Thus, it is our focus of assessment and intervention for persons with ID. As defined by the AAIDD, "adaptive behavior is the collection of conceptual, social, and practical skills that people have learned so they can function in their everyday lives" (AAIDD, 2010). Significant limitations in adaptive behavior impact a person's daily life and affect the ability to respond to a particular situation or to the environment. Table 4.1 provides specific examples of these three areas, which are published by the AAIDD.

Limitations in adaptive behavior can be determined by using standardized tests referenced to the general population, including people with disabilities and people without disabilities. On these standardized measures, significant limitations in adaptive behavior are operationally defined as performance that is at least two standard deviations

TABLE 4.1   Adaptive Skills

Conceptual Skills	Social Skills	Practical Skills
Receptive and expressive language	Interpersonal	Personal activities of daily living such as eating, dressing, mobility, and toileting
Reading and writing	Social Responsibility	
	Self-esteem	Instrumental activities of daily living such as preparing meals, taking medication, using the telephone, managing money, using transportation, and doing housekeeping activities
Money concepts	Gullibility (likelihood of being tricked or manipulated)	
Time concepts		
Number concepts	Naivete (wariness)	
	Following rules/obeying laws	Occupational skills
	Social problem solving	
	Avoiding victimization	Maintaining a safe environment

below the mean. In contrast to IQ scores for determining intellectual abilities, adaptive behavior is measured with the focus on typical performance and not maximum performance. In other words, the criteria critical to measuring limitations in adaptive behavior is *how a person typically performs*, not performance potential.

■ Onset before the Age of 18

The final component of the definition of ID is that it begins early in life, and therefore, a diagnosis of ID is made in childhood. A diagnosis of ID is not considered in adult-onset degenerative diseases such as dementia or those associated with traumatic brain injury. In addition, children under the age of 5 years who have delays in developmental milestones and intellectual functioning are sometimes given a temporary diagnosis of global developmental delay (GDD) that requires reassessment after age 5 (American Psychiatric Association, 2013). This diagnosis recognizes that accurate assessment of intellectual functioning is often not possible during this early childhood period, and therefore, the life-long intellectual functioning prognosis is difficult to determine.

In considering this definition, the AAIDD notes that there are five assumptions that need to be considered in the diagnostic process (American Association on Intellectual Disability, 2010):

1. Limitations in present functioning must be considered within the context of community environments typical of the individual's age peers and culture.
2. Valid assessment considers cultural and linguistic diversity as well as differences in communication, sensory, motor, and behavioral factors.
3. Within an individual, limitations often coexist with strengths.
4. An important purpose of describing limitations is to develop a profile of needed supports.
5. With appropriate personalized supports over a sustained period, the life functioning of the person with ID generally will improve.

ETIOLOGY

The causes of ID may be classified according to when they occurred in the developmental cycle (prenatally, perinatally, or postnatally) or by their origin (biomedical vs. environmental) (Shapiro & Batshaw, 2011). There are hundreds of causes of ID, yet despite knowing the many factors that contribute to ID, in a large proportion of cases the cause remains unknown. The ability to determine cause is highly correlated with the level of the ID. The etiology of ID is much less likely to be known with individuals who are mildly intellectually disabled (IQs of 50 to 70) than with those who are severely affected (IQs of <50) (AAIDD, 2010).

In a large United States population-based study describing probable causes of ID in school-aged children, the following results were obtained (Matilainen, Airaksinen, & Monomen, 1995):

- No defined cause 78.0%
- Prenatal conditions 12.4%
- Genetic 7.1%
- Perinatal conditions 5.9%
- Intrauterine/intrapartum 5.2%
- Postneonatal events 3.6%
- **Teratogenic** 2.9% (factors that can disrupt fetal development)
- Central nervous system (CNS) birth defects 1.5%
- Other birth defects 0.8%
- Neonatal 0.7%

Prenatal factors that can cause ID include genetic aberrations, birth defects that are not genetic in origin, environmental influences, or a combination of factors (Shapiro & Batshaw, 2011). Up to 50% of the individuals diagnosed with ID may have more than one causal factor (AAIDD, 2010). With genetic aberrations, the problem is either with the genes, which are the basic unit of heredity, or the chromosomes, which carry the genes. Each nongerm cell (cells other than the ovum and spermatozoa) contains 23 pairs of chromosomes, including one pair of sex chromosomes that determine the sex of the person. Males have an X and a Y chromosome, and females have two X chromosomes (Shapiro & Batshaw, 2011).

In many cases of ID, the gene or chromosome that has caused the condition can be identified specifically. In fact, more than 350 inborn errors of metabolism that result from genetic changes have been identified. Many of these metabolic errors lead to ID (Sumar & Lee, 2011). The two most common genetic causes of ID are Down syndrome and fragile X syndrome. **Down syndrome** is generally caused by an extra 21st chromosome, and **fragile X syndrome** is the result of a mutation at what is known as the fragile site on the X chromosome (Sumar & Lee, 2011). In other cases, the specific genetic aberration has not been identified. Factors such as higher incidences of a condition in specific families or increased recurrence rates among siblings suggest that the defect is genetic (Sumar & Lee, 2011).

Birth defects that are not considered genetic in origin also can contribute to or cause ID. These could include such things as malformation of parts of the CNS (e.g., **cortical atrophy, hydrocephaly, spina bifida, craniostenosis**) (Shapiro & Batshaw, 2011), congenital cardiac anomalies (Rogers et al., 1995), or metabolic disorders not associated with a genetic defect (e.g., hypothyroidism) (Reuss, Paneth, & Pinto-Martin, et al., 1996). Environmental factors may also be involved in prenatal development of ID. They may include exposure to chemical agents, such as alcohol or nonprescription drugs ingested by the mother during the pregnancy, maternal conditions such as **hyperphenylalaninemia**, a rare form of phenylketonuria caused by increased levels of phenylalanine amino acid (Mayo Clinic, 2015), **toxemia**, hypertension, and diabetes, or to congenital infections such as **cytomegalovirus**, which is a common herpesvirus infection that has a wide range of symptoms from asymptomatic to fever and to severe signs involving the eyes, brain, or other internal organs; rubella; and syphilis (Taylor, 2003).

■ **Genetic Causes**

Genetic causes can be divided into two types: single gene disorders and chromosomal abnormalities. In single gene disorders, there is a problem with the quality of the genetic material; a specific gene is defective. In chromosomal abnormalities, the problem is with the quantity of material. There is either too much or too little genetic material in a specific chromosome.

SINGLE GENE DISORDERS

Single gene disorders follow specific patterns of transmission: autosomal dominant, autosomal recessive, or sex linked. Table 4.2 presents the transmission patterns and risk factors associated with each type.

The autosomal dominant type is caused by a single altered gene. Either parent may be a carrier, or there may have been a spontaneous mutation of the gene. Dominant inheritance occurs when one parent passes on the defective gene. This occurs even if the other parent passes a healthy gene. Because the defective gene can be passed by either parent, there is a 50% risk of the child being affected in each pregnancy (Rogers, 2008).

TABLE **4.2**	**Single Gene Disorders**		
Type	Autosomal Dominant	Autosomal Recessive	Sex Linked
Transmission pattern	Either parent carries gene or spontaneous transmission	Both parents are carriers	Either parent can transmit gene: mother usually a carrier, father cannot be a carrier but can have the disorder
Risk factors	50% risk of child being affected with each pregnancy	25% risk of child being affected with each pregnancy	If mother has affected gene, 25% risk of having affected son or carrier daughter; if father has affected gene, all his daughters will be carriers and his sons will be normal
Sex distribution	Male and female children equally at risk	Male and female children equally at risk	Primarily male children at risk for having disorder, female children at risk for becoming carriers

An example of this type of inherited disorder is tuberous sclerosis.

In the autosomal recessive type, both parents are carriers but show no outward signs or symptoms of having the disorder. Inheritance occurs when both parents pass the defective gene to their offspring. Each pregnancy has a 25% risk of the child being affected (Rogers, 2008). Examples of this type of disorder are phenylketonuria (PKU) and **Tay-Sachs disease**. With X-linked disorders, the affected gene is on the sex chromosomes, specifically the X chromosome, and can occur in either parent. Because males have only one X chromosome, if the father has an affected gene, he will always have the disorder and cannot be a carrier. Because the female has two X chromosomes, she can either be a carrier of the disorder (if only one X chromosome is affected) or have the disease herself (if both X chromosomes are affected). A carrier mother has a 25% risk of having an affected son. If the father has the affected gene, all his daughters will be carriers, but his sons will not be affected (Rogers, 2008). Examples of X-linked disorders are Duchenne muscular dystrophy, fragile X syndrome, Lesch-Nyhan syndrome, and Hunter's syndrome.

■ Chromosomal Aberrations

Chromosomal aberrations include missing or extra chromosomes, either in part, such as a short arm, or the total chromosome, as is found in the trisomal types. Either the autosomes or sex chromosomes can be affected, with the autosomal type resulting in more serious neuromotor impairments (National Human Genome Research, 2015).The most common are trisomies 21, 18, and 13. The patterns of transmission are not as readily identified as those of specific gene defects.

ENVIRONMENTAL INFLUENCES

■ Prenatal Factors

There are numerous environmental causes of ID in the prenatal period, including maternal infections such as rubella, cytomegalovirus, toxoplasmosis, and syphilis. Low birth weight that results from prematurity or intrauterine growth retardation can also be a contributing factor. Maternal factors associated with low birth weight include smoking, lack of prenatal care, infections, poor nutrition, toxemia, and placental insufficiency. Exposure to industrial chemicals or drugs, including certain over-the-counter (OTC) prescriptions and illegal substances, also can affect birth weight, particularly during the first trimester of pregnancy.

■ Perinatal Factors

Two major causative factors of ID in the perinatal period are mechanical injuries at birth and perinatal **hypoxia**, which refers to reduced oxygen supply. Mechanical injuries are caused by difficulties of labor because of malposition, malpresentation, disproportion, or other labor complications that result in tears of the meninges, blood vessels, or other substances of the brain. Factors that cause perinatal hypoxia or anoxia include premature placental separation, massive hemorrhage from placenta previa, umbilical cord wrapped around the baby's neck, and meconium aspiration. Very premature infants also may have impaired respiration or an intracranial hemorrhage that can result in brain damage.

If a mother has an active case of herpes simplex II and is shedding the virus at the time of delivery, the baby can acquire the infection in the birth canal, which can cause severe developmental disability. This can be avoided by testing to determine whether the mother has an active case and, if so, delivering by cesarean section.

■ Postnatal Factors

Traumas or infections that result in injury or a lack of oxygen to the brain are a major cause of ID during the postnatal period. Traumas include near-drowning or strangulation, child abuse, and closed head injuries. Early severe psychosocial deprivation (i.e., attachment disorder, removal from the family home) is a significant factor ID etiology (Shevell & Sherr, 2008). Infections include encephalitis and meningitis. ID that results from meningitis caused by *Haemophilus influenzae* is now preventable, however, with the introduction of the *Haemophilus influenzae* type B (HiB) vaccine (Baraff, Lee, & Schriger, 1993).

INCIDENCE AND PREVALENCE

ID is one of the most frequently occurring developmental disabilities. Estimates of the prevalence of ID in this country range from 1% to 3%. Most professionals associated with the AAIDD accept a prevalence of 2.5%, and they recognize that the prevalence varies with chronological age (Rogers, 2008). The most recent data in the DSM-5 reports indicate a prevalence rate of approximately 1%, which is lower than previous estimates of 2% to 3%. This reduced number is likely due to the fact that IQ is no longer relied on as the specific factor in diagnosis of ID (American Psychiatric Association, 2013). Boys are 1.5 times more likely to be diagnosed with ID than girls, which may be related to the sex-linked genetic disorders that result in ID (Harbour & Maulik, 2010).

SIGNS AND SYMPTOMS

ID often occurs in tandem with, or as a secondary manifestation of, another diagnosis. One study's results found that two-thirds of the children with severe ID (IQ <50) had an additional neurological diagnosis; <20% of children with mild ID were found to have an additional neurological diagnosis. These diagnoses included conditions such as cerebral palsy, epilepsy, and hearing and visual impairments.

ID is defined by the AAIDD as a condition that is present from childhood (age 18 or younger), with (IQ) two standard deviations below the mean as measured on a standardized test and significant limitations in adaptive skills. Adaptive skills must be two standard deviations below the mean on a standardized test in conceptual, social, or practical skill areas (AAIDD, 2010). As previously stated, adaptive skill areas include communication, self-care, home living, social/interpersonal skills, leisure, health and safety, self-direction, functional academics, use of community resources, and work. Adaptive skills should be assessed in all of the individual's performance contexts. Someone with limited intellectual function who does not have adaptive skill deficits is not considered intellectually disabled (AAIDD, 2010).

There are currently two major systems of classification for ID, and both have similar characteristics. The American Psychiatric Association (APA) publishes the *Diagnostic and Statistical Manual of Mental Disorders (DSM),* and the 5th edition was published in 2013. This system is frequently used for diagnostic purposes. It classifies ID based on two major criteria. The first is intellectual functioning, which is determined by standard IQ testing. A score that is less than two standard deviations below the mean constitutes the cutoff for a cognitive deficit. The second criterion is deficits in adaptive functioning. This means that the individual has difficulty with skills required to live independently in a safe and responsible manner.

In addition to the DSM-5 diagnostic criteria, the AAIDD (previously the American Association on Mental Retardation) developed a system of classification based on adaptive skill levels and supports needed to function (AAIDD, 2010). The AAIDD system, because it focuses on function and supports needed in adaptive skills across performance contexts, is very useful for occupational therapy practice.

In the traditional system, ID is classified according to the severity of the impairment in intellectual functioning. This is determined through standardized intelligence testing. To be considered intellectually disabled, the person's performance on these tests must be two standard deviation units or more below the mean. The levels of ID as identified by IQ tests are mild, moderate, severe, and profound. Approximately 85% of individuals with ID are in the mild range, 10% are in the moderate range, 4.0% are in the severe range, and 2.0% are in the profound range of function (King, Toth, Hodapp, & Dykens, 2009). The *DSM-5* classifies four different degrees of mental retardation: *mild, moderate, severe,* and *profound.* These categories are based on the functioning level of the individual (American Psychiatric Association). It is important to remember that not all individuals in a particular classification will function at exactly that level.

The classification system developed by the AAIDD involves a three-step process. The first step is to have a qualified person administer standardized intelligence and adaptive skills assessments that are appropriate for the individual's age, communication abilities, and cultural experience. The second step is to describe the individual's strengths and weaknesses across the dimensions of (1) intellectual and adaptive behavior skills, (2) psychological/emotional considerations, (3) physical/health/etiological considerations, and (4) environmental considerations. The third step is to have the interdisciplinary team determine needed supports across these four dimensions. Supports are classified based on level of intensity and include intermittent, limited, extensive, and pervasive. Intermittent support is provided on an "as-needed" basis. Limited support occurs over a limited time span. Extensive support is assistance provided on a daily basis in a life area. Pervasive support refers to the need for support in all life areas across all environments on a daily basis (AAIDD, 2010).

In addition to the performance deficits produced by ID and the associated conditions already mentioned, a high proportion of individuals with ID also have some form of mental illness. Estimates of prevalence of mental illness among people with ID range from 10% to 20% to 40% to 70% (King et al., 2009). Some of the common types of mental illness seen in people with ID include personality disorders, affective disorders, psychotic disorders, avoidant disorder, paranoid personality disorder, and severe behavior problems that may include self-injurious behavior (Einfeld, Ellis, & Emerson, 2011). Several misconceptions about people with ID may complicate or prevent appropriate care for their mental illness, including the beliefs that people who are intellectually disabled cannot also be mentally ill, do not experience normal feelings and emotions, and are not affected by changes in their environment. Substance abuse problems, especially with alcohol, may be overlooked. Because of limited communication skills and limitations in abstract thinking caused by the ID, the diagnosis of mental illness and mental health problems can be a very difficult process and is frequently inexact. Good communication with caregivers and significant others in the life of the individual with ID is essential.

COURSE AND PROGNOSIS

ID is generally considered a lifelong condition, but the course and prognosis will vary depending upon the cause(s) of the disability and access to resources (Beers & Berkow, 1997; Behrman, Kliegman, & Nelson, 1992). In terms of life expectancy, people with mild ID live as long as the general population (Shevell & Sherr, 2008). However, people with more profound ID are less likely to reach old age. This is likely due to more serious neurological deficits and associated disorders.

Most cases of ID are nonprogressive, that is, once the initial insult to the brain occurs, there is no further damage (Beers & Berkow, 1997; Behrman et al., 1992). The emphasis is on managing the medical aspects of the condition and helping individuals to achieve their highest potential. However, certain genetic conditions (e.g., muscular dystrophy and Tay-Sachs disease) are progressive, with incremental loss of function and, in some cases, associated early death. Those with Down syndrome experience degenerative changes in the brain, beginning at about age 40 years, that eventually result in progressive dementia similar to Alzheimer's (Carr, 2012). The goal for these individuals is to help them achieve the highest level of independence and maintain it as long as possible.

One significant issue that can impact prognosis in people with ID is the presence of stigma in our society. This group often encounters negative stereotypes and prejudice from society that can lead to isolation and discrimination (Werner, 2015). Lower self-esteem and social exclusion can result. In addition, self-reported stigma from people with ID is strongly associated with symptoms of anxiety and depression in this population (Ali, King, Styrdom, & Hassiotis, 2015). However, social inclusion can mediate the impact of stigma and support psychological well-being (Simplican, Leader, Kosciulek, & Leahy, 2015). For example, membership in organizations like the Special Olympics can increase self-esteem, increase quality of life, and reduce stress (Crawford, Burns, & Fernie, 2015).

Another important factor in the improvement of the prognosis for people with ID is access to services that focus on strengths and increase adaptive functioning. With these services, it is possible for individuals with mild ID to gain adaptive behavior skills through remedial programs to the extent that they no longer meet the diagnostic criteria for being intellectually disabled, although their intellectual function has probably not changed significantly (AAIDD, 2010).

DIAGNOSIS

An evaluation must be performed to determine whether a person meets the criteria for being intellectually disabled. Besides ascertaining that the onset of the condition occurred before age 18, there are two main aspects to this process. The first part involves administration of appropriate standardized intelligence tests by a qualified individual. The selection of the specific standardized instrument should be based on factors such as the individual's social, linguistic, and cultural background (AAIDD, 2010). The individual's IQ is interpreted in the context of their level of adaptive behavior.

The second aspect of the process is the evaluation of adaptive behavior as it relates to the targeted adaptive life skill areas. Adaptive functioning is an individual's ability to cope with life demands and meet societal expectations for independence depending on age group (AAIDD, 2010). The skills needed for adaptive behavior become more complex and varied as the person ages. For instance, eating and dressing independently are major skills for the young child, but the child does not need to be able to use a telephone or manage money. Evidence for deficits and strengths in adaptive function should be gained from one or more independent, reliable sources who are familiar with the individual's abilities in different performance contexts. This information should be used to complete a standardized scale designed to provide a composite "picture" of the individual's adaptive function. As with the selection of an intelligence test, care should be taken that the Adaptive Behavior Scale chosen is appropriate for the individual's sociocultural background, education, associated handicaps, motivation, and cooperation level (AAIDD, 2010). There are more than 200 adaptive behavior measures and scales. The most common scale is the Vineland Adaptive Behavior Scales, Second Edition (VAB-II) (Sparrow, Balla, & Cicchetti, 2005), which purports to assess the personal and social skills needed for everyday living. It is an indirect assessment in that the respondent is not the individual in question but someone familiar with the individual's behavior. The VAB-II measures four domains: communication, daily living skills, socialization, and motor skills, and an optional Maladaptive Behavior Index. An Adaptive Behavior Composite is a combination of the scores from the four domains. A second scale frequently used to assess adaptive behavior is the Diagnostic Adaptive Behavior Scale (DABS) formerly titled the Adaptive Behavior Scale (AAIDD, 2010). This measure was developed by the AAIDD to assess conceptual, social,

and practical skills and focuses on the critical "cutoff area" for the purpose of ruling in or ruling out a diagnosis of ID.

MEDICAL/SURGICAL MANAGEMENT

There is no drug treatment for the condition of ID; however, medications may be needed for some of the conditions that may occur in tandem. In the past, psychotropic medications, and particularly antipsychotics, were often used in an attempt to manage challenging behaviors (Glover, Bernard, Brandord, Holland, & Strydom, 2014). However, due to negative side effects and limited evidence that these medications actually decreased these target behaviors, this practice has declined. Instead, psychotropic medications are now often used to treat diagnosed concomitant mental health problems (Tsiouris, Kim, Brown, Pettinger, & Cohen, 2013). A large-scale study of psychotropic drug use in people with ID by Tsiouris et al. (2013) revealed that 45% were receiving an antipsychotic (e.g., risperidone, olanzapine) to treat psychosis and bipolar disorder, 23% were receiving an antidepressant (e.g., Prozac, Zoloft) for an affective disorder, and 16% were receiving an antianxiety agent (e.g., clonazepam).

In addition to medications for treatment of mental health disorders, approximately 30% people with ID also have epilepsy, which may require the use of medications to reduce seizure activity (Lewis et al., 2000). Medications include Tegretol for generalized tonic-clonic seizures and tranquilizers like clonazepam for short-term emergency treatment. Unfortunately, diagnosis of epilepsy in people with ID can be complicated by communication and tolerance issues in this population that make standard testing like electroencephalogram magnetic resonance imaging difficult (McCarron, O'Dwyer, Burke, McGlinchey, & McCallion, 2014). Misdiagnosis can increase the risk for serious, sometimes life-threatening consequences of untreated seizure activity. Vigilance and professionals that are trained in recognizing symptoms of seizures in this population can increase appropriate medication dosage and seizure management.

Finally, neuromuscular dysfunction (e.g., spasticity) is seen in children with ID who have comorbid cerebral palsy. Several medications are sometimes helpful for increasing active and/or passive range of motion for increased function and prevention of contractures (Smith & Kurian, 2012). For example, botulinum toxin (e.g., Botox) is injected directly into the muscle group and will provide a short-term reduction in tone that can be used to strengthen antagonist muscle groups and facilitate the development of functional movement patterns. One longer-lasting medication for tone reduction is intrathecal baclofen. This medication is sometimes delivered by a pump directly into the spinal fluid and can relax spastic muscle groups. All medications have potential side effects and, when given, require close monitoring by the prescribing physician.

IMPACT OF OCCUPATIONAL PERFORMANCE

Virtually all areas of occupational performance and many client factors can be affected by ID, depending on the cause and severity of the ID. As stated previously, the diagnostic criteria for individuals with ID included three categories of adaptive behavior (conceptual, social, and practical skills) (AAIDD, 2010). These areas (communication, language, interpersonal skills, social responsibility, recreation, friendships, daily living skills, work, and travel) fall into all occupational performance areas including (basic) activities of daily living, instrumental activities of daily living, work, play, leisure, and social participation.

Although all of the occupational performance areas and client factors can be influenced by ID, those that are affected will depend on factors such as the presence of additional medical diagnoses and the severity of the diagnosis. It is imperative that the clinician be informed about the specific diagnosis that accompanies the identification of ID to determine the associated client factors that are involved.

For example, occupational therapists often work with persons who have Down syndrome. Babies with Down syndrome often have hypotonia, or poor muscle tone (National Down Syndrome Society, 2012). Because they have a reduced muscle tone, which results in oral motor dysfunction such as protruding tongue, feeding babies with Down syndrome is often difficult. Hypotonia may also affect the muscles of the digestive system, in which case constipation may be a problem. Atlantoaxial instability, a malformation of the upper part of the spine located under the base of the skull, is present in some individuals with Down syndrome. This condition can cause spinal cord compression as well as craniovertebral instability (Brockmeyer, 1992). Additionally, half of children with Down syndrome are diagnosed with a congenital heart defect (National Down Syndrome Society, 2012). In addition to hearing disorders, visual problems also may be present early in life. Cataracts occur in approximately 3% of children with Down syndrome but can be surgically removed.

Approximately half of the children with Down syndrome have congenital heart disease and associated early onset of pulmonary hypertension or high blood pressure in the lungs (National Down Syndrome Society, 2012). Echocardiography may be indicated to identify any congenital heart disease. If the defects have been identified before the onset of pulmonary hypertension, surgery has provided favorable results. Seizure disorders, though less prevalent than some of the other associated medical conditions, still affect between 5% and 13% of individuals with Down syndrome, a 10-fold greater incidence than in the general population. Congenital hypothyroidism, characterized by a reduced basal metabolism, an enlargement of the thyroid gland, and disturbances in the autonomic nervous system, occurs slightly more frequently in babies with Down syndrome. Recent studies indicate that 66% to 89% of children with Down syndrome have a hearing loss of >15 to 20 decibels in at least one ear, due to the fact that the external ear and the bones of the middle and inner ear may develop differently in children with Down syndrome (NIH, 2006). Given that 85% of all ID cases fall in the mild range of cognitive impairment, global and specific mental functions will be most affected with this population. The following case studies illustrate how ID affects an individual's area of occupational performance in different stages of the life cycle.

K.R. is a 21-year-old young woman with Down syndrome. Despite the fact that she has reached the legal age of adulthood, she is still in the process of transitioning from the developmental stage of adolescence to young adulthood. She still receives special education services but is also working on developing work and job skills through traditional vocational services. Her "disability" is expected to be lifelong.

K.R.'s condition was identified at birth. She has received continuous support and direct services to facilitate development of her abilities since then. She has always lived at home with her parents and still does so. She has her own room and bathroom at home and generally has exclusive use of the family room for her leisure pursuits. Her parents are professionals who are actively involved in their professions and the community. They are very realistic about her abilities and extremely supportive, allowing her to make most of her life choices. K.R. has a younger sister who is now away at college. K.R. has always been exposed to and involved in many social and cultural opportunities in the community, both with her family and on her own. Her social circle includes friends with and without disabilities, and she has several close friends as well as many social acquaintances.

K.R. has recently declared her life goals to be getting a job, getting an apartment of her own, and spending leisure time at the local community drop-in/recreational center for individuals with disabilities. Her mother feels that with appropriate supports, all of these goals are attainable.

K.R. is independent in most areas of personal care. As a result of limited fine motor coordination that seems to be complicated by visual-perceptual deficits, she needs assistance with regulating the water temperature for her bath, fastening zippers and buttons, and tying her shoes. She also occasionally needs reminders to straighten her clothing and brush the back of her hair. She has a speech impediment that makes it difficult for individuals who are unfamiliar with her to initially understand her. K.R. has learned to adapt to this limitation and works very hard to make people understand what she is trying to communicate. When cued, she will slow down and work on enunciating her words. She is independent in functional mobility, but because of problems with depth perception, she is very cautious when climbing steps and negotiating between different surface levels. She is able to travel independently in community areas she is familiar with and can ride the community "Dial-a-Ride" bus if the ride is arranged for her. Her mother feels that K.R. would be aware of danger in her home, such as a fire, and would get out of the house. She does not consistently answer the phone when it rings, although she is capable of doing so. For this reason, she is generally not allowed to be at home alone because her parents have no way of checking in with her if she does not answer the phone.

K.R. is able to perform many home management tasks and has recently become motivated to attempt more activities given her desire to have an apartment of her own. She generally dislikes "housework" but knows it is necessary in order to be a good roommate. She folds laundry and puts it away, and is learning to sort light and dark clothing and operate the washing machine. Her mother questions her ability to make judgments about what should or should not go into the dryer, however. She is able to sweep, vacuum, and dust but is not thorough, and this may be a result of her lack of interest and/or her visual-perceptual impairment. She keeps her bathroom clean and makes her bed. She is currently dependent in meal preparation, and this is the area that will probably require the most support for her to live in her own apartment. She cannot safely regulate stove and oven temperatures because of her fine motor problems. At the current time, K.R. attends school in a self-contained special education classroom in the local high school for half a day, focusing on vocational and prevocational skills, and spends the other half-day at Goodwill Industries in a work adjustment trial placement. K.R. has told her mother that she no longer enjoys going to school and would rather go to Goodwill. In addition to school and vocational activities, K.R. volunteers at the local community theater and at her church office doing clerical tasks. She is very interested in obtaining employment and would prefer to work at a video store, a music store, at the mall, or Pizza Hut. She is very interested in clerical tasks and has been working at her father's medical practice putting monthly billings in envelopes to be mailed. K.R. has many leisure interests and activities. She enjoys music and videos, likes to eat out, participates in Special

Olympics, goes to a community center for structured activities, and socializes with her friends. She prefers not to do strenuous physical activities, probably because of the difficulty she has as a result of generalized hypotonia. She has participated in team sports at the center but does so mostly for the social interaction. K.R. is very aware of her limitations and takes herself out of situations that she knows will be difficult or where she might not succeed.

CASE STUDY 2

F.B. is a 60-year-old man who is intellectually disabled. He has a history of behavior problems, including **PICA** and obsessive-compulsive–type behaviors of picking at his skin and clothing and stuffing toilets. He was retired from a sheltered workshop approximately 18 months ago when the emphasis of the program shifted to work readiness for community placement. It was determined that he would not be a good candidate for community work because of his age and lack of necessary supports (e.g., transportation). He currently attends a day program for social/leisure activities. F.B. has no known family and has spent most of his life in public residential institutions or in adult foster care (AFC) homes. He currently has a court-appointed guardian who makes most significant life decisions for him, including those regarding medical care and living arrangements. His guardian supports and encourages F.B. to make his wishes known about how he would like to spend his leisure time and allowed him input into his last housing change. In addition to his intellectual limitations, F.B. also experiences fairly frequent medical problems related to his obsessive-compulsive behaviors (e.g., skin infections). Medical problems, which may be age related, are emphysema and frequent fractures of bones in his lower extremities. F.B. currently lives in an AFC with 11 other adults who are developmentally disabled. His home is only required by law to provide basic care, and so it does not offer training in or support for participation in many home management tasks. His social groups generally consist of other adults with developmental disabilities or paid paraprofessional staff, either at home or the day program. His cultural experiences have been very limited because of his background.

F.B. is independent in most self-care tasks but needs supervision when using the bathroom because of his history of stuffing the toilet. He needs assistance and supports for taking medication owing to his cognitive limitations. He also needs very close monitoring of health status because he has a very high pain tolerance. He tends to prefer solitary activities but has become more verbal, social, and outgoing since going to the day program. He generally seeks out staff to interact with, and this usually takes the form of teasing. He will share activities with day program peers if prompted and has shown protective behaviors toward clients who are more limited and vulnerable than he is. Although he is verbal, he has a speech impediment that makes it difficult for people who are unfamiliar with him to understand what he is saying. He is independently ambulatory; however, he has reduced endurance as a result of an old hip fracture and neuropathy of the right lower extremity caused by a degenerative disease in the lumbar spine. He is dependent for all community mobility as a result of cognitive limitations and lack of experience and training. It is not clear whether he understands emergency situations, but he is cooperative with emergency drill procedures at the day program. It is likely that he would need ongoing supervision to maintain his personal safety.

Because of a lack of experience and opportunity, F.B. is dependent in all home management tasks. He has no responsibility for caring for others but seems to be very aware when one of his peers needs assistance or protection and alerts staff to these needs. He has been retired from the vocational arena for 18 months and now attends a day program that emphasizes social and leisure activities.

F.B. is generally not open to exploring new activities and has to be coaxed and teased by staff to try them. He generally prefers solitary activities and appears to enjoy assembly activities that result in a finished product like picture puzzles and building with Erector Set components. He does not seem to be very interested in watching television or listening to music but does enjoying going on automobile rides with his guardian, especially when she drives her convertible with the top down.

RECOMMENDED LEARNING RESOURCES

American Association on Intellectual and Developmental Disabilities
444 No. Capitol St., NW, Suite 846
Washington, DC, 20001

The American Association on Intellectual and Developmental Disabilities (AAIDD)
501 3rd Street, NW Suite 200
Washington, D.C. 20001
Telephone: (202) 387-1968
Fax: 202-387-2193

Baker, B., Brightman, A., Blacher, J., et al. (2004). *Steps to independence: Teaching everyday skills to children with special needs* (4th ed.). Baltimore, MD: Paul H. Brookes.

The Arc
500 E. Border St., Suite 300
Arlington, TX, 76010
Tel: (817) 261-6003; TTY: (817) 277-0553
Fax: (817) 277-3941

Behrman, R., & Kliegman, R. (Eds.) (2012). *Nelson essentials of pediatrics* (4th ed.). Philadelphia, PA: WB Saunders.

Case-Smith, J. (2015). *Occupational therapy for children* (7th ed.). St. Louis, MO: Mosby.

The Council for Exceptional Children
1920 Association Drive
Reston, VA 22091-1589

National Down Syndrome Congress
1605 Chantilly Dr., Suite 250
Atlanta, GA, 30324
Tel: (800) 232-NDSC

National Down Syndrome Society
666 Broadway
New York, NY, 10012
Tel: (212) 460-9330; toll free: (800) 221-4602

President's Committee for People with Intellectual Disabilities
US Department of Health & Human Services
330 Independence Ave., SW
Washington, DC, 20201
Tel: (202) 619-0634

People First International (self-advocacy group)
1340 Chemeketa St., NE
Salem, OR, 97301
Tel: (503) 588-5288

Special Olympics International, Inc.
1350 New York Ave., NW, Suite 500
Washington, DC, 20005
Tel: (202) 628-3630

REFERENCES

Ali, A., King, M., Styrdom, A., & Hassiotis, A. (2015). Self-reported stigma and symptoms of anxiety and depression in people with intellectual disabilities: Findings from a cross sectional study in England. *Journal of Affective Disorders, 187*, 224–231. http://dx.doi.org/10.1016/j.jad.2015.07.046

American Association on Intellectual and Developmental Disabilities. (2010). *Diagnostic adaptive behavior scale*. Retrieved from http://aaidd.org/intellectual-disability/diagnostic-adaptive-behavior-scale#.VfgnZn1No4I, on September, 2015.

American Association on Intellectual Disability. (2010). *Intellectual disability: Definition, classification, and systems of supports* (11th ed.). Washington, DC.

American Psychiatric Association. (2013). *Diagnostic and statistical manual of mental disorders* (5th ed.). Washington, DC.

Baraff, L., Lee, S., & Schriger, D. (1993). Outcomes of bacterial meningitis in children: A meta-analysis.

Pediatric Infectious Disease Journal, 12, 389–394.

Beers, M., & Berkow, R. (Eds.) (1997). *The Merck manual of diagnosis and therapy* (17th ed.). Rahway, NJ: Merck Sharp & Dohme Research Laboratories.

Behrman, R., Kliegman, R., & Nelson, W. (Eds.). (1992). *Nelson's textbook of pediatrics* (14th ed.). Philadelphia, PA: WB Saunders.

Brockmeyer, D. (1992). Down syndrome and craniovertebral instability: Topic review and treatment recommendations. *Pediatric Neurosurgery, 31*(2), 71–77.

Carr, J. (2012). Six weeks to 45 years: A longitudinal study of a population with Down syndrome. *Journal of Applied Research in Intellectual Disabilities, 25*(5), 414–422. doi: 10.1111/j.1408-3148.2011.00676,x

Crawford, C., Burns, J., & Fernie, B. A. (2015). Psychosocial impact of involvement in the Special Olympics. *Research in Developmental Disabilities, 45–46*, 92–102.

Einfeld, S., Ellis, L., & Emerson, E. (2011). Comorbidity of intellectual disability and mental disorder in children and adolescents: A systematic review. *Journal of Intellectual and Developmental Disability, 36*(2), 137–143. doi: 10.1080/13668250,2011.5725458

Glover, G., Bernard, S., Brandord, D., Holland, A., & Strydom, A. (2014). Use of medication for challenging behavior in people with intellectual disability. *The British Journal of Psychiatry, 205*, 6–7. http://doi.10.1192/bjp.bp.113.141267

Harbour, C., & Maulik, P. K. (2010). History of intellectual disabilities. In: J. Stone & M. Blouin (Eds.), *International encyclopedia of rehabilitation*. New York: Springer.

Hauser, M., & Ratey, J. (1994). *The patient with mental retardation*. In: Hyman, S.

King, B., Toth, K., Hodapp, R., & Dykens, E. (2009). Intellectual disability. In: B. Sadock, V. Sadock, & P. Ruiz (Eds.), *Comprehensive textbook of psychiatry* (9th ed., pp. 3444–3474). Philadelphia, PA: Lippincott Williams & Wilkins.

Lewis, J. N., Tonge, B. J., Mowat, D. R., Einfeld, S. L., Siddons, H. M., & Rees, V. W. (2000). Epilepsy and associated psychopathology in young people with intellectual disability. *Journal of Paediatric Child Health, 36*, 172–175.

Matilainen, R., Airaksinen, E., & Monomen, T. (1995). A population-based study on the causes of mild and severe mental retardation. *Acta Paediatrica, 84*, 261–266.

Mayo Clinic. (2015). *Diseases and conditions: Phenylketonuria*. Retrieved from http://www.mayoclinic.org/diseases-conditions/phenyl-ketonuria/resources/CON-20026275, On December 5, 2015.

McCarron, M., O'Dwyer, M., Burke, E., McGlinchey, E., & McCallion, P. (2014). Epidemiology of epilepsy in older adults with an intellectual disability in Ireland: Associations and service implications. *American Journal on Intellectual and Developmental Disabilities, 119*(3), 253–260. doi: 10.1352/1944-7558-119.3.253

National Down Syndrome Society. (2012). Retrieved from http://www.ndss.org/Search/?query=heart&section=14, on September 24, 2015.

National Human Genome Research. (2015). *Chromosomal abnormalities*. Retrieved from http://www.genome.gov/11508982. on November 5.

National Institutes of Health. *Facts about Down syndrome*. Retrieved from http://www.nichd.nih.gov/publications/pubs/downsyndrome/down, on February 12, 2006.

Reuss, M.,Paneth, M., Pinto-Martin, J., Lorenz, J. M., & Susser, M. (1996). The relation of transient hypothyroxinemia in preterm infants to neurologic development at two years of age. *New England Journal of Medicine, 334*, 821–827.

Rogers, H. (2008). Genetics of intellectual disabilities. *Current Opinion in Genetics and Development, 18*(3), 241–250.

Rogers, B., Msall, M., Buck, G., Lyon, N., Norris, M., Roland, J. M., … Pieroni, D. R. (1995). Neurodevelopmental outcome of infants with hypoplastic left heart syndrome. *Journal of Pediatrics, 126*, 496–498.

Shapiro, B., & Batshaw, M. (2011). Intellectual disability. In: R. Kliegman, B. Stanton, J. St. Geme, N. Schor, & R. Behrman (Eds.), *Nelson textbook of pediatrics* (19th ed.). Philadelphia, PA: Elsevier Saunders.

Shevell, M., & Sherr, E. (2008). Global developmental delay and mental retardation. In: K. Swaiman, S. Ashwal, & D. Ferreira (Eds.), *Pediatric neurology: Principles and practice* (4th ed.). Philadelphia, PA: Mosby Elsevier.

Simplican, S., Leader, G., Kosciulek, J., & Leahy, M. (2015). *Research in developmental disabilities, 38*, 18–29. http://dx.doi.org/10.1016/j.ridd.2014.10.008

Smith, M., & Kurian, M. (2012). The medical management of cerebral palsy. *Paediatrics and Child Health, 22*, 9.

Sparrow, S., Balla, D., & Cicchetti, D. (2005). *Vineland adaptive behavior scales*. San Antonio, TX: PsychCorp.

Sumar, K., & Lee, B. (2011). Down syndrome and other abnormalities of chromosome number. In: R. Kliegman, B. Stanton, N. Shore, J. Geme, & R. Behrman (Eds.), *Nelson textbook of pediatrics* (19th ed.). Philadelphia, PA: Sanders.

Taylor, G. (2003). Cytomegalovirus. *American Family Physician, 67*(3), 519–524.

Tsiouris, J. A., Kim, S., Brown, W. T., Pettinger, J., & Cohen, I. L. (2013). Prevalence of psychotropic drug use in adults with intellectual disability: Positive and negative findings from a large scale study. *Journal of Autism and Developmental Disabilities, 43*, 719–731. http://doi:10.1007/s10803-01201617-6

Werner, S. (2015). Public stigma and the perception of rights: Differences between intellectual and physical disabilities. *Research in Developmental Disabilities, 38*, 262–271. http://doi:10.1016/j.ridd.2014.12.030

5 Muscular Dystrophy

Jennifer L. Forgach and Andrea L. Washington

J.B. is 6 years old and has a 3-year-old brother and a 1-year-old sister. J.B.'s mother is concerned because he does not seem to be "keeping up" with his peers. He gets tired quickly, has had an increased number of falls, and has never learned how to jump. J.B. recently had to quit his soccer team due to increased fatigue. J.B.'s mother takes him to his pediatrician who notes that J.B. has enlarged calves, has proximal muscle weakness, and uses **Gower's maneuver** to rise off the floor. Gower's maneuver refers to the inability to rise up off the floor without using the upper extremities to walk up the thighs to assist with hip extension. This is often seen in multiple types of muscular dystrophy.

The pediatrician refers J.B. and his siblings for blood work, for genetic testing, and to neurology/muscular dystrophy (MD) specialty clinic for further assessment.

J.B. arrives to the MD clinic, and the neurologist meets with J.B. and his family. His blood work shows elevated **creatine kinase** (CK) levels >6,500 IU/L, while his 3-year-old brother's are normal at around 150 IU/L. CK is a steroid hormone produced by the adrenal cortex or synthesized for medical purposes; administered as drugs, they reduce swelling and decrease the body's immune system. Genetic testing reveals that J.B. is positive for Duchenne muscular dystrophy. His younger brother tests negative, and his 1-year-old sister is found to be a carrier. J.B. is referred to occupational and physical therapy and is recommended to follow up with the physician in 6 months. Although the above scenario illustrates one type of MD, MD is not strictly *one* disease.

MD is one of the most prolific **neuromuscular disorders**, which include a number of conditions that affect the muscles and/or direct nervous system control. It is actually a grouping of 9 different disorders with more than 30 different subtypes. MD can broadly be defined as a group of hereditary diseases that weaken the muscles. They are characterized by progressive muscle weakness, defects in muscle protein, and/or the death of muscle cells and tissues. The progressive muscle weakness is caused

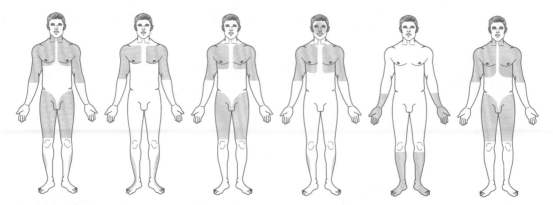

Figure 5.1 Typical distribution of muscle weakness seen in different types of muscular dystrophy. Left to right: Duchenne/Becker, Emery-Dreifuss, limb-girdle, facioscapulohumeral, distal, oculopharyngeal.

by the lack, or absence, of the structural protein dystrophin. **Dystrophin** is a vital part of the intracellular protein complex that is responsible for maintaining the shape and structure of the muscle fiber. In general terms, dystrophin acts as the "glue" to hold the muscle together. Without this "glue," the muscle breaks down causing the progressive weakness that is the hallmark characteristic of MD (Emery, 1994, 2001; http://www.mda.org 2015). It is the distribution and the progression of the muscle weakness that is used to distinguish between the nine types (Fig. 5.1). The nine main types of MD that have been identified are (http://www.mda.org 2015) as follows:

- Duchenne muscular dystrophy (DMD)
- Becker muscular dystrophy (BMD)
- Emery-Dreifuss muscular dystrophy (EDMD)
- Limb-girdle muscular dystrophy (LGMD)
- Facioscapulohumeral muscular dystrophy (FSHD)
- Myotonic muscular dystrophy (MMD)
- Oculopharyngeal muscular dystrophy (OPMD)
- Distal muscular dystrophy (DD)
- Congenital muscular dystrophy (CMD)

Although there are currently nine identified forms of the disease, this chapter will highlight six types of MD most commonly seen by occupational therapists.

DESCRIPTION AND DEFINITIONS

■ Duchenne Muscular Dystrophy

Although DMD is genetically present at birth, symptoms of the disease may not present themselves until the child is 3 to 4 years of age. DMD affects only males and, as will be discussed later, is an **X-linked** recessive inherited condition (Biggar, 2006). This is a type of inheritance, also referred to as sex linked, that occurs when a mother who carries the affected gene passes it onto her son.

DMD is caused by an absence, or deficiency, of dystrophin. Initial symptoms include delayed

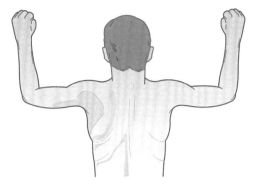

Figure 5.2 The valley sign: Note the depressed area of the left posterior axillary region seen beneath the deltoid when the individual abducts shoulders to 90 degrees, elbows flexed to 90 degrees, with bilateral hands pointing upward.

motor development, proximal weakness, and increased fatigue. These symptoms manifest themselves as a waddling gait, enlarged calf muscles, increased falls, and failure to develop the ability to run or jump (Emery, 1994, 2001). Also present in 90% of males with DMD is the "**valley sign**." This is a depressed area on the posterior axillary fold that can be seen when the patient abducts shoulders to 90 degrees, elbows flexed to 90 degrees, with bilateral hands pointing upward (Fig. 5.2).

The pattern of muscle weakness is always bilateral and symmetrical. It progresses from proximal to distal and affects the lower extremities prior to upper extremities. The rate of progression varies from person to person. The individual can alternately go through periods of both rapid progression and slowed or no progression. Most individuals with DMD will be wheelchair dependent by 12 years of age. DMD affects all voluntary skeletal muscles, as well as cardiac and pulmonary muscles (Emery, 2001). Of note, up to one-third of the individuals with DMD may have cognitive impairments. Current research indicates that this *may* also be related to the lack of dystrophin (Ashraf & Wong, 2005; Emery, 1994, 2001).

As muscle wasting progresses, active range of motion decreases, and the individual can be left with **contractures**, which result in abnormal shortening of muscle tissue that renders the muscle highly resistant to stretching at the elbows, hips, and knees, as well as severe spinal deformities. The joint contractures are often at a 90-degree angle later in the disease process, indicative of prolonged wheelchair use.

Becker Muscular Dystrophy

Like Duchenne, BMD is characterized by progressive muscle weakness, affecting primarily males, as an X-linked recessive inherited condition. While DMD mutations cause virtually no functional dystrophin production, BMD produces dystrophin that is partially functional. BMD is also genetically present at birth, but onset of symptoms can vary widely from 2 to 40 years of age. Symptoms most often appear, however, between 6 and 18 years of age. Individuals with BMD often demonstrate delayed ambulation, difficulty climbing stairs, "toe walking," muscle cramps, and fatigue as their early symptoms (Emery, 1994, 2001; http://www.mda.org 2015; Stockley, Akber, Bulgin, & Ray, 2006).

Muscle wasting/weakness progresses proximal to distal and generally occurs at a slower rate than in DMD (Stockley et al., 2006). It is usually symmetric, starting in the muscles of the pelvic girdle and thighs. Eventually, it extends to the trunk and upper extremities. The calves and forearms remain preserved until later stages of the disease. Facial muscles are not affected. Eventually, heel cord contractures (from toe walking) and **lumbar lordosis**, which is an inward curvature of the lower vertebral column, are seen due to the individual attempting to compensate for pelvic weakness (Emery, 2001).

Affected men can become wheelchair dependent in their 30s. Some may never require the use of a wheelchair, managing daily life with the use of compensation and adaptations.

Limb-Girdle Muscular Dystrophy

Limb-girdle muscular dystrophy accounts for approximately half of the identified subtypes of MD (Cardamone, Darras, & Ryan, 2008). LGMD is classified based on age of onset, rate of progression, and type of inheritance. Most forms of LGMD are of **autosomal recessive** inheritance that occurs when both parents carry and pass on the affected gene to their children. Up to 10% of cases are **autosomal dominant**, which refers to a type of inheritance that occurs when a child inherits a normal gene from one parent and an affected gene from the other parent.

The autosomal recessive forms exhibit more severe symptoms with a faster decline and loss of function, with an onset usually in childhood (Emery, 2001; http://www.mda.org 2015).

Other forms of limb-girdle muscular dystrophy have their onset in later adolescence, or even into adulthood. Adult-onset forms of LGMD are less severe and progress more slowly. Childhood forms can clinically resemble DMD. Males and females are equally affected. Dystrophin levels are normal; however, there is a lack of structural, dystrophin-associated glycoproteins. There are no associated cognitive deficits with LGMD (Bonnemann, 2005).

Progression of muscle weakness is not always symmetrical. It first affects the muscles of the pelvis and shoulders, "the limb girdle." Clinical symptoms are often first identified by a "waddling" gait. Muscle wasting is usually slow, however variable. While individuals with severe cases can lose the ability to ambulate in their early adolescence, others may never have more than complaints of muscle cramping in their lower extremities. Cardiopulmonary complications may appear in later stages of the disease (Bonnemann, 2005; Emery, 2001; http://www.mda.org 2015).

Typical presentation includes enlarged calves, severe lordosis with scoliosis, proximal muscle weakness, and a positive Gower's sign. Gower's maneuver can be described as the inability to rise off the floor without using the upper extremities to "walk up" the thighs to assist with hip extension (Fig. 5.3). When a person is observed to use this technique to get up off the floor, it is documented as having a positive **Gower's sign** (Bonnemann, 2005).

■ Myotonic Muscular Dystrophy

MMD is marked by teen or adult onset. Only 50% of the individuals affected live beyond 50 years of age. MMD is an autosomal dominant inherited disorder, affecting both males and females. Progression of muscle weakness is slow (Emery, 1994; http://www.mda.org 2015).

Muscle wasting/weakness begins in the face, lower legs, forearms, hands, and neck. Delayed relaxation after muscle contraction is a common symptom. This can be seen by "locking up" of the muscles, followed by a slowed relaxation (Emery, 1994; McNally & Pytel, 2007). In addition, MMD affects the gastrointestinal system, vision, heart, and/or respiratory system. Thirty percent of individuals affected with MMD will die from cardiac complications. Cardiac symptoms often precede neurological symptoms. Cognitive impairments may also be associated with this type of MD (McNally & Pytel, 2007).

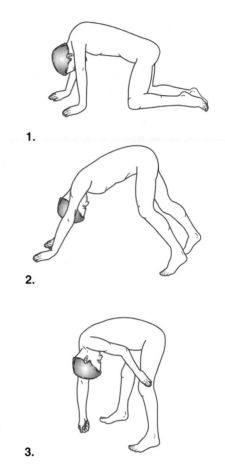

1.

2.

3.

Figure 5.3 The Gower's maneuver: The sequence of movements utilized by individuals with proximal weakness needed to rise off the floor. Named for William Richard Gower who first described this technique in 1879.

■ Facioscapulohumeral Muscular Dystrophy

Facioscapulohumeral muscular dystrophy is the third most common type of the dystrophies (Padberg & van Engelen, 2009). It is an autosomal dominant inherited disorder, affecting both males and females. Onset of symptoms is quite variable, appearing anywhere from the age of 7 to the age of 20. The earlier the disease onset, the more severe the symptoms, and the faster the disease will typically progress (Van der Maarel, Frants, & Padberg, 2007).

It initially affects the facial, shoulder, and upper arm muscles with progressive weakness. Weakness begins with the facial muscles and progresses down the body (Padberg & van Engelen, 2009). Weakness, unlike the other dystrophies, is not usually symmetrical, with one side more affected than the other. Presentation of facial symptoms include the inability or difficulty with closing the eyes, asymmetry of the mouth with smiling, drooping of the corners of the mouth at rest, and inability to whistle or pucker, and **atrophy**, a wasting of tissue that results in decreased muscle mass of the facial muscles, is clearly present (Emery, 1994; Wohlgemuth et al., 2006). As the disorder progresses into the shoulder region, **winged scapula** with severe muscle atrophy is present (Van der Maarel et al., 2007). A winged scapula is a physical symptom when the medial border of a person's scapula is abnormally positioned outward and backward. It is directly an indication of shoulder girdle weakness.

Shoulders appear depressed due to severe muscle weakness (especially in the biceps and triceps), and the individual is ultimately unable to raise his or her arms against gravity. With some individuals, the disease can progress to pelvic muscles and eventually affect their gait. This is most often seen in individuals with early onset of the condition. Many others never have any pelvic involvement and never lose the ability to ambulate (Iosa et al., 2007; Padberg & van Engelen, 2009). This type of MD is not associated with any cardiac complications or cognitive impairments (Emery, 1994).

■ Emery-Dreifuss Muscular Dystrophy

EDMD is a less statistically common form of MD. Like BMD and DMD, it is most often of X-linked recessive inheritance. EDMD primarily affects boys and usually present by the age of 10. Individuals with EDMD display a unique pattern of muscle weakness characterized by the formation of muscle contractures before any significant muscle weakness is recognized by the individual. Contractures of the heel cords, elbows, and muscles of the posterior neck are most common. Tightness of the heel cords may result in toe walking and an increased number of trips and/or falls. Elbows that are contracted to a 90-degree angle are the "most important diagnostic clue" of EDMD to physicians (Brown, Piercy, Muntoni, & Sewry, 2008). Eventually, rigidity of the spine and posterior neck prevents an individual from flexing the body forward. Formation of contractures and the subsequent muscle weakness is generally symmetrical on the body (Brown et al., 2008; Emery, 1994; http://www.mda.org 2015; Yazdanpanah, Javan, Nadimi, & Ghaffarain Shirazi, 2007).

Significant cardiac complications are also highly characteristic of EDMD. It is often necessary to surgically implant a pacemaker to regulate heart and pulse rate. Similar to the other forms of MD, it is often the cardiac and pulmonary complications that cause death in mid-adulthood (Gayathri, Taly, Sinha, Suresh, & Gorai, 2006). It is important to note, however, that with early intervention and proper medical management, individuals with EDMD may live an average life span (Emery, 1994).

ETIOLOGY

Most muscular dystrophies are **familial**, meaning there is some family history of the disease. All of the muscular dystrophies are inherited genetic disorders. Muscular dystrophies can be inherited in one of three ways as listed below. It is important to note, however, that some forms may be inherited in multiple ways; http://www.mda.org 2015;

1. X-linked recessive
   - Also referred to as sex linked, occurs when a mother who carries the affected gene passes it onto her son. Although the mother carries the affected gene on one of her X chromosomes, she may never show symptoms since it is a recessive trait.
   - Muscular dystrophies inherited this way: Duchenne, Becker, Emery-Dreifuss
2. Autosomal recessive
   - Occurs when both parents carry and pass on the affected gene
   - Muscular dystrophies inherited this way: Emery-Dreifuss, limb-girdle, oculopharyngeal, distal, congenital
3. Autosomal dominant
   - Occurs when a child inherits a normal gene from one parent and an affected gene from the other parent
   - Muscular dystrophies inherited this way: Emery-Dreifuss, limb-girdle, facioscapulohumeral, myotonic, oculopharyngeal, distal, congenital

INCIDENCE AND PREVALENCE

It is estimated that at least 1 in every 5,000 people in the population are currently affected with some form of MD. The actual prevalence of the disease is

TABLE 5.1	Incidence and Prevalence of Specific Types of Muscular Dystrophy	
Type of MD	**Incidence**	**Prevalence**
Duchenne MD	1 in 5,300 males	1 in 4,000 males
Becker MD	1 in 30,000 males	1 in 20,000 males
Facioscapulohumeral MD	1 in 22,000 males and females	1 in 50,000 males and females
Myotonic MD	1 in 8,000 males and females	1 in 20,000 males and females
Limb-Girdle MD	Statistically unknown	1 in 25,000 males and females
Emery-Dreifuss MD	Statistically unknown	1/100,000

most likely higher than this as many forms of MD are often misdiagnosed, not yet identified, or overlap clinical symptoms with other disorders. Therefore, specific current statistical information is difficult to obtain (Cardamonne et al., 2008; Emery, 1994, 2001; Kohler et al., 2009; McNally & Pytel, 2007). Table 5.1 is an *approximation* of available statistical figures in research literature today. It should be used only as a tool to compare the occurrence of one type of MD to another.

It is most important to recognize from Table 5.1 that Duchenne and Becker MD are by far the most common types and affect only males. Other forms, like limb-girdle and Emery-Dreifuss, have statistically unknown or unreliable data. This may be due to Emery-Dreifuss being less common than the other forms, and the many different subtypes of limb-girdle. MD occurs worldwide affecting all races, ages, and genders. Depending on the region of the world, or country, a certain form of MD may be very common or very rare (Mah et al., 2014).

SIGNS AND SYMPTOMS

Refer to each of the individual descriptions of the different types of MD for specific signs and symptoms as it relates to each of the various subtypes. As mentioned, decreased strength, muscle cramping, and decreased gross motor skills are the common link between all forms, with each form having its own unique presentation. As previously defined, the Gower's maneuver and the "valley sign" are two key clinical indicators that may be evident in any form of MD with proximal muscle weakness (Emery, 1994, 2001).

There are other progressive neuromuscular disorders that mimic MD and are often mistaken for MD in their early stages. Some of these include **spinal muscular atrophy (SMA)** (a **progressive** or worsening motor neuron disease that results in generalized muscle weakness and is most severe in the muscles closest to the center of the body), myasthenia gravis (MG), Pompe disease, and **Charcot-Marie-Tooth (CMT) disease** (a hereditary, slowly progressing disease of the peripheral nerves). An individual may present with muscle weakness and wasting and some loss of sensation in the feet, legs, hands, and forearms. This often results in contractures and scoliosis mitochondrial myopathy and **amyotrophic lateral sclerosis (ALS)**. These disorders exhibit the same symptoms at onset including muscle cramping, generalized progressive weakness, and joint stiffness and are often treated in neurological clinics alongside individuals with MD (http://www.mda.org 2015).

DIAGNOSIS

MD is often first suspected by a primary care physician when a patient presents with complaints of muscle weakness, increased falls, muscle cramps, or increased fatigue. It is at that point that clinical assessment becomes a vital part of the diagnostic process.

The patient is physically assessed by the physician. Based on the distribution of the weakness in conjunction with other aforementioned physical symptoms, MD may be suspected. At this point, the physician will begin to order more testing to confirm diagnosis.

The following three diagnostic tests are typically used to confirm or rule out an MD diagnosis (Emery, 1994, 2001; Stockley et al., 2006):

- Blood work to perform genetic testing and reveal CK levels. CK levels become elevated when there is muscle damage in the body;

therefore, elevated levels will indicate that there is muscle wasting occurring. Normal CK levels average around 100 to 200 IU/L. The levels in Duchenne MD, in comparison, can be elevated 50 to 100 times this amount (Biggar, 2006; Emery, 1994, 2001).

- **Electromyography (EMG)** is a diagnostic tool used for testing the electrical activity of muscle to evaluate the current electrical activity produced by the skeletal muscles. An EMG examination can be used to confirm the diagnosis of dystrophy and distinguish this from other types of neuromuscular diseases. It cannot reveal what type of dystrophy a patient may have (Emery, 2001).
- **Muscle biopsy** is used to examine the cellular makeup of the muscle tissue and look at the differences in muscle fibers, fiber size, fiber splitting, and fiber necrosis. Muscle biopsy can be used to distinguish the type of dystrophy, based on subtle differences in the muscle tissues (Emery, 1994).

These are not stand-alone tests; therefore, it is important to complete a thorough clinical and neurological exam to identify any patterns of muscle weakness, test reflex responses and coordination, and identify contracted muscles (Wren, Blumi, Tseng-Ong, & Gilsanz, 2007). If one child is diagnosed with MD, all siblings and parents should be tested for the condition as well.

COURSE AND PROGNOSIS

Each of the muscular dystrophies follows its own unique course. Each type has a variable prognosis with most ultimately resulting in a shortened life span. Prognosis will depend on not only the primary diagnosis but also what specific subtype of the disorder is present. For instance, limb-girdle MD has up to 15 different subtypes. Some of these subtypes have a normal life expectancy, while others have a shortened life span. The course and prognosis of each of the muscular dystrophies examined in this chapter are discussed individually below. While the figures represent an average of current statistical data, research and medical advances are beginning to extend life expectancies (http://www.mda.org 2015).

Duchenne muscular dystrophy: Males affected with DMD have an average life expectancy of late teens to early 20s.

The cause of death is usually secondary to respiratory and/or cardiac complications (Biggar, 2006; Emery, 1994; 2001; Kohler et al., 2009).

Becker muscular dystrophy: Less severe than DMD, males affected with BMD demonstrate a much slower progression. Life expectancy varies greatly, but average is between middle and late adulthood, approximately 25 to 30 years after onset of the condition (Emery, 2001; Stockley et al., 2006). If cardiac aspects are minimal, or adequately controlled, a normal life span is possible.

Emery-Dreifuss: Disease progresses slowly, often with cardiac and respiratory complications. Individuals may live an average life span if proper cardiac management is received (Cardamonne et al., 2008; Chen, 2008).

Limb-girdle muscular dystrophy: Progresses slowly. Although symptoms may appear in childhood, they often do not appear until adolescence or even adulthood. In the most severe form, muscles deteriorate rapidly, and life expectancy may be only into the early 30s. Otherwise, an individual may live a normal life span. The course of limb-girdle is by far the most variable of the dystrophies (Bonnemann, 2005; Emery, 1994, 2001; http://www.mda.org 2015).

Facioscapulohumeral: Symptoms appear around age 20. Disease progresses slowly with some periods of rapid decline. Course of disease may spread over many decades, with life expectancy being normal (Padberg & van Engelen, 2009; Van der Maarel et al., 2006).

Myotonic: Disease progresses slowly with course spanning up to 50 to 60 years. Life expectancy typically into late adulthood (Cardamonne et al., 2008).

MEDICAL/SURGICAL MANAGEMENT

Currently, there is no cure or specific treatment that can reverse or stop the progression of any form of MD; however, vast amounts of research is being conducted in this area. Symptom management will have the greatest impact on enhancing a person's quality of life and possibly increasing their life expectancy. The primary goal of treatment with MD is maintenance of independence for as long as possible (Emery, 2001).

Respiratory Maintenance

As mobility and muscle functioning decreases, respiratory maintenance becomes increasingly difficult. The individual will have decreased ability to use the voluntary muscles of the thorax to fully inhale, or cough, causing inability to keep the lungs clear. The individual may require suctioning, cough assist, or antibiotics to preserve lung function. They are high risk for pneumonia and other respiratory infections. Monitoring for signs/symptoms of aspiration is an important part of pneumonia prevention (Kohler et al., 2009; Thompson, 1999).

Skin Integrity

Skin integrity becomes a risk factor with decreased mobility. When skin integrity is compromised, the individual is at increased risk for infection, further tissue damage and loss of joint mobility. Careful skin inspection should be incorporated into one's daily routine. Severe infections can lead to death if not properly managed.

Pain

Pain should be assessed in all individuals with MD. While most types of MD are not directly associated with pain, some physical symptoms may contribute to discomfort (Emery, 1994). Initial feelings of muscle cramping or spasms may occur. The pain cycle may initially worsen when a stretching or strengthening program is initiated. It is advantageous to complete these exercises on a regular basis as the body will tolerate the stretches with less discomfort. In fact, it is common for an individual with MD to request joint stretching as a source of pain relief. As the disease progresses, pain levels should be continually monitored and assessed as increased or localized pain could be indicative of further concerns. Adequate pain management is essential for enhancing quality of life as well as promoting maximum participation in daily tasks.

Nutrition

Good nutrition and hydration are essential to maintain overall health and can aid in the maintenance of skin integrity. Nutrition can also assist in controlling obesity, which can be detrimental to function and mobility. People with MD are at high risk for obesity, secondary to lack of mobility and loss of muscle function. *Safe* maintenance of nutrition becomes a priority as oral and pharyngeal musculature may also be weakened in some forms of MD. As a result, swallowing can become unsafe. Individuals should be closely monitored for signs of dysphagia so that diet can be modified or a feeding tube inserted (Cardamonne et al., 2008; Thompson, 1999).

Occupational and/or Physical Therapy

Therapy should be initiated as soon as the diagnosis is confirmed to train the patient and family in an extensive home exercise program. A baseline of activities of daily living (ADL) skills and mobility performance should also be obtained. It is important to initiate therapy prior to the formation of contractures or muscle tightness (Thompson, 1999). Therapy is an essential component in preventing or slowing loss of strength, range of motion, and function. Another major role of therapy is to assess current equipment needs for home and community use. The role of occupational or physical therapy becomes increasingly important as the disease progresses and specific individual needs change. Evaluation and provision of splints and orthotics as needed to prevent joint contracture formation should further be considered at the time of the evaluation.

Drug Intervention

Corticosteroids are steroid hormones produced by the adrenal cortex or synthesized for medical purposes. When these hormones are administered as drugs, they reduce swelling and decrease the body's immune system *may* decrease muscle damage and assist with preserving respiratory function. Although they present possible benefits, they are often associated with side effects that must be closely monitored, including the tendency to gain weight. While corticosteroids are widely used, there continues to be controversy. Significant research is being conducted regarding whether the use of steroids has any effect on life expectancy. In addition to corticosteroids, there are other medications that are often prescribed by a physician for treatment of MD. Immunosuppressant drugs can be used to delay muscle degeneration. Anticonvulsants can be used to control muscle activity. Antibiotics can be used to control respiratory infections. Over-the-counter analgesics can be used for pain management and cramping (Biggar, 2006).

■ Surgical Management

Surgical management often includes corrective and/or preventative surgeries. Some of these may include, but are not limited to, contracture release, scoliosis repair, cardiac stability, respiratory assist, or spinal stabilization. Spinal deformities can physically reduce a person's ability to breathe and should be closely monitored. Pacemakers can be surgically implanted to control heart rhythms as needed. Tracheostomies may need to be performed if a person requires ventilator assistance or suctioning of secretions. Feeding tubes, either temporary or permanent, may need to be considered if dysphagia is a concern (Kohler et al., 2009; Thompson, 1999).

■ Advances in Medical Management

Current scientific research is being conducted seeking the causes of and treatments for neuromuscular diseases. There are currently three main research methodologies being completed: gene replacement therapy, genetic modification therapy, and drug-based therapy. Gene replacement therapy directly addresses the lack of dystrophin by "replacing" it with a closely related protein that is not affected by the gene mutation. Genetic modification therapy, however, acts to "skip" or "read through" the genetic mutation by manipulating the protein to result in a partially functional dystrophin. Lastly, drug-based therapy (i.e., steroids) seeks to delay muscle wasting by promoting muscle growth or reducing the damage caused by inflammation. As research and clinical trials continue to advance, there is expected to be a greater impact on prognosis and overall quality of life (Braun, Wang, Mack, & Childers, 2014; Mah et al., 2014; Ulane, Teed, & Sampson, 2014).

IMPACT ON OCCUPATIONAL PERFORMANCE

As described in the *Occupational Therapy Practice Framework*, 3rd edition, occupations, client factors, performance skills, performance patterns, context, and environment may all be affected by MD. These are most dependent on the type and the stage of the disease. As previously mentioned, each type of MD has its own unique progression and variable severity. Each individual may have any combination of these different occupational deficits.

■ Activities of Daily Living (ADL)/ Instrumental Activities of Daily Living (IADL)

The individuals with MD may initially be independent with their ADL/IADLS skills; however, a decline in function is anticipated, especially with more severe forms. Maintaining the basic underlying skills of strength and ROM will keep the individual independent longer. As active movement becomes more difficult, the person will require assistance from a caregiver to complete basic tasks such as dressing, grooming, and bathing. Toileting may become a cumbersome task. This can be due to physical limitations making toilet transfers difficult or due to loss of muscle control causing incontinence. Often with more severe forms of MD, the individual is required to wear protective toileting garments.

Eventually, the use of adaptive equipment such as commode chairs, shower chairs, bathing aides, mechanical lifts, ADL equipment, and wheelchairs/mobility equipment may be necessary. These pieces of equipment will help increase independence and make caring for the individual easier and safer. Home modifications such as ramps, grab bars, and bedrails should be considered to promote independence and safety within an individual's home environment. In less severe forms, the individuals may maintain the ability to complete the task themselves but may require increased time to do so. Energy conservation, or task adaptation, should be a consideration for these individuals (Kohler et al., 2009). Tasks such as driving, community mobility, health management and maintenance, meal preparation, and shopping may also require adaptation or modification to allow for some level of participation. This will most likely be an area of dependence for most individuals in later stages of the disease.

■ Education

School is a major concern as the majority of MD cases are diagnosed in early childhood or early adolescence. Most forms of MD do not involve cognitive impairments, and therefore, physical limitations ultimately become the barrier at school (Donders & Taneja, 2009; Thompson, 1999). Often the child with MD fatigues quickly, has difficulty keeping up with peers, and may require physical assistance to get through the school day. A one-on-one aid may be necessary to assist with maneuvering the wheelchair, toileting, assisting with meals, and completing basic educational tasks.

Increased absences due to illness may be common. This, combined with wheelchair/adaptive equipment use and the decreased physical ability to participate in the same activities as peers, may contribute to social isolation.

■ Work

Older individuals may face many of the same barriers as children in school. Social isolation, environmental barriers, fatigue, an inability to keep up with work activities, and requiring physical assistance for some basic tasks may be common in the workplace.

Obtaining and maintaining employment and having the ability to change jobs are more difficult for these individuals due to physical limitations, decreased job opportunities, and employer misperceptions. Some individuals with severe MD may lose, or never have, the physical ability to work. Others may maintain employment with altered responsibilities/adaptations or with relatively little interruption at all.

■ Play/Leisure

A child's primary responsibility is to play. Many individuals diagnosed with MD are children, and this area becomes a significant area of concern. It is important to encourage play, in any capacity, to ensure pleasure, learning, and development. A child with physical impairments may require

modifications to his or her leisure activities to promote success and enjoyment.

For individuals of all ages, leisure activities such as computer and video game play, text messaging, and reading are commonly enjoyed as hand function is often preserved well enough to complete these tasks. It is beneficial to also incorporate and encourage gross motor movements into leisure activities (i.e., balloon volleyball, painting on an easel, etc.) as a means to preserve muscle strength and function (Thompson, 1999).

■ Psychosocial

MD affects everyone within the family, not solely the affected individual. The emotions, fears, and anxieties experienced by the individual are shared by the entire family. Parents often face feelings of guilt, helplessness, and fear over the anticipated loss of their child. Fear and anxiety are often a concern for the younger sibling as they watch the deterioration of their older sibling, with the anticipation that they will soon, too, face the same fate.

As the affected individual loses function, and the loss of independence becomes more evident, the individual often struggles with anger and frustration. Individuals who face severe functional loss often experience feelings of depression. Suicidal ideations may become a concern as the individual faces the loss of his or her perceived role (Bostrom & Ahlstrom, 2005; Chen, 2008; Poysky & Kinnett, 2008).

CASE STUDY 1

A.F. is 32 years old. When she was 13 years old, she began to notice that her hips and lower back would fatigue quickly and that she was having minor trouble with her balance. Her primary care physician felt that it was "growing pains" and told her that he was sure it would pass. A year later, A.F. continued to have problems, and her symptoms worsened. A.F. returned to her physician and, at that time, blood work and a muscle biopsy were conducted. A.F. was eventually diagnosed with limb-girdle muscular dystrophy.

On this day, A.F. presents to the muscular dystrophy clinic per recommendation of her primary care physician. The occupational therapist

evaluates A.F. It was revealed that A.F. has had significant functional decline in the last year. She was previously walking with a walker for household distances. She is now using a borrowed wheelchair for all ambulation. A.F. can independently complete a stand-pivot transfer from her wheelchair to the examining table with increased time allotted. Manual muscle testing scores as follows: grossly 3/5 bilateral shoulder strength, 3+/5 strength at bilateral elbows, and 4/5 in the wrists and hands.

A.F. currently has a shower chair in the bathtub that she borrowed from her grandmother. However, A.F. further reports that she is no longer able to step over the side of the tub. She is now wearing a diaper due to her inability to get to the toilet quickly enough. She attempts to dress herself seated at the edge of the bed but is unable to don her socks or shoes as a result of leg weakness and poor sitting balance. A.F. currently lives alone and does not have family close by to assist her. She has hired a maid to keep the house clean and assist with weekly laundry. She recently had to quit her job as a school teacher due to her physical decline. She is now significantly concerned about her finances.

She reports that she is feeling isolated at home. She does not identify any leisure interests other than watching television. She states that it is too much work to get out of the house, so she just stays home. A.F. is anxious about her recent decline and is not knowledgeable about her condition or prognosis. She is not currently taking any medications except an over-the-counter analgesic, as needed.

CASE STUDY 2

H.M. is a 12-year-old male diagnosed with Duchenne muscular dystrophy. He is currently an inpatient at a children's hospital. He presented to the ER with complaints of difficulty breathing. He subsequently required intubation and eventually a tracheostomy.

Occupational therapy was consulted to evaluate H.M. and to provide recommendations to his family. A review of the medical record reveals that H.M. was diagnosed with muscular dystrophy at the age of 3. He is currently on prednisone, digitalis, a multivitamin, a diuretic, and an analgesic as needed. He is the oldest of four children, with two other brothers also diagnosed with DMD. He had spinal stabilization surgery approximately 1 year ago and releases of bilateral knee contractures about 6 months ago.

Upon entering H.M.'s hospital room, the occupational therapist completes a parent interview and receives the following information: H.M. is currently in the 7th grade in a POHI classroom. He lives in a two-story home, with first floor bedroom and bathroom. They have a ramp outside to enter the home. H.M. has not received therapy in almost a year. Parents are concerned that H.M. has outgrown his current wheelchair and is not properly supported by his seating system. Parents also report that H.M. has been gaining weight, making all wheelchair and surface transfers increasingly difficult. Prior to admission, H.M. required variable assistance for all ADL, IADL, and transfers. There is no current home exercise program in place.

Upon interviewing H.M., he appears to be delayed cognitively, requiring simple questions and multiple cues to follow one-step commands.

He reports no pain throughout his day. He spends his time watching television, playing video games, and texting his friends on his cell phone. H.M. states that he would like to be more independent within his school and home environments.

Evaluation findings as follows: H.M. presents with decreased upper extremity active range of motion and strength, as he is unable to raise his arms over his head or fully straighten his elbows. He also presents with contractures of bilateral shoulders, elbows, and wrists. H.M. demonstrates the ability to isolate all fingers and thumb movements. He presents with decreased grip strength bilaterally. He currently demonstrates the ability to feed himself with a spoon; however, he is observed to lower his head to the plate. H.M. is coughing and choking during meals with minimal chewing observed. He currently requires maximal assistance for all bathing/dressing tasks, which is being completed in bed at this time. Bed mobility is impaired. He requires maximum assistance to transfer from supine to edge of bed and is unable to maintain sitting balance without support.

The inpatient occupational therapist made the following recommendations to H.M. and his family: Referrals were made to outpatient occupational and physical therapy following discharge. A thorough feeding evaluation is recommended with possible feeding tube placement, as he is showing signs/symptoms of aspiration. A new wheelchair and seating system evaluation is to be completed. H.M.'s parents were also provided an initial home exercise program for safe positioning, daily stretching, and mobilization. The social work department was contacted to address possible psychosocial and coping needs.

ACKNOWLEDGMENTS

We would like to thank Lawrence C. Banko for his contributions. Lawrence was responsible for drawing all sketches/illustrations used in this chapter.

ONLINE RESOURCES

Muscular Dystrophy Association
www.mda.org
Centers for Disease Control and Prevention
www.cdc.gov
Parent Project Muscular Dystrophy
www.parentprojectmd.org
National Institute of Health
www.nih.gov
Muscular Dystrophy Canada
www.muscle.ca

Muscular Dystrophy Family Foundation
www.mdff.org
Mayo Clinic Web site
www.mayoclinic.org
Patient and family support group
www.dailystrength.org/muscular-dystrophies/
    support-group
Cincinnati Children's Hospital Web site
www.cincinnatichildrens.org

REFERENCES

America Occupational Therapy Association. (2014). Occupational therapy practice framework: Domain and process (3rd ed). *American Journal of Occupational Therapy, 68*(S1), 1–51. doi:10.5014/ajot.2014.682006

Ashraf, E. A., & Wong, B. L. (2005). The diagnosis of muscular dystrophy. *Pediatric Annals, 34*, 525–528.

Biggar, W. D. (2006). Duchenne muscular dystrophy. *Pediatrics in Review, 27*, 83–88. doi:10.1542/pir.27-3-83

Bonnemann, C. G. (2005). Limb girdle muscular dystrophy in childhood. *Pediatric Annals, 34*, 569–577.

Bostrom, K., & Ahlstrom, G. (2005). Living with a hereditary disease: Persons with muscular dystrophy and their next of kin. *American Journal of Medical Genetics, 136A*, 17–24. doi:10.1002/ajmg.a.30762

Braun, R., Wang, Z., Mack, D., & Childers, M. (2014). Gene therapy for inherited muscle diseases where genetics meets rehabilitation needs. *American Journal of Physical Medicine & Rehabilitation, 93*(Suppl), S97–S107.

Brown, S., Piercy, R., Muntoni, F., & Sewry, C. (2008). Investigating the pathology of Emery-Dreifuss muscular dystrophy. *Biochemical Society Transactions, 36*, 1335–1338. doi:10.1042/BST0361335

Cardamone, M., Darras, B., & Ryan, M. (2008). Inherited myopathies and muscular dystrophies. *Seminars in Neurology, 28*, 250–259. doi:10.1055/s-2008-1062269

Chen, J. Y. (2008). Mediators affecting family function in families of children with Duchenne muscular dystrophy. *Kaohsiung Journal of Medical Sciences, 24*, 514–521.

Donders, J., & Taneja, C. (2009). Neurobehavioral characteristics of children with Duchenne muscular dystrophy. *Child Neuropsychology, 15*, 295–304. doi:10.1080/09297040802665777

Emery, A. E. H. (2001). *The muscular dystrophies*. New York, NY: Oxford University Press.

Emery, A. E. H. (1994). *Muscular dystrophy: The facts*. New York, NY: Oxford University Press.

Gayathri, N., Taly, A. B., Sinha, S., Suresh, T. G., & Gorai, D. (2006). Emery Dreifuss muscular dystrophy: A clinico-pathological study. *Neurology India, 54*, 197–199.

Iosa, M., Mazza, C., Frusciante, R., Zok, M., Aprile, I., Ricci, E., & Cappozzo, A. (2007). Mobility assessment of patients with facioscapulohumeral dystrophy. *Clinical Biomechanics, 22*, 1074–1082. doi:10.1016/j.clinbiomech.2007.07.013

Kohler, M., Clarenbach, C. F., Bahler, C., Brack, T., Russi, E. W., &Bloch, K. E. (2009). Disability and survival in Duchenne muscular dystrophy. *Journal of Neurology, Neurosurgery & Psychiatry, 80*, 320–325. doi:10.1136/jnnp.2007.141721

Mah, J., Kornut, L., Dykeman, J., Day, L., Pringsheim, T., & Jette, N. (2014). A systematic review and meta-analysis on the epidemiology of Duchenne and Becker muscular dystrophy.

Neuromuscular Disorders, 24(6), 482–491. http://dx.doi.org/10.1016/j.nmd.2014.03.008

McNally, E. M., & Pytel, P. (2007). Muscle diseases: The muscular dystrophies. *The Annual Review of Pathology: Mechanisms of Disease, 2,* 87–109. doi:10.1146/annurev.pathol.2.010506.091936

Padberg, G. W., & van Engelen, B. G. (2009). Facioscapulohumeral muscular dystrophy. *Current Opinion in Neurology, 22,* 539–542. doi:10.1097/WCO.0b013e328330a572

Poysky, J., & Kinnett, K. (2008). Facilitating family adjustment to a diagnosis of Duchenne muscular dystrophy. *Neuromuscular Disorders, 19,* 733–738. doi:10.1016/j.nmd.2009.07.011

Stockley, T., Akber, S., Bulgin, N., & Ray, P. (2006). Strategy for comprehensive molecular testing for Duchenne and Becker muscular dystrophies. *Genetic Testing, 10,* 229–243. doi:10.1089/gte.2006.229-243

Thompson, C. E. (1999). *Raising a child with a neuromuscular disorder. A guide for parents, grandparents, friends, and professionals.* New York, NY: Oxford University Press.

Ulane, C., Teed, S., & Sampson, J. (2014). Recent advances in myotonic dystrophy type 2. *Current Neurology and Neuroscience Reports, 14*(2), 429.

Van der Maarel, S. M., Frants, R. R., & Padberg, G. (2007). Facioscapulohumeral muscular dystrophy. *Biochimica et Biophysica Acta, 1772*(2), 186–194. doi:10.1016/j.bbadis.2006.05.009

Wohlgemuth, M., de Swart, B. J. M., Kalf, J. G., Joosten, F. B. M., Van der Vliet, A. M., & Padberg, G. W. (2006). Dysphagia in facioscapulohumeral muscular dystrophy. *Neurology, 66,* 1926–1928.

Wren, T. A. L., Blumi, S., Tseng-Ong, L., & Gilsanz, V. (2007). Three-point technique of fat quantification of muscle tissue as a marker of disease progression in Duchenne muscular dystrophy: Preliminary study. *AJR. American Journal of Roentgenology, 190,* W8–W12. doi:10.2214/AJR.07.2732

Yazdanpanah, P., Javan, A., Nadimi, B., & Ghaffarain Shirazi, H. R. (2007). Genetic pattern of 3 cases of Emery-Dreifuss muscular dystrophy in a family. *Eastern Mediterranean Health Journal, 13,* 201–205.

6

Attention Deficit Disorder

Shelley Mulligan

Samuel is 7 years of age and lives at home with his parents and 12-year-old sister. Samuel just completed his first few months of second grade and had begun to come home from school often in tears, and stating that he hates school. A phone call to his teacher revealed that he was struggling with math, reading, and writing. His teacher also said that he has trouble sitting still, and concentrating, and that he was not getting along well with the other children. His mother recognized that Samuel tended to be impulsive and rarely would sit still, unless he was playing his favorite video game. She found that he was easily frustrated and often irritable with frequent temper outbursts, which had gotten worse over the past few months.

As an infant and very young child, Samuel was quite easy to care for, although he was always full of energy and had trouble following bedtime routines and sleeping through the night. His mother felt that Samuel needed more help than did other children his age to complete basic self-care skills like dressing and bathing or putting his belongings away. He liked playing outside with his bike, scooter, and any type of ball play and preferred gross motor games including rough and tumble play, although he was accident-prone. Samuel had joined a baseball team the previous spring, which did not go well. He had trouble following directions, often pushed or bothered the other children, and was often just running around. Eventually, he withdrew from the program. Samuel is a healthy boy, and his medical history is unremarkable with the exception of a fractured radius, caused by a fall off of his bike 2 years prior. He had not ever received therapy or special education services.

Based on his second grade teacher's concerns, and parent concerns, he was referred for an evaluation by the school district's special education team including a school psychologist, special education teacher, and occupational therapist. Outside of school, he was evaluated by a developmental pediatrician known for her expertise with children with learning and attention disorders, and she diagnosed him with attention deficit hyperactivity disorder (ADHD), combined presentation. The label of ADHD combined is given to adults and children who exhibit both attention and hyperactive-impulsive symptoms. Samuel's evaluation by the school team indicated that Samuel had a poor attention span and that he needed frequent one-on-one assistance to initiate and complete tasks. He tended to interrupt the conversations of others, and the volume of his speech was loud. **Executive function** deficits consistent with the ADHD-combined presentation were noted, including inattention, disorganization, and poor awareness and problem solving. Standardized testing revealed that he had normal intelligence with IQ scores falling in the low-average range (88 to 92), with a slightly higher verbal than performance IQ. However, his math and reading skills were below average. Sensory and motor deficits were identified with respect to auditory processing, and motor planning, and were believed to contribute to his challenges with fine and gross motor skills, and social play.

His mother was most concerned regarding Samuel's school performance, and she was also worried about his emotional well-being and self-esteem. Samuel was determined to be eligible for special education and related services based on his ADHD diagnosis and his challenges at school, and subsequently, an individualized education program (IEP) was developed and implemented. His pediatrician recommended that he begin a trial of Ritalin, but his parents wanted to gather more information about the use of stimulant medication prior to agreeing to a trial of medication.

DEFINITION AND DESCRIPTION

ADHD is the most common neurobiological disorder that manifests in childhood, and it often continues into adolescence and adulthood (Wolraich et al., 2011). ADHD is characterized by persistent and maladaptive symptoms of inattention, hyperactivity, and impulsivity (APA, 2013). The average age of onset is 7 years of age, and boys are four times more likely than girls to have the disorder. ADHD is placed in the latest edition of the *Diagnostic and Statistical Manual for Mental Disorders, Fifth Edition* (DSM-5) by American Psychological Association, (2013) within the section describing neurodevelopmental disorders. This is a change from previous versions of the DSM, which had placed ADHD within the disruptive behavior disorders. ADHD includes three subtypes: combined, predominantly inattentive, and predominately hyperactive-impulsive, which in the DSM-5 are referred to as **clinical presentations** rather than subtypes. This subtle change in semantics from previous versions shifts the disorder from one with distinctly delineated subtypes to one that is more fluid, which better accommodates the changes in presentation or symptoms that often occur over time in the same individuals with ADHD. A helpful addition in the DSM-5 is that examples of how symptoms of the disorder may present in adolescents and adults are included, which gives a little more recognition of the disorder in older children and adulthood. A summary of the symptoms are listed below, and a more thorough and detailed description is available in the DSM-5 (APA, 2013).

■ Inattentive Symptoms of ADHD

- Often fails to give close attention to details or makes careless mistakes in schoolwork, work, or other activities (e.g., overlooks or misses details)
- Often has difficulty sustaining attention in tasks or play activities and remaining focused during activity
- Often does not appear to listen when spoken to directly (e.g., mind seems to wander)
- Has difficulty following through on instructions with task completion; often gets sidetracked
- Has poor organizational skills and has difficulty managing sequential tasks

- Avoids or is reluctant to engage in tasks that require sustained mental effort such as schoolwork
- Often loses necessary items like a cell phone, keys, or glasses
- Is often easily distracted by extraneous or unimportant stimuli
- Is often forgetful in daily activities

■ Hyperactive-impulsive symptoms of ADHD

- Often fidgets with hands, taps hand or feet, or squirms in a chair

- Often gets up and out of one's seat when remaining seated is expected
- Often runs about, or feels restless
- Often has difficulties engaging in leisure activities quietly
- Is often "on the go" or is uncomfortable being still for an extended time
- Often talks excessively
- Often blurts out answers before questions have been completed
- Often has difficulty waiting or taking turns

In addition to the criteria listed above related to symptomatology, there are other factors to consider when evaluating an individual for the possibility of an ADHD diagnosis. In the DSM-5, criteria state that several inattentive or hyperactive-impulsive symptoms must be present prior to 12 years of age (which is 5 years later than what was previously used as a criterion). In order to be diagnosed with ADHD, five or six inattentive or hyperactive-impulsive symptoms as listed above must be observed in two or more settings (e.g., home or school). Thus, symptoms must be evident in more than one context, but not necessarily so severe as to result in impairments in an individual's functioning in multiple contexts. There also must be clear evidence that symptoms interfere with or reduce the quality of the individual's social functioning, academic performance, and/or ability to perform their desired and necessary occupations (APA, 2013). This requirement relates to the negative impact that the clinical symptoms must have on an individual's daily functioning.

DSM-5 criteria are slightly more lenient than are earlier versions of the manual, which required evidence of *clinically significant impairment* in social, academic, or occupational functioning.

Removing the need for clinically significant impairment may make it easier for an individual to meet full diagnostic criteria for ADHD under the new DSM-5 criteria and perhaps will potentially increase the percentage of the population who qualify for the diagnosis. Diagnosticians must also rule out alternative explanations for core symptomatology as an individual's ADHD symptoms cannot be accounted for by another mental disorder. Symptoms consistent with an ADHD diagnosis cannot occur only in conjunction with or be better accounted for by another mental disorder such as schizophrenia or other psychotic disorder (APA, 2013). Although ADHD can certainly be diagnosed in conjunction with other disorders (e.g., autism spectrum disorders), the diagnosis of ADHD should not be used if the symptoms are better accounted for by another existing condition. Finally, DSM-5 criteria require that the level of severity of an individual's ADHD be specified when the diagnosis is made, as mild (few symptoms beyond those needed to make the diagnosis; only minor impairment in functioning), moderate (between mild and severe), or severe (many symptoms in excess of those needed for the diagnosis, and marked impairments in functioning resulting from symptoms).

TYPES OF ADHD

■ ADHD Combined

The label of ADHD combined is given to adults and children who exhibit both attention and hyperactive-impulsive symptoms. Children younger than 17 years of age must exhibit at least six inattentive and six hyperactive-impulsive symptoms, while individuals who are 17 years of age or older require only five symptoms of each category. Therefore, an important change in the DSM-5 diagnostic criteria reflects the understanding that a reduction in symptoms often occurs with increasing age and that a slightly lower threshold in symptoms is sufficient to reliably diagnose the disorder in adults.

■ ADHD Predominately Inattentive

This clinical presentation is given to individuals with sufficient inattentive symptoms (six symptoms if under 17 years of age; five symptoms if 17 years of age or older) but insufficient hyperactive-impulsive symptoms.

■ ADHD Predominately Hyperactive-Impulsive

This clinical presentation is given to adults and children who have sufficient hyperactive-impulsivity symptoms (six symptoms if under 17 years of age; five symptoms if 17 years of age or older) and insufficient inattention symptoms.

■ ADHD: Other Specified or Unspecified

This ADHD category is reserved for individuals who show some symptoms characteristic of the disorder, but who do not meet diagnostic criteria for any of the other three clinical presentations.

ETIOLOGY OF ADHD

The specific underlying causes of ADHD remain largely unknown, although many studies suggest that genetics play a significant role (Williams, Franke, Mick, & Faraone, 2012). Like many other neurobiological disorders, ADHD most likely results from a combination of genetic factors and environmental factors with nutrition, brain injuries, or characteristics of the social environment being possible contributing factors (NIMH, 2012). Many regions of the brain, and chemicals (neurotransmitters) within the brain, have been implicated in ADHD, with the neurotransmitter dopamine receiving the most attention (Antshel et al., 2011). The prefrontal cortex, which serves many cognitive and **executive functions** (e.g., attention, concentration, inhibition), has a high concentration of dopamine, and it has been hypothesized that individuals with ADHD may not produce sufficient levels of dopamine (Antshel et al., 2011). Identifying the specific gene or genes that contribute to ADHD has proven difficult because any single gene variant among the hundreds or thousands of implicated genes makes only a very small contribution to genetic vulnerability (Ross, 2012).

INCIDENCE AND PREVALENCE

The prevalence of ADHD has steadily increased over the past 20 years and is now reported as affecting 11% of children across the United States (APA, 2013). Therefore, supports and clinical services for individuals with ADHD continue to be an important area for health care professionals including occupational therapy. Prevalence estimates for ADHD in children have, however, fluctuated over time and as a result of survey (data gathering) methodologies ranging from as low as 3% to as high as 20% of children. From 1997 to 2012, there was quite a steady 3% to 5% increase per year (retrieved from the Center for Disease Control, 2013). The Centers for Disease Control and Prevention (2014) estimates that ADHD impacts the lives of 9.5% of school-aged children. The National Institutes of Health (NIH) estimates that ADHD currently affects about 4% to 5% of adults. Wolraich and colleagues (2011) reported that approximately 8% of children have ADHD. Although studies have consistently shown that the number of children being diagnosed with ADHD is increasing, the reasons for this upward trend are unclear (Wolraich et al., 2011). Visser et al. (2013) did an extensive review and analysis of parent report data from surveys conducted by the National Survey of Children's Health between 2003 and 2011, which also showed the increasing prevalence of ADHD. In 2011, according to Visser et al., 11% of children 4 to 17 years of age from the United States had received an ADHD diagnosis (6.4 million) at some time, and among those who had been given an ADHD diagnosis, 83% were reported as still having the disorder (Visser et al., 2013). Visser and colleagues also reported that 69% of children with ADHD were taking medication for their symptoms; this equates to 6.1% of the US population or approximately 3.5 million children. These authors noted an overall increase of 42% in diagnosis of ADHD from 2003 to 2011 and a 28% increase in the use of medications to treat the disorder from 2007 to 2011. Taken together, these multiple data sources estimate the prevalence of ADHD at between 8% and 12% of children and from 4% to 6% of adults. Approximately 50% of children continue to meet the criteria for ADHD as adults.

It is important to keep in mind that normal child behavior often includes having a high activity level, being easily distracted, and acting impulsively. All children mature at different rates, and their personalities, temperaments, and energy levels are variable, which makes it challenging to discern true ADHD from normal behavior. At what point does one begin to perceive child behavior as a medical condition or pathological, rather than just as a variant of normal behavior?

This is a fascinating and important question, and the idea that ADHD represents the extreme end of a normal continuum for behaviors related to attention, inhibition, and the regulation of activity level (rather than psychopathology) has been considered by some researchers (Holmberg, Sundelin, & Hjern, 2013). When considering the diagnosis, it is often helpful to be reminded that ADHD symptoms usually appear prior to age seven, and for a diagnosis to be made, symptoms must be significant enough that they negatively impact one's daily functioning in more than one setting or context.

■ Co-occurring or Comorbid Conditions

ADHD is often comorbid with motor, sensory, learning, mood, anxiety, and disruptive behavior disorders in children and adults, and it has also been found to be associated with substance abuse in older adolescence and adults (Antshel et al., 2011). Kaplan and colleagues (2001) reported that as many as 80% of children with ADHD are at risk of having at least one other disorder, such as learning disorders, developmental coordination disorder (DCD), oppositional behavior disorder, depression, and/or anxiety.

Motor disorders have been reported in as many as 40% to 60% of individuals representing all three subtypes of ADHD, with slightly more representation in the combined clinical presentation (Egeland, Ueland, & Johansen, 2012; Piek & Dyck, 2004). Despite the high rate of movement problems in children with ADHD, the DSM-5 (APA, 2013) does not explicitly recognize the comorbidity between **developmental coordination disorder**, which is difficulty coordinating movements (DCD) and ADHD. Rather, it is suggested that the motor skill problems in children with ADHD most likely are due to their ADHD symptoms, namely, distractibility and impulsiveness, rather than a true motor disorder. However, many children with ADHD meet criteria for DCD, which is characterized by a marked impairment motor coordination that is not due to a medical condition or developmental disorder and which interferes significantly with academic achievement or activities of daily living. Piek, Pitcher, and Hay (1999) found an association between inattentive symptoms and fine motor ability, and Pitcher, Piek, and Hay (2003) provided evidence to suggest that motor deficits in ADHD were a result of a specific motor deficit rather than of ADHD symptomatology.

Disorders of attention and learning have also been associated with sensory processing disorders or sensory integration dysfunction (Dunn & Bennett, 2002; Mangeot et al., 2001; Pfeiffer, Daly, Nicholls, & Gullo, 2015). Yochman, Parush, and Ornoy (2004) conducted an investigation comparing the sensory processing abilities of preschool children aged 4 to 6 years with and without ADHD. Results indicated that children with ADHD had an increased risk of sensory processing difficulties such as overresponsivity and/or underresponsivity to sensory input, as well as deficits with visual perception (Yochman, Parush, and Ornoy, 2004). Studies have also shown that ADHD is associated with deficits in somatosensory processing (Parush, Sohmer, Steinberg, & Kaitz, 1997), including adverse reactions to tactile stimuli, and motor planning. More recently, Pfeiffer, Daly, Nicholls, and Gullo (2015) found that children with ADHD were much more likely to exhibit sensory processing challenges in all areas of sensory processing than neurotypical children. Furthermore, their study suggested that children with ADHD were more likely to display problems with higher level functions believed to be dependent in part on efficient sensory processing, including social participation and motor planning. The close association between attention deficits and impairments with sensory, motor, and perceptual functions is further supported by the work of Gillberg (2003) and Hellgren and colleagues (1993, 1994) who have published widely on what they refer to as a condition called **DAMP**, or deficits in attention, motor control, and perception. Researchers over the years have questioned whether individuals with this common clustering of problems represent a single disorder or whether they represent an attention disorder with co-occurring disorders.

A number of mental health disorders are also commonly seen in children and adults with ADHD including mood, anxiety, and disruptive behavior disorders. In adults with bipolar disorder, the incidence of co-occurring ADHD has been reported to be between 10% and 21% (Perroud et al., 2014; Perugi et al., 2013; Wingo & Ghaemi, 2007). Consistent with these reports, epidemiological studies of adults with ADHD have shown bipolar disorder to approximately 20% of subjects (Halmoy et al., 2010). Several hypotheses have been raised to explain this higher-than-chance association ranging from overlapping dimensions, such as impulsivity and increased activity level, to shared genetic vulnerability (Youngstrom, Arnold, & Frazier, 2010). Comorbidity between ADHD and bipolar disorder has been associated with early-life onset of bipolar, with higher numbers of depressive and mixed episodes, fewer asymptomatic periods, and with worse outcomes (Karaahmet et al., 2013; Tamam, Karakus, & Ozpoyraz, 2008). In addition, individuals with both disorders show higher rates of other psychiatric comorbidities, such as anxiety and substance abuse (Tamam, Karakus, & Ozpoyraz, 2008).

comorbid oppositional defiant disorder are at higher risk for deficient driving habits and other risk-taking behavior (Barkley, 2006; Kent et al., 2011; Kuriyan et al., 2013).

On a more positive note, despite these findings, many individuals who have symptoms into adulthood learn to cope with and manage their symptoms well and live productive, happy lives. Levrini and Prevatt (2012) provide a number of helpful strategies, including suggesting that adults with ADHD harness their excess energy and creativity positively with careers that require a lot of stamina or multitasking and that fit well with whatever they excel at and find most interesting.

COURSE AND PROGNOSIS

ADHD is considered a lifelong disorder although studies suggest that only approximately 50% of children continue to meet the criteria for ADHD into adulthood (Visser et al., 2013), and the clinical presentation of the disorder changes over time. Overt behaviors associated with overactivity or **hyperactivity** and impulsivity tend to subside gradually with age, while difficulties with attention and sustained focus and disorganization more often continue into adulthood. In adulthood, a more inward type of hyperactivity has been reported such as restlessness and difficulty sleeping, and impulsivity may present as impatience or being ill tempered. However, it is important to note that relatively little is known about the course of the disorder in adulthood, as there have been few longitudinal studies examining long-term outcomes, and the course of the disorder throughout adulthood.

There is some evidence to suggest that predictors of ADHD recovery in adults include severity of the ADHD symptoms at age 21 and level of education (Barkley, 2006; Kuriyan et al., 2013). Education outcomes of older children with ADHD are somewhat discouraging, with 30% to 50% of children with ADHD receiving special education. Children with ADHD have higher school dropout rates (23% to 40%) and lower grade point averages than do neurotypical peers, and fewer students with ADHD enter college (Kent et al., 2011). As adults, they engage in more risk-taking behaviors, have poorer driving records, and have more problems in the workplace. Individuals with

DIAGNOSIS

No single test is available to diagnose a child or adult as having ADHD, and diagnosis is made based on observations and reports of behavior, rather than on medical or biologically based tests. This process inherently involves a degree of subjectivity, which may account for some of the discrepancies in data related to incidence and prevalence estimates. A licensed health professional or team of professionals typically gathers information about the individual and his or her behavior and environment. For children, parents often first bring their concerns to their child's pediatrician who may refer the family to a mental health specialist with experience in childhood mental disorders, such as a pediatric neurologist, clinical psychologist, developmental pediatrician, or child psychiatrist.

Clinical practice guidelines for diagnosing ADHD from the American Academy of Pediatrics relative to ADHD describe the diagnostic process as involving ruling out other possibilities for the ADHD symptoms or behaviors such as undetected hearing problems, learning disorders, or other medical problems that might affect thinking and behavior (Wolraich et al., 2011). Sensory integration deficits have also been identified as resulting in a similar clinical presentation as ADHD (Miller, Neilson, & Schoen, 2012; Parush, Sohmer, Steinberg, & Kaitz, 2007). Information gathered throughout the evaluation process includes a detailed description of the individual's symptoms; when they began; how severe, excessive, and persistent they are; and how they affect aspects of the person's daily life and activities. Caregivers are asked if they perceive that their child's behaviors happen more often than do those of the child's peers and if they are present across multiple contexts such as school, home, and community settings (NIMH, 2012). Specialists conducting evaluations pay close attention to the individual's behavior in highly structured versus unstructured situations, performance when situated in environments that are busy versus quiet, and behavior when the individual is engaged in activities he or she enjoys versus those the individual does not particularly like.

Main methods of gathering information for a diagnostic evaluation of a child for ADHD include review of relevant medical and education records, interviewing the parent and child (if old enough), administering child **behavior rating scales**, parent self-report measures, and psychological testing (Wolraich et al., 2011). Descriptive, qualitative information about parental concerns regarding the child's behavior helps to narrow the focus of the evaluation, and presents the degree of distress that the child's behaviors are having on the family unit. Parents provide essential demographic information, relevant family medical history, an overview of the child's developmental course and skills, and medical and school history, as well as a detailed history of the child's ADHD symptoms. Purposes of interviewing children vary depending on the age and developmental level of the child, but they always provide an opportunity to observe the child's behavior and to learn about the child's temperament, personality, interests, and daily activities.

A number of well-researched assessment tools or scales that offer normative data across age groups and that are valid and reliable for quantifying the opinions of those who know the child well are available. Two commonly used scales that have been validated with children are the Behavior Assessment System for Children (BASC-2; Reynolds & Kamphaus, 2005) and the Achenbach System of Empirically Based Assessment (ASEBA; Achenbach, 2014). For adults, the ADD Rating Scale (Brown, 2001) and the Adult Self-Report Scale (Adler, Kessler, & Spencer, 2003) are commonly used. Psychological testing to determine an individual's learning style, levels of cognitive functioning, or intelligence testing such as the administration of a test that yields an intelligence quotient or

IQ is another component of the evaluation process. Tests of academic achievement in specific subject areas such as math and reading may also be administered to school-aged children, while other psychological tests might focus psychosocial-emotional skills and other mental processes or behaviors. Often, such testing is conducted to identify coexisting conditions such as learning disorders and to supplement the other sources of data used to diagnose an individual with ADHD.

Finally, standard medical evaluation procedures including genetic testing may be necessary to rule out other medical conditions and childhood psychiatric disorders that might produce ADHD-like symptoms. Allied health, discipline-specific evaluations may be recommended such as those that address vision and hearing, speech/language, auditory processing, sensory and motor skills, and occupational functioning and adaptive behavior. Such evaluations not only provide useful information that contribute to the diagnostic process but also are useful for guiding intervention recommendations and plans.

Professionals working with adults need to consider a wider range of symptoms because symptoms in adults tend to be more varied and less clear-cut as those seen in children and coexisting conditions are often present. As noted earlier, diagnostic criteria include that ADHD symptoms must appear prior to age 12 and continue into adulthood (APA, 2013). Therefore, gathering reliable retrospective accounts of childhood ADHD symptoms is necessary and may be challenging. Spouses or partners, parents, or others who know the adult well are sometimes interviewed. Clinical symptoms of inattention and hyperactivity/impulsiveness are explored in detail to gauge the severity and pervasiveness of the symptoms and how ADHD symptoms impact the individual's functioning in work and leisure pursuits and social relationships. Finally, similar to the evaluation process for children, adults should go through appropriate psychological testing, behavior rating scales, and medical evaluations to rule out other possible explanations for their symptoms and to identify any comorbid conditions. In addition to common comorbidities such as learning, anxiety, and mood disorders, adult ADHD has been associated with conditions such posttraumatic stress disorder, substance abuse, and obsessive-compulsive disorder (Knouse, Cooper-Vince, Sprich, & Safren, 2008).

Medical, Pharmacological, Behavioral, and Educational Interventions for Individuals with ADHD

Although the management of individuals with ADHD has progressed significantly over the past 20 years, considerable work remains to help children and adults with this disorder. There is no cure for ADHD, but interventions can significantly reduce the negative effects of ADHD symptoms. The presentation of ADHD can be markedly different among children and adults, necessitating intervention programs to be individualized. A number of intervention options are considered, and a **multimodal approach** using a number of different interventions in an effort to reduce ADHD symptoms and enhance daily functioning is typically applied. Intervention programs consider the most current and effective research-based therapies, as well as caregiver/individual preferences and concerns. All care plans should include education about ADHD and its various treatment options (medication and behavior, psychotherapies, and other treatments), linkage with community supports and resources, and school-based interventions for school-aged children. Specific medical and nonmedical intervention approaches are discussed in more detail below.

■ Medical and Pharmacological Interventions for ADHD

Pharmacotherapy remains the cornerstone for ADHD intervention for all age groups, with advances in long-lasting stimulant medications being the most common (DeSousa & Kalra, 2012). Earlier research emphasized pharmacological interventions as being most efficacious, with little additional value placed on behavioral and other nonpharmacological interventions (American Academy of Pediatrics, 2011). However, more recent literature suggests that the interpretations of earlier studies may have undervalued these interventions, and recommendations clearly continue to support a multimodal approach to care (American Academy of Pediatrics, 2011). Stimulant medications such as **methylphenidate** (MPH), more commonly known by the trade name Ritalin, and mixed amphetamine salts (MAS) are the most commonly used drugs for treating ADHD in both children and adults (Barkley, 2006). They

work by increasing levels of dopamine and norepinephrine in the brain, and the medication has a calming effect, which improves inattention, impulsivity, and overactivity (DeSousa & Kalra, 2012). Stimulant medications come in different forms, such as a pill, capsule, liquid, or skin patch and may be short-acting, long-acting, or have extended-release capacities. In each of these varieties, the active ingredient is the same, but it is released differently in the body. For example, long-acting or extended-release forms often allow a child to take the medication just once a day before school, so they don't have to make a daily trip to the school nurse for another dose. Trade names of some of the more commonly used FDA-approved medications for children include Adderall, Concerta, Dexedrine, and Ritalin. Side effects of the medication tend to be minor such as decreased appetite, sleep problems, anxiety, mild head ache or stomach upset, and irritability (DeSousa & Kalra, 2012). Side effects can often be managed by modifying dosage or may subside over time.

Clinical research trials have been conducted to measure the effects of long-acting forms of MPH such as Concerta, Daytrana, and Ritalin and mixed salts amphetamine such as Adderall XR with older children (DeSousa & Kalra, 2012). Long-acting formulations have been found to be equally as efficacious as immediate-release forms for adolescents and older children (Biederman et al., 2007; Faraone & Buitelaar, 2010; Greenhill et al., 2002; McGough et al., 2005; Spencer, Greenbaum, Ginsberg, & Murphy, 2009). Overall, single daily dosing is associated with greater compliance for all kinds of medications. In studies in which individuals were treated with both amphetamine and MPH, approximately 50% of participants responded equally to both MPH and amphetamine, whereas almost half responded preferentially to one of the classes of stimulants, with the overall positive response rate being as high as 85% (DeSousa & Kalra, 2012). Unfortunately, there is no way to predict which drug will work for a particular individual, emphasizing the importance of tailoring interventions, using a trial-and-error approach, and a process of careful monitoring with ongoing modifications as needed.

Stimulant medications, including extended-release forms, are also frequently prescribed for adults with ADHD, although not all stimulant medications have been FDA approved for adults. Antidepressants, including tricyclics, such as amitriptyline, and atypical antidepressants, such as Wellbutrin, are also sometimes used to treat adults with ADHD (Barkley, 2006). Adult prescriptions for ADHD medications require special considerations because adults are more likely than children to be taking other medications for conditions such as diabetes or heart disease, which may interact negatively with their ADHD medications. Children and adults who are prescribed medication should be monitored carefully, because a one-size-fits-all approach does not apply for all individuals with ADHD and much remains to be learned regarding the long-term effects of these medications. More information on dosage and management of medication are provided by the American Academy of Child and Adolescent Psychiatry (2007) and by DeSousa and Kalra (2012) and are presented in the clinical practice guidelines for ADHD issued by the American Academy of Pediatrics (2011).

■ Nonpharmacological and Behavioral Interventions for ADHD

Nonpharmacological and **behavioral interventions** include psychological counseling and other therapy services for targeting disruptive or challenging behaviors. Specific skills are also often addressed such as social and organizational skills, executive and other cognitive functions, coping skills, and sensory-motor and/or language skills. Specific occupational performance challenges may also be addressed Therapy programs and counseling services for individuals with ADHD often focus on teaching problem-solving strategies and suggesting and implementing accommodations for managing the challenges of everyday life in work, school, or other community settings. Education on important topics that can be addressed in group and individual sessions with older teens or adults might include relevant neurobiology and neurophysiology, medication management, motivation and initiation of activities, and strategies to enhance attention, concentration, self-esteem, and emotional regulation.

Behavior and psychosocial therapies represent a broad set of interventions that are typically delivered by psychologists or other child behavior specialists. These therapies aim to alter the individual's behavior by modifying either the environment or an individual's patterns of interaction

with others or patterns of thinking (American Academy of Pediatrics, 2011). Specific behavioral techniques may be taught and applied by parents, teachers, peers, or the individual with ADHD himself or herself. Such techniques typically involve the application of consistent consequences to desired behavior (rewards) and to undesirable behavior (negative reinforcement, or punishment). For example, a program described and evaluated by Curtis, Chapman, Dempsey, and Mires (2013) targeted children ages 7 to 10 years with ADHD and their families. The program emphasized parent training, instruction in self-regulation strategies, goal setting, and rehearsal of targeted behaviors for improving the child's understanding of behavioral expectations.

Cognitive-behavioral therapies (CBT) focus on modifying dysfunctional thought patterns and are based on the idea that cognitive thought processes can be monitored and adapted and that they do affect an individual's behavior (Antshel et al., 2011). For example, an individual may be taught to use a process of "stop and think" before acting, or to focus on the positive consequences of task completion for enhancing persistence and motivation. Programs often include training in organizing and planning such as the use of a day planner, strategies for reducing distractibility, enhancing coping strategies especially in stressful situations, and the development of problem-solving skills (Safren et al., 2010). A specific type of cognitive-behavioral therapy called meta-cognitive therapy is sometimes applied with older teens or adults (see Josman & Rosenblum, 2011; Solanto and colleagues, 2010). This intervention applies cognitive-behavioral principles in conjunction with techniques such as reflection, evaluation, and adaptation of ways of thinking and problem solving.

Finally, another nonmedical intervention, peer or life coaching, is becoming a popular intervention for adults with ADHD (Knouse, Cooper-Vince, Sprich, & Safren, 2008). Peer coaching is an individualized approach that focuses largely on personal goal setting, strategy selection, and accountability. Advocates of coaching distinguish it from "traditional" therapy by describing coaching as more action oriented rather than insight oriented, as the adult works through specific problems or strives to reach concrete goals. Coaching sessions tend to be briefer than sessions using cognitive-behavioral therapies and can be delivered on as "as needed basis," rather than on a more regular basis. Specific goals might be targeted such as finding a more satisfying job or living a healthier more balanced lifestyle. Exercises or activities might be implemented to determine what brings the most meaning to one's life as a process of discovery, followed by the development of a plan for engaging in those meaningful activities.

■ Parent Education and Training Programs

Parent training programs are designed for parents of preschool- and school-aged children with ADHD. They focus on teaching strategies for fostering positive child-parent relationships and for managing challenging or disruptive behaviors and provide parents with support and education about the disorder (Charach et al., 2013). While different programs have some unique attributes, they all aim to help parents manage their child's problem behavior by emphasizing the use of effective discipline strategies involving rewards and nonpunitive consequences. Parent training programs also promote positive child-parent relationships by increasing parents' understanding of their child's temperament, and awareness of their own parenting style. Helping parents understand why their children behave the way that they do is a first important step in the process. Parents learn how their child's symptoms interact with their own parenting styles/ways of interacting and with unique stress factors. Specific problem behaviors are then targeted typically through the teaching and application of behavioral techniques, primarily associated with positive reinforcement (Sanders, Bor, & Morawska, 2007). Parent training programs aim to promote a positive and caring relationship between parents and their child, reduce the child's problem behaviors, and enhance overall parenting skills (Charach et al, 2011; Matos, Bauermeister, & Bernal, 2009; Thompson et al., 2009).

■ Educational and Classroom Interventions

School-related interventions are a critical component of a comprehensive intervention program for school-aged children with ADHD, as children with ADHD are more likely to have poorer grades, higher dropout rates, and higher absenteeism as compared to their peers without

the disorder (DuPaul & Weyandt, 2009; DuPaul, Weyandt, & Janusis, 2011). School-aged children whose ADHD symptoms affect their ability to participate fully and benefit from public education programs in the United States are eligible to receive an IEP, including special education and related support services through the Individuals with Disabilities Education Act (IDEA; U.S. Department of Education, 2004). Under the U.S. Rehabilitation Act of 1973, federal legislation that extended civil rights protection to people with disabilities, children with ADHD who need only reasonable accommodations (rather than specialized instruction) to succeed in school may receive such accommodations through a 504 plan rather than through an IEP.

Behavioral programs are commonly implemented in schools and follow the same basic behavioral principles of reinforcement that are used in other settings. Teacher praise or token reinforcements in the form of stickers or points that can be exchanged for rewards such as time spent in preferred activities (e.g., computer time or recess) are commonly used (DuPaul, Weyandt, & Janusis, 2011). Alterations in curricula, environmental adaptations, or academic interventions, which facilitate a child's interest, motivation, and ability to persist when challenged can also be implemented. For example, teachers might provide their ADHD students with clear expectations and rules, give students choices, or reduce task demands by breaking assignments into smaller or shorter components. Preferential seating (seating the child in a place that is relatively free from distraction or close to the teacher for frequent monitoring or cueing) or creating a designated quiet area is often helpful (DuPaul, Weyandt, & Janusis, 2011).

Training in specific skills such as general study and organizational skills, note taking, self-regulation, and social skills has also been found to be effective (DuPaul, Weyandt, & Janusis, 2011). There are a number of computer-assisted math, reading, and writing programs that have been shown to enhance the on-task behavior and overall performance of children with ADHD (DuPaul, Weyandt, & Janusis, 2011). Peer tutoring or other peer-mediated interventions have also been used successfully in school-based settings and have been found not only to positively impact school performance but also to improve social skills and friendships. Typically, this intervention involves pairing a child with ADHD with a higher achieving student who provides instruction and feedback to the student with ADHD (Daley & Birchwood, 2010; Plumer & Stoner, 2005).

IMPACT ON OCCUPATIONAL PERFORMANCE

For young preschool-aged children, symptoms of ADHD often hinder their ability to play effectively with peers, control and manage their behavior in the home and community, participate in a variety of learning activities, and perform basic self-care skills. For older children, challenges in their roles as students are particularly common, as well as the quality of their performance of basic and instrumental activities of daily living. For adults with ADHD, social and community participation, sustaining meaningful relationships, and functioning in the workplace may be negatively affected by symptoms of the disorder. It is also important to note that common coexisting conditions, such as learning, sensory, motor, mood, and/or anxiety disorders when present, also impact one's ability to perform one's daily occupations, and it is often difficult to discern what condition is most responsible for certain problems.

The main occupations of humans include activities of daily living (such as personal self-care activities like bathing, dressing, and eating), instrumental activities of daily living (such as homemaking tasks and money management tasks), rest and sleep, education, work, play, leisure, and social participation (American Occupational Therapy Association, 2014). For individuals living with ADHD, symptoms affecting the ability to attend, concentrate, adapt, plan, organize, and control emotions may impair performance in any of these occupational areas. School performance and student roles have probably received the most attention for individuals with ADHD (DuPaul & Weyandt, 2009) with challenges noted with academic work, classroom behavior, study skills, and motor skills including handwriting.

Children and adolescence with ADHD may exhibit problems with learning, initiating, organizing basic self-care tasks such as completing a morning routine of grooming, and dressing in a timely and thorough manner (Dunn, Coster, Cohn, & Orsmond, 2009; White & Mulligan, 2005). For adults, instrumental activities of daily living, social participation, and work occupations are most often impacted. Adults with ADHD have been shown to have greater risk for lower socioeconomic status and lower rates of professional employment (Cermak & Maeir, 2011). Driving is also an area that has been given attention in the ADHD population, as teens and adults with ADHD have been shown to be at a higher risk for accidents and violations than drivers without the disorder (Reimer, Mehler, D'Ambrosio, & Fried, 2010).

Participation in leisure activities and play skills is also often compromised in children and adults with ADHD. Shimoni, Engel-Yeger, and Tirosh (2010), for example, found that boys with ADHD reported less enjoyment from their leisure activities than did their typical peers. Cordier, Bundy, Hocking, and Einfeld (2009) studied the play behaviors of children 5 to 11 years of age with ADHD and found that they had more difficulties in social play and had less interpersonal empathy in comparison with typical peers. Habits, routines, and roles supporting one's engagement in his or her occupations may also be disrupted in individuals with ADHD. Interventions targeting these areas may help those with ADHD overcome poor habits such procrastination or change disruptive behavioral patterns characterized by beginning many new projects, but then not following through with them to completion. Environmental and contextual factors such as clutter and crowds, poor lighting, and/or excessive noise hinder the performance of all individuals. However, the negative influence of these environmental factors on one's occupational performance may be exaggerated in individuals with ADHD. Sociocultural environments or expectations within a particular context may also be particularly challenging for individuals for ADHD such as those that are highly unstructured, require long periods of sedentary work, or lack of interesting activity or stimulation. Successful engagement of their occupations may therefore be enhanced by modifying or addressing environmental and/or contextual elements

SUMMARY

This chapter has provided information on the diagnosis, etiology, clinical presentation, prevalence, and prognosis of ADHD. The many ways in which ADHD symptoms commonly impact one's occupational performance or the ability to successfully participate in one's daily life was also described, along with an overview of methods of evaluation and treatment for both children and adults. It is important to emphasize that ADHD is a complex condition and every client with the disorder is unique. Best practice is described as implementing a **multimodal intervention** approach that is individually tailored to meet the unique presentation of each client, with consideration of the client's own goals and priorities, and in concert with the other medical, pharmacological, psychological, and/or educational interventions that the individual might be receiving. Despite continual advances in our understanding of the disorder, and its typical course throughout one's life, there is still much to be learned about the nature of the disorder and how best to treat children and adults with ADHD.

An adult case study and a child case study are presented below to illustrate how ADHD may present in specific individuals, and to provide an opportunity for you to work through possible evaluation methods, models of intervention, and potential outcomes. As you read through the case studies, it may be helpful to address and be thinking about the following questions: (1) What type of ADHD does this individual present with, and how do ADHD symptoms affect his or her ability to carry out their required and desired occupations? (2) Was the evaluation conducted comprehensive, or would there be other information that would have been helpful to gather to assist in guiding intervention? (3) What medical, psychological, educational, or occupational intervention strategies or approaches would be appropriate to consider for this individual?

CASE STUDY 1

Cory, at 5 years of age, was recently diagnosed with ADHD-combined presentation by his pediatrician. His parents were having difficulty managing his behavior in the home including frequent temper outbursts, hyperactivity, and perceived immaturity in his play skills and inability to carry out basic self-care tasks. He was started on Dexedrine to help manage his symptoms, and he was planning to start kindergarten in the fall, in 4 months time. He had not ever received therapy or support services in the past, although he had attended a community preschool program two mornings a week for 3 months when he was 4 years of age. His medical history included frequent ear infections and upper respiratory infections and was otherwise unremarkable. Height and weight were average, and he was followed regularly by his pediatrician. Cory lived at home with his parents and two siblings, 2 and 8 years of age. His mother stayed at home to manage the household and care for the children, and his father worked as a university professor. His father had a history of ADHD, and both parents were quite knowledgeable about the disorder. Interviews with his parents revealed that Cory was full of energy and protested consistently when he did not get his way, often to the point of being aggressive. Medication had settled his behavior

somewhat, although his mother was concerned regarding side effects including loss of appetite and sleep problems.

During the weekdays, he spent most of his time playing with his 2-year-old sister. He usually got up in the morning around 7:00 and had an afternoon nap early afternoon for 2 to 3 hours. He enjoyed playing with construction toys like big blocks and with his train set. He liked playing outside on the swing set, playing with balls of any kind (running and kicking), and riding his two-wheeled bike with training wheels. Cory needed assistance with his self-care including dressing and toileting and only recently was toilet trained, although he continued to have occasional accidents. His mother reported that Cory was able to assist with brushing his teeth and washing his face. He was able to eat using a spoon and fork, although his mother stated that he was a very messy and picky eater and rarely would sit at the dining room table for more than about 5 minutes. Cory often protested when it was time to get dressed or during grooming tasks. His mother said that helping Cory with basic self-care tasks and taking the children out on the weekends to the park, the mall, or other community settings were very exhausting, and she was hoping to get some ideas on how to better manage Cory's behavior.

Cory was referred for occupational therapy at an outpatient pediatric clinic, and his occupational therapy evaluation consisted of informal interview with his mother; observations of sensory processing, play, and motor skills; and administration of the three standardized assessments including the Sensory Processing Measure, Preschool Home Form (Parham, Ecker, Kuhaneck, Henry, & Glennon, 2010); the Miller Function and Participation Scale, Home Form (Miller, 2006); and the Brief Rating Inventory of Executive Functions, Preschool Form, by Giola, Isquith, Guy, and Kenworthy (2000). The evaluation revealed that Cory presented as a happy, talkative child who was full of energy with an increased activity level. Instructions often needed to be repeated during standardized testing, and Cory experienced difficulty persisting at a task when challenged, often saying "No I can't. I am all done." Cory tended to move quickly from one activity to the next with limited productive and sustained play at any one activity, and he behaved impulsively. His gross motor skills fell within the low-average range, and visual-motor and fine motor skills both fell significantly below average. Sensory processing concerns on the Sensory Processing Measure were noted in the hearing, touch, balance, and social participation areas and included sensation-seeking behaviors (especially excessive movement), tactile hypersensitivity, and not being able to adequately filter irrelevant noise and other stimuli.

His mother reported that she wanted assistance with managing Cory's impulsivity, lack of attention to tasks, and noncompliance. Her requests of him were often ignored, or he would have a temper outburst that involved screaming and sometimes hitting or pinching her. She was also concerned that he did not share and take turns well when playing with peers and was fearful that Cory might hurt his younger sister when interacting with her at home. His lack of independence with basic self-care skills and fine motor skills was also of concern, and she was worried that he would experience difficulties when starting kindergarten. His assessment revealed that during play, Cory insisted on controlling the play situation, always wanting to assume the leader role. Observations of play indicated limited problem-solving strategies, minimal creative and goal-directed play, and need for control and for immediate gratification.

In summary, the occupational therapy evaluation indicated that Cory had some coexisting sensory integration deficits, including decreased visual-motor integration and sensory modulation deficits. Executive function deficits consistent with the ADHD-combined presentation were noted, including inattention, disorganization, increased activity level, impulsivity and lack of self-control, and poor problem solving. His executive functioning and sensory motor problems impacted his ability to perform many of his daily occupations including play, his performance of basic self-care skills, and, most importantly, his ability to cope with stress, regulate his behavior, and exhibit self-control especially when asked to perform an undesirable or challenging task. Despite these challenges, Cory was very interested in his environment and seemed eager to please others, and many developmental areas and skills were progressing typically, such as use of language and gross motor skills.

CASE STUDY 2

Amanda was diagnosed with ADHD predominately inattentive presentation when she was a high school student and had been taking stimulant medication off and on since then. At 26 years of age, she was referred for occupational therapy by her counselor, a clinical psychologist, to address some challenges she was having in the workplace and with community living skills. She was living in an apartment with a roommate and was receiving counseling for anxiety and to assist in managing her symptoms associated with ADHD. Occupational therapy evaluation methods included informal interviews with Amanda and her mother, which were conducted separately; a workplace observation; administration of the Canadian Occupational Performance Measure (Law et al., 2005); and administration of the Behavior Rating Inventory of Executive Function, Adult Form (Roth, Isquith, & Gioia, 2006).

Evaluation results revealed that Amanda was employed full time as an administrative assistant for a property management company. Her parents lived about an hour away in a neighboring town; she had two adult siblings who lived in other states.

Socially, she spent leisure time with her roommate and reported having a few other friends whom she saw regularly. She worked out at a gym regularly and enjoyed listening to music and watching movies. Aside from ADHD, her medical history was unremarkable with no major illness or hospitalizations. During the weekdays, she typically worked 10 AM to 6 PM. She typically got up at 9 AM and took public transit (bus) to and from work. Although she had a driver's license, she did not have a car. She enjoyed cooking dinner and often would prepare dinner for both her and her roommate. In the evenings, she often went to the gym and watched TV. On weekends, she often visited her parents and enjoyed catching up on her sleep. Evaluation results indicated that Amanda wanted to perform better with her job, and she expressed a need to improve her organizational skills. She reported that she always felt busy doing things and had a lot of energy but that tasks never seemed to get done. She enjoyed starting new projects in the home and at work, but often, there was little follow-through to completion. She was easily distracted and had not developed effective ways of prioritizing and organizing her time. Results from the Behavior Rating Inventory of Executive Function, Adult Version (BRIEF-A; Roth, Isquith, & Gioia, 2006), indicated some executive function deficits in the ability to plan and organize tasks and with working memory. Her ability to self-monitor her behavior was scored in the dysfunctional range, while emotional control, inhibition, and ability to shift and adapt were scored within the average range.

A worksite, 1-hour observation revealed that Amanda had a demanding job that required her to frequently multitask (talk on the phone, schedule appointments, meet with clients, problem solve tenant complaints and concerns, assist contractors, organize records, etc.). She would often begin a task, get interrupted, and then forget to go back and complete what she was doing. The office space was very open, bright, and cheery, although the reception area and her space were very close to the waiting area, which was noisy most of the time. Amanda said that she always felt stressed at work and felt as though she was always behind and not meeting expectations. She was capable of doing the tasks asked of her, but just did not have the time to get everything done, and she was fearful of getting fired. There was one other person who worked in the front office area. They seemed to have a good, comfortable working relationship, and each had their own responsibilities and also shared some responsibilities. Amanda reported that she most wanted to improve her financial situation and improve her time management and efficiency at work and ability to cope with work. Evaluation results suggested deficits in her ability to sustain focus and attention to tasks and decreased organizational and problem-solving skills.

RECOMMENDED LEARNING RESOURCES

Recommended Books

Taking charge of ADHD, revised edition: The complete authoritative guide for parents, by Russell Barkley

Taking charge of adult ADHD, by Russell Barkley with Christine Benton

ADHD answer book: Professional answers to 275 of the top questions parents ask, by Susan Ashley

Overcoming ADHD without medication: A parent and education's guide association for youth, children, and natural psychology

The disorganized mind: Coaching your ADHD brain to take control of your time, tasks and talents, by Nancy Ratey

Rethinking ADHD: Integrated approaches to helping children at home and at school, by Ruth Schmidt Neven

Succeeding with adult ADHD: Daily strategies to help you achieve your goals and manage your life, by Levrini and Prevatt (2012), American Psychological Association.

Recommended Organizations and Web sites

National Institutes of Mental Health
www.nimh.nih.gov/health/publications/attention-deficit-hyperactivity-disorder/index.shtml

Center for Disease Control
www.cdc.gov/ncbddd/adhd/research.html

Children and Adults with Attention deficit/ Hyperactivity Disorder (CHADD)
www.chadd.org

Attention Deficit Disorder Association
www.add.org

ADHD Aware
www.adhdaware.org

American Psychiatric Association
www.psych.org

REFERENCES

Achenbach, T. (2014). *Achenbach System of Empirically Based Assessment (ASEBA)*. Retrieved from www.aseba.org

Adler, L., Kessler, R., & Spencer, T. (2003). *Adult Self Report Scale, ASRS-VI.I Screener*. New York, NY: World Health Organization.

American Academy of Child and Adolescent Psychiatry. (2007). Practice parameters for the assessment and treatment of children and adolescents with Attention-Deficit/Hyperactivity Disorder. *Journal of the American Academy of Child and Adolescent Psychiatry, 46*(7), 894–921, Retrieved from http://dxdoi.org/10.1097/chi.0b013e318054e724

American Academy of Pediatrics. (2011). ADHD: Clinical practice guideline for the diagnosis, evaluation, and treatment of attention-deficit/hyperactivity disorder in children and adolescents. *Pediatrics, 128*(5), 1–16. doi: 10.1542/peds.2011-2654

American Occupational Therapy Association. (2014). Occupational Therapy Practice Framework: Domain & Process, 3rd edition. *American Journal of Occupational Therapy, 68*(Suppl. 1), S2–S51. Retrieved from http://dx.doi.org/10.5014/ajot.2014.682006

American Psychiatric Association. (2000). *Diagnostic and statistical manual of mental disorders (IV-text revision)*. Washington, DC: Author.

American Psychiatric Association. (2013). *Diagnostic and statistical manual of mental disorders* (5th ed.). Washington, DC: Author.

Antshel, K. M., Hargrave, T., Simonescu, M., Kaul, P., Hendricks, K., & Faraone, S. V. (2011). *Advances in studying and treating ADHD*. Retrieved from http://www.biomedcrentral.com/1741-7051/9/72

Barkley, R. A. (2006). *Attention-deficit hyperactivity disorder: A handbook for diagnosis and treatment*. New York, NY: Guildford Press.

Biederman, J., Boellner, S. W., Childres, A., Lopez, F. A., Krishnan, S., & Zhang, Y. (2007). Lisdexamfetamine dimesylate and mixed amphetamine salts extended-release in children with ADHD: A double-blind, placebo-controlled, crossover analog classroom study. *Biological Psychiatry, 62*, 970–976. doi: https://dxdoi.org/10.1016/j.biopsych.2007.04.015

Brown, T. E. (2001). *Brown ADD rating scales for children, adolescents and adults*. San Antonio, TX: Pearson Inc.

Centers for Disease Control and Prevention. (2014). *Fast stats: Attention deficit hyperactivity disorder*. Retrieved from http://www.cdc.gov/nchs/fastats/adhd.htm

Cermak, S., & Maeir, A. (2011). Cognitive rehabilitation of children and adults with attention deficit hyperactivity disorder. In N. Katz (Ed.), *Cognition, occupation, and participation across the lifespan* (3rd ed., pp. 249–276). Bethesda, MD: AOTA Press.

Charach, A., Carson, P., Fox, S., Ali, M. U., Beckett, J., & Lim, C. G. (2013). Interventions for preschool children at high risk for ADHD: A comparative effectiveness review. *Pediatrics, 131*(5), 51584–51604. doi: 10.1542/peds.2012-0974

Charach, A, Dashti, B., Carson, P., Booker, L., Lim, C. G., Lillie, E., … Schachar, R. (2011). Attention deficit hyperactivity disorder: Effectiveness of treatment in at-risk preschoolers; Long-Term effectiveness in all ages, and variability in prevalence, diagnosis, and treatment. *Comparative Effectiveness Review, 44*. Retrieved from www.effectivehealthcare.ahrq.gov/reports/final.cfm

Cordier, R., Bundy, A., Hocking, C., & Einfeld, S. (2009). A model for play-based intervention for children with ADHD. *Australian Occupational Therapy Journal, 56*, 332–340. doi: 10.1111/j.1440-1630.2009.00796.x

Curtis, D. F., Chapman, S., Dempsey, J., & Mire, S. (2013). Classroom changes in ADHD Symptoms following clinic-based behavior therapy. *Journal of clinical Psychology and Medical Settings, 20*(1), 114–122. doi 10.1007/s10880-012-9307-2

Daley, D., & Birchwood, J. (2010). ADHD and academic performance: Why does ADHD impact on academic performance and what can be done to support ADHD children in the classroom? *Child: Care, Health and Development, 36*(4), 455–464. doi: 10.1111/j.1365-2214.2009.01046.x

DeSousa, A., & Kalra, G. (2012). Drug therapy of attention deficit hyperactivity disorder: Current trends. *Mens Sana Monograph, 10*, 45–69. doi: 10.4103/0973-1229.87261

Dunn, W., & Bennett, D. (2002). Patterns of sensory processing in children with attention deficit hyperactivity disorder. *Occupational Therapy Journal of Research, 22*, 4–15. doi: 10.1177/153944920202200102

Dunn, W., Coster, L., Cohn, E., Orsmond, G. I. (2009). Factors associated with participation in children with and without ADHD in household tasks. *Physical and Occupational Therapy in Pediatrics, 29*(3), 274–294. doi: 10.1080/01942630903008327

DuPaul, G. J., & Weyandt, G. M. (2009). School-based intervention for children with attention deficit hyperactivity disorder: Effects on academic, social, and behavioral functioning. *International*

Journal of Disability, Development and Education, *53,* 161–176. doi: 10.1080/10349120600716141

DuPaul, G. J., Weyandt, L., & Janusis, G. (2011). ADHD in the classroom: Effective intervention strategies. *Theory Into Practice, 50,* 35–42. doi: 10.1080/00405841.2011.534935

Egeland, J., Ueland, T., & Johansen, S. (2012). Central processing energetic factors mediate impaired motor control in ADHD combined subtype but not in ADHD inattentive subtype. *Journal of Learning Disabilities, 45*(4), 361–370. doi: 10.1177/0022219411407922

Faraone, S. V., & Buitelaar, J. (2010). Comparing the efficacy of stimulants for attention deficit hyperactivity disorder in children and adolescents using meta analyses. *European Child and Adolescent Psychiatry, 19,* 353–364. doi: 10.1007/s00787-009-0054-3

Gillberg, C. (2003). Deficits in attention, motor control, and perception: A brief review. *Archives of Disability in Children, 88,* 904–910. doi: 10.1136/adc.88.10.904

Giolo, G. A., Isquith, P. K., Guy, S., & Kenworthy, L. (2000). *Brief Rating Inventory of Executive Functions (BRIEF).* Lutz, FL: Psychological Assessment Resources.

Greenhill, L. L., Beyer, D. H., Finkleson, J., Shaffer, D., Biederman, J., Conners, C. K., … Volkow, N. (2002). Guidelines and algorithms for the use of methylphenidate in children with Attention-Deficit/Hyperactivity Disorder. *Journal of Attention Disorders, 6*(Suppl 1), S89–S100.

Halmoy, A., Halleland, H., Dramsdahl, M., Bergsholm, P., Fasmer, O. B., & Haavik, J. (2010). Bipolar symptoms in adult attention-deficit/hyperactivity disorder: A cross-sectional study of 510 clinically diagnosed patients and 417 population-based controls. *Journal of Clinical Psychiatry, 71*(1), 48–57. doi: 10.4088/JCP.08m04722ora

Hellgren, L. Gillberg, C., Gillberg, I. C., et al. (1993). Children with deficits in attention, motor control, and perception (DAMP) almost grown up: General health at 16 years, *Developmental Medicine and Child Neurology, 35,* 881–892. doi: 10.1111/j.1469-8749.1993.tb11565.x

Hellgren, L., Gillberg, I. C., Bagenholm, A. et al. (1994). Children with deficits in attention, motor control, and perception (DAMP) almost grown up: Psychiatric and personality disorders at age 16. *Journal of Child Psychology and Psychiatry, 35,* 1255–1271. doi: 10.1111/j.1469-7610.1994.tb01233.x

Holmberg, K., Sundelin, C., & Hjern, A. (2013). Screening for attention deficit/hyperactivity disorder (ADHD): Can high risk children be identified in first grade? *Child: Care, Health and Development, 39*(2), 268–276. doi: 10.1111/j.1365-2214.2012.01382.x

Josman, N., & Rosenblum, S. (2011). A metacognitive model for children with atypical brain development. In N. Katz (Ed.), *Cognition, occupation, and participation across the lifespan* (3rd ed., pp. 223–247). Bethesda, MD: AOTA Press.

Kaplan, B., Wilson, B., Dewey, D., & Crawford, S. G. (2001). DCD may not be a discrete disorder. *Human Movement Science, 17,* 471–490.

Karaahmet, E., Konuk, N., Dalkilic, A., Saracli, O., Atasoy, N., Kurcer, M. A., & Atik, L. (2013). The comorbidity of adult attention-deficit/hyperactivity disorder in bipolar patients. *Comprehensive Psychiatry, 54*(5), 549–555. doi: 10.1016/j.comppsych.2012.11.005

Kent, K., Pelham, W. E., Molina, B. S. G., Waschbush, D., Yu, J., Sibley, M. H., & Karch, K. (2011). The academic experience of male high school students with ADHD. *Journal of Abnormal Child Psychology, 39,* 451–462. doi: 10.1007/s10802-010-9472-4

Knouse, L. E., Cooper-Vince, C., Sprich, S., & Safren, S. A. (2008). Recent developments in the psychosocial treatment of adult ADHD. *Expert Review of Neurotherapies, 8*(10), 1537–1548. doi: 10.1586/14737175.8.10.1537

Kuriyan, A. B, Pelham, W. E., Molina, B., Waschbusch, D. A., Gnagy, E., Sibley, M. H., … Kent, K. M. (2013). Young adult educational and vocational outcomes of children diagnosed with ADHD. *Journal of Abnormal Child Psychology, 41*(1), 27–41. doi: 10.1007/s10802-012-9658-z

Law, M., Baptist, S., Carswell, S., McColl, A., Polatajko, H., & Pollock, N. (2005). *Canadian occupational performance measure* (4th ed.). Toronto: CAOT Publications, Canadian Occupational Therapy Association.

Levrini, A., & Prevatt, F. (2012). *Succeeding with adult ADHD: Daily strategies to help you achieve your goals and manage your life.* Washington DC: American Psychological Association.

Mangeot, S. D., Miller, L. J., McIntosh, D. N., McGrath-Clarke, J., Simon, J., Hagerman, R. J., & Goldson, E. (2001). Sensory modulation dysfunction in children with attention-deficit–hyperactivity disorder. *Developmental Medicine & Child Neurology, 43*(06), 399–406. doi: 10.1111/j.1469-8749.2001.tb00228.x

Matos, M., Bauermeister, J. J., & Bernal, G. (2009). Parent–child interaction therapy for Puerto Rican preschool children with ADHD and behavior problems: A pilot efficacy study. *Family Process, 48*(2), 232–252. doi: 10.1111/j.1545-5300.2009.01279.x

McGough, J. J., Biederman, J., Wigal, S. B., Lopez, F. A., McCracken, J. T., Spencer, T., … Tulloch S. J. (2005). Long-term tolerability and effectiveness of once-daily mixed amphetamine salts

(Adderall XR) in children with ADHD. *Journal of the American Academy of Child and Adolescent Psychiatry*, *44*, 530–538. doi: 10.1097/01. chi.0000157550.94702.a2

Miller, L. J. (2006). *Miller function and participation scales*. San Antonio, TX: Pearson.

Miller, L. J., Neilson, D. M., & Schoen, S. (2012). Attention deficit hyperactivity disorder and sensory modulation disorder: A comparison of behavior and physiology. *Research in Developmental Disabilities*, *33*, 804–818. doi: 10.1016.j.ridd.2011.12.005

National Institutes of Mental Health (NIMH). (2012). *Attention Deficit Hyperactivity Disorder (ADHD)*. National Institutes of Health, U.S. Department of Health and Human Services, publication no. 12-3572.

Parham, D., Ecker, C., Kuhaneck, H. M., Henry, D. A., Glennon, T. J. (2010). *Sensory processing measure (SPM)*. Torrance, CA: Western Psychological Services.

Parush, S., Sohmer, H., Steinberg, A., & Kaitz, M. (1997). Somatosensory functioning in children with attention deficit hyperactivity disorder. *Developmental Medicine & Child Neurology*, *39*(7), 464–468. doi: 10.1111/J.1469-8749.1997. tb07466.x

Parush, S., Sohmer, H., Steibnerg, A., & Kaitz, M. (2007). Somatosensory function in boys with ADHD and tactile defensiveness. *Physiology and Behavior*, *90*, 553–558. doi: 10.1016/j. physbeh.2006.11.004

Perroud, N., Cordera, P., Zimmermann, J., Michalopoulos, G., Bancila, V., Prada, P., … Aubry, J. M. (2014). Comorbidity between attention deficit disorder (ADHD) and bipolar disorder in a specialized mood disorders clinic. *Journal of Affective Disorders*, *168*, 161–166. doi: 10.1016/j. jad.2014.06.053

Perugi, G., Ceraudo, G., Vannucchi, G., Rizzato, S., Toni, C., & DelOsso, L. (2013). Attention deficit/ hyperactivity disorder symptoms in Italian bipolar adult patients: A preliminary report. *Journal of Affective Disorders*, *149*(1–3), 430–434. doi: 10.1016/j/jad.2012.12.010

Pfeiffer, B., Daly, B. P., Nicholls, E. G., & Gullo, D. F. (2015). Assessing sensory processing problems in children with and without attention deficit hyperactivity disorder. *Physical & Occupational Therapy in Pediatrics*, *35*(1):1–12. doi: 10.3109/01942638.2014.904471

Piek, J. P., & Dyck, M. J. (2004). Sensory-motor deficits in children with developmental coordination disorder, attention deficit hyperactivity disorder and autistic disorder. *Human Movement Science*, *23*(3/4), 475–488. doi: 10.1016/j. humov.2004.08.019

Piek, J. P., Pitcher, T. M., & Hay, D. A. (1999). Motor coordination and kinaesthesis in boys with attention deficit-hyperactivity disorder. *Developmental Medicine and Child Neurology*, *41*, 159–165. doi: 10.1111/j.1469-8749.1999.tb00575.x

Pitcher, T. M., Piek, J. P., & Hay, D. A. (2003). Fine and gross motor ability in males with ADHD. *Developmental Medicine and Child Neurology*, *45*, 525–535. doi: 10.1017/ S0012162203000975

Plumer, P. J., & Stoner, G. (2005). The relative effects of classwide peer tutoring and peer coaching on the positive social behaviors of children with ADHD. *Journal of Attention Disorders*, *9*(1), 290–300. doi: 10.1177/1087054705280796

Reimer, B., Mehler, B., D'Ambrosio, L. A., & Fried, R. (2010). The impact of distractions on young adult drivers with attention deficit hyperactivity disorder (ADHD). *Accident Analysis and Prevention*, *42*(3), 842–851. doi: 10.1016/j. aap.2009.06.021

Reynolds, C., & Kamphaus, R. W. (2005). *The behavior assessment system for children-2*. Circle Pines, MN: American Guidance Service.

Ross, R. G. (2012). Advances in the genetics of ADHD. *American Journal of Psychiatry*, *169*(2), 115–177. doi: 10.1176/appi. ajp.2011.11111647

Roth, R., Isquith, P., & Gioia, G. (2006) Behavior Rating Inventory of Executive Function®–Adult Version (BRIEF®-A). Lutz, FL: Par Psychological Assessment Resources, Inc.

Safren, S., Sprich, S., Mimiaga, M. J., Surman, C., Knouse, L., Groves, M., & Otto, M. W. (2010). Cognitive behavioral therapy vs relaxation with educational support for medication-treated adults with ADHD and persistent symptoms: A randomized controlled trial. *Journal of the American Medical Association*, *304*(8), 875–117. doi: 10.1001/jama.2010.1192

Sanders, M. R., Bor, W., & Morawska, A. (2007). Maintenance of treatment gains: A comparison of enhanced, standard, and self-directed Triple P-Positive Parenting Program. *Journal of Abnormal Child Psychology*, *35*(6), 983–998. doi: 10.1007/s10802-007-9148-x

Shimoni, M., Engel-Yeger, B., & Tirosh, E. (2010). Executive dysfunctions among boys with Attention Deficit Hyperactivity Disorder (ADHD): Performance-based test and parents report. *Research in Developmental Disabilities*, *33*(3), 858–865. doi: 10.1016/j.ridd.2011.12.014

Solanto, M. V., Marks, D. J., Wasserstein, J., Mitchell, K., Abikoff, H., Alvir, J. M., & Kofman, M. D. (2010). Efficacy of meta-cognitive therapy for adult ADHD. *American Journal of Psychiatry*, *167*, 958–968. doi: 10.1176/appi.ajp.2009.09081123

Spencer, T. J., Greenbaum, M., Ginsberg, L. D., & Murphy, W. R. (2009). Safety and effectiveness of coadministration of guanfacine extended release and psychostimulants in children and adolescents with attention-deficit/hyperactivity disorder. *Journal of Child and Adolescent Psychopharmacology, 19*, 501–510. doi: 10.1089/cap.2008.0152

Tamam, L., Karakus, G., & Ozpoyraz, N. (2008). Comorbidity of adult attention-deficit hyperactivity disorder and bipolar disorder: Prevalence and clinical correlates. *European Archives of Psychiatry and Clinical Neuroscience, 258*(7), 385–393. doi: 10.1007/s000406-008-x

Thompson, M. J., Laver-Bradbury, C., Ayres, M., Le Poidevin, E., Mead, S., Dodds, C., ... Sonuga-Barke, E. J. (2009). A small-scale randomized controlled trial of the revised New Forest Parenting Programme for preschoolers with attention deficit hyperactivity disorder. *European Child and Adolescent Psychiatry, 18*(10), 605–616. doi: 10.1007/s00787-009-0020-0

U.S. Department of Education. (2004). Individuals with Disabilities Education Improvement Act of 2004, P.L. 108–446, 120 USC.

Visser, S. N., Danielson, M. L., Bitsko, R. H., Holbrook, J., Kogan, M. D., Ghandour, R. M., ... Blumberg, S. J. (2013). Trends in the parent-report of health care provider-diagnosed and medicated attention-deficit/hyperactivity disorder: United States, 2001–2011. *Journal of the American Academy of Child and Adolescent Psychiatry*, doi: 10.1016/j.jaac.2013.09.001

White, B., & Mulligan, S. (2005). Behavioral and physiologic response measures of occupational task performance: A preliminary comparison between typical children and children with attention disorder. *American Journal of Occupational Therapy, 59*(4), 426–436. doi: 10.5014/ajot.59.4.426

Williams, N. M., Franke, B., Mick, E., & Faraone, S. V. (2012). Genome-wide analysis of copy number variants in attention deficit hyperactivity disorder: The role of rare variants and duplications at 15q13.3. *American Journal of Psychiatry, 169*, 195–204. doi: 10.1176/appi.ajp.2011.11060822

Wingo, A. P., & Ghaemi, S. N. (2007). A systematic review of rates and diagnostic validity of co-morbid adult attention deficit/hyperactivity disorder and bipolar disorder. *Journal of Clinical Psychiatry, 68*(11), 1776–1784. doi: 10.4088/JCP.v68n1118

Wolraich, M., Brown, L., Brown, R. T., DuPaul, G., Earls, M., Feldman, H. M., ... Visser, S. (2011). Subcommittee on Attention-Deficit/Hyperactivity Disorder; Steering Committee on Quality Improvement and Management ADHD: Clinical practice guideline for the diagnosis, evaluation and treatment of attention deficit/ hyperactivity disorder in children and adolescents. *Pediatrics, 128*(5), 1007–1022. doi: 101542/peds.2011-2654

Yochman, A., Parush, S., & Ornoy, A. (2004). Responses of preschool children with and without ADHD to sensory events in daily life. *American Journal of Occupational Therapy, 58*(3), 294–302. doi: 10.5014/ajot.58.3.294

Youngstrom, E., Arnold, E., & Frazier, T. (2010). Bipolar and ADHD comorbidity: Both artifact and outgrowth of shared mechanisms. *Clinical Psychology Science Practice, 17*, 350–359. doi: 10.1111/j.1468-2850.2010.01226.x

Sensory Processing Disorder

Ben J. Atchison and Brandon G. Morkut

Since the age of two, it seemed that 4-year-old Thomas responded to stimuli around him in a way that was unusually intense. For example, when a sudden noise occurred, such as turning on the vacuum or the blender or when someone knocked on the door or rang the doorbell, he would stop and fall to the ground with excessive outbursts of emotion, with his hands over his ears crying "Stop, stop." Consoling him after this happened was very difficult. After being dressed for the day, he would often remove his clothing, preferring to play in his diaper, and often took that off as well. Attempts to put his clothing back on were always a battle as he fussed and cried and took his clothes off after being dressed again. Mealtimes were increasingly challenging as well as his food preferences were limited to smooth and soft textures. Clearly, it was going to be a challenge for Thomas to begin his preschool program in a few months. After describing his behaviors to a close friend whose child had similar difficulties, Thomas' parents were advised to look into the possibility that he was experiencing something called a sensory processing disorder (SPD).

DESCRIPTION AND DEFINITIONS

In the early 1960s, the late Dr. A. Jean Ayres, an occupational therapist and neuroscientist at the University of Southern California, reported a series of clinical studies that emphasized the connection between the important roles of sensory processing in learning and behavior. Beginning with this statement in her classic textbook, Sensory Integration and Learning Disorders, published in 1972, Ayres noted: "Learning is a function of the brain; learning disorders are assumed to reflect some deviation in neural function" (p. 1). Ayres described a theoretical model of sensory integration that included treatment guidelines. She was insistent that while her theory was built on brain and behavioral research, it was formative as theories must be and that her findings were tentative and not to be considered conclusive. From her pioneering work in the mid 20th century to the present time, a series of scientific investigations have been published, mostly by occupational therapists, to expand theoretical constructs of sensory processing as well as develop informal and formal assessment procedures and intervention guidelines for children and adults with what Ayres initially identified as sensory integration dysfunction (SID).

Miller, Anzalone, Lane, Cermak, and Osten (2007) published the seminal article Concept Evolution in Sensory Integration: A Proposed Nosology for Diagnosis. Based on input from focus groups of occupational therapy scholars and empirical evidence, the authors proposed that the term SID be replaced with SPD. Further, three SPD phenotypes were described: sensory modulation disorder (SMD), sensory-based motor disorder (SBMD), and sensory discrimination disorder (SDD), each with subtypes (as shown in Fig. 7.1). These typologies will be described in detail in the section on signs and symptoms.

In conjunction with this proposed SPD **nosology**, a term used to classify medical conditions, Miller and her colleagues also recommended a more well-defined distinction regarding terminology. They proposed that the theory be identified as sensory integration theory, the disorder as SPD, and that intervention be referred to as occupational therapy using a sensory integration approach (OT-SI). It is important to note that Miller and her colleagues were explicit, as was Ayres, that further scholarly dialogue and research on the proposed nosology were to be expected and required for continued evolution of SPD concepts.

ETIOLOGY

While there is no specific identified cause of SPD, there are a number of studies that point to extrinsic and intrinsic factors that result in the difficulty of the central nervous system (CNS) to detect, register, and process sensory information. Preliminary research continues to hypothesize that heredity, environmental factors, prenatal conditions, and perinatal complications (e.g., jaundice, forceps/vacuum delivery, and fetal distress) are strong factors for SPD. Miller (2014) designed a small research pilot ($N = 26$) to identify possible correlation between heredity and SPD and found a relationship between SPD and heredity as evidenced by 92% of the sample children having at least one parent who identified that his or her own behaviors were indicative of SPD. Forty percent of the participant's mothers recognized personal attributes associated with SPD in comparison to 37% of fathers.

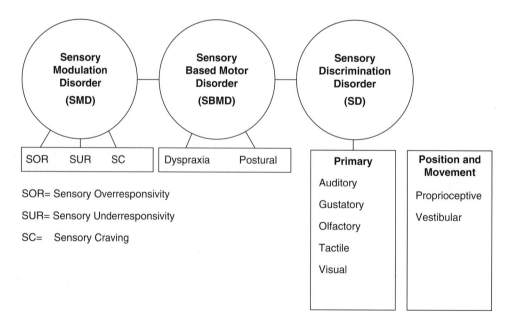

Figure 7.1 Typologies of sensory processing disorder. (Adapted from Sensory Processing Disorder: A Conceptual Model. From Miller, L. J., Anzalone, M. E., Lane, S. J., Cermak, S. A., & Osten, E. T. (2007). Concept evolution in sensory integration: A proposed nosology for diagnosis. American Journal of Occupational Therapy, 61(2), 135–140.)

One of the most significant environmental factors believed to influence SPD is **sensory deprivation** or a considerable lack of quality sensory stimulation, as evidenced by children living in Eastern European orphanages (Miller, 2014). As a result of immature sensory systems at birth (e.g., tactile, proprioceptive, visual, auditory, and vestibular), substantial alterations take place postnatally for all humans. During infancy, connections between sensory neurons continue to be established to allow sensory systems develop functionally by way of appropriate modifications in neural pathways. Early repetitive exposure to nonthreatening environmental events, which promote sensory processing and spontaneous activity, is required to facilitate the maturation of neuronal circuits. Studies have also shown that exposure to sensory-rich experiences during childhood is essential in the exponential speed of and overproduction of neuronal development. This overproduction, in turn, promotes neuronal pruning. **Neuronal pruning** is a necessary process to eliminate the overproduction of sensory neurons that are generated mostly in infancy through middle childhood. This allows better efficiency in learning new information and explains, in part, the neuroplasticity of brain development (Fox, Levitt, & Nelson, 2010). When infants are deprived of sensory enrichment, the natural process of overproduction and pruning does not occur. By way of example, it was discovered that children living in the former communist bloc within Eastern European orphanages were not often provided adequate conditions for typical sensory development to occur, which resulted in poor developmental and atypical behavioral outcomes (Lin, Cermak, Coster, & Miller, 2005). Research data suggest that internationally adopted children who were institutionalized 12 months or more demonstrated severe SPD patterns of dysfunction when compared to those adopted at <8 months with minimal or no institutional placement. Those in the former group experienced higher reactivity and aversion to tactile, vestibular, proprioceptive, visual, and auditory input as well as difficulty with motor planning skills, or dyspraxia (Wilbarger, Gunnar, Schneider, & Pollak, 2010).

Other significant factors that are believed to contribute to SPD are chronic exposure to pre- and postnatal stressors and neurodevelopmental difficulties. Studies have shown that chronic prenatal stress and alcohol exposure have been identified to impact sensory processing in primates. Furthermore, studies of humans have indicated that maternal stress hormones (e.g., adrenaline and cortisol) can cross the placental barrier resulting in altered neurotransmitter activity, thus facilitating abnormal sensory modulation in offspring (Brunton, 2013). Research outcomes reported by Atchison (2007) identified significant SMDs in children who experienced prenatal exposure to alcohol in conjunction with postnatal abuse. Among the same population, Henry, Sloane, and Black-Pond (2007) found severe neurodevelopmental deficits in language, memory, visual processing, motor skills, attention, and behavior.

Presently, there is a lack of strong empirical evidence to determine a definitive etiology for SPD. However, emerging evidence continues to suggest that SPD reduces a child's ability to engage in daily activities, such as social interaction, self-care, learning, and play (Schaaf et al., 2010). Hypothesized risk factors associated with SPD include the following (Ben-Sasson, Carter, & Briggs-Gowan, 2009; Keuler, Schmidt, Van Hulle, Lemery-Chalfant, & Goldsmith, 2011; May-Benson, Koomar, & Teasdale, 2009; Schneider et al., 2007, 2008, 2009; Wickremasinghe et al., 2013):

- Low birth weight (<4.5 lb)
- Prematurity (<36 weeks gestation)
- Maternal illness
- Maternal use of medications
- Living with a single parent
- Lower socioeconomic status

The search continues for evidence that SPD is a unique disorder with distinct etiologic factors and pathomechanics. At the time of this publication, research scientists at major centers around the world, from a variety of scientific disciplines, are conducting primate studies, rat studies, and anatomical and genetic studies. Studies of specific patterns of sensory modulation, using precise measures such as electroencephalography, neuroimaging, and **electrodermal reactivity**, which is a measure of stress and emotion, are being conducted and reported in the literature (Miller, 2014). For example, recent research (2013) discovered, by way of specialized neuroimaging technology, that the brains of boys with SPD were found to have unique abnormalities in the posterior white matter including the posterior corpus callosum, posterior corona radiata, and posterior thalamic radiations. These structures are implicated in interconnections of auditory, visual, and tactile systems as well as the two cortical hemispheres (Owen et al., 2013). An excellent resource for recent and current studies are archived and continually updated at: www.spdfoundation.net.

INCIDENCE AND PREVALENCE

Performance dysfunction related to sensory processing has been identified in all age groups, intellectual levels, and socioeconomic groups. In a systematic review of the literature related to prevalence of SPD, Ahn, Miller, Milberger, and McIntosh (2004) examined the prevalence of SPD among 1,800 kindergartners attending a Colorado suburban public school for the 1999–2000 school year. The Short Sensory Profile (SSP) (Dunn, 1999) was administered to 1,796 parents, which resulted in 703 surveys completed and returned, yielding a 39% return rate. Of the 703 children, results indicated 96 children (13.7%) met criteria for an SPD evaluation. Based on the study's empirical evidence, researchers cautiously suggest that approximately 220,000 kindergartners in the United States may demonstrate a critical threshold of symptoms to warrant an evaluation to rule out SPD (Miller, 2014). In addition, a longitudinal study ($N = 1,312$) (Ben-Sasson et al., 2009) investigated the prevalence of sensory overresponsivity (SOR) in a demographically proportionate Connecticut elementary school. Data collection methods included the Sensory Over-Responsivity Scales (SensOR; Schoen, Miller, & Green, 2008) in conjunction with additional parent-report instruments. Parent-rated surveys were distributed at three predetermined periods among the sample population beginning at (1) 11 to 42 months of age, (2) 22 to 56 months, and (3) 7 to 11 years old. Final data analysis indicated 148 (16.5%) children of the sample population acquired notably elevated SOR scores, as defined by identifying four or more unsettling sensations on the SensOR (Schoen et al., 2008). Investigation of demographic risk factors that may influence SOR symptoms identified the population with elevated SOR results ($N = 148$). They were more likely to be of minority ethnicity, of lower economic status, and living with a single parent and to have experienced considerably lower birth weight and gestational period. In addition, 76.4% ($N = 113$) of the population with elevated SOR results identified tactile input as the most bothering sensation (Ben-Sasson et al., 2009). Even though evidence supports the existence of SPD as an isolated disorder, Miller (2014) and colleagues validated SPD as a "combination disorder" (p. 267) reflective of more than one SPD pattern and/or subtype. In an additional study, Miller (2014) investigated the existence of co-occurrence among the subtypes of SMD and patterns of SPD in children ages three to 12 years old (N=200). Results indicated that 59% of the sample population possessed combined subtype symptoms of SMD in conjunction with 70% of subjects validating combined patterns of SPD. The most frequent SPD pattern/subtype combinations involve motor planning difficulty with sensory craving (SC), motor postural disorder, and sensory underresponsivity (SUR) with postural disorder (Miller, 2014).

Disruption in sensory processing has also been most frequently recognized in children with autism spectrum disorders (ASDs), attention deficit hyperactivity disorder (ADHD), learning disabilities, fragile X syndrome, and developmental/complex trauma. Tomchek and Dunn (2007) investigated sensory processing dysfunction in children between ages 3 and 6 years ($N = 281$) diagnosed with ASD. Results indicated that 95% of the children with ASD displayed some degree of sensory processing dysfunction in the pattern of SMD in conjunction with SOR as the co-occurrence subtype most frequently identified with ADHD (i.e., 40% to 60%) and fragile X.

SIGNS AND SYMPTOMS

Participation in daily activities requires the CNS complex process of organizing internal and external sensations to allow for a functional response that is meaningful and appropriate to a given demand. Sensory processing includes the detection, modulation, integration, interpretation, and organization of sensory sensations (Bialer & Miller, 2011). It is postulated that individuals who display SPD symptoms encounter errors in the analysis of sensory information in the brain. Since all humans experience interpretation errors in sensory processing, it is the deficiency of habituation and adaptation to these sensations that results in chronic manifestations of poorly organized behavior responses. Therefore, intervention is only recommended when the inability to process and organize sensory input significantly impacts one's capability to facilitate a functional response toward a daily occupation. Schaaf and Miller (2005, p. 1) note, "The goal of intervention is to improve the ability to process and integrate sensory information and to provide a basis for improved independence and participation in daily life activities." Furthermore, three patterns of SPD have been identified, each with subtypes as described below and illustrated in Figure 7.1.

■ Pattern 1: Sensory Modulation Disorder

Sensory modulation allows for purposeful and successful participation in activities of daily living, which is dependent on the central and autonomic nervous system's ability to maintain "system harmony" through a complex process of regulating and organizing the intensity of sensory input to facilitate a functional graded response. However, a disorder in sensory modulation occurs when difficulty with regulating and organizing external or internal sensory stimuli results in a maladaptive emotional or motor response. Evidence suggests that SMD can impact one or more of the seven sensory systems: vestibular, tactile, visual, proprioception, auditory, olfactory, and/or gustatory as supported by laboratory measures of altered physiological responses to specific stimuli (James, Miller, Schaaf, Nielsen, & Schoen, 2011). Within SMD, three subtypes have been identified including SOR, SUR, and SC.

Subtype 1: Sensory Overresponsivity

This subtype is characterized by responses to stimuli that are more intense or have a longer duration than typically expected and may occur in only one or among multiple sensory modalities. Oftentimes, the behaviors that children demonstrate are judged to be intentional because the response sets are often context dependent. For example, the same type of auditory stimulus that sets off an adverse behavioral reaction in the classroom but is not observed at home will often lead to the conclusion that the child can control the behavior when in fact it is automatic and unconscious. At home, the child may have more control of an auditory stimulus where, in the classroom,

the same stimulus occurs without expectation. Repetition of this unexpected stimulus can create a cumulative effect, resulting in a range of aggressive reactions to complete avoidance or shutdown in the stimulus environment. Miller et al. (1999) demonstrated, in a laboratory model, that activation of the sympathetic nervous system is a marker of SOR, specifically noted in the exaggeration of the fight or flight responses typically experienced in stressful situations. Persons with SOR often demonstrate inflexibility and hypervigilance and tend to be difficult to console when they are in "overresponsive" mode. SOR is often seen in children with autism, fragile X syndrome, ADHD, and mood disorders (Schaaf et al., 2010).

Subtype 2: Sensory Underresponsivity

Children who experience SUR experience challenges in the feed-forward mechanism of the CNS, lacking a central predictive set of actions in given situations (Miller, 2014). It is as if there is a lack of ability to detect incoming sensory information, which is often misinterpreted as the child having "lazy" tendencies and being unmotivated. The infant and toddler with SUR are often considered to be "an easy baby" as there seems to be less demands on the caregiver. However, this same child shows less interest in active exploration of the environment, which can best be explained by a hypoaroused manner, which manifests in a lack of natural, exploratory sensory behavior and may be manifested in inefficient tactile and proprioceptive sensory responses, which are typically robust in developing infants and toddlers (Quake-Rapp & Atchison, 2011). It is soon discovered that the child with SUR requires a more intense and extended duration of sensory stimuli to reach an optimal level of arousal. Most caregivers will intuitively "turn up the volume" of sensory stimuli to address this behavior. A child with SUR often demonstrates difficulty with sustained task performance as the lack of a consistent interaction with sensory input, which can lead to SDDs, motor planning difficulty, or both (Miller, 2014).

Subtype 3: Sensory Craving

While it is clear in the human growth and development literature, including teratologic studies, that humans seek sensory input to make meaning of the external environment, children with this subtype of SMD seek sensory input with an approach that results in erratic, disorganized behavior. The child in the physician's office who wants to touch the reflex hammer, stethoscope, and other available items within reach is different than the child who runs about the office, turning things over and generally creating concern among those in the room. The behavior appears to be impulsive, unsafe, and boundary-free, and the child will energetically engage in physical actions that add to his or her craving for sensory input. Oftentimes, this child is considered to be "fearless" as he or she engages in constant spinning, jumping, and running into objects with a "crashing and bashing" approach. When the necessary boundaries are enforced and thus unable to meet sensory needs, children with SC may become highly agitated and explosive. With extreme cases, the ability to learn is compromised, interpersonal relationships become very difficult to sustain, and activities of daily living are disrupted (Quake-Rapp & Atchison, 2011).

Miller describes SC as an active seeking of sensation that is "insatiable" and often results in significant disorganization and less-than-acceptable behavior (Miller, 2014). These are children who are removed from the classroom for behavioral concerns as early as preschool. Other children often complain of the child with SC behaviors due to their aggressive social interaction and intrusive interruption of others' play space. Children who crave sensation often have a need for increased volume when viewing a video and will speak in a loud voice or shrill, frenetic pattern of verbal communication. When on the playground, these children cannot get enough of the varied stimulation from the equipment whether it be rotation or angular or vertical stimulation that comes from jumping, climbing, swinging, and twirling. Oftentimes, these children are described as being very active, yet this high activity is beset with disorganized and less purposeful outcomes than a child engaged in typical, robust play. Miller (2014) suggests that there are two distinct groups of sensory cravers with the first being more common, with an observed need for "more and more" stimulation that is difficult to control, or self-regulate. The second type is less common but includes those who seek out extreme sensory experiences and experience self-regulation of their craving tendencies. This group of sensory cravers has outcomes that are less disorganized, with more purpose as seen in "extreme sports" activities such as cliff diving, parachuting, high-speed auto racing, and snowboarding.

Pattern 2: Sensory-Based Motor Disorder

Subtype 1: Postural Disorders

Those body functions that are dependent on smooth and efficient processing of vestibular and kinesthetic input are often disrupted among children with SPD, resulting in difficulty with maintaining normal postural tone. Smooth control of movement and endurance may be compromised, particularly in antigravity activity. Poor balance between agonist and antagonist muscle groups, poor balance reactions in both static and dynamic challenges, poor weight shifting and trunk mobility, and deficits in smooth oculomotor control may be present in children with sensory-based motor disorder (SBMD). Children with either sensory seeking or underresponsivity may demonstrate behaviors associated with SBMD. The arousal level of the person, whether it is SOR or SUR, may result in postural control problems and difficulty with motor planning. The child who typically maintains a slumped position while attempting to complete a handwriting task and quickly losing a sustained effort to do so is typical of a child with this pattern of SPD (Miller, 2014).

Subtype 2: Dyspraxia

Dyspraxia, or difficulty with motor planning, is the inability to plan unfamiliar or novel tasks, resulting in a clumsy, awkward, maladaptive response. The key idea here is that the task is *novel*. Asking a person to perform a task that is done routinely, such as buttoning a button on a shirt, would be an evaluation of fine motor coordination and less motor planning ability. When attempting a motor task that is not in one's repertoire of acquired skills, the person with dyspraxia will demonstrate significant awkwardness in the use of hands and body to perform the task. It is clearly a sensory-based problem in that persons with dyspraxia appear to be unsure of where their body is in space and may have difficulty with timing, grading, and executing movement to complete the task with success. Most people have experienced the awkwardness of learning new dance steps. After a series of repetitions, a more accurate use of the body is felt and observed in most individuals. It is true, of course, that some of us will never learn to dance! That, however, may be tied to a lack of interest rather than poor somatosensory processing. Usually, there are other motor planning challenges that one can succeed in, unless dyspraxia prevents success in every new motor activity attempted. Many children with dyspraxia are creative and highly verbal and are safe when engaged in fantasy games that don't require "doing" something specific. Children with dyspraxia often prefer passive activity such as watching television, playing on computers, or reading to the exclusion of any activities that challenge motor planning abilities. The fear that emerges when being required to participate in physical education activities at school or other settings is real for a child. This may result in repeated feelings of failure, leading to significant impairment of confidence and self-esteem.

■ Pattern 3: Sensory Discrimination

SDDs are reflected by difficulty with qualitative processing of sensory stimuli (Miller, 2014). It is not uncommon to have a combination of strengths and weaknesses in sensory discrimination, which leads to the idea that one is a "visual" or "auditory" learner or learns best "by doing." Commonly, descriptions of sensory discrimination and assessments emphasize visual, auditory, and tactile perception. Visual discrimination includes such skills as pattern recognition and visual-spatial analysis. Pattern recognition problems include difficulty in the recognition of differences in similar shapes such as ovals versus circles or in the reversal of letters and numbers that persists after the age of six. Problems in visual-spatial analysis are observed in attempts to solve simple puzzles and replicate simple designs and can ultimately impact on the ability to adequately develop handwriting skills. Auditory discrimination includes the ability to differentiate similar sounds such as b and d and words such as with and which, while tactile perception is often described as the ability to identify an object with vision occluded, using the integration of tactile and visual discrimination to do so, such as reaching into one's pocket and retrieving a quarter, rather than a penny, for the parking meter.

A unique feature of the SDD typology is the inclusion of the somatic senses, which includes proprioceptive and vestibular discrimination and referred in sensory processing language as somatosensation. Normal **somatosensation**, a term to describe the combination of tactile, proprioceptive, and vestibulary sensory processing, provides for a foundational body scheme, which Ayres (1972) classically described as the "blueprint for movement," enabling adequate processing of feed-forward skills for planning movement and postural stability. The awareness of where one's body is in space in relation to the external environment, and the excursion, speed, precision, and gradation of movement needed to complete a motor task is a function of somatosensory discrimination. Children who experience SOR as well as SUR may have difficulty with this aspect of sensory discrimination, which can create difficulties in body scheme and motor planning.

COURSE AND PROGNOSIS

The course and prognosis of SPD are impacted by recognition by the child's healthcare providers that the behaviors observed are not willful misbehavior on the part of the child. Oftentimes, children who demonstrate behaviors associated with SPD are immediately determined to have a behavioral disorder or something that is a result of ineffective parenting. Recognizing that SPD is a neurological disorder is critical in meeting the needs of the child. At the very least, providing a comprehensive effort to rule out SPD when behaviors suggest this diagnosis is essential. The child with SPD is different than the typical child, and the associated behaviors are not merely a matter of "noncompliance" or "oppositional defiance." Attempts to use a behavioral modification approach or a "talk therapy" approach to change difficult behaviors or at worst using capital punishment will very likely result in escalation of difficult behaviors.

Comorbidity studies have been published, which provide some understanding of the course of SPD. Children diagnosed with ADHD experience a diminished cortical response to sensory input as compared to typical children (Reynolds, Lane, & Gennings, 2009). Children with a dual diagnosis of ADHD and the SOR have been found to demonstrate anxiety more than do children with only ADHD as indicated by higher scores on the Revised Children's Manifest Anxiety Scale (Reynolds & Lane, 2007). Children with ASD with higher degrees of sensory overresponsivity were found to have less competence in daily activities including school performance (Reynolds, Bendixen, Lawrence, & Lane, 2011). Atypical sleep patterns were found to relate to atypical sensory behaviors among children with ASD with predictive accuracy of 87.5% by way of behavioral and physiologic measures (Reynolds, Lane, & Thacker, 2011).

A common question among caregivers of children diagnosed with SPD is whether the challenges identified will be resolved as the child ages. The general answer is that we learn to adapt or compensate for these challenges but the challenges remain. A review of the literature by Abernathy (2010) suggests that while adults with a history of SPD will develop compensatory strategies to manage the specific challenges, quality of life can be compromised, yet there are strategies that an occupational therapist with expertise in OT-SI can suggest to bring positive results. Dunn's work in the last two decades has been helpful in providing an understanding of how SPD can be described and evaluated across the lifespan. Her most recent work has resulted in the development of a set of standardized tools to determine both caregiver-generated and self-report data to provide a way in which occupational therapists can document and identify specific sensory processing challenges (Dunn, 2014).

DIAGNOSIS

It is important to note that three different diagnostic manuals include SPD or very close descriptions of this disorder, as a legitimate diagnosis. These include the Diagnostic Classification of Mental Health and Developmental Disorders of Infancy and Early Childhood, Revised (DC: 0-3R) (Zero to Three, 2005), the *Diagnostic Manual for Infancy and Early Childhood* of the Interdisciplinary Council on Developmental and Learning Disorders (ICDL, 2005), and the *Psychodynamic Diagnostic Manual* (PDM Task Force, 2006).

While the efforts to include SPD in the fifth edition of the Diagnostic and Statistical Manual (DSM-5) was not successful, the application process resulted in an exponential increase in the recognition of the term SPD as well as facilitating the most significant degree of research on SPD in history (Miller, 2014). Funding by the Wallace Research Foundation has resulted in the formation of the collaborative SPD Scientific Work Group, composed of investigators with strong records of NIH-funded research at world-renowned centers, which has led to major contributions to the knowledge base of SPD including work toward

the validation of the SPD diagnosis (Brett-Green, Miller, Gavin, & Davies, 2008; Brett-Green, Miller, Schoen, & Nielsen, 2010; Davies & Gavin, 2007; Schoen, Miller, Brett-Green, & Nielsen, 2009).

The most common tools used to diagnose SPD are behavioral measures including clinical observations, caregiver-generated sensory profiles, and standardized assessments to determine challenges as well as strengths in sensory processing. A key to the diagnostic process is to clearly identify the impact of sensory challenges on adaptive behavior. Clearly, everyone can identify an idioscyncratic behavior that interferes with optimal efficiency in daily living, yet compensatory strategies are typically deployed to lessen the impact on function. This would not be considered an SPD. However, when that perceived challenge overwhelms a person's ability to engage and participate in everyday occupations, an analysis of sensory processing is necessary to identify not only the source of the challenge but also the support needed to potentially enable better adaptation.

Despite recognition by the American Academy of Pediatrics that occupational therapy for SPD is a promising and effective intervention, there is a lack of consensus among healthcare providers that a distinct diagnosis of SPD exists (Zimmer et al., 2012). In an effort to produce evidence for a distinct, stand-alone condition, several important studies have been published that suggest this. A longitudinal study of all infants born in New Haven, Connecticut were followed from birth to their eighth birthday. After excluding all cases of developmental delays, autism, and genetic disorders, it was determined that 75% of the remaining group of children presented with SPD signs and symptoms only, suggesting a stand-alone condition (Carter, Ben-Sasson, & Briggs-Gowan, 2011). A study by Van Hulle, Schmidt, and Goldsmith (2012) completed a phenotypic and behavior-genetic analysis on 970 seven-year-old children to delineate comorbidity between childhood psychopathology and SOR. Diagnostic surveys included ADHD, conduct disorder, oppositional defiant disorder, agoraphobia, general anxiety, obsessive-compulsive disorder, panic disorder, separation anxiety, social phobia, specific phobia, depression, enuresis, trichotillomania, selective mutism, and pica behavior. Fifty-eight percent (58%) of children who screened positive for SOR did not qualify for one of the diagnosis included, and 68% of those who screened positive for psychopathologic diagnoses did not screen positive for SOR, suggesting that SOR exists independent of childhood psychiatric disorders.

MEDICAL AND SURGICAL MANAGEMENT

Early identification of SPD by a pediatrician, family doctor, or other health provider is essential so that referral to a qualified occupational therapist can occur. Historically, it has not been uncommon for a child who presented with SPD signs and symptoms to be given a medical diagnosis due to the lack of any diagnostic criteria for SPD. Interestingly enough, the policy paper published by the American Academy of Pediatrics suggested that pediatricians not diagnose children with SPD until further evidence of a distinct diagnosis was validated. In the same statement, however, the authors indicated that intervention was potentially effective, which initiated an increased frequency of diagnosis of SPD by pediatricians (Miller, 2014). It is essential that occupational therapists educate ephysicians and other health care providers about SPD and provide screening checks that can be used to identify children who could benefit from an assessment of sensory processing to rule out SPD. Children who demonstrate signs and symptoms of SPD have often already been medically diagnosed with ADHD, which may result in being prescribed stimulant medications such as Adderall and Ritalin. These medications can reduce impulsiveness and hyperactivity, leading to improved concentration, sustained time on task, and more purposeful responses.

However, not all physicians necessarily select medication as the primary regimen of treatment for children with SPD. In some cases, they may prescribe an initial trial of OT-SI to determine if the child's response lessens or even negates the need for medication. It is not uncommon for children with SPD who experience sleep difficulties to be prescribed melatonin, which is an over-the-counter natural supplement that can enable the child to acquire an improved state of sleep. It has been suggested that children with SPD may not naturally generate and regulate adequate levels of melatonin due to an inefficiency of serotonin, a neurotransmitter that regulates the natural release of melatonin (M. Sloane, *personal communication*, February 15, 2016).

IMPACT ON OCCUPATIONAL PERFORMANCE

The end result of typical sensory processing is effective participation and engagement in occupation. As noted earlier, unless analysis of sensory processing impacts on the child's functional abilities in occupational performance, further intervention is not felt to be necessary. However, for most children, the presence of one type of SPD can indeed impact on occupational performance. Each area of occupation is significantly impacted when the ability to process sensory information and produce an adaptive, meaningful, and efficient response is compromised.

◼ Play

Play is the main occupation of children and requires skills that are grounded in all sensory modalities. Knox, an occupational therapist, developed a comprehensive analysis of play for ages 0 to 72 months and is useful in creating a play profile based on four dimensions including management of space, management of materials, symbolic and pretense, and social participation in play. Each dimension, when analyzed from a sensory processing framework, clearly requires modulation, sensory-based motor functions, and sensory discrimination in order for purposeful play to develop. By way of example, the following describes some of the specific tasks within the first three dimensions for a child 36 to 48 months that are all dependent upon sensory processing to acquire.

Space Management: Gross Motor and Interest (Intentionality)

- Gross motor includes smooth walking, jumping, climbing, running with graded acceleration and deceleration of movement, hopping on one foot, and catching and throwing a ball using shoulder movements. Effective modulation of the visual, vestibular, and proprioceptive sensory mechanisms is foundational to anticipation, initiation, and maintenance of gross motor activities. The more success a child feels, the higher the degree of interest in engaging and participating in gross motor play, which of course leads to development of new and more challenging gross motor activities.

Transitional, quality movement is dependent upon the child's ocular-postural function that is dependent on smooth modulation of vestibular-visual dyad. The need for acceleration and deceleration, holding and placing of the extremities in isolated positions, along with smooth execution of gross motor movement is the direct result of tactile-kinesthetic integration superimposed on vestibular-ocular mechanisms.

- Strong interest in novelty and drawn fine motor activities. With developing intersensory skills, the child is clearly drawn to try out new tasks as he or she receives feedback from the outcomes of earlier engagement and participation.

Material Management: Manipulation, Construction, Purpose, and Attention

- Small muscle activity—hammers, sorts, and inserts small objects
- Makes simple objects, takes apart objects, and combines play materials
- Shows interest in a completed project
- Plays with single object for about 10 minutes

Interest in a variety of fine motor activities is further facilitated by the emergence of precision hand prehension and manipulation patterns integrated with higher-level visual discrimination tasks that allow for improved pattern recognition and spatial relation skills

Pretense-Symbolic; Imitation and Dramatization

- Increased mimicry in play, for example, domestic play; past experiences are dramatized
- Pretending with toys; develops story sequence with toys
- Creates and enacts multiple characters with feelings that primarily include anger and crying

Pretense requires motor planning skills to express ideation of observations and past experiences. It's not uncommon for parents to enjoy observing their toddlers trying to "help" when they are engaged in household tasks through imitation of their actions. Sequential storytelling, typically by way of doll play, demonstrates motor planning abilities as the child sequences actions and verbal exchanges between the objects that become personified.

Difficulty with these developmental tasks can be often be tied to challenges in sensory modulation including hyperresponsive and hyporesponsive, dyspraxia and postural integrity, and difficulty with higher-order visual-perceptual and cognitive skills that are grounded in sensory discrimination.

■ Basic Activities of Daily Living

Basic activities of daily living (BADLs) are primarily habitual and predictive. Thus, these tasks are typically less challenging for someone with intact sensory processing. However, for a person with SPD, the multisensory components of bathing/showering, dressing, eating, feeding, personal hygiene and grooming, and toileting can be significantly challenging. For example, SOR to visual, tactile, proprioceptive, olfactory, auditory, and gustatory sensations can create severe food selectivity issues when the ability to detect, register, and modulate incoming stimuli is compromised. Difficulty with dressing for children and adults can be related to tactile sensitivity to texture, tags in shirt collars, and wearing hose, ties, and clothing that is too lightweight but also includes problems with motor planning as can often be observed with children who cannot sequence and organize their bodies in space to put on clothing, use fasteners, or tie shoes independently. Bathing can be significantly challenging for a child with SOR who becomes increasingly distressed at the sound of water rushing from the faucet as well as discomfort from being washed with a face cloth and having hair shampoo applied, all of which can be perceived as threatening and cause significantly negative reactions in a child with SOR.

■ Instrumental Activities of Daily Living

Instrumental activities of daily living (IADLs) require more complex cognitive level skills that emerge primarily from sensory-based motor and sensory discrimination abilities. Persons with dyspraxia may experience difficulty with planning and organizing steps to accomplish basic life skills due to poor sensory discrimination across all sensory mechanisms. Going shopping, which can result in being in a crowded facility, having to use an escalator or elevator, and standing in line to wait for checking out, can be distressing for someone with SOR. Dining out can be difficult due to the sounds, smells, and crowded sensation to which a person with SOR is particularly sensitive or can be very challenging for parents of a child with SS who can't regulate in the midst of opportunities to explore by running around the restaurant, going up to guest's tables, throwing items from the table, and needing to be in constant motion while at a table. Riding in an automobile may result in complaints of feeling nauseated, especially when riding in the back seat. The crowded, rapid movement of a crowded airport can be intolerable for those with SOR as the sensory chaos that ensues from entrance to takeoff overwhelms the sensory responsivity of a person with SPD.

■ Rest and Sleep

The lack of a balance of rest and other areas of occupation can lead to sleep problems in all people. The cycle of the "4 As (awake, alert, attending, and asleep)" is compromised when factors in the environment interfere with this cycle. The need for a consistent "diet" of sensory enrichment is key to healthy rest and sleep as it helps the nervous system maintain a modulated state. The child with SOR to movement, along with proprioceptive and tactile stimuli, will more likely prefer to engage in much more passive visual activity as opposed to outdoor play. Alternatively, the child who tends to crave sensory input, resulting in overstimulation—especially in the evening hours—may have difficulty with reduction of an arousal state, creating sleep disturbance. External factors, such as direct and ambient auditory, visual, and even olfactory sensation, can impact significantly on sleep patterns as well.

■ Education

Supporting the educational needs of children with various disabilities has historically been a major focus of occupational therapists who work with school-age children and adolescents. Ayres' early work was directed toward children with learning disabilities (Ayres, 1972). Five decades after initiating her pioneering work focused on this population, occupational therapists continue to rule out SPD as a factor in readiness for specific academic skills among a variety of educational diagnoses. All three typologies have implications for educational competencies. Common problems include a child's inability to attend to classroom demands and difficulty being in one position without tran-

sition. There are varied demands that a child needs to be able to consistently show competence in order to succeed in school. These include performing self-care tasks without assistance, maintaining care of personal belongings, moving through the day without significant fatigue, organizing and sequencing oral and written directions, ability to correctly interpret social and environmental cues from teachers and peers, and staying "on task" without being consistently distracted. SPD can easily compromise these and other educational-related tasks that can be addressed with working on "just right" challenges that are at the level of the child's developmental level.

■ Work

The antecedent behaviors and aptitudes necessary for the occupational performance of work can be significantly impacted by SPD. Due to modulation difficulty, fatigue from poor postural stability, motor planning problems, and higher-level discrimination difficulties, even mainstream jobs can be a challenge for a person with SPD.

May-Benson (2009) described the impact of SPD on adults, noting that functional limitations secondary to SPD impacts on an adult's occupational performance. Studies by Pfieffer (2002) and Moore and Henry (2002) reported on the negative influence of poor sensory processing and motor coordination problems on occupational choices, including the ability to obtain employment and engage in leisure activities (as cited by May-Benson, 2009). May-Benson and Patane (2010) found more than half of their study participants chose to be homemakers specifically because of their sensory processing difficulties, even though all had advanced educational degrees. In their study, it was noted that respondents indicated that sensory processing problems impacted on intimate relationships, leading in one case to problems having children. Lastly, driving a car was commonly reported as being severely restricted by sensory processing problems (May-Benson, 2009) and poor motor performance (Cousins and Smyth, 2003, as cited in May-Benson, 2011). By way of interview data, Heufner, Cohn, and Koomar (2010) reported on the negative impact of mothers' sensory processing problems on parenting their children with SPD during mealtimes, waking and bedtime routines, and participation in child-selected leisure activities, creating disruption that impacted the entire family.

■ Social Participation

Persons with modulation difficulty, whether it be sensory overresponsiveness, sensory underresponsiveness, or sensory craving, will experience significant challenges in developing and maintaining socially acceptable behaviors. Examples of challenging behaviors include aggressive reactions to sensory stimuli, particularly tactile sensation, and avoiding interaction due to fear and discomfort with particular types of environmental stimuli, that is, sounds, smells, lights, and colors derail. Embedded in play development is the ability to develop and sustain interpersonal relationships that are apparent very early on with the first episode of infant regard for a caregiver by way of eye contact, "molding," or positive physical response to being gentling by a caregiver through later stages of group interaction skills that develop in early childhood. While reporting on a small sample ($N = 12$), a study by Cosbey, Johnston, and Dunn (2010) suggests that boys with SPD demonstrate some variation in social participation that differs from those of peers without a diagnosis of SPD. By way of a case study report of an adult male with sensory defensiveness and dyspraxia, ADLs and work performance were compromised by organizational and sequential abilities along with challenges experienced in dating and social interactions. These difficulties were found to impact on positive self-esteem as well.

CASE STUDY

Hector and Anna were very pleased when their first child, Jose, was born. Even though Hector expressed his neutrality about having a boy or a girl, he was elated to have a son. For the first year, Hector and Anna understood now what their friends with children had told them about having to expect being "sleep deprived" as they continued to have difficulty with establishing a regulated state after he was fed, held for a while, and beginning to fall asleep. It was unexpected that Jose would resist a pacifier when he would be returned to his crib, which they had been told was often necessary and helpful to help calm a baby, especially after having been fed and diapered. He cried for long periods of time when put down in his crib. Attempts to provide a pacifier was met with complete resistance as he would eject it from his mouth and cry with increasing intensity. They would pick him up and rock him, which would eventually result in his falling asleep. However, soon after they returned him to his crib, he would cry with increasing intensity until he was held again. While calming quickly, attempts to quietly, slowly, and carefully lay him down again after falling asleep again were frequently unsuccessful. Attempts to console Jose with a pacifier was unsuccessful. He simply would not retain it. The fact that Jose simply could not tolerate or accept the pacifier was troubling. Exhausted, Hector and Ana were at a loss as to why Jose could not be consoled with a pacifier. All their friends with infant children were often distraught when a pacifier went missing as they could not calm their baby without it. During a well-infant appointment with their nurse practitioner, she ruled out problems with his oral intake as his weight gain was within the normal curve. Recently, she had worked with another case similar to Jose in which an occupational therapist has provided suggestions for calming. Jose had always been able to latch when breast-feeding, and while it took longer than expected to finish the process as Jose took "breaks" throughout the feeding process, he did acquire enough intake to allow for proper nutritional needs. He was beginning to take in cereal, but this was very time consuming even though the reflexive tongue protrusion was diminished. Ruling out a physical problem, the PNP provided them with a referral for an evaluation to obtain a sensory profile of Jose and determine challenges in specific sensory modulation that would indicate both internal and external factors that were possibly creating Jose's dysregulation. In addition, she advised Jose's parents that the occupational therapist would provide strategies to support his challenges with oral motor regulation.

CASE STUDY 2

Robert has just started his first semester at his local community college and is feeling increasingly anxious about whether or not he will make it in college. Throughout his educational experiences from K to 12, Robert had always experienced difficulty with being in large groups, and sitting and listening to his teacher's presentations that went beyond 20 minutes. He would often become restless and fidgety, sometimes feeling like his body, in his words, "was about to explode." At times, he noticed that his discomfort was heightened if there were smells coming out of the school cafeteria, if his teachers or other students had perfume or cologne, or if there were ambient noises in the room or outside the classroom that others didn't seem to notice or in which they were not bothered. He dreaded classes in which the instructors used PowerPoint presentations—especially those that were mostly text based with minimal graphics to illustrate points presented. He would easily get distracted and miss important points that were likely to be on exams. Furthermore, if the teacher had a high, grating voice—like the professor of his English Literature course—he literally would get up, grab his things, and leave the room. She had already asked him to come to her office when this happened for the third time and advised him that his grade would suffer significantly if he continued to leave her class. Robert knew that he was at risk for failing if he did not figure out how to cope and adapt to his challenges. He made an appointment with his advisor who readily recognized that Robert could benefit from consultation with an occupational therapist who was working with high school and college students who had sensory processing disorders. He provided Robert with general information about SPDs and suggested that it would be helpful to have an assessment. He provided Robert with a survey to fill out in advance of his visit with the OT: the Adolescent Adult Sensory Profile, which would begin to identify the sensory modulation typology that interfered with Robert's ability to succeed in his classroom activities as well as his participation in classroom group activities. Most importantly, as he suggested to Robert, the assessment could lead to some supportive strategies that might alleviate the challenges he was experiencing.

RECOMMENDED BOOKS

Miller, L. J. (2011). *No longer a secret: Unique common sense strategies for with sensory or motor challenges.* Arlington, TX: Sensory World.

Sensory Integration and Learning Disorders, by A. Jean Ayres Published in 1972. This is the classic textbook of Dr. Ayres in which she presents the neuroscience of sensory integration, evaluation, and intervention approaches for what is now termed sensory processing disorder. Western Psychological Disorders.

Kranowitz, C. (2006). *The out-of-sync child: Recognizing and coping with sensory processing disorder.* New York: Perigee.

Kranowitz, C. (2006). *The out of sync child has fun: Activities for kids with sensory processing disorder.* New York: Perigee.

Miller, L. J. (2006). *Sensational kids: Hope and help for children with sensory processing disorders.* New York: Perigee.

Sensoryplanet.com. A social network community for persons with SPD.

SPDFoundation.net. The "gold standard" for resource information on sensory processing including the theory of sensory integration, the diagnosis of sensory processing disorder, and the treatment of SPD known as occupational therapy using a sensory integration approach (OT-SI), research archives, bibliographies, and all other resources for the professional community.

SPDFoundation.net/families.html. Resource site that provides information for parents of children with SPD as well as for anyone wanting to know more about sensory processing disorder and treatment.

SPDUniversity.org. A comprehensive site for online courses, webinars, and links to educational resource for professionals.

REFERENCES

Abernathy, H. (2010). The assessment and treatment of sensory defensiveness in adult mental health. A literature review. *British Journal of Occupational Therapy, 73*, 210–218.

Ahn, R. R., Miller, L. J., Milberger, S., & McIntosh, D. N. (2004). Prevalence of parents' perceptions of sensory processing disorders among kindergarten children. *American Journal of Occupational Therapy, 58*, 287–293.

Atchison, B. (2007). Sensory modulation disorders among children with a history of trauma: A frame of reference for speech pathologists. *Language, Speech, and Hearing Services in Schools, 38*, 109–116.

Ayres, J. A. (1979). *Sensory integration and the child.* Los Angeles, CA: Western Psychological Services.

Ben-Sasson, A., Carter, A. S., & Briggs-Gowan, M. J. (2009). Sensory over-responsivity in elementary school: Prevalence and social-emotional correlates. *Journal of Abnormal Child Psychology, 37*(5), 705–716. doi: 10.1007/s10802-008-9295-8

Bialer, D., & Miller, L. J. (2011). *No Longer A SECRET: Unique common sense strategies for children with sensory or motor challenges.* Arlington, TX: Future Horizons.

Brett-Green, B. A., Miller, L. J., Gavin, W. J., Davies, P. L. (2008). Multisensory integration in children: A preliminary ERP study. *Brain Research, 1242*, 283–290. doi: 10.1016/j.brainres.2008.03.090

Brett-Green, B., Miller, L. J., Schoen, S. A., & Nielsen, D. M. (2010). An exploratory event related potential study of multisensory integration in sensory over-responsive children. *Brain Research, 1321*, 67–77. doi: 10.1016/j.brainres.2010.01.043

Brunton, P. (2013). Effects of maternal exposure to social stress during pregnancy: Consequences for mother and offspring. *Reproduction, 146*, 175–189. doi: 10.1530/REP-13-0258

Carter, A., Ben-Sasson, A., & Briggs-Gowan, M. (2011). Sensory overresponsivity, psychopathology, and family impairment in school-aged children. *Journal of the American Academy of Child Adolescent Psychiatry, 50*(12), 1210–1219. doi: 10.1016/j.jaac.2011.09.010

Collins, B. & Miller, L. (2012, May–June). Focus on sensory craving. *Autism Aspergers Digest*, 16–17.

Cosbey, J., Johnston, S. S., & Dunn, M. L. (2010). Sensory processing disorders and social participation. *American Journal of Occupational Therapy, 64*, 462–473. doi: 10.5014/ajot.2010.09076

Cousins, M., & Smyth, M. (2003). Developmental coordination impairments in adulthood. *Human Movement Science, 22*, 433–459.

Davies, P. L., & Gavin, W. J. (2007). Validating the diagnosis of sensory processing disorders using EEG technology. *American Journal of Occupational Therapy, 61*, 176–189. doi: 10.5014/ajot.61.2.176

Dunn, W. (1999). *Sensory profile user's manual.* San Antonio, TX: Psychological Corporation.

Dunn, W. (2014). *Sensory profile 2: Users manual.* San Antonio, TX: Pearson, Inc.

Fox, S., Levitt, P., & Nelson, C. (2010). How the timing and quality of early experiences influence the development of brain architecture. *Child Development, 81*(1), 28–40. doi: 10.1111/i.1467-8624.2009.01280.x

Henry, J., Sloane, M., & Black-Pond, C. (2007). Neurobiology and neurodevelopmental impact of childhood traumatic stress and prenatal alcohol exposure. *Language, Speech, and Hearing Services in Schools, 38*, 99–108.

Heufner, K., Cohn, E., & Koomar, J. (2012). Mothering when mothers and children both have sensory processing challenges. *British Journal of Occupational Therapy, 75*, 449–455.

Interdisciplinary Council on Developmental and Learning Disorders. (2005). *Diagnostic manual for infancy and early childhood: Mental health, developmental, regulatory–sensory processing and language disorders and learning challenges (ICDL–DMIC).* Bethesda, MD: Author.

James, K., Miller, L. J., Schaaf, R., Nielsen, D. M., & Schoen, S. (2011). Phenotypes within sensory modulation dysfunction. *Comprehensive Psychiatry, 52*, 715–724. doi: 10.1016/j.comppsych.2010.11.010

Keuler, M. M., Schmidt, N. L., Van Hulle, C. A., Lemery-Chalfant, K., & Goldsmith, H. H. (2011). Sensory overresponsivity: Prenatal risk factors and temperamental contributions. *Journal of Development & Behavioral Pediatrics, 32*(7), 533–541. doi: 10.1097/DBP.0b013e3182245c05

Lin, S. H., Cermak, S., Coster, W. J., & Miller, L. (2005). The relation between length of institutionalization and sensory integration in children adopted from Eastern Europe. *American Journal of Occupational Therapy, 59*, 139–147. http://dx.doi.org/10.1100/2012/375436

May-Benson, T. (2010, June 15). Occupational therapy for adults with sensory processing disorder. *OT Practice*, 15–19.

May-Benson, T. (2011). Understanding the occupational therapy needs of adults with sensory processing disorders. *OT Practice, 16*(10), 13–18.

May-Benson, T. A., Koomar, J. A., & Teasdale, A. (2009). Incidence of pre-, peri, and post-natal birth and developmental problems of children with sensory processing disorder and children with autism spectrum disorder. *Frontiers in Integrative Neuroscience, 3*, 31. doi: 10.3389/neuro.07.031.2009. eCollection 2009.

Miller, L. J. (2014). *Sensational kids: Hope and help for children with sensory processing disorder* (revised ed.). New York, NY: Penguin Group.

Miller, L. J., Anzalone, M. E., Lane, S. J., Cermak, S. A., & Osten, E. T. (2007). Concept evolution in sensory integration: A proposed nosology for diagnosis. *American Journal of Occupational Therapy, 61*(2), 135–140.

Miller, L. J., McIntosh, D. N., McGrath, J., Shyu, V., Lampe, M., Taylor, A. K., Tassone, F., Neitzel, K., Stackhouse, T., & Hagerman, R. (1999). Electrodermal responses to sensory stimuli in individuals with fragile X syndrome: A preliminary report. *American Journal of Medical Genetics, 83*(4), 268–279.

Moore, K., & Henry, A. (2002). Treatment of adult psychiatric patients using the Wilbarger Protocol. *Occupational Therapy in Mental Health, 18*(1), 43–46.

Owen, J., Marco, E., Desai, S., Fourie, E., Harris, J., Hill, S., … Mukherjee, P. (2013). Abnormal white matter microstructure in children with sensory processing disorders. *NeuroImage Clinical, 2*, 844–855. doi: 10.1016/j.nicl.2013.06.009

PDM Task Force. (2006). *Psychodynamic diagnostic manual.* Silver Spring, MD: Alliance of Psychoanalytic Organizations.

Pfieffer, B. (2002). The impact of dysfunction in sensory integration on occupations in childhood through adulthood: A case study. *Sensory Integration Special Interest Section Quarterly, 25*(1), 1–2.

Quake-Rapp, C., & Atchison, B. (2011). Sensory processing disorder and treatment. In D. Greydanus, D. Patel, H. Pratt, & J. Calles (Eds.). *Behavioral pediatrics* (3rd ed.). Happauge, NY: Nova Science Publishers.

Reynolds, S., & Lane, S. J. (2007). Diagnostic validity of sensory over-responsivity: A review of the literature and case reports. *Journal of Autism and Developmental Disorder, 38*(3), 516–529.

Reynolds, S., Bendixen, R. M., Lawrence, T., & Lane, S. J. (2011a). A pilot study examining activity participation, sensory responsiveness, and competence in children with autism spectrum disorder. *Journal of Autism and Developmental Disorders, 41*, 1496–1506.

Reynolds, S., Lane, S. J., & Gennings, C. (2009). The moderating role of sensory over-responsivity in HPA activity: A pilot study with children diagnosed with ADHD. *Journal of Attention Disorders, 13*, 468–478. doi: 10.1177/1087054708329906

Reynolds, S., Lane, S. J., & Thacker, L. (2011b). Sensory processing, physiological stress, and sleep behaviors in children with and without autism spectrum disorder. *OTJR: Occupation, Participation, and Health, 31*(2), 246–257. http://dx.doi.org/10.5014/ajot.2012.004523

Schaaf, R. C., & Miller, L. J. (2005). Novel therapies for developmental disabilities: Occupational therapy using a sensory integrative approach. *Journal of Mental Retardation and Developmental Disabilities, 11*, 143–148. doi: 10.1002/mrdd.20067

Schaaf, R. C., Schoen, S. A., Smith Roley, S., Lane, S. J., Koomar, J., & May-Benson, T. A. (2010). A frame of reference for sensory integration. In P. Kramer & J. Hinojosa (Eds.), *Frames of reference for pediatric occupational therapy* (3rd ed., pp. 99–186). Baltimore, MD: Lippincott Williams & Wilkins.

Schneider, M. L., Moore, C. F., Gajewski, L. L., Larson, J. A., Roberts, A. D., Converse, A. K., & DeJesus, O. T. (2008). Sensory processing disorder in a primate model: Evidence from a longitudinal study of prenatal stress effects. *Child Development, 79*(1), 100–113.

Schneider, M. L., Moore, C. F., Gajewski, L. L., Laughlin, N. K., Larson, J. A., Gay, C. L., … DeJesus, O. T. (2007). Sensory processing disorders in a nonhuman primate model: Evidence for occupational therapy practice. *The American Journal of Occupational Therapy, 61*, 247–253.

Schneider, M. L., Moore, C. F., Larson, J. A., Barr, C. S., DeJesus, O. T., & Roberts, A. D. (2009). Timing of moderate level of prenatal alcohol exposure influences gene expression of sensory processing behavior in rhesus monkeys. *Frontiers in Integrative Neuroscience, 3*, 30.

Schoen, S. A., Miller, L. J., Brett-Green, B., & Nielsen, D. M. (2009). Physiological and behavioral differences in sensory processing: A comparison of children with Autism Spectrum Disorder and Sensory Modulation Disorder. *Frontiers in Integrative Neuroscience, 3*, 29.

Schoen, S. A., Miller, L. J., & Green, K. (2008). A pilot study of the Sensory Over-Responsivity Scales: Assessment and inventory. *American Journal of Occupational Therapy, 62*, 393–406.

Tomchek, S. D., & Dunn, W. (2007). Sensory processing in children with and without autism: A comparative study using the Short Sensory Profile. *American Journal of Occupational Therapy, 61*, 190–200.

Van Hulle, C., Schmidt, N., & Goldsmith, H. (2012). Is sensory overreponsivity distinguishable from childhood behavioral problems? A phenotypic and genetic analysis. *Journal of Child*

Psychology and Psychiatry, 53(1), 64–72. doi: 10.1111/j.1469-7619.2011.02432.x

Wickremasinghe, A., Rogers, E., Johnson, B., Shen, A., Barkovich, A., & Marco, E. (2013). Children born prematurely have atypical sensory profiles. *Journal of Perinatology, 33*(8), 631–635.

Wilbarger, J., Gunnar, M., Schneider, M., & Pollak, S. (2010) Sensory processing in internationally-adopted post-institutionalized children. *Journal of Child Psychology and Psychiatry, 51*(10), 1105–1114.

Zero to Three. (2005). *Diagnostic classification of mental health and developmental disorders of infancy and early childhood, revised (DC:0–3R).* Arlington, VA: National Center for Clinical Infant Programs.

Zimmer, M., Desch, L., Rosen, L., Bailey, M., Becker, D., Culbert, T., & Adams, R. C. (2012). Sensory integration therapies for children with developmental and behavioral disorders. *Pediatrics, 129*(6), 1186–1189. doi: 10.1542/peds.2012-0876

Mental Conditions

The Mental Conditions Unit includes mental conditions as specified by the Diagnostic and Statistical Manual of Mental Disorders, 5th Edition. These chapters focus on conditions that are diagnosed in both adults and pediatrics. People with these conditions may be referred to occupational therapy for the specified mental condition or have the mental condition as a secondary diagnosis. Each chapter provides information about the etiology, incidence and prevalence, signs and symptoms, course and prognosis, diagnosis, medical/surgical management, and impact on occupational performance of these conditions. Case illustrations are used to provide examples of lives affected by the conditions. The conditions included in this unit are the following:

Chapter 8: Mood Disorders
Chapter 9: Schizophrenia and other Psychotic Disorders
Chapter 10: Anxiety Disorders
Chapter 11: Neurocognitive Disorders
Chapter 12: Complex Trauma
Chapter 13: Obsessive-Compulsive and Related Disorders
Chapter 14: Somatic Symptoms and Related Disorders
Chapter 15: Feeding and Eating Disorders
Chapter 16: Substance-Related and Addictive Disorders

8

Mood Disorders

Ann Chapleau and Jennifer Harrison

Helen sits in her rocking chair in her small living room, smoking a cigarette. The room is dimly lit by the television screen. Her silver hair is disheveled, and her sweat suit is stained and dirty. She has several days' worth of Meals on Wheels containers on the coffee table, mostly uneaten. A picture of her deceased husband is on the end table, as are various photos of her grown daughter, who lives in another state. Helen has not left her home in over 6 months, except for doctor visits. She worked as a tool and die operator for 14 years after her daughter went to kindergarten, but quit after she was hospitalized for depression for the second time when her daughter left for college. She thinks of these two times in the hospital as her "change of life" difficulties, but realizes that her symptoms have continued off and on for the last two decades. She has early-stage emphysema, but has not been able to stop smoking. She no longer knits or bakes, two of her favorite hobbies.

Ten years ago, she tried a newer antidepressant at the behest of her daughter. It seemed to help, but her mouth was too dry and she had difficulty feeling alert in the morning when she woke up. That, paired with the high co-pay for the medication, led to her decision to stop taking it after 4 months. At her last doctor's visit, her physician asked her if she was feeling depressed again, but Helen was too ashamed to tell him how sad and lonely she had been feeling for months. She wanted to tell him that there wasn't any point in living anymore and that her life doesn't have any meaning, but she remained silent. At home, she is overwhelmed by feelings of guilt. She had been raised to keep a tidy home and be active, and not to feel sorry for oneself, but she feels too tired to do anything except watch television.

Mood disorders are among the most disabling and prevalent illnesses worldwide. The World Health Organization (WHO) estimates that major depressive disorder (MDD) and bipolar disorder (BPD) are among the leading causes of disability, and depression is the leading cause of disability worldwide in terms of years lost to disability (WHO, 2012a). Depression often strikes people younger than do other chronic illnesses and impacts an estimated 350 million worldwide (WHO, 2012b). Despite the prevalence and impact on global health care costs, as well as quality of life for individuals and their families, mood disorders often go undetected and untreated.

DESCRIPTION AND DEFINITION

Mood disorders represent a spectrum of mood disturbances, from the extremely low mood of **depression** to the extremely elevated mood of **mania**. The American Psychiatric Association (APA) provides a classification system known as the Diagnostic and Statistical Manual of Mental Disorders, now in its fifth edition (DSM-5; APA, 2013), to identify symptoms using universal terminology. Depressive disorders include MDD and dysthymic disorder, which are often referred to as **unipolar depression**, as they do not include mood variances on the other end of the mood spectrum. MDD, often referred to as major depression, is characterized by symptoms such as sadness, hopelessness, guilt, irritability, and cognitive impairments, like poor concentration and difficulty making decisions. A diagnosis of MDD requires the presence of a **major depressive episode**, which is a period of depressed or irritable mood, with additional symptoms lasting at least 2 weeks, resulting in severe impairments in functioning.

The BPD spectrum includes BPD I, BPD II, and **cyclothymia**, which all involve some degree of elevated mood and usually a history of at least one major depressive episode. In addition, the DSM-5 includes substance-induced BPD and BPD related to a medical condition (APA, 2013). BPD I is characterized by mood swings from extremely high (mania) to extremely low (depression). Manic behaviors include **euphoria**, irritability, **grandiosity**, decreased sleep, impulsivity, and distractibility, which significantly interfere with daily functioning. A diagnosis of BPD I is warranted when an individual presents with either a manic or **mixed episode**. A **manic episode** is a highly elevated or irritable mood lasting at least 1 week, with or without psychotic symptoms such as delusions and hallucinations. Severity of symptoms results in significant impairment in functioning, which may require hospitalization. A mixed episode is characterized by the presence of both manic and major depressive symptoms almost daily for at least 1 week, resulting in rapid mood cycling with or without psychotic symptoms.

BPD II can be characterized by the presence or history of an MDD and at least one **hypomanic episode**. Hypomania involves similar but less intense mood and energy elevation than does mania.

Cyclothymia represents a chronic (at least 2 years), but less severe, mood disturbance involving both hypomanic behaviors and depressive symptoms that do not meet the criteria for either a manic or major depressive episode (Fig. 8.1).

Terms to describe the clinical symptoms of mood disorders include

- **Affect**: the display of emotion, particularly facial expression
- **Anhedonia**: lack of interest in previously pleasurable activities
- **Avolition**: lack of drive or ambition to complete goal-directed tasks or activities
- **Dysphoria**: a depressed or negative mood state
- **Euphoria**: highly elevated, exaggerated mood

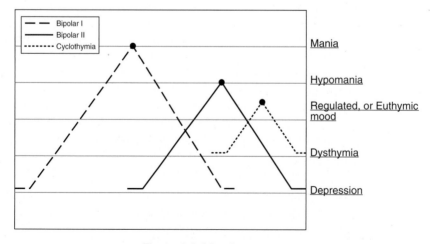

Figure 8.1 Mood spectrum.

- **Flight of ideas**: rapidly changing, disconnected thoughts
- **Grandiosity**: inflated sense of self-esteem or importance
- **Hypomania**: elevated mood that is less intense than full mania
- **Psychomotor agitation**: increased physical movements that are purposeless and reflective of an agitated or anxious state (e.g., wringing hands, fidgeting, pacing)
- **Psychomotor retardation**: abnormally slowed or reduced movements or speech
- **Psychosis**: the presence of delusions or hallucinations without insight

ETIOLOGY

Despite ongoing research, there is still no one known cause of mood disorders.

Both MDD and BDP are widely believed to result from a complex combination of biological, genetic, and psychosocial factors. Many factors can influence the development of mood disorders, including an individual's genetic makeup, biology, other co-occurring medical and psychiatric conditions, cognitive abilities, personality, support systems, personal history, exposure to stress, and coping strategies. Additionally, mood disorders can be triggered by childbirth, seasonal changes, substance use, and other medical conditions.

■ Biological Factors

Much of the research over the past 50 years has focused on biological changes in brain function (National Institute of Mental Health, 2014; U.S. Department of Health and Human Services, 1999). Current research using advanced technologies of brain imaging to examine structures and brain activity provides evidence that mood disorders are disorders of the brain. Functional magnetic resonance imaging (fMRI), positron emission tomography (PET), photon emission computer tomography (PECT), and magnetic resonance spectroscopy (MRS) studies reveal abnormal functioning in regions of the brain that regulate mood, sleep, thinking, appetite, and behavior (Franklin, Carson, & Welch, 2015).

In studies of MDD, functional abnormalities have been found in limbic system, the brain region that represents centers of emotion. These parts of the limbic system include the amygdala, hippocampus, insula, regions of the anterior cingulate cortex, and the dorsolateral prefrontal cortex (Cole et al., 2010; Gos et al., 2010; McKinnon et al., 2009). Functional abnormalities, including reduced cortical thickness of the frontal and temporal lobes and within the limbic system, have also been found in studies of BPD (Kruger, Seminowicz, Goldapple, Kennedy, & Mayberg, 2003; Oertel-Knöchel et al., 2015). In a systematic review of controlled studies with BPD, changes in the hippocampus were also found (Otten & Meeter, 2015). These abnormalities are consistent with studies in which both MDD and BPD subjects demonstrated blunted or decreased behavioral and physiological reactivity to sad or negative stimuli, such as pictures and videos (Foti, Olvet, Klein, & Hajcak, 2010; Miklowski & Johnson, 2006).

The role of neurotransmitters, such as serotonin, acetylcholine, and melatonin, in mood disorders has been studied for several decades. Neuroimaging and genetic studies have focused on the role of genes that may predispose an individual to dysregulated levels of neurotransmitters. Current research focuses on neurotransmitter systems, such as the effects of dysregulated dopamine, noradrenaline, and serotonin transporters and receptors in the brain and research related to the improvement of primary and augmented medication therapies for MDD and BPD (O'Leary, Dinan, & Cryan, 2015; Owenby, Brown, & Brown, 2011).

Biological abnormalities of the brain, however, may not necessarily be the cause of a mood disorder, but may develop as a result of the disorder. For example, some researchers believe that chronic stress can trigger depression, as the body continually responds to stress through neurochemical changes (Hennessy, Schiml-Webb, & Deak, 2009; Kumar et al., 2015). One such stress response is the excessive secretion of cortisol, which can interfere with the limbic-cortical systems. The challenge for researchers is to differentiate which abnormalities are causal factors and which develop in response to environmental factors that trigger neurochemical changes.

Both MDD and BPD are known to run in families as heritable traits, but researchers have had minimal success in isolating any specific responsible genes. Genetic variations associated with both MDD and BPD support the growing belief among researchers that mood disorders involve a combination of altered genes that interact with environmental factors, such as stress, to explain why some family members with a known genetic risk develop either MDD or BPD while other family members do not (McMahon et al., 2010). The research on biomarkers for MDD and BPD also shows promise, which could lead to improved diagnosis in primary care and other first-line providers based on laboratory testing and not simply clinical presentation or family history (Redei & Mehta, 2015).

Twin studies also support the genetic link in mood disorders (Gillespie et al., 2015). In studies of MDD, heritability was found to contribute 30% to 40% of the risk for depression, with as much as 60% in adolescent depression (Dolan, de Kort, van Beijsterveldlt, & Boomsma, 2014; Kendler, Gatz, Gardner, & Pedersen, 2006; Kendler et al., 2011; Nivard et al., 2015). In studies of BPD, heritability is even higher. Identical twins have a concordance rate of 57%, while the concordance rate for fraternal twins is 14% (Miklowitz & Johnson, 2009).

■ Psychosocial Risk Factors

In addition to the role of biological and genetic factors in the development of mood disorders, the role of stressful life events has been widely studied. For example, traumatic events, such as childhood sexual, physical, or emotional abuse, increase the risk of both MDD and BPD (Maniglio, 2010; Miklowitz & Johnson, 2009). Other risk factors include exposure to war, disaster, displacement, parental mental illness, domestic violence, physical or sexual assault, involvement in a serious accident, death of a loved one, chronic work stress, and caregiver stress (Maniglio, 2010; Wingo et al., 2010). This relationship appears to be related to stress and inflammatory processes in the brain, which are associated with depression (Bufalino, Hepgul, Aguglia, & Pariante, 2013; Denson, Spanovic, & Miller, 2009; Irwin & Cole, 2011). However, it is important to remember that the majority of people who experience life stressors do not develop a mood disorder and that not all mood disorders are triggered by a traumatic event. For those who experience traumatic life events, it is estimated that 20% will develop MDD and that estimate is higher for those who experience more profound trauma (Monroe & Reid, 2009).

INCIDENCE AND PREVALENCE

MDD is both common and widespread, with a 12-month prevalence rate of 7%, a lifetime prevalence of 20%, and a relapse rate of more than 50% (APA, 2013; Gotlib & Hamilton, 2008). The 12-month prevalence for BPD is much lower. Community samples in the United States can range from 0.4% to 0.6% (APA, 2013), or from 3.9% to 10%, based on inclusion criteria of the full bipolar spectrum (Miklowitz & Johnson, 2009).

In any given year, 20.9 million (9.5%) adults in the United States will experience a mood disorder, with 14.8 million suffering from MDD and 5.7 million suffering from BPD (Kessler, Chiu, Demler, & Walters, 2005; Kessler et al., 2010). Women are more frequently diagnosed with MDD than are men (Gavin et al., 2010; Kessler et al., 2010). Additionally, lower socioeconomic status is associated with both MDD and BPD (Dijkstra-Kersten, Biesheuvel-Leliefeld, van der Wouden, Penninx, & van Marwijk, 2015; Schoeyen et al., 2011). Low socioeconomic status is also related to lower rates of treatment and higher rates of medication nonadherence (Alekhya et al., 2015).

SIGNS AND SYMPTOMS

Both MDD and BPD are marked by a complex set of symptoms that interfere with daily functioning. Moreover, both disorders are associated with high rates of suicide, the 14th leading cause of death worldwide (Clements et al., 2013; O'Connor & Nock, 2014), making a proper diagnosis essential for treatment purposes.

■ Major Depressive Disorder

According to the APA (APA, 2013), the following are the typical symptoms of MDD:

- Depressed mood
- Anhedonia
- Weight loss
- Altered sleep
- Change in psychomotor behavior
- Fatigue/loss of energy
- Feelings of worthlessness or guilt
- Impaired cognition
- Thoughts of death or suicide

Children with depressive disorders may not exhibit the same set of symptoms as do adults.

Symptoms may include irritability, negativity, acting clingy or overly needy, behavioral problems in school, refusing to attend school, and fear of a parent's death (U.S. Department of Health and Human Services, 2014).

■ Bipolar Disorder

According to the APA (2013), the following are the typical symptoms of BPD:

- Grandiosity
- Minimal need for sleep
- Excessively talkative or having pressured speech
- Racing thoughts or flight of ideas
- Distractibility
- Excessive goal-directed activity or psychomotor agitation
- Impulsivity or participation in dangerous or risky activities

COURSE AND PROGNOSIS

The course of illness and prognosis of both MDD and BPD is varied and is complicated by co-occurring conditions such as anxiety, cardiovascular and pulmonary disease, diabetes, and obesity, which can be related to lifestyle, limited access to care, and the effects of long-term psychotropic medication use (Carnethon et al., 2007; Colton & Manderscheid, 2006). In addition, individuals with mood disorders are more likely to abuse alcohol and/or drugs, which can negatively impact prognosis (Boschloo et al., 2010; Conway, Compton, Stinson, & Grant, 2006).

■ Major Depressive Disorder

Average age of onset for MDD is in the mid- to late-20s (Beesdo et al., 2009). Approximately one-third of those diagnosed with MDD will develop a chronic course of the illness, often lasting throughout their lifetime (Institute of Medicine, 2009). Although MDD is commonly regarded as an adult illness, there is growing evidence that depressive symptoms meeting diagnostic criteria can be present in adolescence, childhood, and even early childhood/preschool years (Hammen, 2009; Luby, 2010). Childhood depression carries a higher risk for recurrence (30% to 50%) during adolescent years and early adulthood (Costello et al., 2002; Thapar, Collishaw, Pine, & Thapar, 2012) and can also be a risk factor for more severe depression in adulthood, as well as among the children

of depressed adults (Mars et al., 2015; Weissman et al., 1999).

During adolescence, rates for depression are equally common among boys and girls, but after age 13, the rate doubles or triples for girls. This higher rate continues into adulthood for women until after middle age (Costello et al., 2002; Mars et al., 2015; Thapar et al., 2012). Adolescents who experience an initial depressive or manic episode are at a higher risk of conversion to BPD (Beesdo et al., 2009).

MDD among older adults is common, representing approximately 10% of older adults (Lyness, Caine, King, Cox, & Yoediono, 1999). While the prevalence of diagnosed depression appears to decline with age, risk of depression and suicide increases when co-occurring physical illness or pain affects ability to function (National Institute of Mental Health, 2007). About one in three older adults with MDD develops a chronic course of the illness (Licht-Strunk et al., 2007; Penkunas & Hahn-Smith, 2015).

■ Bipolar Disorder

Age of onset for BPD is earlier than in MDD, with an average age of 17.5 years (Beesdo et al., 2009). BPD can occur in childhood and early adolescence, as well. A **prodromal** period, ranging from 1.8 to 7.3 years, before full onset of BPD, has been noted in a number of studies (Skjelstad, Malt, & Holte, 2010). Symptoms of dysregulated mood and fluctuations in energy increase in intensity during this period.

Longitudinal studies of BPD indicate that a full, functional recovery from a first episode is uncommon. There is a high risk of relapse, recurring episodes, and mood cycling during the first 2 years of the illness. In addition, suicidal behavior is higher during this early phase (Clements et al., 2015; Nordentoft, Mortensen, & Pedersen, 2011; Salvatore et al., 2007). Sixty percent of people with BPD will experience a recurrence within the first 2 years, while as many as 75% will experience recurrences within the first 5 years. In addition, many will suffer residual symptoms, such as depression, between these episodes (Miklowitz, 2007).

Those who experience an initial depressive or mixed episode are at greater risk for more severe depression and morbidity later in the illness than are those who initially experience a manic episode. In general, the course of the BPD is highly variable, but early treatment is associated with a better prognosis (Clements et al., 2015).

Rates of suicide among people with BPD are higher than in any other psychiatric condition: four times higher than among those with MDD and 15 times higher than among the general population. As many as 60% of people with BPD attempt suicide at least once during the course of the illness, and 5% die as a result of suicide (Clements et al., 2015; Miklowski & Johnson, 2006).

DIAGNOSIS

■ Major Depressive Disorder

A diagnosis of MDD can be determined when an individual has experienced at least one major depressive episode, in the absence of any manic, mixed, or hypomanic episodes (APA, 2013). Symptoms must represent a significant change in typical functioning that interferes with daily living. According to the APA (2013), a depressive episode must include at least five of the symptoms listed previously during a 2-week period, and at least one of the symptoms observed must be either depressed mood or loss of interest or pleasure.

■ Bipolar Disorder

The BPDs can be differentiated by the experience of either a depressive or manic episode. A diagnosis of BPD I is warranted when an individual has experienced at least one manic or mixed episode, with manic mood as the dominant presentation. The individual may have had at least one major depressive episode, as well. A classification of BPD II is determined when the individual has had at least one depressive episode and at least one hypomanic episode, but no manic or mixed episode. BPD II features a predominantly depressed mood. As in MDD, symptoms of BPD must represent a change from previous level of functioning. The disturbed mood must last a minimum of 1 week and include at least three of the symptoms listed previously (APA, 2013).

MEDICAL/SURGICAL MANAGEMENT

■ Pharmacology for Major Depressive Disorders

Antidepressant medications work to regulate neurotransmitters, particularly serotonin and norepinephrine. The newest and most widely prescribed category is the "second-generation" antidepressants called selective serotonin reuptake inhibitors (SSRIs) and serotonin and norepinephrine reuptake inhibitors (SNRIs). SSRIs and SNRIs are the current medications of choice due to lesser side effects than seen with "first-generation" tricyclics and monoamine oxidase inhibitors (MAOIs).

Unfortunately, side effects of all antidepressants can range from minor to life threatening, depending on the individual, and can result in medication noncompliance. Side effects can include nausea, headache, agitation, sexual dysfunction or loss of drive, dry mouth, constipation, blurred vision, and sedation.

MAOIs require strict adherence to diet and medication restrictions, as certain foods and medicines can interact with the MAOIs, resulting in increased risk of stroke.

■ Pharmacology for Bipolar Disorder

Medications for mood stabilization can vary, based on the need to treat acute symptoms versus maintenance treatment. Monitoring of medication use is important to ensure that the mood stabilizer does not cause an episode at the opposite end of the spectrum. Lithium was the first approved medication for BPD and has been the most commonly used medication for mood stabilization for decades. Extensive research still supports its efficacy (Miklowski & Johnson, 2006).

Other mood stabilizers found to be effective include valproic acid or divalproex sodium, known as Depakote, and anticonvulsant medications, such as lamotrigine (Lamictal), gabapentin (Neurontin), topiramate (Topamax), and oxcarbazepine (Trileptal). Potential side effects include sedation; weight gain; tremors; dry mouth; excessive thirst, or polydipsia; restlessness; acne; gastric irritation; and kidney problems.

A treatment regime for acute mania may consist of a combination of lithium, divalproex, or carbamazepine and an atypical antipsychotic medication (Spielmans et al., 2013). Atypical antipsychotic medication side effects can include extensive weight gain, sedation, dizziness, blurred vision, skin rash, and sun sensitivity (Table 8.1).

■ Electroconvulsive Therapy

Convulsive, or shock, therapy has been used in psychiatry for decades. Early use was often associated with tragic results, including permanent severe blunting of affect, permanent memory loss,

TABLE 8.1 Common Medications and Side Effects

Medications	Potential Side Effects
Mood Stabilizers	• Sedation • Weight gain • Tremors • Dry mouth • Excessive thirst (polydipsia) • Restlessness • Acne • Gastric irritation • Kidney malfunction
Atypical Antipsychotics	• Sedation • Dizziness • Blurred vision • Skin rash • Sun sensitivity • Weight gain
Antidepressants • SSRIs • SNRIs • "First-generation" tricyclics • MAOIs	• Sedation • Nausea • Headache • Agitation • Sexual dysfunction or loss of drive • Dry mouth • Constipation • Blurred vision • Increased risk of stroke (MAOIs)

and even death. Electroconvulsive therapy (ECT) has evolved over time, as medical advances have increased our knowledge of the intricacies of the brain. Currently, ECT is considered a safe, effective treatment for MDD and BPD, but is primarily used with those who are treatment resistant to pharmacology (Ottosson & Odeberg, 2012; Taylor, 2007; Travino, McClintock, & Hussain, 2010). The mortality rate for ECT is about 2 deaths per 100,000 treatments and is associated with complications from anesthesia (Fink & Taylor, 2007).

The ECT procedure involves the use of anesthesia prior to induction of a controlled seizure. The seizure is evoked by administration of an electrical shock using electrodes attached to the scalp. ECT is usually administered in a series, over the course of several days or weeks, depending on the individual and severity of symptoms. Although effective, it is still not clear how ECT works. Researchers believe the antidepressive effects may result from an increase in monoamines and serotonin levels, increases in neurotrophic factors that can include cellular improvements and norepinephrine and serotonin receptor expression, and/or increases in anticonvulsant action, which can increase opioids (Ottosson & Odeberg, 2012; Trevino et al., 2010).

■ Repetitive Transcranial Magnetic Stimulation

Repetitive transcranial magnetic stimulation (rTMS) is a newer intervention for treatment-resistant depression (Gross et al., 2007). rTMS involves a noninvasive procedure of creating a magnetic field that passes through the skull inducing electrical currents in the brain that activate specific nerve cells. The procedure can be repeated daily over a period of days or weeks. It has proven successful in reducing depressive symptoms and improving remission rates (George et al., 2010; Holtzheimer et al., 2010; McGirr, Van den Eynde, Tovar-Perdoma, Fleck, & Berlim, 2015). Based on recent successful clinical trials, an rTMS device for the treatment of MDD has been approved by the U.S. Food and Drug Administration. rTMS is used either singly or in combination with pharmacotherapy and is associated with fewer cognitive and memory side effects when compared with ECT (George et al., 2010; McGirr et al., 2015).

IMPACT ON OCCUPATIONAL PERFORMANCE

Mood disorders, particularly those at the extreme ends of the mood spectrum, can significantly interfere with daily functioning. Symptoms of both MDD and BPD interfere with one's ability to work, socialize, recreate, sleep, eat, and learn. The impact on occupational performance, however, can vary greatly based on factors such as severity of symptoms, responsiveness to treatment, number of episodes, co-occurring conditions, and age of onset. For example, an adult with a high level of premorbid functioning, who experiences a single episode and responds well to intervention, may successfully return to work and family roles. For many individuals, however, there are numerous barriers to occupational performance once symptoms occur.

■ Activities of Daily Living

The ability to care for personal health such as eating well, following a healthy diet, sleeping, and exercising regularly can be impaired. Previously maintained daily routines can be disrupted. Symptoms of avolition and anhedonia seen in depressive episodes can decrease motivation for exercise, proper nutrition, grooming, and hygiene. Symptoms of distractibility, impulsivity, and psychomotor disturbances that are characteristics of a manic or hypomanic episode can interfere with the quality of self-care. Additionally, sleep patterns are often disturbed, with individuals not getting adequate sleep, sleeping excessively, or experiencing poor sleep quality. Weight gain or loss is common and can be related to either changes in daily habits or long-term medication use.

■ Instrumental Activities of Daily Living

Early onset in childhood or adolescence, a time of developing skills and interests, coupled with high rates of recurrence throughout adulthood, can limit one's ability to develop educational, social, and work skills. For individuals who continue to experience residual symptoms between episodes, it can be even more difficult to re-engage in meaningful life roles. The individual dealing with recurring depressed, manic, or cycling moods has great difficulty managing daily tasks that can include work, school, parenting/caregiving, home maintenance, and healthy leisure.

Many individuals with mood disorders lack the educational and training requirements needed for a successful career. Moreover, persons suffering from depressive episodes are likely to experience symptoms of anhedonia, avolition, and cognitive difficulties, which decrease motivation and ability to work. Studies reveal that those diagnosed with MDD or BPD are less likely to work outside the home, either full- or part-time (Mojtabai et al., 2015; Substance Abuse and Mental Health Services Administration [SAMHSA], 2009), and those who do work experience lowered productivity and increased absenteeism (Kessler et al., 2006; Mojtabai et al., 2015; SAMHSA, 2011). An evidence-based practice for supported employment for adults with mental illness including MDD and BPD has demonstrated substantial improvements in employment outcomes as well as decreased hospitalization, arrest, and incarceration (SAMHSA, 2011).

Children and adolescents with early onset of a mood disorder may experience symptoms that can negatively impact school performance, such as lower scores on achievement tests and impaired peer interactions, including social withdrawal or fighting and disruptive behavior. Studies have shown that high school students with depression, particularly females, are more likely to drop out of high school and are less likely to enroll in college (Fletcher, 2007). Young adults with depression are also more likely to disenroll in college especially when engaged in substance use (Arria et al., 2013).

Involvement in healthy leisure activities is usually limited, as well. Those with MDD are likely to socially isolate and cease participation in activities due to symptoms of anhedonia and avolition. During a manic or hypomanic episode, individuals may experience an initial burst of creative, goal-directed energy, but they are more likely to engage in risky or dangerous activities and, over time, to become more unable to organize time and activities. Interventions such as the best practice IMPACT (Improving Mood—Promoting Access to Collaborative Treatment) have substantial evidence of effectiveness in combating avolition and anhedonia in older adults with MDD or BPD (Penkunas & Hahn-Smith, 2015).

In general, those who experience recurring episodes, limited treatment success, co-occurring medical or psychiatric conditions, and lack of healthy support systems are more likely to demonstrate an overall decline in functioning. Early intervention and ongoing access to treatment and other support networks can improve one's ability to maintain meaningful and productive roles and to experience a greater quality of life through social participation.

CASE STUDY 1

Phyllis spent excessive hours at her new human resources job, planning how to take over the company. She was visibly irritated with what she perceived as organizational inefficiencies and spoke about her concerns to her employers. Her grandiosity was evident to all of her coworkers. She drafted numerous versions of detailed proposals to "take the company to the next level." Despite working long hours at her computer each day, she failed to complete the tasks she was hired to do. She was continually distracted by her big plans. In addition, she began shopping for new clothes that she felt would be in keeping with her elevated status. She ran up large credit card bills and was in financial trouble. Phyllis found it difficult to sleep regularly and often stayed up until 3:00 or 4:00 AM working on her computer, although she rarely accomplished what she set out to do. She tried using over-the-counter sleep aids and Melatonin and started drinking a few glasses of wine before bed, but she worried that she would develop a dependency. For these same reasons, she was reluctant to see a physician about her mood issues, even though she began to recognize that her behavior was perceived as odd by her colleagues.

When she shared her business ideas with family members, they gave her feedback about how unrealistic she was being and urged her to focus on her job. She responded defensively, unable to recognize how her behavior was negatively affecting her work. Although she was highly talented in her field, she was fired after 3 months on the job. After she was fired, the other areas of her life began to spiral out of control. She missed two job interviews related to not being able to sleep because she was up all night preparing. Phyllis felt this lack of sleep was associated with beginning to have visions at night that she could communicate directly with leaders of industry with her thoughts. When she disclosed these thoughts to her best friend, her friend convinced her to talk to her family doctor. Her family doctor referred her to a psychiatrist, and she was diagnosed with BPD with psychotic features. She began treatment with medication and cognitive-behavioral therapy and, within 4 months, was able to return to the job market where she obtained a job in a similar industry as she had worked before. Although she still had times when her mood shifted outside of her "normal bandwidth," she found that medication, therapy, regular yoga, checking in with three good friends at least weekly for check-ins, and avoiding alcohol allowed her to live the kind of life she was proud of.

CASE STUDY 2

Justin is a 9-year-old boy who was admitted to the child and adolescent psychiatric inpatient unit at the local community mental health center. He had been living in a foster home since being removed from his biological parents' home at age 7, due to neglect.

His foster parents describe Justin as quiet and passive in his interactions with others, avoiding eye contact and wearing his hair long, over his eyes. They reported that Justin spends most of his free time in his room, alone, watching television or playing video games. Schoolwork is a daily struggle for Justin's foster parents, as they indicate he is disinterested in school and avoids completing his assignments. They report he "throws temper tantrums" when they make him do home-work. He frequently complains of having an upset stomach when it is time to get ready for school in the morning. During the initial interview with the occupational therapist, Justin shared that he felt he was "bad" and that was why he had been removed from his biological parents' custody.

During his stay in the inpatient unit, Justin completed a more comprehensive evaluation. He reported that he has times when he feels like he does not want to wake up and has considered hanging himself in his room. He described times when he cut himself on his thighs or calves to feel a sense of relief and calm. He reported a lack of motivation and energy and that he feels unworthy of friendship or the love that his foster parents and grandparents give to him. Justin talked about

wanting to sleep all day most weekends, often not eating except when someone was watching him or would notice his lack of appetite.

Once stable and no longer considered a sui-cide risk, Justin was discharged from the hospital. He continues to work with an occupational thera-pist, a social worker, and his family physician. In addition, he joined a group at school focused on resiliency. He gradually started talking to a few boys in his grade and joined an Olympics of the Mind group after school. Within 2 years, he and his foster parents decided to pursue adoption, and he happily reported to his support team that he understood that he was a really cool kid and that "my parents are pretty lucky to be able to adopt me...they got that going for them....so there's that."

RECOMMENDED LEARNING RESOURCES

National Alliance on Mental Illness (NAMI)
3803 N. Fairfax Dr., Ste. 100
Arlington, VA 22203
Phone: 703-524-7600
Fax: 703-524-9094
www.nami.org

National Institute of Mental Health (NIMH)
Science Writing, Press, and Dissemination Branch
6001 Executive Boulevard, Room 8184, MSC 9663

Bethesda, MD 20892-9663
Phone: 1-866-615-6464
Fax: 301-443-4279
www.nimh.nih.gov

NARSAD
60 Cutter Mill Road, Suite 404
Great Neck, NY 11021
Phone: 516-829-0091
Fax: 516-487-6930
www.narsad.org

REFERENCES

Alekhya, P., Sriharsha, M., Venkata Ramudu, R., Shivanandh, B., Priya, T., Darsini, P., … Hrushikesh Reddy, Y. (2015). Adherence to antidepressant therapy: Sociodemographic fac-tor wise distribution. *International Journal of Pharmaceutical and Clinical Research*, 7(3), 180–184. ISSN-0975 1556

American Psychiatric Association. (2013). *Diagnostic and statistical manual of mental disorders* (5th ed.). Washington, DC: Author. ISBN-13: 9780890425558

Arria, A. M., Caldeira, K. M., Vincent, K. B., Winick, E. R., Baron, R. A., & O'Grady, K. E. (2013). Discontinuous college enrollment: Associations with substance use and mental health. *Psychiatric Services*, 64(2), 165–172. doi: 10.1176/appi. ps.20120016

Beesdo, K., Hofler, M., Leibenluft, E., Lieb, R., Bauer, M., & Pfenning, A. (2009). Mood epi-sodes and mood disorders: Patterns of inci-dence and conversion in the first three decades of life. *Bipolar Disorders*, 11, 637–649. doi: 10.1111/j.1399-5618.2009.00738.x

Boschloo, L., Vogelzangs, N., Smit, J. H., van den Brink, W., Veltman, D. J., Beekman, A. T. F., & Penninx, B. W. J. H. (2010). The performance of the Alcohol Use Disorder Identification Test (AUDIT) in detecting alcohol abuse and depen-dence in a population of depressed or anxious per-sons. *Journal of Affective Disorders*, 126, 441–446. doi: 10.1016/j.jad.2010.04.019

Bufalino, C., Hepgul, N., Aguglia, E., & Pariante, C. M. (2013). The role of immune genes in the asso-ciation between depression and inflammation: A review of recent clinical studies. *Brain, Behavior, and Immunity, 31*, 31–47. doi: 10.1016/j.bbi.2012.04.009

Carnethon, M. R., Biggs, M. L., Barzilay, J. I., Smith, N. L., Vaccarino, V., Bertoni, A. G., & Siscovich, D. (2007). Longitudinal association between depressive symptoms and incident type 2 diabetes mellitus in older adults: The cardiovascular health study. *Archives of Internal Medicine, 167*, 802–807. doi: 10.1001/archinte.167.8.802.

Clements, C., Jones, S., Morriss, R., Peters, S., Cooper, J., While, D., … Kapur, N. (2015). Self-harm in bipolar disorder: Findings from a prospective clinical database. *Journal of Affective Disorders, 173*, 113–119. doi: 10.1016/j.jad.2014.10.012

Clements, C., Morriss, R., Jones, S., Peters, S., Roberts, C., & Kapur, N. (2013). Suicide in bipolar disorder in a national English sample, 1996–2009: Frequency, trends and characteristics. *Psychological Medicine, 107*, 1–10. doi: 10.1017/S0033291713000329

Cole, J., Toga, A. W., Hojatkashani, C., Thompson, P., Costafreda, S. G., Cleare, A. J., … Fu, C. H. Y. (2010). Subregional hippocampal deformations in major depressive disorder. *Journal of Affective Disorders, 126*, 272–277. doi: 10.1016/j.jad.2010.03.004

Colton, C. W., & Manderscheid, R. W. (2006). Congruencies in increased mortality rates, years of potential life lost, and causes of death among public mental health clients in eight states. *Prevention of Chronic Diseases, 3*(2), 1–14.

Conway, K. P., Compton, W., Stinson, F. S., & Grant, B. F. (2006). Lifetime comorbidity of DSM-IV mood and anxiety disorders and specific drug use disorders: Results from the National Epidemiologic Survey on Alcohol and Related Conditions. *Journal of Clinical Psychiatry, 67*, 247–257. doi: 10.4088/JCP.v67n0211

Costello, E. J., Pine, D. S., Hammen, C., March, J. S., Plotsky, P. M., Weissman, M. M., … Leckman, J. F. (2002). Development and natural history of mood disorders. *Social and Biological Psychiatry, 52*, 529–542. doi: 10.1016/S0006-3223(02)01372-0

Denson, T. F., Spanovic, M., & Miller, N. (2009). Cognitive appraisals and emotions predict cortisol and immune responses: A meta-analysis of acute laboratory social stressors and emotion inductions. *Psychological Bulletin, 135*, 823–853. doi: 10.1037/a0016909

Dijkstra-Kersten, S. M. A., Biesheuvel-Leliefeld, K. E. M., van der Wouden, J. C., Penninx, B. W. J. H., & van Marwijk, H. W. J. (2015). Associations of financial strain and income with depressive and anxiety disorders. *Journal of Epidemiology and Community Health, 69*(1), 1–14. doi: 10.1136/jech-2014-205088

Dolan, C. V., de Kort, J. M., van Beijsterveldt, C. E. M., Bartels, M., & Boomsma, D. I. (2014). GE Covariance through phenotype to environment transmission: An assessment in longitudinal twin data. *Behavioral Genetics, 44*, 240–253. doi: 10.1007/s10519-014-9659-5

Fink, M., & Taylor, M. A. (2007). Electroconvulsive therapy: Evidence and challenges. *Journal of the American Medical Association, 298*, 330–332. doi: 10.1001/jama.298.3.330

Fletcher, J. M. (2007). Adolescent depression: Diagnosis, treatment, and educational attainment. *Health Economics, 17*, 1215–1235.

Foti, D., Olvet, D. M., Klein, D. N., & Hajcak, G. (2010). Reduced electrocortical response to threatening faces in major depressive disorder. *Depression and Anxiety, 27*, 813–820. doi: 10.1002/da.20712

Franklin, G., Carson, A. J., & Welch, K. A. (2015). Cognitive behavioural therapy for depression: Systematic review of imaging studies. *Acta Neuopsychiatrica, 27*(5), 1–14. doi: 10.1017/neu.2015.41

Gavin, A. R., Walton, E., Chae, D. H., Alegria, M., Jackson, J. S., & Takeuchi, D. (2010). The associations between socio-economic status and major depressive disorder among Blacks, Latinos, Asians and non-Hispanic Whites: Findings from the Collaborative Psychiatric Epidemiology Studies. *Psychological Medicine, 40*, 51–61. doi: 10.1017/S0033291709006023

George, M. S., Lisanby, S. H., Avery, D., McDonald, W. M., Durkalski, V., Pavlicova, M., … Sackeim, H. A. (2010). Daily left prefrontal transcranial magnetic stimulation therapy for major depressive disorder. *Archives of General Psychiatry, 67*, 507–516. doi: 10.1001/archgenpsychiatry.2010.46

Gillespie, N. A., Eaves, L. J., Maes, H., & Silberg, J. L. (2015). Testing models for the contribution of genes and environment to developmental change in adolescent depression. *Behavioral Genetics, 45*, 382–393. doi: 10.1007/s10519-015-9715-9

Gos, T., Krell, D., Bielau, H., Steiner, J., Mawrin, C., Trubner, K., … Bogerts, B. (2010). Demonstration of disturbed activity of the lateral amygdaloid nucleus projection neurons in depressed patients by the AgNOR staining method. *Journal of Affective Disorders, 126*, 402–410. doi: 10.1016/j.jad.2010.04.006

Gotlib, I. H., & Hamilton, J. P. (2008). Neuroimaging and depression: Current status and unresolved issues. *Current Directions in Psychological Sciences, 17*, 159–163. doi: 10.1111/j.1467-8721.2008.00567.x

Gross, M., Nakamura, L., Pascual-Leone, A., & Fregni, F. (2007). Has repetitive transcranial magnetic stimulation (rTMS) treatment for depression improved? A systematic review and meta-analysis comparing the recent vs. the earlier rTMS studies. *Acta Psychiatria Scandinavia, 116*, 165–173.

Hammen, C. (2009). Adolescent depression: Stressful interpersonal contexts and risk for recurrence. *Current Directions in Psychological Sciences, 18*, 200–204.

Hennessy, M. B., Schiml-Webb, P. A., & Deak, T. (2009). Separation, sickness, and depression: A new perspective on an old animal model. *Current Directions in Psychological Sciences, 18*, 227–231. doi: 10.1111/j.1467-8721.2009.01636.x

Holtzheimer, P. E., McDonald, W. M., Mufti, M., Kelley, M. E., Quinn, S., Corso, G., & Epstein, C. M. (2010). Accelerated repetitive transcranial magnetic stimulation for treatment-resistant depression. *Depression and Anxiety, 27*, 960–963. doi: 10.1002/da.20731

Institute of Medicine, National Research Council. (2009). *Depression in parents, parenting, and children: Opportunities to improve identification, treatment, and prevention.* Washington, DC: The National Academies Press. ISBN 978-0-309-12178-1

Irwin, M. R., & Cole, S. W. (2011). Reciprocal regulation of the neural and innate immune systems. *Nature Reviews Immunology, 11*, 625–632. doi: 10.1038/nri3042

Kendler, K. S., Gatz, M., Gardner, C. O., & Pedersen, N. L. (2006). A Swedish national twin study of lifetime major depression. *American Journal of Psychiatry, 163*, 109–114. doi: 10.1176/appi.ajp.163.1.109

Kendler, K. S., Eaves, L. J., Loken, E. K., Pedersen, N. L., Middeldorp, C. M., Reynolds, C, ... Gardner, C. O. (2011). The impact of environmental experiences on symptoms of anxiety and depression across the life span. *Psychological Science, 22*, 1343–1352. doi: 10.1177/0956797611417255

Kessler, R. C., Akiskal, H. S., Ames, M., Birnbaum, H., Greenberg, P., Hirschfeld, R. M. A., ... Wang, P. S. (2006). Prevalence and effects of mood disorders on work performance in a nationally representative sample of U.S. workers. *American Journal of Psychiatry, 163*, 1561–1568.

Kessler, R. C., Chiu, W. T., Demler, O., & Walters, E. E. (2005). Prevalence, severity, and comorbidity of twelve-month DSM-IV disorders in the National Comorbidity Survey Replication (NCS-R). *Archives of General Psychiatry, 62*, 617–627.

Kessler, R. C., Green, J. G., Gruber, M. J., Sampson, N. A., Bromet, E., Cuitan, M., ... Zaslavsky, A. M. (2010). Screening for serious mental illness in the general population with the K6 screening scale: Results from the WHO World Mental Health (WMH) survey initiative. *International Journal of Methods in Psychiatric Research, 19*, 4–22. doi: 10.1002/mpr.310

Kruger, S., Seminowicz, S., Goldapple, K., Kennedy, S. H., & Mayberg, H. S. (2003). State and trait influences on mood regulation in bipolar disorder: Blood flow differences with an acute mood challenge. *Biological Psychiatry, 54*, 1274–1283. doi: 10.1016/S0006-3223(03)00691-7

Kumar, P., Slavich, G. M., Berghorst, L. H., Treadway, M. T., Brooks, N. H., Dutra, S. J., ... Pizzagalli, D. A. (2015). Perceived life stress exposure modulates reward-related medial prefrontal cortex responses to acute stress in depression. *Journal of Affective Disorders, 180*, 104–111. doi: 10.1016/j.jad.2015.03.035

Licht-Strunk, E., van der Windt, D. A. W. M., van Marwijk, H. W. J., de Haan, M., & Beekman, A. T. F. (2007).The prognosis of depression in older patients in general practice and the community: A systematic review. *Family Practice, 24*, 168–180. doi: 10.1093/fampra/cml071

Luby, J. L. (2010). Preschool depression: The importance of identification of depression early in development. *Current Directions in Psychological Science, 19*, 91–95. doi: 10.1177/0963721410364493

Lyness, J. M., Caine, E. D., King, D. A., Cox, C., & Yoediono, Z. (1999). Psychiatric disorders in older primary care patients. *Journal of General Internal Medicine, 14*, 249–254.

Maniglio, R. (2010). Child sexual abuse in the etiology of depression: A systematic review of reviews. *Depression and Anxiety, 27*, 631–642. doi: 10.1002/da.20687

Mars, B., Collishaw, S., Hammerton, G., Rice, F., Harold, G. T., Smith, D., ... Thaper, A. (2015). Longitudinal symptom course in adults with recurrent depression: Impact on impairment and risk of psychopathology in offspring. *Journal of Affective Disorders, 182*, 32–38. doi: 10.1016/j.jad.2015.04.018

McGirr, A., Van den Eynde, F., Tovar-Perdoma, S., Fleck, M. P. A., & Berlim, M. T. (2015). Effectiveness and acceptability of accelerated repetitive transcranial magnetic stimulation (rTMS) for treatment-resistant major depressive disorder: An open label trial. *Journal of Affective Disorders, 173*, 216–220. doi: 10.1016/j.jad.2014.10.068

McKinnon, M. C., Yucel, K., Nazarov, A., & MacQueen, G. M. (2009). A meta-analysis examining clinical predictors of hippocampal volume in patients with major depressive disorder. *Journal of Psychiatry and Neuroscience, 34*, 41–54.

McMahon, F. J., Akula, N., Schulze, T. G., Muglia, P., Tozzi, F. Detera-Wadleigh, S. D., … Rietschel, M. (2010). Meta-analysis of genome-wide association data identifies a risk locus for major mood disorders on 3p21.1. *Nature Genetics, 42,* 128–131. doi: 10.1038/ng.523

Miklowitz, D.J. (2007). The role of the family in the course and treatment of bi-polar disorder. *Current Directions in Psychological Science, 16,* 192–196.

Miklowitz, D. J., & Johnson, B. S. L. (2009), Social and familial factors in the course of bipolar disorder: Basic processes and relevant interventions. *Clinical Psychology: Science and Practice, 16,* 281–296. doi: 10.1111/j.1468-2850.2009.01166.x

Mojtabai, R., Stuart, E. A., Hwang, I, Susukida, R., Eaton, W., Sampson, N., & Kessler, R. C. (2015). Long-term effects of mental disorders on employment in the national comorbidity survey ten-year follow-up. *Social Psychiatry and Psychiatric Epidemiology, 1–12.* doi: 10.1007/s00127-015-1083-5

Monroe, S. M., & Reid, M. W. (2009). Life stress and major depression. *Current Directions in Psychological Science, 18,* 68–72. doi: 10.1111/j.1467-8721.2009.01611.x

Nordentoft, M., Mortensen, P. B., & Pedersen, C. B. (2011). Absolute risk of suicide after first hospital contact in mental disorder. *Archived of General Psychiatry, 68*(10), 1058–1064. doi: 10.1001/archgenpsychiatry.2011.113

National Institutes of Health, National Institute of Mental Health. (2014). *Statistics: Any disorder among adults.* Retrieved from http://www.nimh.nih.gov/statistics/1ANYDIS_ADULT.shtml

National Institute of Mental Health. (2007). *Older adults: Depression and suicide facts.* (NIH Publication No. 4593). Retrieved from http://www.nimh.nih.gov/health/publications/older-adults-listing.shtml

Nivard, M. G., Dolan, C. V., Kenlder, K. S., Kan, K. J., Willemsen, G., van Beijsterveldt, C. E. M., … Boomsma, D. I. (2015). Stability in symptoms of anxiety and depression as a function of genotype and environment: A longitudinal twin study from ages 3 to 63 years. *Psychological Medicine, 45,* 1039–1049. doi: 10.1017/S003329171400213X

O'Connor, R. C., & Nock, M. K. (2014). The psychology of suicidal behaviour. *Lancet Psychiatry, 1,* 73–85. doi:10.1016/S2215-0366(14)70222-6

Oertel-Knöchel, V., Reuter, J., Reinke, A., Marbach, K., Feddern, R., Alves, G., Prvulovic, D, … Knöchel, C. (2015). Association between age of disease-onset, cognitive performance and cortical thickness in bipolar disorders. *Journal of Affective Disorders, 174,* 627–635. doi: 10.1016/j.jad.2014.10.060

O'Leary, O. F., Dinan, T. G. & Cryan, J. F. (2015). Faster, better, stronger: Towards new antidepressant therapeutic strategies. *European Journal of Pharmacology, 753,* 32–50. doi: 10.1016/j.ejphar.2014.07.046

Otten, M., & Meeter, M. (2015). Hippocampal structure and function in individuals with bipolar disorder: A systematic review. *Journal of Affective Disorders, 174,* 113–125. doi: 10.1016/j.jad.2014.11.001

Ottosson, J.-O., & Odeberg, H. (2012). Evidence-based electroconvulsive therapy. *Acta Psychiatry Scandinavia, 125,* 177–184. doi: 10.1111/j.1600-0447.2011.01812.x

Owenby, R. K., Brown, L. T., & Brown, J. N. (2011). Use of risperidone as augmentation treatment for major depressive disorder. *Annals of Pharmacotherapy, 45*(1), 95–100. doi: 10.1345/aph.1P397

Penkunas, M. J., & Hahn-Smith, S. (2015). An Evaluation of IMPACT for the treatment of late-life depression in a public mental health system. *Journal of Behavioral Health Services & Research, 42*(3), 334–345. doi: 10.1007/s11414-013-9373-8

Redei, E. E., & Mehta, N. A. (2015). The promise of biomarkers in diagnosing depression in Primary Care: the present and future. *Current Psychiatry Reports, 17,* 64–73. doi: 10.1007/s11920-015-0601-1

Salvatore, P., Tohen, M., Khalsa, H. M., Baethge, C., Tondo, L., & Baldessarini, R. J. (2007). Longitudinal research on bipolar disorders. *Epidemiologia E Psichiatria Sociale, 16,* 109–117. doi: 10.1017/S1121189X00004711

Schoeyen, H. K., Birkenaes, A. B., Vaaler, A., Auestad, B. H., Malt, U. F., Andreassen, O. A., & Morken, G. (2011). Bipolar disorder patients have similar levels of education but lower socioeconomic status than the general population. *Journal of Affective Disorders, 132*(1-2), 209–215. doi:10.1016/j.jad.2010.08.012

Skjelstad, D. V., Malt, U. F., & Holte, A. (2010). Symptoms and signs of the initial prodrome of bipolar disorder: A systematic review. *Journal of Affective Disorders, 126,* 1–13. doi: 10.1016/j.jad.2009.10.003

Substance Abuse and Mental Health Services Administration. (2009). *The NSDUH Report: Employment and major depressive episode.* Retrieved from http://www.oas.samhsa.gov/2k9/162/Employment.htm

Substance Abuse and Mental Health Services Administration. (2011). *Supported employment: Evidence-based practices toolkit.* Rockville, MD: Center for Mental Health Services,

Substance Abuse and Mental Health Services Administration, U.S. Department of Health and Human Services.

Spielmans, G. I., Berman, M. I., Linardatos, E., Rosenlicht, N. Z., Perry, A., & Tsai, A. C. (2013). Adjunctive atypical antipsychotic treatment for major depressive disorder: A meta-analysis of depression, quality of life, and safety outcomes. *Public Library of Science Medicine*, *10*(3), 1–24. doi: 10.1371/journal.pmed.1001403

Taylor, S. (2007). Electroconvulsive therapy: A review of history, patient selection, technique, and medication management. *Southern Medical Journal*, *100*, 494–498.

Thapar, A., Collishaw, S, Pine, D. S., & Thapar, A. K. (2012). Depression in adolescence. *Lancet*, *379*, 1056–1067. doi:10.1016/S0140-6736(11)60871-4

Trevino, K., McClintock, S. M., & Husain, M. M. (2010). A review of continuation electroconvulsive therapy: Application, safety, and efficacy. *Journal of ECT*, *26*(3), 186–195. doi: 10.1097/YCT.0b013e3181efa1b2

U.S. Department of Health and Human Services, National Institutes of Health, National Institute of Mental Health. (2014). *Depression*. (NIH Publication No. 08-3561). Retrieved from http://www.nimh.nih.gov/health/publications/depression/nimhdepression.pdf

U.S. Department of Health and Human Services, Substance Abuse and Mental Health Services Administration, Center for Mental Health Services, National Institutes of Health, National Institute of Mental Health. (1999). *Mental health: A report of the Surgeon General*. Retrieved from http://www.surgeongeneral.gov/library/mentalhealth/home.html

Weissman, M. M., Wolk, S., Goldstein, R. B., Moreau, D., Adams, P., Greenwald, S., … Wichramaratne, P. (1999). Depressed adolescents grown up. *Journal of the American Medical Association*, *281*, 1701–1713. doi: 10.1001/jama.281.18.1707

Wingo, A. P., Wrenn, G., Pelletier, T., Gutman, A. R., Bradley, B., & Ressler, K. J. (2010). Moderating effects of resilience on depression in individuals with a history of childhood abuse or trauma exposure. *Journal of Affective Disorders*, *126*, 411–414. doi: 10.1016/j.jad.2010.04.009

World Health Organization. (2012). *Depression: A global health concern*. Retrieved from http://www.who.int/mental_health/management/depression/who_paper_depression_wfmh_2012.pdf?ua=1

World Health Organization. (2012). *Depression fact sheet no. 369*. New York, NY: Author. Retrieved from http://www.who.int/mediacentre/factsheets/fs369/en/

Schizophrenia and Other Psychotic Disorders

Ann Chapleau

Megan is a 12-year-old girl, in the 6th grade at middle school. She was born in Texas, but moved with her mother and four siblings to Michigan when she was five. Megan's father was jailed in Texas for running a methamphetamine laboratory in their family home. The family moved in with Megan's grandmother in the Detroit area, and her mother was able to find part-time employment in hotel housekeeping. Megan had difficulty adjusting to her new living situation and starting school for the first time. She had trouble following classroom rules such as sharing supplies and toys. In the second and third grade, she struggled with learning to read and write. Her IQ score was 85. She did not develop any close friendships. She struggled academically with most subjects, but excelled in art, often drawing or painting very dark and strange images that she could not explain. She became increasingly withdrawn and disinterested in peer-related activities such as participating in sports and going to the movies.

When Megan was 12, she was referred for psychological testing, which revealed that she had the clinical symptoms of psychosis. Megan revealed to the psychologist that Satan had appeared to her on multiple occasions. She was tormented by voices telling her that she was evil and should commit suicide. She was seen by a psychiatrist who diagnosed her with early-onset schizophrenia, admitting her to a local child and adolescent psychiatric hospital for medication and psychotherapy.

DESCRIPTION AND DEFINITION

Schizophrenia is one of the most severe, complex, and debilitating of all mental health disorders. It is a progressive disorder that can be treated, but not cured. This lifelong brain disorder is characterized by periods of **psychosis**, which is the presence of delusions or hallucinations without insight, and/or disorganized thoughts/speech, abnormal motor behavior, and diminished volition and emotional expression. It is also marked by a progressive decline in daily living skills, including work and education skills, social/relationship skills, and basic self-care abilities (American Psychiatric Association [APA], 2013). This chapter will focus primarily on the disorder of schizophrenia. A brief overview of other psychotic disorders considered part of the schizophrenia spectrum will be provided at the end of the chapter.

ETIOLOGY

There is no one single factor found to be the cause of schizophrenia. There are a number of models that attempt to explain the multiple factors that can contribute to the development of the disorder. Current research supports a genetic vulnerability as well as environmental triggers (Karl & Arnold, 2014; Kaur et al., 2014; Leask, 2004). Findings from advanced brain imaging suggest the presence of genetic markers, reduced brain activity in the frontal and temporal regions, and structural abnormalities in all regions of the brain, including enlarged ventricles, reduced volume of gray matter in the cerebral cortex, and decreased size of the hippocampus and thalamus (De Peri et al., 2012; Lieberman et al., 2008). The role of key neurotransmitters, including dopamine, glutamate, and serotonin, is being explored to determine their role in genetic alterations (Choi & Tarazi, 2010; Sawa & Snyder, 2002). Emerging research also suggests that abnormal cortical-subcortical brain connectivity may play a key role (Woodward & Cascio, 2015).

Complications in prenatal development or during delivery, affecting brain development, have also been associated with schizophrenia (Brown & Derkits, 2010; Cannon, Jones, & Murray, 2002; Gyllenberg et al., 2015; Walker, Kestler, Bollini, & Hochman, 2004). Additionally, complications in later brain development, including chronic cannabis use and exposure to trauma or other stress, have also been linked to schizophrenia (Duhig et al., 2015; Veen et al., 2004). Longitudinal studies have focused on the pattern of structural changes in the brain and have found progressive anatomical changes both prior to and following onset of the illness (Arango et al., 2008; Kempton, Stahl, Williams, & DeLisi, 2010; Sun et al., 2009).

Despite major progress in research, the cause of schizophrenia and other psychotic disorders remains a mystery. With new technology including molecular genetics, in vivo brain imaging, and advancements in psychopharmacology, there is hope for discovering the cause or causes of schizophrenia that can ultimately lead to advancements in prevention and treatment.

INCIDENCE AND PREVALENCE

Schizophrenia affects more than 21 million people worldwide (World Health Organization [WHO], 2014) and 2.5 million American adults (Treatment Advocacy Center, 2009). The incidence of schizophrenia is low, with a median value of 15.2/100,000 people. The lifetime prevalence is estimated to be 0.3% to 0.7% (APA, 2013). Schizophrenia crosses all racial, geographical, and socioeconomic boundaries. Some studies, however, indicate that migrant status, lower economic status, residing in a higher latitude or urban setting, and male gender are factors associated with a higher incidence and prevalence (McGrath, Saha, Chant, & Welham, 2008; Schmitt, Malchow, Hasan, & Falkai, 2014).

SIGNS AND SYMPTOMS

Despite scientific advancements that reveal neurobiological abnormalities of the brain, schizophrenia continues to be misunderstood in the general public. Negative stereotypes are reinforced by the unique nature of the signs and symptoms of this disorder. Schizophrenia affects the brain, which regulates impulse control, judgment, affect, and social skills. Perhaps most important, schizophrenia affects one's self-awareness. As a result, people with schizophrenia are more likely to have difficulty recognizing and accepting that they have the disorder. This lack of self-awareness is similar to anosognosia, a lack of awareness of neurological damage, often seen in individuals following stroke or other acquired brain injuries. Lack of self-awareness can lead to resistance to treatments that could help reduce or eliminate symptoms.

Symptoms of schizophrenia vary greatly, but fall within the following five categories: delusions, hallucinations, disorganized thinking/speech, grossly disorganized or abnormal motor behavior, and negative symptoms (APA, 2013).

- **Delusions** are fixed beliefs that, even in the face of contradictory evidence, are typically due to a misinterpretation of an event or experience. People with schizophrenia may experience more than one type of delusion at a time or at different points in time during the course of the illness. Delusions are categorized as bizarre or nonbizarre. Bizarre delusions are characterized by beliefs or events that are clearly impossible and not related to everyday life experiences, such as a belief that aliens have impregnated the person while he/she was asleep. An example of a nonbizarre delusion is the belief that all coworkers are talking about the person. The individual may interpret all private conversations observed at work to be about him or her. Delusional content can include any of the following types:
  - Persecutory: The most common of all delusions are delusions in which one believes himself or herself to be victimized, ridiculed, or placed under surveillance by known or unknown persons. Some people who suffer from persecutory delusions, such as **paranoia**, believe that someone is attempting to poison them, leading to a refusal to eat or drink. Another example is thought broadcasting, in which the individual is convinced that outside forces are able to transmit, or broadcast to others, his or her inner thoughts.
  - Referential: These are also fairly common forms of delusions. In this form of delusion, one believes that common cues from the environment, such as facial expressions of celebrities on television, casual comments in daily conversations, or newspaper stories, are specifically targeted to the individual, holding special meaning or a message for him or her.
  - Somatic: This form of delusion is marked by beliefs that involve the person's body. For example, a person may believe he or she has received a secret operation while under anesthesia or that she is pregnant, despite evidence to the contrary.
  - Religious: People who suffer from religious delusions may believe they are Jesus Christ or are acting out direct orders from God.
  - Grandiose: Examples of this delusion include believing that one is all-powerful or important, believing that one is acting on secret orders from the President of the United States, or believing oneself to be a genius or multimillionaire.
  - Erotomania: This is a belief that another person, often one unknown to the individual, is in love with the individual.
- **Hallucinations** are the experience of particular sensations that are not real to others and that are experienced while awake. The most common form is auditory, in which an individual hears voices or sounds. The individual may perceive voices in the external environment, or inside his or her head, often more than one voice conversing, or speaking directly to the person. Voices can be taunting and cruel, sometimes commanding the individual to perform certain acts, such as harming self or others, or can be familiar voices that are perceived as friendly companions. Visual hallucinations involve seeing images of people or objects in the environment. The individual may describe seeing shadowy figures or the image of a dead body. Other less commonly seen forms of hallucinations include olfactory (smell), tactile (touch), and gustatory (taste) hallucinations.
- **Disorganized thinking**: Speech content, which can provide clues about thought processes, may encompass any of the following types of disorganized thinking:
  - Loose associations: answers that begin to veer "off track" of the original questions
  - Tangential: unrelated comments or answers
  - Incoherent: often referred to as "word salad" and is seen in more severe cases
- **Grossly disorganized behavior or catatonia** is unpredictable, socially inappropriate

behavior that interferes with daily activities. Examples of disorganized behavior include agitated or angry outbursts with no known provocation, sexually acting out in public (e.g., masturbation), and difficulties performing goal-directed tasks such as meal preparation or grooming. **Catatonia** is an abnormal motor behavior characterized by a loss of responsiveness to environmental cues. The individual may assume rigid or bizarre postures and resist attempts made to move or reposition him or her. Excessive, nonpurposeful motor activity may also be observed. In extreme cases, the individual appears to be completely unresponsive, as in a catatonic stupor.

- **Negative symptoms** are features that represent an absence of function or experience. Two prominent features of schizophrenia include **diminished emotional expression** and **avolition**. Diminished emotional expression is restricted facial expressions, eye contact, speech intonations, and movements that are typically used to convey meaning or emphasize speech. Avolition is a lack of motivation to engage in social or productive activities. Other negative symptoms include **alogia** (impoverished speech), **anhedonia** (loss of pleasure in previously enjoyed activities), and **asociality** (decreased interest in socialization and maintenance of relationships).

Cognitive Symptoms

Memory, attention, language, and executive function, such as abstract reasoning and planning skills, are affected by schizophrenia. Use of neuroimaging and cognitive tests has revealed impaired neurocognitive functioning in completing tasks requiring use of frontal and temporal lobes (Keefe & Harvey, 2012; Lieberman et al., 2008). Individuals with schizophrenia demonstrate reduced ability to process visual stimuli (Koethe et al., 2009) and to respond to environmental stimuli, due to motor skills deficits (Walker et al., 2004). This limited visual processing may lead to deficits in social cognition, which is the ability to recognize, interpret, and act upon social cues during social interactions. There is a substantial body of research supporting the social cognitive deficits in this disorder (Chung, Mathews, & Barch, 2011).

Mean IQ scores range from 80 to 85, which is significantly lower than the norm of 100 for the general population (Jibson, Glick, & Tandon, 2004). People with schizophrenia also lack skills in identifying social cues and solving social problems. In general, research has not yielded any specific cognitive deficit present in all individuals with schizophrenia. Impairments appear generalized and vary greatly from person to person.

Affective Symptoms

Flattened or inappropriate **affect** is a common symptom of schizophrenia, and people with schizophrenia are more likely to demonstrate difficulties in identifying and expressing emotions. Studies have found that people with schizophrenia have a limited ability to scan and recognize facial expressions of others (Bediou et al., 2007). This, coupled with a limited ability to identify social cues, can lead to maladaptive social functioning.

Mood disturbances are also commonly seen. **Dysphoria**, depressed, anxious, or angry mood can be present during or following a psychotic episode and may require intervention. Individuals who develop insight into the severity of their illness are at greater risk of becoming depressed or experiencing demoralization.

COURSE AND PROGNOSIS

Onset of symptoms can be gradual or acute, but there are usually earlier signs of dysfunction in both **premorbid functioning**, the period from birth to the **prodromal phase**. The prodromal phase can range from weeks or months to years before full onset of symptoms. Studies of premorbid functioning reveal subtle signs of problems in motor development, affect, and school performance. Impairments in cognitive functioning are often documented in school records and formal testing much earlier in life (MacCabe et al., 2013; Russell et al., 1997). Some individuals do not present with significant premorbid "clues," but begin to show early signs of psychosis and unusual behavior in the prodromal phase. Nonspecific clinical symptoms seen in the prodromal phase can include affective changes such as depressed or anxious mood, irritability, insomnia, and cognitive changes such as impaired concentration and difficulty attending to tasks. Late-emerging symptoms in the prodromal phase can include suspiciousness, brief hallucinations, and perceptual difficulties (Kulhara, Banerjee, & Dutt, 2008).

The course of the illness varies greatly, with multiple episodes and changeable symptoms. The APA provides a classification of the longitudinal course that can be applied 1 year after initial onset. The course can be classified as a first, multiple, or continuous episode, in either an acute episode or in partial or full remission.

Some individuals are able to maintain independent living and work competitively, while others experience a chronic decline in functioning resulting in the need for 24-hour supervision and care. Approximately 10% to 20% of individuals are able to maintain remission for 5 years after the first psychotic episode, but the majority experience continued relapses (Jibson et al., 2004). Noncompliance with medication and chronic substance abuse significantly increase the risk for relapse (Alvarez-Jimenez et al., 2012). Relapses, which are associated with deterioration in daily functioning, can also be triggered by lack of available psychosocial treatment and support, noncompliance with psychosocial treatment, and environmental stressors (Jibson et al., 2004). Over time, with multiple psychotic episodes, negative and cognitive symptoms may become more prominent while delusions and hallucinations are more likely to decrease in intensity in late middle age (Lieberman et al., 2008).

Other factors that can negatively impact prognosis include male gender, having a gradual and early onset of symptoms, a family history of schizophrenia, poor premorbid functioning, dysfunctional family relationships, and experience of abuse or neglect (Jibson et al., 2004; Walker et al., 2004). Even when medication has been shown to reduce or even stop symptoms such as hallucinations and delusions, cognitive impairments, such as decreased executive functioning and abstract reasoning, are more likely to persist. Individuals with more severe cognitive loss are apt to experience decreased occupational performance and quality of life than do those who demonstrate cognitive improvements (Jibson et al., 2004; Tolman & Kurtz, 2012).

People with schizophrenia die, on average, 12 to 25 years earlier than do those in the general population. These deaths are usually related to pulmonary, cardiac, and infectious diseases and cancer (Colton & Manderscheid, 2006; Crump, Winkleby, Sundquist, & Sundquist, 2013). Complications from antipsychotic medications, self-neglect, fear of health institutions, lack of access to health care, and increased suicide rate (Meltzer, 2002) are all contributing factors to this disparity in life expectancy. Individuals with schizophrenia are also at a higher risk of death from a motor vehicle accident or when killed by a car as a pedestrian (Treatment Advocacy Center, 2009).

DIAGNOSIS

The criteria for a diagnosis of schizophrenia require the presence of symptoms for a period of at least 1 month, with some clinical signs present for at least 6 months (APA, 2013). The age of onset for schizophrenia is between 16 and 30 years of age and is typically earlier for males than for females. Diagnosis after age 45 is unusual (National Institute of Mental Health [NIMH], 2009). Early-onset schizophrenia, however, can be diagnosed in childhood or adolescence. Childhood onset refers to a diagnosis of schizophrenia before the age of 13 and is characterized by an insidious onset, rather than a clear first episode, with multiple neurodevelopmental impairments present prior to onset of psychotic or negative symptoms (Arango et al., 2008). Adolescent onset usually has a clear first episode, with a mean onset age of 15 (Arango et al., 2008).

MEDICAL/SURGICAL MANAGEMENT

The focus of treatment is to reduce or eliminate symptoms and to provide environmental supports to enhance quality of life. The primary treatment for symptom reduction continues to be medication, although technological advances show promise for other medical or surgical approaches to treatment.

■ Pharmacological Treatment

Prior to the 1950s, treatment consisted of institutionalization, including physical restraints, seclusion, and even lobotomy. There was no medication for relief of clinical symptoms. Thorazine was the first **antipsychotic medication** introduced in the 1950s. Other similar medications, referred to as "first-generation" or "typical" antipsychotics, were also quickly developed. This first group of medications, which included Haldol, Prolixin, and Navane, proved effective in decreasing positive symptoms of schizophrenia by blocking dopamine receptors. Unfortunately, the side effects were often severe, including **extrapyramidal syndrome** (abnormal movements similar to Parkinson's disease), **tardive dyskinesia** (motor abnormalities such as writhing movements), cardiac problems, and heavy sedation.

The first atypical antipsychotics were introduced in the late 1980s. Atypical antipsychotics differ from the typical or first-generation antipsychotics in that they occupy different neurotransmitter receptors. Clozapine (Clozaril) was introduced in 1989 and received FDA approval in 1990. It is considered to be effective in treating psychotic symptoms for individuals who were previously unresponsive to other first-generation medications. A major drawback, however, is the potential for serious side effects, including development of agranulocytosis, which requires regular blood work to monitor white blood cell count. Despite its effectiveness, it is not a favored medication among people with schizophrenia due to the medical risk, additional side effects, inconvenience, and excessive cost (Jibson et al., 2004).

Other atypical antipsychotics introduced since the 1990s include risperidone (Risperdal), olanzapine (Zyprexa), quetiapine (Seroquel), ziprasidone (Geodon), aripiprazole (Abilify), and paliperidone (Invega). They also are less likely to cause motor abnormalities such as extrapyramidal effects, but there can be other side effects including sedation, mild hypotension, weight gain, akathisia (restlessness), dry mouth, and constipation (Lieberman et al., 2005; NIMH, 2009).

Serious side effects from medications contribute to a decreased quality of life. In addition to symptoms such as constipation, blurred vision, and impaired sleep, individuals may also experience motor impairments such as tardive dyskinesia, which is characterized by involuntary facial and body movements. For some, tardive dyskinesia remains a permanent condition even when medications are stopped.

■ Repetitive Transcranial Magnetic Stimulation

While medications have been successful in reducing symptoms such as hallucinations and delusions, there has been no proven treatment for negative symptoms. Transcranial magnetic stimulation (TMS) was developed in the 1980s to study brain function. It involves creating a magnetic field that passes through the skull, creating a current in the brain that activates nearby nerve cells. A coil of wire, wrapped in plastic, is held to the head, while a capacitor is discharged to create the magnetic field. Researchers learned that repeated applications (repetitive transcranial magnetic stimulation [rTMS]) over the course of several days appear to affect brain activity. The magnetic field can be targeted to specific regions of the brain where nerve cells are associated with psychiatric symptoms. Recent studies of rTMS, while inconclusive, show promise in reducing negative symptoms of schizophrenia (Diabac-de Lange, Knegtering, & Aleman, 2010; Matheson, Green, Loo, & Carr, 2010). Other studies of rTMS have also shown effectiveness in reducing positive symptoms of auditory hallucinations, when used in conjunction with antipsychotic medication (Bagati, Haque Nizamie, & Prakash, 2009).

■ Electroconvulsive Therapy

Electroconvulsive therapy (ECT) is a medical procedure that consists of inducing a seizure by administration of electrical shock using electrodes attached to the scalp. Anesthesia is used for this brief procedure. It is generally administered in a series over the course of days or weeks. The mortality rate for ECT is approximately 2 deaths per 100,000 treatments and usually are associated with anesthesia complications (Fink & Taylor, 2007). ECT is used for treating severe symptoms, such as catatonia, that do not respond to medication. Studies indicate some short-term benefits in global functioning when used in conjunction with antipsychotic medication (Tharyan & Adams, 2005). A more recent systematic study, however, examined randomized controlled trials of ECT compared to sham ECT (Poublon & Haagh, 2011), a placebo treatment, and found that the sham ECT group also demonstrated some improvements over time, suggesting a placebo effect. Side effects of ECT include confusion, experienced immediately after the procedure, as well as short-term memory loss for about 1 to 2 weeks.

OTHER PSYCHOTIC DISORDERS

In addition to schizophrenia, there are several other psychotic disorders as classified by the APA (2013). Schizophrenia and the following disorders all share the common feature of active psychosis.

■ Schizophreniform Disorder

Clinical features are nearly identical to schizophrenia with the exception of two differences: (1) Total duration of the illness is more than 1 month but less than 6 months, and (2) occupational performance deficits may not be present. About one-third of all people diagnosed with schizophreniform disorder will experience remission within the 6-month period, but the remaining two-thirds are likely to eventually be diagnosed with either schizophrenia or schizoaffective disorder.

■ Schizoaffective Disorder

Clinical symptoms of schizophrenia are present, including delusions or hallucinations, but at some point in the course of the illness, a major depressive, manic, or mixed episode occurs. There are two subtypes of schizoaffective disorder, depending on the mood presentation: bipolar type, which includes a manic or mixed episode, and depressive type. Age of onset is typically in early adulthood, but can range from adolescence to late life.

■ Delusional Disorder

Symptoms include the presence of delusions lasting at least 1 month. Auditory or visual hallucinations may be present, but are not prominent. Olfactory or tactile hallucinations may be both present and prominent if they relate to the delusion. For example, if a person believes he or she has an unknown infectious disease, the person may experience related body sensations or odors. Activities of daily living skills are not significantly impaired, although work, social, and relationship problems can occur as a result of the delusional beliefs. For example, those who experience jealous or persecutory delusions may demonstrate angry or violent behavior. Age of onset for delusional disorders is highly variable, from adolescence to late life. The course of the illness can also be variable, from chronic to full remission within several months.

■ Brief Psychotic Disorder

While symptoms can emerge in adolescence or early childhood, the average age of onset is mid-30s. The disorder is characterized by a sudden onset of psychotic symptoms or highly disorganized or catatonic behavior lasting between 1 day and 1 month. The brief episode is followed by a return to premorbid functioning. There may or may not be a precipitating stressor, such as death of a loved one or a traumatic experience in war combat. Individuals experience great confusion and dramatic mood shifts. Occupational performance can be significantly impaired, and there is an increased risk of suicide due to impulsivity.

■ Psychotic Disorder Due to Another Medical Condition

In this disorder, delusions or hallucinations are a direct result of a general medical condition, such as epilepsy, brain lesions, Huntington's disease, hepatic or renal disease, lupus, or auditory or visual nerve injuries. The course can be varied, from a single episode to recurrent. Even when the underlying medical condition is resolved, psychotic symptoms can continue, particularly in cases of brain injury.

■ Substance/Medication-Induced Psychotic Disorder

Clinical features include hallucinations or delusions directly due to effects of a drug or exposure to a toxin. In cases of intoxication or withdrawal from an abused drug, the hallucinations and delusions are more severe and present well beyond what would be expected during the intoxication/withdrawal/detoxification stages. Onset can result from a single use of a substance or following prolonged use.

■ Catatonia Specifier

The presence of multiple catatonia symptoms may be present in a number of disorders. When it accompanies another mental disorder (Catatonia Associated with Another mental disorder) or is the result of a medical condition (Catatonic Disorder Due to Another Medical Condition), the diagnostic code will be included. A category of Unspecified Catatonia is used when some catatonic symptoms are present and disruptive to daily functioning but do not meet full criteria or there is not enough clinical information to make a more thorough diagnosis.

■ Other Specified Schizophrenia Spectrum and Other Psychotic Disorder

This diagnostic category is used when individuals present with some psychotic symptoms and significant functional impairments that do not meet the full criteria for any specific psychotic disorder. For example, the individual may present with only auditory hallucinations. In documenting the diagnosis, the healthcare provider specifies this as the reason for the "other" diagnosis.

■ Unspecified Schizophrenia Spectrum and Other Psychotic Disorder

Similar to the "other" diagnostic category described above, this diagnosis applies to individuals whose symptoms do not meet full criteria for any of the other schizophrenia spectrum disorders. It differs in that the healthcare provider cannot specify the reasons for the limited diagnosis due to a lack of thorough clinical information.

IMPACT ON OCCUPATIONAL PERFORMANCE

Because schizophrenia typically presents in early adulthood, a period of developing new roles and responsibilities such as career, life partnership, independent living, and parenthood, its lifelong effects are profound. Functional abilities vary greatly, but can be positively affected by environmental factors such as the presence of social support systems, financial assistance, and opportunities for housing or work.

Overall, quality of life is significantly lower for people with schizophrenia, as they represent lower socioeconomic status, are typically unemployed or underemployed, and are at higher risk of homelessness and incarceration (WHO, 2009). They are more likely to be victims of crime, especially violent crimes, and to abuse alcohol and/or drugs. Approximately 50% of all people with schizophrenia have a co-occurring diagnosis of substance abuse or dependence (Volkow, 2009). Smoking rates are also high among those with schizophrenia, estimated as high as 60% to 90% (Hahn et al., 2012), and as high as three times the general population (Williams & Foulds, 2007). One reason for the increased smoking rates may be self-medication. Nicotine has been found to stimulate the brain's dopamine receptors, positively impacting sensory processing abilities, including decreased startling response and eye-tracking deficits (Winterer, 2010).

■ Basic Activities of Daily Living

The ability to manage personal health is significantly compromised. Antipsychotic medications can cause weight gain, cardiac problems, and other health risks. Many individuals have impaired motor functioning, visual processing

deficits, and cognitive deficits, which, coupled with avolition and anhedonia symptoms, can limit interest or ability to participate in traditional exercise, nutrition, or smoking cessation programs.

Avolition, anhedonia, and disorganized behavior can also affect one's ability to initiate and complete self-care tasks such as grooming and hygiene. Impaired visual processing and difficulty interpreting visual stimuli can be associated with excessive application of makeup or ineffective attempts to bathe or shave thoroughly.

■ Instrumental Activities of Daily Living

The majority of people with schizophrenia do not live or work independently. The ability to work or succeed in school; to manage a household including cooking, cleaning, laundry, and budgeting; or to function as a caregiver requires multiple skills such as higher level cognitive processes, sensorimotor skills, and social interaction skills, all of which can be affected by the symptoms of schizophrenia. Those who experience repeated relapses over time, which often involve hospitalization, demonstrate an overall decline in functioning, which limits opportunities for independent living.

■ Education

There is some evidence of impaired academic performance in premorbid functioning as well as during the prodromal phase, with standardized testing and general IQ scores in a significantly lower range than the general population (Fuller et al., 2002; Jibson et al., 2004). Many individuals experience their first acute onset in young adulthood, which can derail plans for post–high school education or graduation. In fact, worldwide, about one-third of all people with schizophrenia do not graduate from high school (WHO, 2009). While antipsychotic medication can be effective in treating symptoms such as hallucinations and delusions, there is no intervention that has been shown to create meaningful improvements in cognitive functioning. For the vast majority of those with schizophrenia, ongoing cognitive impairments persist and can have a major impact on academic success.

■ Work

Competitive work situations require multiple job-specific skills, the ability to learn new information quickly, and the ability to interact effectively with coworkers, customers, and superiors. Individuals with schizophrenia are more likely to lack college education or other technical or skilled trade certifications. Even with supported employment assistance, people with schizophrenia are more likely to be placed in minimum wage jobs such as fast-food work, which requires the ability to process and respond quickly while maintaining effective communication with coworkers. These work environments are often too demanding for the individual with active symptoms of schizophrenia. Successful work environments provide structured tasks, additional time allotted to complete work, the ability to work part-time hours, and opportunities for job coaching, particularly when new expectations are introduced.

■ Leisure and Social Participation

Symptoms of anhedonia and avolition can play a crucial role in limiting involvement in leisure activities. Psychosocial functioning may be impaired by both symptoms of asociality and affective symptoms, such as flattened affect and the ability to recognize and reciprocate appropriate social cues. People with schizophrenia typically have less financial and transportation resources for recreation, fewer social contacts, and less interest in leisure activities. As a result, they are more likely to be socially isolated. In fact, those living in independent or semi-independent apartments with fewer opportunities for social participation and support report higher levels of loneliness than do those living in group homes (Schwartz & Gronemann, 2009). Additionally, engagement in physically active forms of leisure has been found to be associated with lower negative emotion (McCormick, Snethen, Smith, & Lysaker, 2012).

CASE STUDY 1

Joe, a thin, middle-aged man, can often be seen walking about downtown, wearing a cap fashioned out of aluminum foil, pulling a handcart loaded with assorted household items and clothing. He is well known to the mental health community and is a familiar sight to local residents. Joe grew up in a middle class family, the only child of parents who were both accountants. His parents described him as a happy baby and a bright student, who had attended college to study engineering. But things began to change for Joe and his family when he moved 1 hour away to the state university when he was 19. Although his teen years were marked by a gradual withdrawal from friends and family, he began to demonstrate more socially bizarre behaviors while at college and when home on weekends. He started dressing in dark, heavy, hooded clothing even in warm weather and developed an intense preoccupation with watching the C-SPAN television channel. His parents were concerned about his behavior, but hoped it was a temporary phase of adapting to his changing life.

During winter break of his sophomore year in college, while his parents were vacationing in Mexico, Joe was seen by neighbors in the park near his family home wearing camouflage and sleeping in a small pup tent. Police were called, and Joe hid in his tent, refusing to speak to them. He was forcibly removed and taken to the local psychiatric hospital for emergency admission. During his evaluation by the on-call psychiatrist, he revealed that he had moved out of his home because he had discovered "bugs" planted throughout the house. He believed that he was under surveillance by the CIA and was worried that his parents had been arrested. He reported that he had been suspicious of a plot against him for quite some time, but that this final "discovery" was the confirmation for which he was waiting. When the staff arranged for him to speak to his parents, who reassured him they were only on vacation, Joe was convinced that CIA agents were impersonating their voices. A physical exam including blood testing was conducted to rule out any medical or drug-related cause of the psychosis. His parents were interviewed to obtain pertinent social and medical history. They shared that he had experienced some problems over the past 2 years in getting along with roommates and was only sporadically attending his classes, resulting in low grades. Joe was diagnosed with schizophrenia, first episode, currently in acute episode and admitted to the inpatient program under court order. He was given antipsychotic medications and discharged to his parents upon their return home. He was not able to return to college as planned. He attempted to enroll at the local community colleges for various classes, but was never able to complete the courses.

Joe has been in and out of the psychiatric hospital numerous times in the past 25 years. His admissions are typically preceded by him not taking his medications, which results in a return of delusions that he is under CIA surveillance. He has never been employed and has never had a significant-other relationship. He is suspicious of others, and so he will not consent to living in a room and board facility or group home. His attempts at independent living in community apartments are usually short-lived. He has been evicted for inability to pay rent as well as for unsafe conditions in the residence, such as hoarding and not cleaning. He resides for brief periods with his parents and has had numerous episodes of street homelessness.

CASE STUDY 2

Maggie was diagnosed with schizoaffective disorder, depressive type, at age 20, during her last year of college, when she began hearing voices telling her she was ugly and stupid. She became increasingly depressed and eventually attempted suicide. She was hospitalized at a local medical hospital as there was no mental health inpatient facility or program in the area. The attending doctor prescribed an aggressive course of psychotropic medication. After a 48-hour stay, when Maggie was no longer actively suicidal, she was discharged with a prescription and a referral to follow up with outpatient counseling. She took the medication as prescribed for 3 months, but experienced serious side effects such as gaining 20 lb, abnormal eye movements, and eventually developing diabetes. Although she had only been an occasional cigarette smoker, she began chain-smoking and began smoking marijuana almost daily. She described her cigarette and marijuana smoking as a way to cope with her constant anxiety.

During this initial 3-month period, Maggie was unable to return to school or her 10-hour-per-week work-study job she had held at the college bookstore. She told her parents she would take the medication but that she wasn't going to counseling "with all those crazy people." She moved back in with her parents and no longer socialized with her dorm roommates or college friends. She summarized her feelings during that time stating, "I felt so lonely and isolated. I was embarrassed about how I looked and I was too nervous to be around anyone. I mostly watched TV and ate a lot of junk food. I was so afraid I was going to be like this for the rest of my life. I thought about suicide, too." After talking with a family friend who was a mental health case manager, Maggie researched the Recovery Center, a community drop-in support program in a nearby town, and she began attending regularly. With help from the staff and peer support specialists over the past 2 years, Maggie has learned to advocate for herself, working with a psychiatrist to find a better medication at a lower dosage with fewer side effects. She participates in cognitive-behavioral therapy, focusing on learning healthier coping strategies. She would also like to learn yoga and be more active physically.

Maggie returned to school part-time and completed her bachelor's degree. While she still has what she calls her "bad days," she has been stable and has not been rehospitalized. She continues to live at home but has a goal to get her own apartment. She is now passionate about helping others and has been hired as a peer leader at the Recovery Center. The people she has met there have become a strong support system for her. She often speaks to community groups as part of a panel of peer support specialists, working to end the stigma of mental illness. Maggie says of her mental illness, "This is not the road I envisioned for myself, but it has shaped who I am and I am a better person for it."

RECOMMENDED LEARNING RESOURCES

National Alliance on Mental Illness (NAMI)
3803 N. Fairfax Dr., Ste. 100
Arlington, VA 22203
Phone: 703-524-7600
Fax: 703-524-9094
www.nami.org

National Institute of Mental Health (NIMH)
Science Writing, Press, and Dissemination Branch
6001 Executive Boulevard, Room 8184, MSC 9663
Bethesda, MD 20892-9663

Phone: 1-866-615-6464
Fax: 301-443-4279
www.nimh.nih.gov

Brain and Behavior Research Foundation
90 Park Avenue, 16th Floor
New York, NY 10016
Phone: 800-829-8289
https://bbrfoundation.org

Torrey, E. F. (2001). *Surviving schizophrenia: A manual for families, consumers, and providers.* New York: Harper Collins Publishing.

REFERENCES

Alvarez-Jimenez, M., Priede, A., Hetrick, S. E., Bendall, S., Killackey, E., Parker, A. G., … Gleeson, J. F. (2012). Risk factors for relapse following treatment for first episode psychosis: A systematic review and meta-analysis of longitudinal studies. *Schizophrenia Research.* doi:10.1016/j.schres.2012.05.007

American Psychiatric Association. (2013). *Diagnostic and statistical manual of mental disorders: DSM-5.* Washington, DC: Author.

Arango, C., Moreno, C., Martinez, S., Parellada, M., Desco, M., Moreno, D., … Rapoport, J. (2008). Longitudinal brain changes in early-onset psychosis. *Schizophrenia Bulletin, 34,* 341–353.

Bagati, D., Haque Nizamie, S., & Prakash, R. (2009). Effect of augmentatory repetitive transcranial magnetic stimulation on auditory hallucinations in schizophrenia: Randomized controlled study. *Australian and New Zealand Journal of Psychiatry, 43,* 386–392. doi:10.1080/00048670802653315

Bediou, B., Asri, F., Brunelin, J., Krolak-Salmon, P., D'Amato, T., Saoud, M., & Tazi, I. (2007). Emotion recognition and genetic vulnerability to schizophrenia. *British Journal of Psychiatry, 191,* 126–130. doi: 10.1192/bjp.bp.106.028829

Brown, A. S., & Derkits, E. J. (2010). Prenatal infection and schizophrenia: A review of epidemiologic and translational studies. *The American Journal of Psychiatry, 167,* 261–280. doi: 10.1176/appi.ajp.2009.09030361

Cannon, M., Jones, P. B., & Murray, R. M. (2002). Obstetric complications and schizophrenia: Historical and met-analytic review. *American Journal of Psychiatry, 159,* 1080–1092.

Choi, Y. K., & Tarazi, F. I. (2010). Alterations in dopamine and glutamate neurotransmission in tetrahydrobiopterin deficient spr–/– mice: Relevance to schizophrenia. *Biochemistry and Molecular Biology Reports, 43,* 593–598. doi:10.5483/BMBRep.2010.43.9.593

Chung, Y. S., Mathews, J. R., & Barch, D. M. (2011). The effects of context processing on different aspects of social cognition in schizophrenia. *Schizophrenia Bulletin, 37,* 1048–1056. doi:10.1093/schbul/sbq012

Colton, C. W., & Manderscheid, R. W. (2006). Congruencies in increased mortality rates, years of potential life lost, and causes of death among public mental health clients in eight states. *Preventing Chronic Disease, 3,* 1–14. Retrieved from http://www.cdc.gov/pcd/issues/2006/apr/05_0180.htm

Crump, C., Winkleby, M. A., Sundquist, K., & Sundquist, J. (2013). Comorbidities and mortality in persons with schizophrenia: A Swedish national cohort study. *American Journal of Psychiatry, 170,* 324–333. doi:10.1176/appi.ajp.2012.12050599

Diabac-de Lange, J. J., Knegtering, R., & Aleman, A. (2010). Repetitive transcranial magnetic stimulation for negative symptoms of schizophrenia: Review and meta analysis. *Journal of Clinical Psychiatry, 71,* 411–418. doi: 10.4088/JCP.08r04808yel

De Peri, L., Crescini, A., Deste, G., Fusar-Poli, P., Sacchetti, E., & Vita, A. (2012). Brain structural abnormalities at the onset of schizophrenia and bipolar disorder: A meta-analysis of controlled magnetic resonance imaging studies. *Current Pharmaceutical Design, 18,* 486–494. doi:10.2174/138161212799316253

Duhig, M., Patterson, S., Connell, M., Foley, S., Capra, C., Dark, F., … Scott, J. (2015). The prevalence and correlates of childhood trauma in patients with early psychosis. *Australian and New Zealand Journal of Psychiatry, 49*, 651–659. doi:10.1177/0004867415575379

Fink, M., & Taylor, M. A. (2007). Electroconvulsive therapy: Evidence and challenges. *Journal of the American Medical Association, 298*, 330–332.

Fuller, R., Nopoulos, P., Arndt, S., O'Leary, D., Ho, B. C., & Andreason, N. C. (2002). Longitudinal assessment of premorbid cognitive functioning in patients with schizophrenia through examination of standardized scholastic test performance. *American Journal of Psychiatry, 159*, 1183–1189.

Gyllenberg, D., Sourander, A., Surcel, H. M., Hinkka-Yli-Salomaki, S., McKeaque, I. W., & Brown, A. S. (2015). Hypothyroxinemia during gestation and offspring schizophrenia in a national birth cohort. *Biological Psychiatry.* Advance online publication. doi: 10.1016/j.biopsych.2015.06.014

Hahn C., Hahn E., Dettling, M., Gunturkun, O., Ta, T. M., & Neuhaus, A. H. (2012). Effects of smoking history on selective attention in schizophrenia. *Neuropharmacology, 62*, 1897–1902. doi:10.1016/j.neuropharm.2011.12.032

Jibson, M. D., Glick, I. D., & Tandon, R. (2004). Schizophrenia and other psychotic disorders. *Focus, 2*(1), 17–30.

Karl, T., & Arnold, J. C. (2014). Schizophrenia: A consequence of gene-environment interactions? *Frontiers in Behavioral Neuroscience, 8*, 435. doi:10.3389/fnbeh.2014.00435

Kaur, H., Jojodia, A., Grover, S., Baghel, R., Gupta, M., Jain, S., & Kukreti, R. (2014). Genetic variations of PIP4K2A confer vulnerability to poor antipsychotic response in severely ill schizophrenia patients. *Public Library of Science, 9*, e102556. doi: 10.1371/journal.pone.0102556

Keefe, R. S., & Harvey, P. D. (2012). Cognitive impairment in schizophrenia. *Handbook of Experimental Pharmacology, 213*, 11–37. doi: 10.1007/978-3-642-25758-2_2

Kempton, M. J., Stahl, D., Williams, S. C. R., & DeLisi, L. E. (2010). Progressive lateral ventricular enlargement in schizophrenia: A meta-analysis of longitudinal MRI studies. *Schizophrenia Research, 120*, 54–62. doi: 10.1016/j.schres.2010.03.036

Koethe, D., Kranaster, L., Hoyer, C., Gross, S., Neatby, M. A., Schultze-Lutter, F., ... Leweke, F. M. (2009). Binocular depth inversion as a paradigm of reduced visual information processing in prodromal state, antipsychotic-naïve and treated schizophrenia. *European Archives of Psychiatry and Clinical Neuroscience, 259*, 195–202. doi:10.1007/s00406-008-0851-6

Kulhara, P., Banerjee, A., & Dutt, A. (2008). Early intervention in schizophrenia. *Indian Journal of Psychiatry, 50*, 128–134.

Leask, S. J. (2004). Environmental influences in schizophrenia: The known and the unknown. *Advances in Psychiatry, 10*, 323–330.

Lieberman, J. A., Drake, R. E., Sederer, L. I., Belger, A., Keefe, R., Perkins, D., & Stroup, S. (2008). Science and recovery in schizophrenia. *Psychiatric Services, 59*, 487–496.

Lieberman, J. A., Stroup, S. T., McEvoy, J. P., Swartz, M. S., Rosenheck, R. A., Perkins, D. O., ... Hsiao, J. K. (2005). Effectiveness of antipsychotic drugs in patient with chronic schizophrenia. *New England Journal of Medicine, 353*, 1209–1223.

MacCabe, J. H., Wicks, S., Lofying, S., David, A. S., Berndtsson, A., Gustafsson, J. E., Allebeck, P., & Dalman, C. (2013). Decline in cognitive performance between ages 13 and 18 years and the risk for psychosis in adulthood: A Swedish longitudinal cohort study in males. *JAMA Psychiatry, 70*(3), 261–270. doi: 10.1001/2013.jamapsychiatry.43

Matheson, S. L., Green, M. J., Loo, C., & Carr, V. J. (2010). A change in the conclusions of a recent systematic meta-review: Repetitive transcranial magnetic stimulation is effective for the negative symptoms of schizophrenia. *Schizophrenia Research.* Advance online publication. doi: 10.1016/j.schres 2010.05 029

McCormick, B. P., Snethen, G., Smith, R. L., & Lysaker, P. H. (2012). Active leisure in the emotional experience of people with schizophrenia. *Therapeutic Recreation Journal, 46*(3), 179–190.

McGrath, J., Saha, S., Chant, D., & Welham, J. (2008). Schizophrenia: A concise overview of incidence, prevalence, and mortality. *Epidemiologic Reviews, 30*, 67–76.

Meltzer, H. Y. (2002). Suicidality in schizophrenia: A review of the evidence for risk factors and treatment options. *Current Psychiatry Reports, 4*, 279–283.

National Institute of Mental Health. (2009). *Schizophrenia* (NIH Publication No. 09-3517). Bethesda, MD: U.S. Department of Health and Human Services.

Poublon, N. A., & Haagh, M. (2011). The efficacy of ECT in the treatment of schizophrenia: A systematic review. *Erasmus Journal of Medicine, 2*(1), 16–19.

Russell, A. J., Munro, J. C., Jones, P. B., Hemsley, D. R., & Murray, R. M. (1997). Schizophrenia and the myth of intellectual decline. *American Journal of Psychiatry, 154*, 635–639.

Sawa, A., & Snyder, S. H. (2002). Schizophrenia: Diverse approaches to a complex disease. *Science, 296*, 692–695.

Schmitt, A., Malchow, B., Hasan, A., & Falkai, P. (2014). The impact of environmental factors in severe psychiatric disorders. *Frontiers*

in Neuroscience, 8, 19, 1–10. doi: 10.3389/
fnins.2014.00019

Schwartz, C., & Gronemann, O. C. (2009). The
contribution of self-efficacy, social support and
participation in the community to predicting loneliness among persons with schizophrenia living in
supported residences. *Israel Journal of Psychiatry
and Related Sciences, 46*(2), 120–129.

Sun, D., Phillips, L., Velakoulis, D., Yung, A.,
McGorry, P. D., Wood, S. J., … Pantelis, C.
(2009). Progressive brain structural changes
mapped as psychosis develops in 'at risk' individuals. *Schizophrenia Research, 108,* 85–92.

Tharyan, P., & Adams, C. E. (2005). Electroconvulsive
therapy for schizophrenia. *Cochrane Database of
Systematic Reviews, 2,* CD000076.

Tolman, A. W., & Kurtz, M. M. (2012). Neurocognitive
predictors of objective and subjective quality of life
in individuals with schizophrenia: A meta-analytic
investigation. *Schizophrenia Bulletin, 38,* 304–315.
doi:10.1093/schbul/sbq077

Treatment Advocacy Center (2009).
Schizophrenia Fact Sheet. Retrieved from:
www.treatmentadvocacycenter.org/problem/
consequences-of-non-treatment/schizophrenia

Veen, N. D., Selten, J. P., van der Tweel, I., Feller, W.
G., Hoek, H. W., & Kahn, R. S. (2004). Cannabis

use and age at onset of schizophrenia. *American
Journal of Psychiatry, 161,* 501–506.

Volkow, N. D. (2009). Substance use disorders in
schizophrenia—Clinical implications of comorbidity. *Schizophrenia Bulletin, 35,* 469–472.

Walker, E., Kestler, L., Bollini, A., & Hochman, K.
M. (2004). Schizophrenia: Etiology and course.
Annual Review of Psychology, 55, 401–430.

Williams, J. M., & Foulds, J. (2007). Clinical Case
Conference: Successful tobacco dependence
treatment in schizophrenia. *American Journal of
Psychiatry, 164*(2), 222–227.

Winterer, G. (2010). Why do patients with schizophrenia smoke? *Current Opinion in Psychiatry, 23,*
112–119. doi: 10.1097/YCO.013e3283366643

Woodward, N. D., & Cascio, C. J. (2015). Resting-
state functional connectivity in psychiatric
disorders. *JAMA Psychiatry.* Advance online publication. doi: 10.1001/jamapsychiatry.2015.0484

World Health Organization. (2014, October).
Schizophrenia Fact Sheet No. 397. Retrieved from:
http://www.who.int/mediacentre/factsheets/fs397/en/

World Health Organization. (2009). *Discussion paper:
Mental health, poverty and development.* Geneva,
Switzerland: World Health Organization. Retrieved
from: http://www.who.int/entity/nmh/publications/
discussion_paper_en.pdf

10 Anxiety Disorders

Christine K. Urish

As the occupational therapist arrives on the inpatient psychiatric unit, she finds Jillian pacing up and down the hallway. Jillian was admitted last evening as a result of her significant functional decline in all areas of occupational performance. She has been diagnosed with generalized anxiety disorder by her psychiatrist. "I know my psychiatrist has written a referral for me to attend occupational therapy; I know all about occupational therapy," she states. "I have worked in this hospital on the pediatrics unit for quite some time. I know the occupational therapists come to the pediatrics unit and play with the children and try to get them to move and interact with their parents. I don't need to play. I am so anxious. I worry all the time, and it seems as if I worry about everything. I don't really think occupational therapy and play will help me at all. I cannot sleep or rest, and I am very worried that I will be fired because I'm not functioning as I should because I am anxious and tired." The occupational therapist suggests Jillian come with her to discuss occupational therapy services and to complete an initial interview. The occupational therapist wants to determine how Jillian's anxiety is impacting her ability to do everyday things. As the occupational therapist walks down the hall, Jillian responds by saying, "I'm not able to be a nurse anymore; then what will I do?" "This play therapy is not going to help my anxiety, I cannot do anything right and I am certain this is not going to help me." "What in the world was my psychiatrist thinking when he ordered me to attend occupational therapy groups?" "How in the world is this going to help me at all?" Jillian is obviously thinking that occupational therapy is one-dimensional. In her mind, occupational therapy is about play. The occupational therapist knows that she will have to explain to Jillian how occupational therapy services on the pediatrics unit differ from an inpatient psychiatric setting. She also knows that she will have to do her best to try and convince Jillian that occupational therapy can be beneficial to her. The occupational therapist feels that this information could assist Jillian in improving her performance skills and decreasing her anxiety. The occupational therapist looks forward to the challenge of working with Jillian both individually and in a group of other patients diagnosed with anxiety disorders.

If Jillian will learn relaxation techniques and mindfulness strategies and develop her skill at using them, through participation in occupational therapy services, her level of anxiety may decrease. She may find that she is better able to sleep at night, and thus, her energy level and concentration may improve. The occupational therapist also has a feeling that Jillian may be overly focused on her success and performance at work, and that Jillian's overall life balance—and more specifically her leisure lifestyle—may be limited. As an occupational therapist, she is concerned about Jillian's overall ability to balance her work, activities of daily living, instrumental activities of daily living (IADLs), continuing education required by her employment status as a nurse, sleep and rest, leisure, and social participation. Although Jillian thinks that all occupational therapy includes is play, this therapist will work with Jillian to assist her in understanding that a balance of occupations, occupational performance and occupational engagement, is essential to being productive.

INTRODUCTION

This chapter discusses anxiety disorders: how they are classified, are diagnosed, and differ from "normal" feelings. Evidence-based research on intervention will be presented throughout the chapter. The impact of anxiety disorders on performance skills in occupation will be examined through the detailed case studies at the end of the chapter. Learning resources for development of additional knowledge are provided at the end of the chapter as well.

DEFINITION AND DESCRIPTION

Anxiety is defined as "apprehension of danger, and dread accompanied by restlessness, tension, tachycardia, and dyspnea unattached to a clearly identifiable stimulus" (Dirckx, 2005). It is important to distinguish fear from anxiety. **Fear** is similar in that it is an alerting response to a known, external, definite threat. Anxiety is a response to a threat that is unknown, vague, and internal, and it can lead to conflicted feelings (Sadock, Sadock, & Ruiz, 2015). It is normal to have some degree of anxiety in our lives: "Will I get a raise during my review with my boss?" "Will my dress be appropriate for the social occasion to which I am driving?" "Will I get a good grade on the test I recently completed?" Most often, someone can be nervous or anxious about a number of life events but be able to perform daily occupations without incident. In our day-to-day existence, we

experience anxiety, whether or not we recognize it as anxiety. Anxiety can motivate us into action. A certain amount of anxiety or anxious feelings is quite normal. For example, "I'm anxious about my performance review at work at the end of the month, so I will go in early or stay late this week to make sure I am caught up on things" or "I think my clothing is getting tighter; I seem to have put on a few pounds. I need to spend more time exercising to lose some weight and improve my physical appearance." Anxiety, however, can also be pathological, when we worry incessantly about things that we cannot control or change. When this incessant worry begins to negatively impact our ability to work, learn, or socialize, anxiety may be considered pathologic. Anxiety symptoms may vary from individual to individual (Sadock et al., 2015).

CLASSIFICATION OF ANXIETY DISORDERS

The *Diagnostic and Statistical Manual of Mental Disorders*, **Fifth Edition (DSM-5)** has established criteria to determine if anxiety or anxiety-related conditions are pathologic (American Psychiatric Association [APA], 2013). The criteria present both physical and psychological symptoms that must be met for a diagnosis to be made. A significant change from DSM IV-TR to DSM-5 was the change from a large category of anxiety disorders in which 11 disorders were classified. The DSM-5 classifies the previous anxiety disorders in three large categories. These include anxiety disorders, obsessive-compulsive and related disorders, and trauma and stress-related disorders. This chapter focuses on the first category, anxiety disorder. For information on obsessive-compulsive and related disorders, refer to Chapter 13. Complex Trauma is addressed in Chapter 12. Occupational therapists treat clients diagnosed with these disorders in a variety of mental health settings including inpatient, partial hospitalization, and outpatient settings. Occupational therapists also treat clients in a variety of nonmental health settings in which they may observe anxiety symptoms in the clients they treat across the life span. If an occupational therapist is observing a client with anxiety symptoms, they should not be overlooked, as they can significantly impact occupational engagement and performance as well as overall health and quality of life.

Although occupational therapists do not make psychiatric diagnoses, a thorough understanding of the criteria for making such a diagnosis is important for the clinician to facilitate clinical observations. When considering the classification of anxiety disorders within the DSM-5, the following diagnoses are included:

- Separation anxiety disorder
- Selective mutism
- Specific phobia
- Social anxiety disorder, previously known as social phobia
- Panic disorder
- Agoraphobia
- Generalized anxiety disorder
- Substance/medication-induced anxiety disorder
- Anxiety disorder due to another medical condition

■ Panic Disorder

Panic disorder includes short, sudden attacks of fear, fear of losing control, or terror (Johns Hopkins, 2016). The diagnosis of panic disorder includes panic attacks, which recur and are unexpected. A **panic attack** is described as an abrupt surge of intense fear/intense discomfort, which can peak within minutes and at which time four (or more) of the following symptoms occur:

- Heart palpations, increased heart rate or pounding heart
- Sweating

- Shaking or trembling
- Sensation of shortness of breath or feeling of smothering
- Feeling of choking
- Chest discomfort or pain
- Nausea or distress in abdomen
- Feelings of dizziness, light-headedness, or faint
- Chills or sensation of increased heat
- Numbness or sensation of tingling
- Feelings of not being in reality or being separate or detached from oneself
- Fear of loss of control
- Fear of death

At least one of the panic attacks has to be followed by 1 month or more of one or both of the following criteria. An ongoing, persistent concern or worry about additional panic attacks or the consequences of having additional panic attacks. The individual fears he or she will lose control, is experiencing a heart attack, or is "going crazy." Further, the individual experiences a significant maladaptive change in behavior related to previous attacks, for example, engaging in behavior in an attempt to facilitate not having an attack such as avoiding exercise or situations in which they are unfamiliar. It is important to note that the symptoms and associated behavior are not able to be attributed to the physiological effects of a substance (street drugs or prescribed medication) or another medical condition such as a heart condition or hyperthyroidism.

■ Phobia

Phobia refers to irrational fears that lead individuals to often avoid certain objects and specific situations all together (Substance Abuse and Mental Health Services Administration [SAMHSA], 2015). The diagnosis of phobia includes the individual presenting with marked and persistent fear or anxiety regarding an object or situation such as flying on an airplane, sight of certain animals, receiving an injection, sight of blood, or being at a certain elevation/height. It is important to note that in children, this fear or anxiety can be expressed through behavior that includes crying, tantrums, clinging, and lack of movement (APA, 2013). The object or situation that is feared by the individual almost always provokes instant fear or anxiety. As a result, the object or situation is *actively* avoided by the individual, or alternatively the individual may endure exposure to the object or situation with intense fear or anxiety. When considering the level of fear or anxiety regarding the object or situation, it is considered out of proportion to the actual danger posed by the specific object or situation and to the sociocultural context (APA, 2013).

Individuals with phobia demonstrate fear, anxiety, or avoidance, which is persistent and must last more than 6 months. The fear, anxiety, or avoidance of the object or situation causes significant distress in social, occupational, or other areas of life function. It is common for individuals to have multiple specific phobias (APA, 2013). It is important to note that agoraphobia is not included in this category of phobia, rather it is a single category of anxiety disorder.

There are five different types of specific phobias most often observed in adult clinical populations (Fadem, 2012). These phobias, in descending order of frequency seen in clinical settings, include situational, natural environment, blood-injection injury, animal, and other types. Situational phobias include fears of tunnels, bridges, using public transportation, flying in an airplane, and being in closed places. Situational phobias are usually more common in adults than in children. Natural environment phobias include fear of natural occurrences such as lightning, thunder, heights, and deep water. These fears often present in childhood. Blood-injection-injury phobias focus on the fear of receiving an injection or treatment, which requires some invasive bodily procedure. The specific phobia of animals is the fourth most frequently seen phobia in adult clinical populations. This phobia includes insects in addition to animals. The final type of specific phobia is categorized as other type that includes loud sounds, falling, contracting an illness, and choking. A fear of costume characters in children is also considered in this category (Fadem, 2012).

The diagnosis of social phobia, now known as social anxiety disorder, is a marked, persistent fear or anxiety regarding being in one or more social situations where the individual has the potential to be scrutinized by others. This can include social interactions such as meeting unfamiliar individuals, engaging in conversation, being observed by others while eating or drinking, and performing in front of others such as giving a speech. It is important to note that in children, the anxiety must occur in settings that include peers, not just adult interactions (APA, 2013). The person with social anxiety disorder has the fear of his or her anxiety showing and as a result being negatively evaluated, which will result in humiliation and embarrassment. As a result of their anxiety and the negative evaluation of others, they will be rejected or offend others (APA, 2013). Persons with social anxiety disorder experience fear or anxiety in nearly all social situations. Therefore, the individual will go to great lengths to avoid social situations or will endure situations with extreme fear or anxiety. The fear or anxiety experienced is out of proportion to the actual threat of the social situation and to the sociocultural context (APA, 2013). Fear, anxiety, or avoidance is persistent and lasts 6 months or longer and causes a significantly negative impact upon social, occupational, or other significant area of life functioning (APA, 2013). It is important to note that the fear, anxiety, or avoidance cannot be attributed to physiological effect of a substance such as a prescribed medication or a drug of abuse, or another medical condition. The fear, anxiety, or avoidance is not better explained by symptoms present in another mental disorder such as panic disorder, body dysmorphic disorder, or autism spectrum disorder. If another medical condition is present, such as Parkinson's disease, obesity, or disfigurement from an injury or serious burn, the fear, anxiety, or avoidance is unrelated or considered excessive (APA, 2013). This diagnosis has one specifier: whether or not the fear is limited to speaking or performing in public.

■ Agoraphobia

Agoraphobia in the past was considered within the DSM IV-TR within the diagnostic category of phobia. Within the DSM-5, agoraphobia is classified as a separate diagnosis. An individual diagnosed with agoraphobia will demonstrate fear or marked anxiety in two of five situations which include the following:

- Use of public transportation (e.g., plane, train, automobile, bus, ship)
- Being in an open space (e.g., bridge, parking lot, open marketplace)
- Being in an enclosed area (e.g., shopping mall, theatre, movie cinema)
- Being in a crowd or standing in line
- Alone outside of the home (APA, 2013)

The individual diagnosed with agoraphobia fears and avoids these situations because of thoughts that escape may be very difficult or that help may not be available in the event of developing panic-like symptoms or other symptoms that would incapacitate or embarrass the individual, such as the fear of falling or the fear of incontinence, common among the elderly. The agoraphobic situations are avoided, a companion is required, or the situation may be endured, however, with great fear or anxiety. The fear or anxiety experienced by the individual is out of proportion to the actual danger posed by the agoraphobic situations and to the sociocultural context (APA, 2013). To be diagnosed with agoraphobia, the symptoms must persist more than 6 months and cause significant distress or impairment in social, occupational, or other important area of life functioning. If the individual has another medical condition (e.g., Parkinson's disease or inflammatory bowel disease), the fear, anxiety, or avoidance is excessive (APA, 2013).

■ Generalized Anxiety Disorder

This disorder is diagnosed when an individual has excessive worry and anxiety, which occurs more often than not for a period of at least 6 months. This excessive worry or anxiety can include a number of events or activities such as school or work performance or family concerns (APA, 2013). Individuals have difficulty controlling their worry, and they characteristically also have three or more of the following six symptoms:

1. Feelings of being on edge, restless, or keyed up
2. Becoming easily fatigued
3. Feeling as if his or her mind is going blank and difficulty with concentration
4. Irritability
5. Tension in muscles
6. Difficulty with sleep, which can include falling asleep, staying asleep, or restless sleep (APA, 2013)

It is important to note that in children only one of the aforementioned items is required for a diagnosis. The concern of the individual with generalized anxiety disorder is not related to another DSM-5 disorder such as OCD (anxiety about contamination) or weight gain as in anorexia nervosa (APA, 2013). Anxiety, worry, or accompanying physical symptoms cause clinically significant distress or impairment in social, occupational, or other important areas of life functioning (APA, 2013). The symptoms cannot be attributable to another medical condition (e.g., hypothyroidism) or due to physiological effects of a substance (e.g., prescribed medication or drug abuse).

When considering generalized anxiety disorder in children, worry tends to focus on competence or quality of performance. Anxiety disorders may coexist with other disorders such as depression, substance abuse, eating disorders, schizophrenia, personality disorders, or other anxiety disorders (National Institute of Mental Health [NIMH], 2016). Comorbidity of another mental illness was high when individuals were diagnosed with social phobia and generalized anxiety disorder (Brown, Campbell, Lehman, Grisham, & Mancil, 2001). It is important to note that comorbidity between depression and anxiety often goes unnoticed (Bouchard & Verrier, 2005). In individuals diagnosed with an anxiety disorder, up to 45% are diagnosed with major depression at some point in time in their lives. The comorbidity between generalized anxiety disorder and panic disorder is known to exceed 55% (Bouchard & Verrier, 2005). It is important to note that individuals diagnosed with depression do not develop a secondary anxiety disorder, rather individuals with anxiety disorder are known to more often develop a comorbidity of depression (Bouchard & Verrier, 2005). Individuals diagnosed with social phobia also had high levels of comorbidity with avoidant personality disorder (Rettew, 2000). When considering anxiety disorders from a comprehensive perspective, it is important to note that anxiety disorders may coexist with cancer and heart disease as well (NIMH, 2016). It is important for clinicians to consider comorbidity to select the most effective intervention for individuals with anxiety disorders and other coexisting conditions in everyday practice.

■ Etiology

The understanding of the causes of anxiety has increased in recent years as neurochemical and physical pathways of fear and anxiety have been critically examined (Brantley, 2007). Despite this, more research is needed as we are far from having a clear understanding of these complex conditions. In examining the causes of anxiety disorders, one must consider the powerful interaction between biology, cognitive/emotional influences, and stress. The likelihood of developing an anxiety disorder includes a combination of life experiences, psychological traits, and genetic factors. Anxiety disorders, such as panic disorder, have a stronger genetic basis than do other disorders, although at this time-specific genes have not been identified (United States Surgeon General [USSG], 1999). Women are more at risk for being diagnosed with anxiety disorders than men, although it is not clear as to why. Some researchers suggest the role of gonadal steroid. Other researchers suggest that women's response to stress and their exposure to a wider range of life events is different from those experienced by men (USSG, 1999). There are three major etiologic considerations in examining anxiety disorders. These include biological factors, genetic factors, and psychosocial factors. Three major schools of psychosocial theory have contributed to the understanding of the causes of anxiety: psychoanalytic, behavioral, and existential. Each of these frameworks presents conceptual and practice applications for the treatment of anxiety disorders. According to the biological theories of anxiety, an excessive autonomic reaction is present with increased sympathetic tone. Increased catecholamines are released in addition to increased production of norepinephrine metabolites. **Gamma-aminobutyric acid** (GABA) levels are decreased, and this causes central nervous system hyperactivity. Additionally, a decrease in serotonin causes anxiety, and increased dopaminergic activity is related to anxiety. The temporal cortex activity in those with anxiety is decreased. The center of the brain, locus caeruleus, is hyperactive when anxiety is present, especially during a panic attack (Sadock et al., 2015). Magnetic resonance imaging evidence indicates that individuals with panic disorder have pathology in the temporal lobes of the brain, in particular, in the hippocampus (Sadock et al., 2015). Biological research into the etiology of generalized anxiety disorder has focused on GABA and serotonin receptors.

There are also indications that genetics may play a role in the etiology of anxiety disorders. Despite the fact that well-controlled research studies into panic disorder are limited, available genetic research has indicated that nearly half the individuals with panic disorder have at least one relative affected with an anxiety disorder (Sadock et al., 2015). Approximately 5% of individuals with high levels of anxiety have a variant of the gene associated with serotonin metabolism (Sadock et al., 2015). Phobias also seem to be more common among family members. More specifically, the blood-injection–type phobia has a significantly high familial tendency. Further, first-degree relatives with social phobia are three times more likely to be diagnosed with social phobia than those who have first-degree relatives without a mental disorder (Sadock et al., 2015).

From a psychoanalytic perspective, anxiety is viewed as developmentally related to childhood fears of disintegration and is related to the fear of loss of a loved one or an object or the fear of castration. Clinicians critically examine possible triggers when working with individuals with anxiety disorders. In people diagnosed with phobias, from a psychoanalytic perspective, the individual attempts to repress. When this fails, other defense mechanisms such as avoidance are called upon (Sadock et al., 2015). Individuals diagnosed with generalized anxiety disorder, according to the psychoanalytic perspective, have unresolved unconscious conflicts. Behavioral theories propose that anxiety is a response that is learned from exposure to parental behavior or through the process of classical conditioning. Anxiety disorders include faulty, distorted, or counterproductive thinking patterns (Sadock et al., 2015).

The success of treating individuals with anxiety disorders using a behavioral approach lends credence to this approach in intervention (Sadock et al., 2015). Anxiety is acquired through classical conditioning and observational learning and maintained through operant conditioning. Learning theory is of significance in the treatment of phobias and provides clear explanation for many symptoms experienced by the phobic individual (Sadock et al., 2015). According to the cognitive-behavioral school of thought, an individual with generalized anxiety disorder has an incorrect and inaccurate perception of danger. This inaccuracy is facilitated by selective attention to negative information within the environment, distortion in information processing, and an inability to cope. From an existential perspective, there is no one specifically identifiable stimulus that facilitates the feeling of chronic anxiety in an individual. Anxiety, according to an existential approach, occurs when the individual becomes aware of profound feelings of a lack of meaning in his or her life. This lack of meaning for some individuals is more fear provoking than are thoughts of death. With increased concerns of bioterrorism and nuclear attacks, existential concerns in society have been noted to be increasing (Sadock et al., 2015). Occupational therapy professionals are well suited to address anxiety from an existential perspective as we critically examine meaning and occupation in an individual's day-to-day existence. The cumulative and long-term effects of stress contribute to the development of anxiety and anxiety disorders (Sadock et al., 2015). Chronic stress places an individual at serious risk for physical illness, emotional, social, and spiritual dysfunction. Clearly, unmanaged chronic stress needs to be identified and addressed (Brantley, 2007).

INCIDENCE AND PREVALENCE

In the United States, 40 million persons experience an anxiety disorder in 1 year (SAMHSA, 2015). Generalized anxiety disorder affects 6.8 million adults, which is approximately 3.1% of the US population (Anxiety and Depression Association of America [ADAA], 2014). Panic disorder affects 6 million individuals, with women being more likely to experience this diagnosis than men. Less than 30% of individuals who suffer from anxiety disorders, however, seek treatment (Lepine, 2002). Phobias affect 19 million individuals, with women being twice as likely to be affected as men (ADAA, 2014; World Health Organization [WHO], 2013). Phobias typically begin in childhood; the median age is 7 years of age at onset (ADAA, 2014). The annual cost of anxiety disorders is estimated to be $42 to $47 billion per year, which is one-third of the total cost of all mental illnesses (ADAA, 2014). Of the total cost, $23 billion (54% of cost) is spent in nonpsychiatric medical costs (physician office visits, emergency room costs). Persons diagnosed with anxiety disorders are three to five times more likely to visit their physician and are six times more likely to be hospitalized. These are significant health care costs, in addition to potential for lost productivity for an employer/company. Approximately $4.1 billion (10%) is spent in indirect workplace costs, $1.2 billion (3%) in mortality costs, and $0.8 billion (2%) in pharmaceutical (prescription) costs. Costs to the workplace are attributed more to lost productivity rather than absenteeism. Other than phobia, all anxiety disorders were found to be associated with impairment in work performance. It is important to note that for every one dollar spent in the United States on the treatment of anxiety and depression, a return of four dollars is realized in improved health and ability to work (World Health Organization [WHO], 2016).

■ Panic Disorder

This diagnosis affects 5 million American adults (NIMH, 2016). Women are two to three times as likely to be diagnosed with panic disorder as men. An underdiagnosis of panic disorder in men, however, may skew this distribution (Sadock et al., 2015). The male-to-female ratio for panic disorder without agoraphobia is 1:1 and agoraphobia is 1:2 (Sadock et al., 2015). The ethnic differences present in panic disorder are small. One social factor contributing to the development of a panic disorder is relational, for example, experiencing separation or divorce. The mean age for diagnosis of a panic disorder is 25 years of age (Sadock et al., 2015). This disorder often begins in late adolescence or early adulthood (NIMH, 2011).

■ Phobia

Overall, phobias are the most common mental disorder in the United States with 19.2 million American adults being diagnosed with a specific phobia (NIMH, 2016). Specific phobia is considered to be more common than social phobia. In women, specific phobia is the most common mental disorder. In men, the most common mental disorder is substance-related disorders, with specific phobia being the second most common mental disorder (Sadock et al., 2015). Despite the fact that phobias are the most common mental disorder, a significant number of persons do not seek help for their phobia(s) or are misdiagnosed upon seeking medical attention (Sadock et al., 2015). In considering social anxiety disorder, 15 million American adults are diagnosed with this disorder. Men and women are equally likely to experience social anxiety disorder that usually begins in childhood or early adolescence (NIMH, 2016).

■ Generalized Anxiety Disorder

Studies indicate 6.8 million American adults experience this disorder (NIMH, 2016), with twice as many men as women impacted (Sadock et al., 2015). The lifetime prevalence for this diagnosis is 5%. In anxiety disorder clinics, approximately 25% of the clients treated are diagnosed with generalized anxiety disorder (Sadock et al., 2015). Lifetime prevalence rate for anxiety disorder is 28.8% (Kessler et al., 2005). When considering individuals older than age 55, the best estimate prevalence rate based on Epidemiologic Catchment Area (ECA) data for anxiety disorders was 11.4%. Prevalence of simple phobia in those older than 55 years of age was 7.3%, and panic disorder was 0.5%. The prevalence rates reported indicate that anxiety disorders are common in the general population, with anxiety disorders having the earliest age of onset of mental disorders (Kessler et al., 2005). Prevalence rates for anxiety disorders according to gender are between one-third and two-thirds higher in women (WHO, 2013). Rates of anxiety disorders in women could be due to the perception women hold regarding stressful life events (USSG, 2005). Further, the World Health Organization (WHO) identified gender-specific risk factors, which include gender-based violence (including sexual violence), subordinate social status, socioeconomic disadvantages specific to women, and responsibilities to care for others (WHO, 2013).

SIGNS AND SYMPTOMS

It is important to consider the messages presented by society as we examine the signs and symptoms of anxiety disorders. Messages such as "Don't Worry, Be Happy" abound. It is something that individuals may subscribe to in trying to keep their symptoms "under control," so no one will recognize they are experiencing a great deal of internal turmoil and distress (Roth & Fonagy, 2004). In making a diagnosis of an anxiety disorder, presenting symptoms are the primary consideration. Many anxiety disorders may present with similar physical symptoms. In some disorders, however, the symptoms are more severe than in others. Although all individuals may experience some degree of fear, worry, and anxiety, health care providers need to critically examine the diagnostic criteria relative to the degree of symptoms present and the duration of symptoms.

■ Panic Disorder

The diagnosis of panic disorder includes experiencing a panic attack. Symptoms of a panic attack include heart pounding; increased sweating; feelings of trembling or shakiness; feeling short of breath; feeling as if choking will occur; chest tightness; pain; discomfort; abdominal discomfort; distress or nausea; feeling faint, light-headed, or dizzy; feelings of unreality or depersonalization; fear of going crazy or losing control; fear of death; sensation of tingling or numbness; hot flashes; or chills. Individuals who experience at least four of these symptoms, which appear quickly and peak within 10 minutes, are said to have experienced a panic attack. To obtain the diagnosis of panic disorder, an individual must have experienced four attacks within 4 weeks or one attack within the last month with ongoing worry or concern of when another attack will strike (SAMHSA, 2015). Panic attacks typically are short lived but can last up to 10 minutes in duration. Rarely, attacks will last up to 1 hour and can occur while sleeping. Individuals with panic disorder who reported childhood physical abuse were more likely to have additional comorbid psychiatric diagnoses including depression and had a higher likelihood of attempting suicide (Friedman et al., 2002).

■ Phobia

Symptoms of a phobia include many of the physical symptoms previously presented in panic disorder, including sweating, increased heart rate, and trembling (SAMHSA, 2015). Phobias are traditionally classified by the specific fear through the use of Greek or Latin prefixes. For example, acrophobia is the fear of heights, ailurophobia is the fear of cats, pyrophobia is the fear of fire, and xenophobia is the fear of strangers (Sadock et al., 2015). Diagnosis of a phobia should indicate which type of phobia (animal, natural environment, blood-injection, situational, other) (APA, 2013). If the person experiences extreme anxiety when faced with the feared situation or object, the individual's daily routine, social activities, and interpersonal relationships are impacted, and, because of these fears, a diagnosis may be made by a qualified and trained professional. Phobias may impact many different areas of occupation depending on the specific feared stimulus of the individual. In social anxiety disorder, the symptoms present are similar to those for specific phobia. In addition, the extreme anticipatory anxiety regarding performance or social situations negatively impacts cognition and leads to actual or perceived poor performance in the situations evoking fear, which only further perpetuates the cycle of anxiety (APA, 2013).

COURSE AND PROGNOSIS

■ Panic Disorder

The age of onset for panic disorder is typically early to middle adulthood (Pigott, 2003). However, onset can occur at childhood, early adolescence, or midlife (Sadock et al., 2015). Panic disorder is associated with increased risk of agoraphobia and depression. One relationship factor identified as contributing to panic disorder is the history of a recent divorce or separation (Sadock et al., 2015). Comorbidity of depression, substance abuse, and other anxiety disorders are associated with poor prognosis. Considered a chronic condition, the course of panic disorder is variable across clients as well as within a single individual. Studies that have examined intervention for panic disorder are not easily interpreted because of the inability of researchers to control for the effects of treatment (Sadock et al., 2015). However, 30% to 40% of individuals have presented as symptom free after long-term follow-up. One-half of individuals with this diagnosis continue to have symptoms, but these symptoms are mild enough to not significantly impact their lives. Approximately 10% to 20% of individuals continue to have symptoms despite treatment (Sadock et al., 2015). It is important that clinicians use a psychometrically sound instrument such as the Panic Disorder Severity Scale to monitor clients and determine if symptoms are recurring to facilitate treatment modification. By responding to recurrence of symptoms, a complete relapse may be avoided (Rouillon, 1996). However, whereas some individuals may experience episodic outbreaks with years of remission between, still others may experience continuous severe symptoms (APA, 2013).

■ Phobia

The most predominant phobias among women are animal, natural environment, and situational-specific phobias; whereas blood-injection injury is experienced equally by both genders (APA, 2013). Females are more frequently affected than males with the ratio of 2:1; however, this varies depending on phobic stimuli (APA, 2013). Phobias are the most common anxiety disorder. Individuals

may commonly avoid the feared stimulus and may go to extreme lengths to avoid the feared stimulus (Sadock et al., 2015). Depression is a comorbid condition in approximately one-third of people with phobia. Animal phobia, natural environment phobia, and blood-injection phobia appear to peak at childhood. Other phobias have a peak onset at early adulthood. Approximately 75% of individuals have phobias about one or more situation or object (APA, 2013). Phobias have been found to run in families, especially blood-injection phobia (Sadock et al., 2015). Limited data exist regarding the course of specific phobia despite being the most common anxiety disorder. Individuals frequently do not seek treatment for this condition and may live with anxiety for many years. The condition appears to remain constant and does not appear to have the waxing and waning progression that is seen in other anxiety disorders. For individuals who do seek treatment, a positive response to intervention was associated with better long-term outcomes (Curtis, Magee, Eaton, Wittchen, & Kessler, 1998). One study that examined outcomes of individuals diagnosed with phobia 10 to 16 years after treatment challenged the notion that recovery from this diagnosis is characterized by complete and lasting remission from symptoms (Curtis et al., 1998).

■ Social Anxiety Disorder

The age of onset for individuals with social phobia is childhood or adolescence, and the individual may experience symptoms of the disorder for many years. Parental psychopathology, including social anxiety disorder, depression, and parenting style (overprotection or rejection), has been associated with development of social anxiety disorder in youth (Judd, 1994). This disorder is commonly associated with substance dependence, depression, avoidant personality disorder, panic disorder, and generalized anxiety disorder (Lieb et al., 2000). Social anxiety disorder is more common in women than in men; however, in clinical samples, the reverse is often true (Sadock et al., 2015). Social anxiety disorder has onset before other psychiatric conditions (Long, 2011). Additionally, psychiatric conditions complicate approximately one-third of those diagnosed with social anxiety disorder. Early intervention of social anxiety disorder may prevent the onset of other psychiatric conditions (Long, 2011). Without intervention, the course of social anxiety disorder is chronic and unremitting. A significant concern relative to this disorder is the strong tendency of society, including mental health professionals, to trivialize this disorder (Lipsitz, Mannuzza, Klein, Ross, & Fyer, 1999).

Generalized Anxiety Disorder

The age of onset for generalized anxiety disorder is variable and difficult to pinpoint. It can occur as early as childhood (Sadock et al., 2015). Individuals, when questioned about their symptoms, often recall feeling anxious as long as they can remember. This condition tends to worsen without treatment and especially during times of increased stress (Fadem, 2012). One-third of individuals with generalized anxiety disorder symptoms seek psychiatric intervention. More often, these individuals present to family practitioners, cardiologists, internists, or gastroenterologists from whom they are seeking relief for the somatic concerns that they are experiencing as a result of this condition (Sadock et al., 2015). Because of a high incidence of comorbidity of generalized anxiety disorder with other psychiatric conditions, a specific course and prognosis are difficult to identify. Generalized anxiety disorder can be viewed as a chronic condition in which the individual may experience symptoms that can be lifelong (Sadock et al., 2015).

■ Medical/Surgical Management

At present, there are no specific laboratory tests that can be used to diagnose anxiety. Society has become more aware and accepting of identification and treatment of mental illness over the last several years. This is apparent through public health initiatives targeted at addressing mental health concerns, such as National Mental Illness Awareness Week, Anxiety Screening Day, and Depression Screening Day, as well as through the increasing amount of information regarding mental illness, diagnosis, and treatment available via the Internet (Long, 2011; NIMH, 2016; SAMHSA, 2015). Current guidelines for treatment of severe mental illness can be found in four different categories (Richards, Klein, & Carlbring, 2003). These categories vary depending on the score and stringency for which the guidelines rely on research evidence. The categories include recommendations, comprehensive treatment options, algorithms, and expert consensus guidelines. In 1998, comprehensive treatment options were

developed for panic disorder by the APA (Mellman et al., 2001). However, the strength of evidence presented in support of these treatment options is less stringent than Patient Outcomes Research Team (PORT) recommendations. PORT treatment recommendations for schizophrenia were developed by the U.S. Agency for Health Care Policy and Research. The PORT project critically examined literature, which was then followed by expert review. The PORT recommendations contain very specific evidence of efficacy of treatment interventions that supported the utilization of these interventions. The APA guidelines developed for panic disorder were by a professional organization and did not require the evidence considered for inclusion to be as stringent as the guidelines used for the development of PORT. As a result, the APA treatment guidelines are less prescriptive than the PORT treatment recommendations. Algorithms, a single rule or set of rules, are used when solving a problem. Medication algorithms are considered within practice guidelines. Algorithms provide practitioners with a step-by-step approach to clinical decisions considering medications. At present, the Texas Medication Algorithm Project has the most extensive collection of medication algorithms for persons with mental illness. Unfortunately, there are no algorithms for anxiety disorder treatment. Algorithms do exist, however, for schizophrenia, bipolar disorder, and major depressive disorder (Mellman et al., 2001). The last category includes expert consensus guidelines. These are recommendations based upon surveys completed by a comprehensive array of experts in the treatment of identified conditions. These guidelines do not rely on critical analysis of research literature. The rationale provided for the development of these expert guidelines is related to the fact that research literature at times does not address specific points in treatment decision making. At present, expert treatment guidelines exist for panic disorder (APA, 2013). In addition to expert treatment guidelines for practitioners, guidelines have been developed for patients and families regarding these diagnoses (APA, 2016). People with anxiety disorders are three to five times more likely to seek the care of a physician and six times more likely to be hospitalized for a psychiatric disorder (Copeland, 2003). From an occupational therapy perspective, their functional abilities would be assessed, and it would be determined how their anxiety was impacting activities of daily living, IADLs, sleep/rest, education, work, play, leisure, and social participation (American Occupational Therapy Association [AOTA], 2014). The occupational therapist may consider administering an activity configuration, role checklist, interest checklist, or self-assessment of occupational functioning to determine functional deficits (Reed, 2014). Assessments such as the Canadian Occupational Performance Measure, Occupational Performance History Interview—2.1, and the Occupational Self Assessment are appropriate considerations (Reed, 2014). The most common treatments for anxiety disorders include a combination of pharmacologic and psychological interventions with the exception of specific phobia for which there is no good pharmacologic treatment (Fadem, 2012). Remission is the ultimate goal for the treatment of anxiety disorders (Kjernisted & Bleau, 2004). Occupational therapy intervention is targeted at changing performance deficits in areas of occupation as a result of the symptoms experienced by the person (Reed, 2014). Occupational therapy intervention may also examine activity demands and modifications that could be made to the activity or environment to assist the individual in independence in areas of occupation (AOTA, 2014). Although some individuals may continue to experience symptoms of anxiety throughout their lives, occupational therapy intervention can be focused toward the development or reestablishment of meaningful daily routines. Engagement in meaningful occupation can serve to facilitate adaptation, which can lead to improved health and wellness, quality of life, and positive life satisfaction. It is important to remain client centered as interventions that may reduce anxiety in one individual may prove ineffective for another. Medications utilized to treat anxiety disorders include anxiolytics and antidepressants, specifically SSRIs (Sadock et al., 2015). One should be cautious when working with clients who are on benzodiazepines who have addiction concerns, as these medications are highly addictive. Further, older adults are at risk of falls when on benzodiazepines because of side effects impacting balance as a result of the half-life of the medication. Side effects of benzodiazepines include sedation and fatigue, cognitive and memory impairments, delayed reaction time, impaired balance and coordination, hangover effects, withdrawal, and abuse potential. For individuals diagnosed with panic disorder, antidepressant

medications such as paroxetine hydrochloride (Paxil), which is a selective SRI, or benzodiazepines such as alprazolam (Xanax) are approved by the Food and Drug Administration and are often prescribed (Fadem, 2012; Sadock et al., 2015). Paxil has been shown to be effective with individuals diagnosed with social phobia. Benzodiazepines may be used for social phobia on a very short-term basis (Sadock et al., 2015). Some research has indicated that cognitive-behavioral interventions are superior to pharmacologic approaches, whereas other research indicates the contrary (Sadock et al., 2015). In considering cognitive-behavioral interventions for anxiety disorders, a variety of interventions exist. Findings from one study indicated that when treating individuals with panic disorder, progress can be obtained through the use of a self-help workbook and brief therapist contact (Hecker, Losee, Robertson-Nay, & Maki, 2004). An emphasis on family and client psychoeducation, focusing on symptomatology, nature and course of panic disorder, and lifestyle modifications, has been suggested as evidence-based interventions that cost less (in Australia) than the cost of drug therapy over a 1-year period of time (Andrews, Oakley-Browne, & Castle, 2003). The efficacy of cognitive-behavioral therapy (CBT) has been examined through evidence-based research. It is important to note that CBT interventions are often coupled with pharmacotherapy; however, within individuals diagnosed with panic disorder, use of medications may interfere with CBT intervention approach (Shearer, 2007). The APA's comprehensive treatment guidelines for panic disorder indicate that most individuals can be treated on an outpatient basis and may rarely require hospitalization (APA, 2013). Cognitive-behavioral interventions suggested by the APA include the use of psychoeducation, panic monitoring, breathing monitoring, anxiety management skill development, cognitive restructuring, and in vivo exposure. Establishing and maintaining a therapeutic alliance with the individual diagnosed with panic disorder is viewed as a key element in successful intervention as well as educating the individual on the early signs of relapse.

Panic Disorder

From an occupational therapy perspective, individuals with panic disorder may need assistance in the area of IADLs. People may be fearful of leaving the house, and therefore, community mobility may be impaired. Systematic desensitization can be useful but very stressful for individuals in addressing this fear (Andrews, Oakley-Browne, Castle, Judd, & Baillie, 2003). Relaxation training, including deep breathing, progressive muscle relaxation, visualization, and autogenic training, is an effective intervention utilized by occupational therapy practitioners for individuals with panic disorder and phobias (Bonder, 2010). Although relaxation therapies such as visualization, deep breathing, meditation, and progressive muscle relaxation have been shown to decrease anxiety, there is limited research (Conrad & Roth, 2007).

Phobia

When considering other available interventions for phobia, 70% to 85% of individuals responded with clinically significant improvement when exposure was used as a behavioral intervention. The addition of cognitive components appeared to add little efficacy (Roth & Fonagy, 2004). Therapist-directed exposure was suggested rather than self-directed exposure to the feared stimulus. Although some studies have used virtual reality techniques as intervention for the treatment of phobias, this may be cost prohibitive and technically challenging but could provide a clinic with the ability to expose the client to a wide range of feared stimuli (North, North, & Coble, 1998).

Social Anxiety Disorder

When considering evidence-based intervention for social anxiety disorder, five cognitive-behavioral treatments including exposure therapy, cognitive restructuring, exposure coupled with cognitive restructuring, social skills training, and relaxation were compared and found to be moderately effective with no differences obtained at the end of the study or at the follow-up (Federoff & Taylor, 2001). Further, both individual and group interventions were found to be equally beneficial to individuals with this diagnosis. Some obstacles to effective treatment for social anxiety disorder are as follows: the individual's avoidance of treatment because of fear, shame, or stigma. Limited screening to assess social anxiety disorder is available at present. Assessment and intervention may be directed toward somatic complaints expressed by the individual rather than the social anxiety disorder. Physicians lack knowledge of effective treatment options or they trivialize the

client's concerns or view them as unchangeable (Bruce & Saeed, 1999). Despite these facts, cognitive-behavioral therapy is useful when treating social phobia (NIMH, 2016). Both cognitive therapy and exposure therapy present good efficacy, and the combination presents the largest effect sizes in meta-analytic reviews (Taylor, 1996).

Limited research has been completed examining the link between sensory defensiveness in adults and increased anxiety (Kinnealey & Fuiek, 1999). It is hypothesized that many symptoms of sensory defensiveness may be interchangeable with psychiatric disorders including generalized anxiety disorder. Research has explored the use of sensory integration interventions for decreasing anxiety levels by using deep pressure, tactile, and proprioceptive activities (Kinnealey, Oliver, & Wilbarger, 1995).

Generalized Anxiety Disorder

Generalized anxiety disorder can be addressed using cognitive therapy focusing on education and lifestyle alterations focusing on how the external environment influences internal feelings. Addressing diet (caffeine intake), medication use (over-the-counter medications may increase anxiety), and the need for regular exercise can also be helpful in addressing generalized anxiety disorder (Kjernisted & Bleau, 2004). Rational/cognitive approaches that focus on assisting the person in replacing negative self-statements with more positive ones can be effective with individuals diagnosed with generalized anxiety disorder. Time management activities that assist the individual in prioritizing activities may assist in decreasing anxiety as well. Expressive activities such as journal writing, drawing, or other craft activities can provide a mechanism for the individual to communicate his or her feelings and may assist in the development of coping skills (Reed, 2014). Clinicians should be mindful regarding the length of intervention provided to individuals with anxiety disorders. Outpatient sessions between 6 and 7 weeks were deemed too short by clients in two different studies (Prior, 1998; Rosier, Williams, & Ryrie, 1998). Structured course content should include opportunities for skill development, communication, and practice with ongoing monitoring by the clinician. Cognitive aspects of intervention such as relaxation training and assertiveness were found to be most beneficial per client report. An 8-week course was felt to allow more time for learning and practice of the cognitive aspects of the course deemed most important by those diagnosed with anxiety disorders (Rosier et al., 1998).

■ Impact on Client Factors and Occupational Performance

The impact of anxiety disorders on client factors is dependent on the specific disorder with which the client is diagnosed. In the area of mental functions, specifically global mental functions, sleep, temperament, and energy can be impacted by the diagnosis of an anxiety disorder. In the area of specific mental functions, the following areas are impacted: attention, reduced recall (memory), impaired ability to make associations, time management, problem solving, decision making, and emotional functions in the area of self-control (Sadock et al., 2015). From a sensory perspective, individuals with an anxiety disorder may demonstrate increased startle response. Physical signs present in anxiety disorder from a neuromuscular and movement-related perspective include feeling shaky, muscle tension, backache, headache, and fatigue. From a cardiovascular and respiratory perspective, symptoms include tachycardia and hyperventilation, which can lead to syncope (passing out). From a gastrointestinal perspective, clients may experience signs of diarrhea and have the feeling of an upset stomach or "butterflies" in the stomach. When considering the genitourinary system and reproductive functions, clients may experience urinary frequency and decreased libido, which could relate to reproduction or lack of desire for sexual relationships (APA, 2013; Fadem, 2012; Sadock et al., 2015).

Panic Disorder

The symptoms an individual may experience during a panic attack can have a negative impact upon the many different areas of occupation, including care of others, care of pets, childrearing, community mobility, safety and emergency maintenance, shopping, sleep/rest, formal educational participation, job performance, and leisure and social participation (AOTA, 2014). A common concern of individuals who experience panic disorder is anticipation of when the next attack will occur. This fear can significantly alter daily roles, habits, routines, and rituals. This can have a negative impact upon their ability to initiate performance in daily activities. The individual who experiences a panic disorder and has children may worry about the well-being of his or her children. He or she may feel as if he or she is dying while having an attack. Those experiencing symptoms of panic disorder may begin restricting themselves to their residence for fear of having a panic attack while in public, and this behavior can facilitate agoraphobia.

Social Anxiety Disorder

Social anxiety disorder impacts the areas of educational participation, such as having to get up in front of class and give a presentation. Job performance, as well as other social roles and responsibilities, may be impaired (Fischler & Booth, 1999). Communication skills may be negatively affected because of the individual's significant level of anxiety. Individuals with social phobia may experience low self-esteem due to their inability to perform up to self-imposed standards, yet they frequently do not seek assistance for their concerns. Individuals with this disorder may be characterized by others as "nervous" or "ineffective" in social situations. To increase the potential for individuals with social anxiety disorder to experience success, the occupational therapist should work toward establishing environmental control to reduce anxiety regarding the unknown. Individuals may benefit from working alone initially to reduce self-consciousness and at their own pace. Positive feedback for effective performance is essential. Working with individuals diagnosed with social phobia to self-disclose diagnosis to supportive individuals may assist in reducing self-consciousness and embarrassment when symptoms arise (Fischler & Booth, 1999).

Generalized Anxiety Disorder

Any area of occupation can be impacted by generalized anxiety disorder. The individual may express excessive worry about himself or herself and his or her own health and well-being (IADLs) or his or her educational participation, job performance, as well as social participation. This anxiety disorder is one that many people express as similar to the gray cloud of worry that follows them everywhere and as such impacts every area of occupation.

Generalized Anxiety Disorder

Jillian is a 44-year-old registered nurse. She has worked in nursing for 20 years on a hospital pediatrics unit. For the last 7 months, for more days than not, Jillian finds it difficult to control her level of anxiety and worry. She is worried about getting along with coworkers, pleasing the physicians with whom she works, and interacting appropriately with the parents of the children for whom she is providing care. Additionally, Jillian has been worrying about her children's school performance and the fact that many companies in her community are downsizing. Although her husband has frequently reassured her that his position is stable, she cannot help but worry that he will lose his job or be demoted. With the economy being on a downhill slide, this serves to increase Jillian's fears regarding employment and finances. Jillian also worries about her difficulty attending to her tasks as a nurse. She finds her mind going blank, and she has difficulty concentrating on what a physician is saying to her while she is doing rounds. Three times during the last month, she has recorded physician's orders incorrectly. The unit secretary has caught these errors and brought them to Jillian's attention. Jillian is demonstrating difficulty responding in an appropriate fashion to safety concerns, which are typically presented in her workplace such as "code blue." She feels others know of her problems. She is concerned about her relationships with her coworkers since she is so preoccupied by her anxiety, and she finds herself irritable at work and has "snapped" at a several coworkers over the last few months. Jillian has been having extreme difficulty falling and staying asleep. She has been awakening 2 to 3 hours early and is not able to fall back to sleep. As a result, she feels fatigued and has been experiencing increased muscle tension, backaches, and frequent headaches. Jillian describes her ongoing keyed-up feelings of restlessness like "walking on eggshells." Jillian expresses frustration in her lack of ability to relax and inability to decrease her anxiety. Jillian expresses little appetite and has experienced noticeable weight loss over the last 7 months. At home, Jillian has not been preparing meals for her family as she had in the past and rather has been relying solely on frozen dinners and takeout food for family dining. Jillian picks up the house but does not clean per se. She used to keep her house immaculate, but for the past several months, she has verbalized feelings of fatigue and lack of desire to keep things clean in her home. Although she expresses numerous interests including scrapbooking, cooking, reading, and walking, she has not been able to participate in these leisure activities because of her anxiety level and accompanying fatigue. Jillian had previously been active as a volunteer at her church and involved in activities of her son's football league, but at this time, she feels so overwhelmed that she is unable to complete these tasks. She has been caring for her children marginally. She has experienced difficulty helping them with their school work and has been distant or short with them in her communication. Jillian's husband and friends too have noticed a change in Jillian's behavior. Although they have been supportive of and encouraging Jillian, they do not know what to do or how to assist her in diminishing her level of worry. Jillian agrees to go on family outings in the community with her husband and children, but at the last minute, she backs out. When asked why, she provides little to no explanation for the last minute change of plans. Jillian's marriage is "on the rocks" because she is experiencing difficulties in communicating to her husband and he is starting to wonder if she may be having an affair as she appears so anxious all of the time. Infrequently, she will speak to friends on the phone but has not gone to social activities with her friends in months. Financially, Jillian and her family have money in their savings, live comfortably, and have been saving for their children's college education and their retirement. Despite these facts, Jillian spends between 4 and 6 hours each weekend reviewing the financial status of the family and constantly worrying about expenses that are considered by many others to be routine expenditures. Jillian has seen a psychiatrist who has prescribed medication and supportive psychotherapy 1 week ago. Despite Jillian's complaints of fatigue, the psychiatrist encouraged her to try to walk one to two times per week as physical exercise is beneficial to those with generalized anxiety disorder. Additionally, deep breathing exercises were reviewed in attempts to decrease her level of anxiety. Jillian plans to continue to pursue therapy on an outpatient basis with a psychologist and occupational therapist for relaxation training and to critically examine life stressors and develop effective coping mechanisms to deal with her current level of anxiety.

Phobia

Emma is a 9-year-old female who is in fourth grade. She lives with her mother, grandmother, and brother Larry. Emma is a high achieving student in school, who has many friends and enjoys a variety of after-school activities such as Girl Scouts, playing soccer, and computer games. Three years ago, Emma's parents divorced and her mother and brother moved from Oregon to Iowa. In Iowa, in the spring and summer when it rains, often times there are severe thunderstorms. Emma had never experienced extreme thunder and lightning until she moved to Iowa. In May of this year, Emma missed 12 school days due to thunderstorms and her ongoing and persistent worry regarding her safety during a severe storm episode. When the weather becomes ominous, Emma will head for the basement of her home and will not come out until she is 100% certain that there is no chance of thunder or lightening. Even when Emma's mother shows her on the Weather Channel on television, there are no storms in the area and the most recent storm is over, Emma will persist in staying in the basement. Emma worries she will be struck by lightning, and her irrational fear keeps her from engaging in many occupations during stormy weather. Not only does Emma's fear negatively impact her engagement in school and extracurricular activities, she will not eat and has been experiencing bouts of constipation. Emma refuses to eat or drink as there is no bathroom in the basement, and she does not want to have to leave the basement due to her extreme fear. Emma's mother after several missed school days due to this behavior contacted the school counselor. The counselor reported Emma's irrational fears have negatively impacted her school performance and peer engagement. At school, if Emma hears thunder, she immediately runs to the bathroom which is in an interior location on the lower level of the school and will not leave. The school counselor stated she is worried as the other children are beginning to "tease" Emma about her phobia of storms. The counselor has tried to work with Emma and has taught her deep breathing but feels that more intervention is needed. Emma too is concerned as her performance and attention at school is "off" as she appears to always be staring out the window, examining the current weather situation. The school counselor suggested that Emma's mother seek assistance at the local mental health center. The mental health center employs an occupational therapist who considers Emma in the context of her school and home environments and how her phobia is negatively impacting her engagement in desired occupations. Together with the psychologist, the OT and client (Emma and her family) develop strategies for Emma to try in an attempt to ally her fears and anxieties. The psychologist utilizes virtual reality technology and the occupational therapist uses behavioral and sensory interventions. The OT works with Emma on developing a sensory box that she can use to self-soothe when her negative thoughts/feelings seem to take over. Further, the OT instructs Emma's mom on strategies she can use at home from a behavioral perspective to reinforce the use of the sensory box and positive coping techniques. The school counselor reported that Emma has appeared more engaged in school, spending less time attending to the weather outside, and was able to remain in her classroom for a longer time period when a storm was occurring. Emma did not rush to the bathroom, rather she was able to leave her classroom and stand/sit in the hallway so she could continue to hear the classroom instruction. Together with the psychologist and OT and the mental health center, the school counselor is hopeful to continue the progress Emma has made in addressing her irrational fears of electrical storms and improve her school performance, after-school activity engagement, and peer relationships.

RECOMMENDED LEARNING RESOURCES

American Occupational Therapy Association (AOTA). (2014). *Occupational therapy practice framework: Domain & process* (3rd ed.). Bethesda, MD: Author.

American Psychiatric Association. (2016). *Treatment Guidelines*. Retrieved from https://www.apa.org/practice/guidelines/index.aspx

American Psychiatric Association. (2013). *Diagnostic and statistical manual of mental disorders V* (5th ed.). Washington, DC: Author.

Andrews, G., Oakley-Browne, M., & Castle, D. (2003). Summary of guidelines for the treatment of panic disorder and agoraphobia. *Australasia Psychiatry, 11*, 29–33.

Anxiety Disorders Association of America. Retrieved from http://www.adaa.org/

Bonder, B. (2015). *Psychopathology and function* (5th ed.). Thorofare, NJ: Slack Inc.

Bourne, E. J. (2011). *The anxiety and phobia workbook* (5th ed.). Oakland, CA: New Harbinger Publications.

Brantley, J. (2007). *Calming your anxious mind* (2nd ed.). Oakland, CA: New Harbinger Publications.

Kase, L., Antony, M. M., & Vitale, J. (2006). *Anxious 9 to 5: How to beat worry, stop second guessing yourself and work with confidence.* Oakland, CA: New Harbinger Publications.

Reinecke, M. A. (2010). *Little ways to keep calm and carry on: Twenty lessons for managing worry, anxiety and fear.* Oakland, CA: New Harbinger Publications.

REFERENCES

American Occupational Therapy Association. (2014). *Occupational therapy practice framework: Domain & process* (3rd ed.). Bethesda, MD: Author.

American Psychiatric Association. (2013). *Diagnostic and statistical manual of mental disorders* (5th ed.). Arlington, VA: Author. Retrieved from https://www.apa.org/practice/guidelines/index.aspx

American Psychiatric Association (2016). *Treatment Guidelines*. Retrieved from https://www.apa.org/practice/guidelines/index.aspx

Andrews, G., Oakley-Browne, M., Castle, D., Judd, F., & Baillie, A. (2003). Summary of guideline for the treatment of panic disorder and agoraphobia. *Australasian Psychiatry, 11*, 29–33. doi: 10.1046/j.1440-1665.2003.00529

Anxiety and Depression Association of America. (2014). *Facts and statistics.* Retrieved from http://www.adaa.org/about-adaa/press-room/facts-statistics

Bonder, B. (2010). *Psychopathology and function* (4th ed.). Th orofare, NJ: Slack Inc

Bouchard, S., & Verrier, P. (2005). *Anxiety disorders & comorbidities.* Retrieved from http://www.anxietycanada.ca/english/pdf/comorbidEn.pdf

Brantley, J. (2007). *Calming your anxious mind* (2nd ed.). Oakland, CA: New Harbinger Publications.

Brown, T. A., Campbell, L. A., Lehman, C. L., Grisham, J. R., & Mancil, R. B. (2001). Current and lifetime comorbidity of the DSM-IV anxiety and mood disorders in large clinical sample. *Journal of Abnormal Psychology, 110*, 585–599.

Bruce, T., & Saeed, A. (1999). Social anxiety disorder: A common under recognized mental disorder. *American Family Physician, 60*, 2311–2320.

Conrad, A., & Roth, W. T. (2007). Muscle relaxation therapy for anxiety disorders: It works but how? *Journal of Anxiety Disorders, 21*(3), 243–264.

Copeland, M. E. (2003). *The worry control workbook.* Dummerston, VT: Peach Press.

Curtis, G. C., Magee, W. J., Eaton, W. W., Wittchen, H. U., & Kessler, R. C. (1998). Specific fears and phobias. Epidemiology and classification. *British Journal of Psychiatry, 173*, 212–217.

Dirckx, J. H. (2005). *Stedman's concise medical dictionary for the health professional* (28th ed.). Philadelphia, PA: Lippincott Williams & Wilkins.

Fadem, B. (2012). *Behavioral science in medicine* (2nd ed.). Philadelphia, PA: Lippincott Williams & Wilkins.

Federoff, I. C., & Taylor, S. (2001). Psychological and pharmacological treatments of social phobia: A meta analysis. *Journal of Clinical Psychopharmacology, 21*, 311–324.

Fischler, G. L., & Booth, N. (1999). *Vocational impact of psychiatric disorders: A guide for rehabilitation professionals.* Gaithersburg, MD: Aspen Publication.

Friedman, S., Smith, L., Fogel, D., Paradis, C., Viswanathan, R., Ackerman, R., & Trappler, B. (2002). The incidence and influence of early traumatic life events in patients with panic disorder: A comparison with other psychiatric outpatients. *Journal of Anxiety Disorders, 16*(3), 259–272.

Hecker, J. E., Losee, M. C., Roberson-Nay, R., & Maki, K. (2004). Mastery of your anxiety and panic and brief therapist contact in the treatment of panic disorder. *Journal of Anxiety Disorders, 18*, 111–126.

Johns Hopkins. (2016). *Health library: Panic disorder.* Retrieved from http://www.hopkinsmedicine.org/healthlibrary/conditions/mental_health_disorders/panic_disorder_85,P00738/

Judd, L. L. (1994). Social phobia: A clinical overview. *Journal of Clinical Psychiatry, 55*(Suppl.), 5–9.

Kessler, R. C., Chiu, W. T., Demler, O., & Walters, E. E. (2005). Prevalence, severity, and comorbidity of twelve-month DSM-IV disorders in the National Comorbidity Survey Replication (NCS-R). *Archives of General Psychiatry, 62*(6), 617–627.

Kinnealey, M., & Fuiek, M. (1999). The relationship between sensory defensiveness, anxiety, depression and pain in adults. *Occupational Therapy International, 6,* 195–206.

Kinnealey, M., Oliver, B., & Wilbarger, P. (1995). A phenomenological study of sensory defensiveness in adults. *American Journal of Occupational Therapy, 49,* 444–451.

Kjernisted, K. D., & Bleau, P. (2004). Long term goals in the management of acute and chronic anxiety disorders. *Canadian Journal of Psychiatry, 49*(Suppl. 1), 51S–63S.

Lepine, J. P. (2002). The epidemiology of anxiety disorders: Prevalence and societal costs. *Journal of Clinical Psychiatry, 63*(Suppl. 14), 4–8.

Lieb, R., Wittchen, H. U., Höfler, M., Fuetsch, M., Stein, M. B., & Merikangas, K. R. (2000). Parental psychopathology, parenting styles, and the risk of social phobia in offspring: A prospective longitudinal community study. *Archives of General Psychiatry, 57,* 859–866.

Lipsitz, J. D., Mannuzza, S., Klein, D. F., Ross, D. C., & Fyer, A. J. (1999). Specific phobia 10–16 years after treatment. *Depression & Anxiety, 10,* 105–111.

Long, P. W. (2011). *Anxiety disorders.* Retrieved from http://www.mentalhealth.com/

Mellman, T. A., Miller, A. L., Weissman, E. M., Crismon, M. L., Essock, S. M., & Marder, S. R. (2001). Evidence-based pharmacologic treatment for people with severe mental illness: A focus on guidelines and algorithms. *Psychiatric Services, 52,* 619–625.

National Institute of Mental Health (NIMH). (2011). *Anxiety disorders.* Retrieved from: http://www.nimh.nih.gov/health/topics/anxiety-disorders/index.shtml

National Institute of Mental Health (NIMH). (2016). *Anxiety disorders.* Retrieved from http://www.nimh.nih.gov/health/topics/anxiety-disorders/index.shtml

North, M. M., North, S. M., & Coble, J. R. (1998). Virtual reality therapy: An effective treatment for psychological disorders. In G. Riva (Ed.), *Virtual reality in neuro-psycho-physiology.* Amsterdam, The Netherlands: IOS Press.

Pigott, T. A. (2003). Anxiety disorders in women. *Psychiatric Clinics in North America, 26*(3), 621–672.

Prior, S. (1998). Determining the effectiveness of short term anxiety management course. *British Journal of Occupational Therapy, 61,* 207–212.

Reed, K. L. (2014). *Quick reference to occupational therapy* (3rd ed.). Austin, TX: Pro-Ed.

Rettew, D. C. (2000). Avoidant personality disorder, generalized social phobia, and shyness: Putting the personality back into personality disorders. *Harvard Review of Psychiatry, 8,* 283–297.

Richards, J., Klein, B., & Carlbring, P. (2003). Internet based treatment for panic disorder. *Cognitive Behavioral Therapy, 32,* 125–135.

Rosier, C., Williams, H., & Ryrie, I. (1998). Anxiety management groups in a community mental health team. *British Journal of Occupational Therapy, 61,* 203–206.

Roth, A., & Fonagy, P. (2004). *What works for whom: A critical review of psychotherapy research* (2nd ed.). New York, NY: Guilford Press.

Rouillon, F. (1996). Epidemiology of panic disorder. *Encephale, 5,* 25–34.

Sadock, B. J., Sadock, V., & Ruiz, P. (2015). *Kaplan & Sadock's synopsis of psychiatry: Behavioral science & clinical psychiatry* (11th ed.). Philadelphia, PA: Lippincott Williams & Wilkins.

Shearer, S. L. (2007). Recent advances in the understanding and treatment of anxiety disorders. *Primary Care Clinics in Office Practice, 34,* 475–504.

Substance Abuse and Mental Health Services Administration. (2015). *Mental disorders: Anxiety disorder.* Retrieved from http://www.samhsa.gov/disorders/mental

Taylor, S. (1996). Meta-analysis of cognitive behavioral treatments for social phobia. *Journal of Behavior Therapy and Experimental Psychiatry, 27*(1), 1–9.

United States Surgeon General (USSG). (1999). *Mental health: A report of the surgeon general.* Retrieved from http://www.surgeongeneral.gov/library/mentalhealth/home.html#topper

United States Surgeon General (USSG) (2005). *Mental health: A report of the surgeon general.* Retrieved: http://www.surgeongeneral.gov/library/mentalhealth/home.html#topper

World Health Organization. (2013). *Gender and women's mental health.* Retrieved from http://www.who.int/mental_health/prevention/genderwomen/en/

World Health Organization. (2016). *Investing in treatment for depression and anxiety leads to a fourfold return.* Retrieved from http://www.who.int/mediacentre/news/releases/2016/depression-anxiety-treatment/en/

Neurocognitive Disorders

Joyce Fraker and Jayne Yatczak

Corrine slowly entered Roland's room and gently awakened him for his morning activities of daily living (ADL). Roland opened his eyes and looked at her with an expression of disorientation and fear. Corrine had known him for almost a year, and though he could never remember her name, he usually greeted her with a smile of recognition. Today was different. Roland appeared tense, with agitated movements of his arms and legs. Corrine sat next to him, stroked his arms rhythmically, and told him her name. "It is such a beautiful day; let's open the curtain and look at the view," she told him. She opened the curtains and handed him his glasses. Roland put them on without difficulty and turned his vacant gaze toward the window. Within moments, Roland relaxed, and his limbs calmed.

Corrine said, "Let's get dressed. I will help you put on your clean pants." She lightly touched a leg to cue him to lift it so she could place his foot in the pant leg. Roland looked at her, anxious and bewildered. "What do you want me to do?" he cried. Corrine lightly touched his foot, directing him to lift it. Roland tightly gripped his upper thighs and he began to shake. He pleaded, louder this time, "I can't move them, what do you want me to do?" Corrine gently took his hand and began stroking his arm. "Let's just rest for a moment," she said. After he had visibly calmed, Corrine gently lifted each foot and placed them into the pant legs. She positioned his walker and said, "You can help us stand." She lightly guided him by the elbow, and he came to a stand. "Thank you for doing such a good job," Corrine told him, and helped him pull on the pants. "Now all we need are shoes, and then we can get some breakfast." Roland looked at her, again without recognition, the fear now replaced with calm.

DESCRIPTION AND DEFINITIONS OF NEUROCOGNITIVE DISORDERS

In 2013, the *Diagnostic and Statistical Manual of Mental Disorders, fifth edition* (DSM-5), redefined dementia and most cognitive disorders as "neurocognitive disorders," abbreviated as NCD. Although dementia is still a recognizable term, officially what was known as vascular dementia, frontotemporal dementia, and dementia with Lewy bodies are now called, respectively, vascular neurocognitive disorder (vascular NCD), frontotemporal neurocognitive disorder (frontotemporal NCD [FTNCD]), and neurocognitive disorder with Lewy bodies (NCDLB). NCD due to Alzheimer's disease can be simply stated as Alzheimer's disease (AD).

NCDs include a range of conditions including delirium, disorders formerly defined as dementias, and NCD due to traumatic brain injury (TBI). This chapter will focus on the types of NCD most commonly seen by occupational therapists with the exceptions of NCD due to TBI, which is more completely covered in another chapter.

■ Delirium

Description and Definition of Delirium

The diagnostic criteria for delirium are as follows: (a) disturbance in attention with decreased ability to focus, sustain, or shift attention; (b) an additional change in cognition (such as memory loss, disorientation, language disturbance) or the development of perceptual disturbance (hallucinations, paranoid thoughts); (c) the disturbance quickly develops, usually within hours or days, and the severity of symptoms fluctuate throughout the course of a day; (d) the changes in attention and cognition cannot be explained by a preexisting or developing NCD; and (e) there is medical evidence that the disturbance is either caused by a medical condition or developed during intoxication or withdrawal from a substance; such substances include alcohol, prescription medication, and illegal substances such as cocaine or hallucinogens (American Psychiatric Association, 2013).

It is not unusual for delirium to occur when a person is being treated, or is in need of treatment, for an acute physical condition. A high fever can bring on delirium, causing the person to be confused, to misinterpret shadows, to be disoriented (especially in a hospital environment, which is unfamiliar and possibly frightening), and to be unable to express thoughts and needs clearly. These symptoms might fluctuate, just as the degree of a fever might fluctuate during the course of a day. An asymptomatic urinary tract infection is often suspected when a delirium occurs without clear signs of a medical problem. The delirium ends after the acute medical condition clears.

Etiology of Delirium

Delirium is caused by one or more underlying medical conditions. Although a fever can bring on a delirium, the rise in body temperature is merely a symptom of an underlying medical condition. Medical conditions associated with delirium are many and varied. They include adverse medication side effects; substance intoxication or withdrawal; infection; metabolic disturbances; traumatic head injury; vascular injury; cancer; and inflammatory disorders (Peterson et al., 2001, 2008). Risk factors for delirium include increased severity and complexity of physical illness, use of many prescription medications, extremes of age (older or younger), and the presence of a baseline cognitive impairment, such as an NCD (Hales & Yudofsky, 2003; Samuals & Neugroschl, 2008).

Delirium can manifest in confusion and disorientation following surgery and, in some cases, may be the first sign of a more serious NCD such as NCD with Lewy bodies (Weiner & Lipton, 2009). In fact, delirium is a frequent finding during recovery from hip fractures, stem cell transplant, acquired immunodeficiency syndrome (AIDS), and terminal cancer (Hales & Yudofsky, 2003).

Incidence and Prevalence of Delirium

Estimating the incidence and prevalence of delirium is difficult because it is often overlooked or left untreated. Sadock, Sadock, and Ruiz (2014) state that delirium is commonly under-recognized by health care workers. In adults aged 55 and older, delirium may be present in as many 1% of dwelling adults, 10% of emergency department patients, 80% of critical care patients and 80% of patients in end of life care. According to the DSM-5, 14% to 24% of individuals admitted to hospitals have delirium as well as up to 60% of individuals in nursing homes or postacute care settings (American Psychiatric Association, 2013).

Signs and Symptoms of Delirium

The **prodromal** symptoms of delirium can include restlessness, anxiety, sleep disturbance, and irritability. Clinical features of delirium include altered arousal and disturbance of the sleep-wake cycle. The person may have daytime sleepiness, nighttime agitation, difficulty falling asleep, or wakefulness throughout the night; in some cases, there may be a complete reversal of the night-day sleep-wake cycle. Perception may be altered, with misperceptions, illusions, delusions, or hallucinations. The wrinkled pattern of a blanket may appear to be an object; a shadow in the corner seems to move and is perceived as threatening. The person will likely have decreased attention, impaired memory, or disorientation to time or place; there can be rapid shifts in emotion as well as periods of agitation (American Psychiatric Association, 2013). Neurological abnormalities can include **dysgraphia** (inability to write a sentence), constructional **apraxia** (evidenced by inability to draw a clock face), **dysnomic aphasia** (difficulty naming objects), motor abnormalities (tremor, **asterixis**, or hand-flapping tremor), myoclonus or muscle spasms, and reflex and tone changes (Hales & Yudofsky, 2003).

The three subtypes of delirium are hyperactive, hypoactive, and mixed. Hyperactive delirium is characterized by agitation, restlessness, and excessive emotional reactivity or emotional lability. Hypoactive delirium has much different features such as **somnolence**, withdrawal, decreased responsiveness, and apathy. Mixed delirium is seen when the person has symptoms of both hyperactive and hypoactive delirium within the same day. The person with hypoactive delirium makes little or no demands on staff and may not be diagnosed or treated for delirium as quickly as the person with hyperactive delirium. The occurrence of delirium, and especially hypoactive delirium, is associated with increased length of hospital stay and increased morbidity (Girard, Pandharipande, & Wesley, 2008).

Course and Prognosis of Delirium

Delirium has a rapid onset. For persons who have delirium, many meet diagnostic criteria within the same day that they developed their first symptoms, and most meet criteria within 48 hours of emergence of symptoms. The course usually fluctuates. There can be lucid intervals as well as periods of confusion and anxiety within the course of a day or even hours. It is not unusual for symptoms to worsen in the evening or at night, and this phenomenon is known as **sundowning** (Sadock, Sadock, & Ruiz, 2014).

Delirium usually has a brief duration of less than a week, though the symptoms will persist as long as any condition causing the delirium is present. After treating the causative factor, symptoms of delirium usually recede in three to 7 days. For older patients, the delirium can last longer and take as many as two weeks to resolve (Sadock, Sadock, & Ruiz, 2014). The possible outcomes for delirium range from full recovery to death (Hales & Yudofsky, 2003). It should be noted that a person does not die from delirium. For a person who is declining with a terminal illness, it is not uncommon for delirium to develop as the body's life-sustaining systems begin to fail. It is also important to note that there is a risk for falls that accompanies delirium. The person hospitalized postoperatively or for a serious illness may attempt to get out of bed even though he or she may not have the needed strength, balance, or coordination. Disturbed thought processes including impulsivity, emotionality, confusion, and fear may also lead a person with delirium to remove lines and tubes necessary for his or her medical treatment or engage in other, potentially dangerous behavior (Schneider & Levenson, 2008).

Medical Management of Delirium

Treatment for delirium involves treating any underlying cause or medical condition. It is important to withdraw any sedatives or most medications that act on the central nervous system (CNS). One exception to this rule is when the delirium is related to withdrawal from alcohol or sedatives, in which case the use of **anxiolytics** is indicated. In other patients with delirium, treatment may include the **neuroleptic** haloperidol (Schneider & Levenson, 2008). Since delirium is thought to be a reflection of a neurotransmitter dysfunction, antipsychotics may restore the acetylcholine/dopamine balance (Seitz & van Zyl, 2006). The person with delirium requires extra supportive physical care, including attention to nutrition and hydration, and maintenance of a safe and quiet environment. If hospitalized, it is also helpful for the person to have positive, orienting cues, such as familiar pictures or things nearby, and frequent contact with family or loved ones (Sadock, Sadock, & Ruiz, 2014).

For a person who is normally alert with intact memory, the symptoms of delirium are a significant cause for concern and should be considered a medical emergency. If the person is recovering from a medical condition that resulted in delirium, care should be taken that long-term decisions, such as guardianship and nursing home placement, be avoided until the delirium has cleared. Consider the possibility of an individual who has a delirium caused by a prescribed medication, such as a sedative. If the delirium is not accurately diagnosed and the medication routine changed, the person could be assessed as being unable to live independently. Delirium is a temporary condition whose course usually ends as the person becomes medically stable.

▪ Dementia: Alzheimer's Disease

Description and Definitions of Dementia: Alzheimer's Disease

Historically, memory impairment has been the hallmark symptom of dementia. Many years of research and technology developments have added to the knowledge base in this field. In 2013, the American Psychiatric Association published the *DSM-5*, which did more than just rename dementia as a NCD. Now, the various types of NCD are differentiated by much more complex symptoms of cognitive impairment, classified as neurocognitive domains. Table 11.1 gives an overview of the neurocognitive domains, which includes complex attention, **executive function**, learning and memory, language, perceptual-motor, and social cognition (American Occupational Therapy Association, 2014; American Psychiatric Association, 2013).

The *DSM-5* differentiates major and mild NCDs within each type of NCD. A significant criterion for this differentiation is the level of function. For the NCD to be a major NCD, independence in instrumental activities of daily living (IADLs) is impaired. In a mild NCD, there may be capacity for independence in IADLs though the person may need more time, more effort, and compensatory strategies (American Psychiatric Association, 2013).

This chapter will focus primarily on the NCD most often seen by the occupational therapist: NCD due to AD. The remaining types of NCDs will be reviewed in a briefer format.

Etiology of Alzheimer's Disease

The cause of AD is poorly understood, and, at present, there is no perfect biological marker that is diagnostic of AD in a living person (Minati, Edinton, Bruzzone, & Giaccone, 2009). The clinical diagnosis is one of exclusion, made after ruling out alternate etiologies, such as cardiovascular disease or Parkinson's disease, and after considering current and past medical and psychiatric conditions, surgeries, metabolic abnormalities, and pharmacotherapy (Burke et al., 2015). The best diagnostic tools for confirming a diagnosis of AD, such as **magnetic resonance imaging** and **spectroscopy** which refer to the measurement of radiation intensity, diffusion tensor imaging, cerebrospinal fluid analysis, positron emission tomography, and electroencephalography, can be difficult and expensive. But even these advanced tests yield only 60% to 90% specificity and sensitivity (Minati et al., 2009). The best tools for diagnosing AD, such as magnetic resonance imaging (MRI) and spectroscopy, diffusion, positron emission tomography, and electroencephalography can be difficult and expensive. However, even these advanced tests yield only 60to 90% specificity development and utilization of superior diagnostic tools have not been a priority to researchers due to the lack of highly effective treatment options following a positive diagnosis (Minati et al., 2009). However, much research has focused on associated features and laboratory findings relevant to AD in an attempt to discover its origin(s). This chapter will review some of the major findings now being studied.

TABLE 11.1 Neurocognitive Domains

	Cognitive Domain	Performance Skill	Examples of Observable Performance
Complex Attention	**Diagnostic and Statistical Manual of Mental Disorders (DSM-5):** Complex attention: Sustained attention; divided attention; selective attention; processing speed **Occupational Therapy Practice Framework (OTPF):** Mental function/attention: Sustained shifting and divided attention; concentration; distractibility	Maintains attention over time; maintenance of attention despite competing stimuli or distractors; attending to two tasks within the same time period	**Mild NCD:** Normal tasks take longer than usual; there are errors in routine tasks; thinking becomes more difficult when competing with stimuli such as radio, TV, other conversations, and driving; neglects minor grooming details **Major NCD:** Increased difficulty in environments with multiple stimuli; information must be kept simple; may not attend to task through to completion, including eating; cannot simultaneously perform two simple tasks such as talking and walking; neglects grooming nonvisible body parts or neglects grooming entirely; at risk for wandering
Executive Function	**DSM-5:** Executive Function: Planning; decision making; working memory; responding to feedback/error correction; overriding habits/inhibition; mental flexibility **OTPF:** Mental function/higher-level cognitive: Judgment; concept formation; metacognition; executive functions; praxis; cognitive flexibility insight	Performs steps in logical order; selects appropriate tools/materials/actions for the task; categorize objects/events/ideas according to similarities; synthesize information; self-assess and correct errors; combines thought and motor planning to fluidly and effectively perform an action; adjusts to unexpected changes in the environment	**Mild NCD:** Increased effort required to perform multistep tasks; difficulty multitasking or returning to task after an interruption; reduced work output; does not anticipate predicted changes, such as increase in property taxes **Major NCD:** Abandons complex tasks; needs to focus on one task at a time; can no longer plan routine IADL; tools and materials may be used in unsafe manner; does not notice or respond to effects of actions, such as brushing only front of teeth

TABLE 11.1 *Continued*

	Cognitive Domain	Performance Skill	Examples of Observable Performance
Learning and Memory	**DSM-5:** Learning and memory: Immediate memory; recent memory; long-term memory **OTPF:** Mental functions/memory: Short term; long term; working memory. Global mental functions: orientation to person, place, and time	Can retain small amount of new information for short period of time; can store and retrieve information over long periods of time, often over the entire lifespan; can manage new and stored information to carry out complex tasks such as learning, reasoning and comprehension	**Mild NCD:** May cope with short-term memory loss by using lists or calendar; difficulty navigating in unfamiliar areas **Major NCD:** Repeats self in conversation; cannot remember plans for the day; poor orientation to time and date; may get lost in familiar environments; cannot retain/follow a directive or cue after a few seconds
Language	**DSM-5:** Language: Expressive language; receptive language **OTPF:** Voice and speech functions: Fluency and rhythm. Mental functions/thought: control and content of thought, awareness of reality vs. delusions, and logical and coherent thought. Performance skills/social interaction skills: produces speech, gesticulates, and speaks fluently	Can understand or comprehend language heard or read; can perform functions of naming, word finding, grammar, and syntax; can put thoughts into words and sentences; uses socially appropriate gestures to communicate or support a message; speaks in a fluent and continuous manner, with an even pace; speech demonstrates logical and coherent thought.	**Mild NCD:** Begins to have word finding difficulty; forgets names of acquaintances; becomes anxious with verbal overload **Major NCD:** Decline in both expressive and receptive language; may forget names of close friends and family; may use "no" as answer to all questions
Perceptual Motor	**DSM-5:** Perceptual-motor: Abilities that include visual perception, visual-constructional, perceptual-motor, praxis, and gnosis **OTPF:** Sensory functions: Visual, hearing, vestibular, and proprioceptive. Movement functions: Motor reflexes, involuntary movement reactions, and control of voluntary movement and gait patterns. Mental functions: Perception	Aware of the environment within the visual field; can detect and discriminate sound; responds to sensation related to position, balance, and movement against gravity; aware of body position and space; postural, body adjustment, and supporting reactions; eye-hand and eye-foot coordination; bilateral integration; fine and gross motor control; productive gait and mobility	**Mild NCD:** May need to rely more on maps or others for directions; less precise in parking; needs greater effort for spatial tasks such as carpentry and sewing **Major NCD:** Significant difficulty with use of tools/operating motor vehicles; more confused at dusk/lower levels of light; gait slows with a tendency to shuffle; poor balance creates fear of falling, which leads to holding on tightly (grab rails, furniture) or pushing something (wheelchair, furniture)

TABLE **11.1** *Continued*			

	Cognitive Domain	**Performance Skill**	**Examples of Observable Performance**
Social Cognition	**DSM-5:** Social cognition: Recognition of emotions; theory of mind **OTPF:** Mental functions: Thought and emotional. Global mental functions: Temperament and personality. Performance skills/ social interaction skills: approaches/starts, concludes/disengages, turns toward, looks, places self, touches, regulates, questions, replies, discloses, expresses emotion, disagrees, thanks, transitions, times response, times duration, takes turns, matches language, clarifies, acknowledges and encourages, empathizes, heeds, accommodates, and benefits	Recognizes and interprets body language; considers another person's emotions; understands rules and concepts for social interaction including rules of etiquette	**Mild NCD:** Subtle changes in personality; less able to read non-verbal cues; decreased empathy or inhibition; disregards priorities/ needs of others **Major NCD:** Insensitive to acceptable social standards or topics of conversation; makes decisions without regard to safety (choosing proper clothing for weather or keeping important information private); continual need for reassurance; poor regulation of emotions

American Psychiatric Association. (2013). *Diagnostic and statistical manual of mental disorders* (5th ed.). Washington, DC: Author.

American Occupational Therapy Association. (2014). *Occupational therapy practice framework: Domain & process* (3rd ed.). Bethesda, MD: Author. doi.org/10.5014/ajot.2014.682006

Neuropathology of Alzheimer's Disease

Neuroimaging tools, such as MRI, are being used to detect the earliest changes of AD, to differentiate AD from other forms of NCDs, and to improve methods for clinical trials in AD and related disorders (Jack, C., et al., 2015; DeCarli, 2001). Some of these physical findings are cortical atrophy, widened sulci, and ventricular enlargement (Hales & Yudofsky, 2003). This shrinking of brain structure is a result of neuronal loss, which seems to be caused by **neurofibrillary tangles** and beta-amyloid plaques which are tau proteins

Amyloid deposits are part of the histopathological definition of AD; therefore, a great deal of weight is put on the biomarkers of amyloid in AD research. **Beta-amyloid** plaques are caused by a chemical accident or the defective breakdown of a benign substance known as **amyloid precursor protein** (APP). APP lives in various

parts of the body, including the brain, and its role in cellular function is unknown. As part of its mysterious function, APP regularly gets broken down into much smaller soluble components and is washed away with other decomposed tissues and chemicals. Under some conditions that are not understood, the breaking apart does not proceed correctly. The outcome produces sticky, insoluble shards of beta-amyloid. These shards stick to each other, attracting fragments of dead and dying neurons, and slowly decline into dense, misshapen plaques (Shenk, 2003). Beta-amyloid plaques collect outside and around the neurons. It is believed that this accumulation causes physical damage to axons and that prolonged neuronal response to this injury ultimately leads to the development of neurofibrillary tangles and neuronal death (Vickers, Dickson, & Adlard, 2000). Amyloid has a preference for depositing in regions of the brain that support complex cognitive function. An active area of AD research is testing the relationship between amyloid levels and cognitive function.

Neurofibrillary tangles are made up of another contaminated protein called tau. **Tau** normally serves as connectors or "railroad ties" for a track-like structure that transports nutrients and other important molecules throughout the cell body of every neuron. The contaminated or tangled tau somehow becomes hyperphosphorylated, a corruption resulting in several extra molecules of phosphorous. Without the stabilizing railroad ties of normal tau, the tracks bend into a twisted mess. Under the weight of the nutrients being transported, the tracks buckle, and the damage increases. Inside the neuron, this twisted debris gets worse as the filaments of track keep twisting around each other. As cell communication and nourishment are lost, the neuron begins to wither. The cell body, axons, and dendrites disintegrate, and as a result, thousands of synapses vanish (Bear, Connors, & Paradiso, 2001; Shenk, 2003). It is well documented that the brains of persons with AD have an abundance of the abnormal structures of beta-amyloid plaques and neurofibrillary tangles (Shenk, 2003). Filamentous structures known as "Hirano bodies" found primarily in the hippocampus are also associated with the disease (Neugroschl, Kolevzon, Samuels, & Marin, 2004).

The structural changes just described do not cause AD but are the end product of a pathological process. The challenge for researchers is to discover what causes this degeneration. The loss of neurons occurs throughout the brain but is significant in the cerebral cortex. The cerebral cortex is responsible for higher brain functions, including thinking, judgment, reasoning, speech, and language. Plaques and tangles are also dense in the hippocampus, which plays a role in attention and memory (Cohen & Eisdorfer, 2001).

It is possible that amyloid has a function as a repair protein. Amyloid levels have been noted to increase when there is some injury to the brain. Some researchers contend that beta-amyloid plaques do not lead to AD but, in fact, might be a by-product of the AD process (Shenk, 2003).

Genetic Predisposition of Alzheimer's Disease

Unlike some diseases, AD is not caused by a single gene. Recent advances in understanding the human genome combined with technologic advances in methods of analysis have revealed new genes associated with AD risk. More than one gene mutation is seen in AD, and multiple genetic loci associated with increased risk have been identified over the past few years. The role of the innate immune system was identified in 2013 by the discovery that rare variants in *TREM2*, a microglial surface receptor, are associated with a significantly increased risk of AD (Ryan, Rossor, & Fox, 2015). In most cases, genes alone are not sufficient to cause AD. The two types of AD are early onset and late onset. Early onset refers to AD that manifests before the age of 65, and late onset refers to AD seen at or after age 65. Less than 5% of AD is early onset, and this form of the disease is often inherited (Rocchi, Pellegrini, Siciliano, & Murri, 2003; U.S. Department of Health and Human Services, 2004).

Three genes have been identified as responsible for the rare, early-onset, familial form of AD. Mutated chromosome 21 causes an abnormal APP to be produced. Mutated chromosome 14 causes an abnormal protein called presenilin 1 to be produced. Mutated chromosome 1 causes yet another abnormal protein, presenilin 2, to be produced (National Institute on Aging, 2003). It appears that these mutations increase the likelihood that beta-amyloid will be snipped from the APP, causing more of the sticky beta-amyloid to be formed (Cohen & Eisdorfer, 2001). Even if only one of these genes inherited from a parent is mutated, the person will almost certainly develop early-onset AD. This means that in these families, children have a 50% chance of developing early-onset AD if one parent has this disease.

In the more common, late-onset AD, the apolipoprotein E genotype is the strongest risk factor (Karch & Goate, 2015). Although the apolipoprotein E genotype is equally common in men and women, it has a much stronger effect in women. The Apolipoprotein E, or APOE allele is an example of a completely biological factor that interacts with biological and gender-related factors such as hormones, education, behavioral preferences, type of occupation, and physical activity and increases the risk of AD (Rocca, Mielke, Vemuri, & Miller, 2014). The apolipoprotein E gene is found on chromosome 19. This gene codes for a protein that helps carry cholesterol in the bloodstream. The apolipoprotein E gene comes in several forms, called alleles. The three most common alleles are apolipoprotein

E 2, apolipoprotein E 3, and apolipoprotein E 4. A person inherits one apolipoprotein E allele from each parent. One or two copies of the 4 allele increases the risk of getting AD. However, having the 4 allele does not mean that AD is certain, as some persons with even two of the 4 allele do not develop the disease. The rarer 2 allele may be associated with having a lower risk for AD and later age at onset (Blazer, Steffens, & Busse, 2004; Karch & Goate, 2015; U.S. Department of Health and Human Services, 2004). AD may also be linked to mutations in the gene that encodes for insulin-degrading enzyme, which helps to break down beta-amyloid. Other genes related to AD include those involved in intracellular APP trafficking and the creation of apolipoprotein neural receptors and transmembrane proteins that influence calcium levels and beta-amyloid production (Minati et al., 2009).

Down's syndrome is a risk factor for AD. Individuals with Down's syndrome carry an extra copy of chromosome 21, which contains the APP gene. As a result, researchers believe that APP processing in neuronal membranes is abnormal leading to the formation of beta-amyloid plaques and eventual AD neuropathology. In fact, the brains of almost all individuals with Down's syndrome over the age of 40 show anatomical changes associated with AD, and as many as 66% will develop clinically detectable dementia in their 50s (Beacher et al., 2009). In another study, it was reported that 32.1% of a sample of individuals with Down's syndrome between the ages of 55 and 59 had dementia, 17.7% between the ages of 50 and 54, and 8.9% between the ages of 45 and 49 (Coppus et al., 2006). Due to preexisting learning disabilities, AD is more difficult to detect and treat in this population (Beacher et al., 2009).

More recently, a possible link between environmental conditions in early brain development and future manifestation of AD has been proposed. The "Latent Early-life Associated Regulation" or "LEARn" model posits that factors such as diet, toxin exposure, and hormones early in one's development may disrupt DNA structure in a manner that influences the way certain genes are regulated. In support of this model, animal studies have shown that exposure to lead early in life may upregulate the expression of APP in old age (Lahiri, Zawia, Sambamurti, & Maloney, 2008; Wu et al., 2008).

Neurotransmitter Abnormalities in Alzheimer's Disease

There are a number of neurotransmitters that are associated with AD. Most changes are related to the glutamatergic system, with most changes in the activation and expression of NMDA and the acetylcholinergic system. Changes are also found in other central neurotransmitter systems including the serotoninergic, dopaminergic, and noradrenalinergic systems. Changes in these systems are most probably the result of global brain atrophy seen as the disease progresses. The neurotransmitter acetylcholine is proposed to be responsible for the cognitive symptoms of AD and is implicated in the progression of AD. Neurons that contain acetylcholine are known as cholinergic neurons, and many of these are bunched together to form tracts. Cholinergic tracts radiate throughout the entire brain. Autopsy shows that for a person with AD, many cholinergic tracts throughout the entire brain have been destroyed. The enzyme choline acetyltransferase (CAT), which is needed to form acetylcholine, is seriously reduced in the brains of persons with AD. This reduction of CAT is greatest in areas of the brain where there is a dense amount of plaques and tangles (U.S. Department of Health and Human Services, 2004). Although the cognitive impairments of AD have been traditionally attributed to the degeneration of cholinergic systems, alterations in the neuronal histaminergic system have been increasingly recognized as contributing to the cognitive impairments seen in AD (Zlomuzica et al., 2015). The neuronal histaminergic system is an area where further research may lead to the development of more effective drugs for the treatment of cognitive symptoms. Other neurotransmitter systems found to be altered in people with AD include norepinephrine, GABA, and glutamate (Neugrosch et al., 2004).

Cardiovascular Risk Factors in Alzheimer's Disease

Although vascular dementia accounts for 15% to 25% of all dementia cases, there is now a concern that cardiovascular disease is also linked to AD. As people are living longer with AD, and living long enough to be diagnosed with AD at age 80 and 90, these groups are also at risk for developing cardiovascular disease. Some see this group as having a "mixed dementia," or a combination of AD and vascular disease (Cohen & Eisdorfer, 2001). Currently, the question is not whether the two disease processes are mixed but whether the vessel damage is causal or consequential to the degeneration of neural tissue (Stone, Johnstone, Mitrofanis, & O'Rourke, 2014). Increasing evidence suggests the neuropathology and cognitive decline of AD is caused by clinically silent bleeding from small cerebral vessels. Studies have established that the presence of infarcts in eersons with AD results in lower cognitive function, especially in the area of episodic memory of specific experiences and events (Gore-lick et al, 2011). (U.S. Department of Health and Human Services, 2004). In autopsy studies, 60% to 90% of AD cases exhibit variable cerebrovascular pathology (Kawas & Brookmeyer, 2001). Researchers have also found the use of statins, the most common type of cholesterol-lowering drug, to be associated with a lower risk of developing AD (Rocchi et al., 2003). Research has linked cases of familial AD with vessel damage indicating that these dementias may possibly be forms of vascular dementia, as well. Recent advance in the resolution of cerebral imaging has made it possible for researchers to detect silent micro bleeds, which do most of the damage in vascular dementia. The vulnerability of the brain to the pulse is linked to the high metabolism of the brain. To enable the high volume of blood flow, the resistance of the brain's vessels is low making it vulnerable to the long-term beat of the heart. Loss of elasticity, vascular remodeling, and arterial stiffness also increase the intensity of the pulse and correlate with cognitive decline in aging. Ways to protect the brain from the long-term effect of the pulse include controlling blood pressure and diabetes and minimizing arteriosclerosis and atherosclerosis.

Other Potential Causes of Alzheimer's Disease

One of the theories of aging suggests that over time, damage from a kind of molecule called a free radical can build up in neurons and cause a loss of function. Free radicals can be helpful in fighting infection, but too many can injure cells by changing other nearby molecules, such as those in the neuron's cell membrane or in DNA. This process can lead to a chain reaction, releasing more free radicals and causing more damage. This is called oxidative damage and may contribute to AD by upsetting the proper flow of substances in and out of cells, by disrupting cell metabolism, and/or by interfering with other cell processes such as protein synthesis, stress response, and enzyme-catalyzed reactions (National Institute on Aging, 2003; Reed, Sultana, & Butterfield, 2010). Some researchers are focusing on a possible connection between oxidative stress and beta-amyloid, the principal component of plaques found in the brain of the person with AD (Varadarajan, Yatin, & Aksenova, 2000). To support the role of oxidative stress in contributing to AD, researchers have found that antioxidant defense is altered in the brains of persons with mild cognitive impairment (MCI), a condition that is often a precursor to AD (Reed et al., 2010).

Researchers are also studying the possible role of inflammation, because cells and compounds that are known to be involved in inflammation are found in AD plaques. Some scientists think that inflammation is harmful and sets off a cycle of events that lead to the death of neurons. Others believe that some aspects of the inflammatory process may be a helpful part of the brain's natural healing efforts (National Institute on Aging, 2003). Research is focused on even more factors that may be related to AD, including trace elements, the role of the immune system, and the possibility of a viral connection. The role of numerous misfolded proteins in the neuropathology of AD along with other neurodegenerative diseases such as Parkinson's disease, Huntington's disease, and amyotrophic lateral sclerosis (ALS/Lou Gehrig's disease) is also a topic of scientific inquiry (Kanehisa, Limviphuvadh, & Tanabe, 2010).

■ Incidence and Prevalence of Alzheimer's Disease

It is estimated that there are 5.3 million Americans with AD. While most persons with AD are 65 or older, there are about 200,000 individuals under age 65 who have younger-onset AD (Alzheimer's Association, 2015). According to population-based studies, 600,000 Americans with AD died in 2010, and in 2011, it was the sixth leading cause of death (Mitchell, 2015). With the aging of the baby boomer population and medical advances, it is predicted that by 2050, there will be 18 million Americans with NCD; within this group, 14 million will have NCD due to AD. AD increases in prevalence with increasing age, and women tend to have a higher incidence of AD. For persons age 85, 11% of men and 14% of women have AD. At age 90, the rate increases to 21% for men and 25% for women. While AD is the most common form of NCD, approximately 10% to 15% of persons with AD have a coexisting vascular dementia (Sadock et al., 2014).

In addition to age and gender, there are numerous factors that appear to create a higher risk for AD (Hales & Yudofsky, 2003; Neugrosch et al., 2004; Reitz et al., 2010; Shah et al., 2009). These factors include the following:

1. Low educational level
2. History of head trauma with loss of consciousness
3. History of depression
4. Late maternal age
5. Environmental and occupational exposure (e.g., to aluminum)
6. History of electroconvulsive therapy (ECT)
7. Alcohol abuse
8. **Analgesic** abuse
9. Long-standing physical inactivity
10. Vascular risk factors (e.g., hypertension, high cholesterol)
11. Type II diabetes
12. Black or Hispanic ethnicity
13. High waist-to-hip ratio

Minati et al. state that TBI is increasingly believed to be a risk factor for the development of AD due to the accumulation of **beta-amyloid** and **tau** pathology that follows neural degeneration. They also indicate that cerebrovascular abnormalities may increase the chances of being diagnosed with AD. However, they assert that the most important risk factors are advanced age and genetic predisposition (Minati et al., 2009).

Related to these risk factors, there also appear to be several variables that may reduce the risk of developing AD (Breitner & Albert, 2009; Neugrosch et al., 2004; Shah et al., 2009). These include the following:

1. Exposure to antioxidants (such as vitamin E)
2. Regular consumption of fish
3. Estrogen replacement therapy in postmenopausal women
4. Use of nonsteroidal anti-inflammatory drugs (NSAIDs)
5. Use of specific antihypertensive drugs

6. Use of statins
7. Use of specific histamine blockers
8. Physical activity
9. Exposure to education, cognitive training, and mental stimulation

However, the effectiveness of some of these agents is still a matter of scientific debate.

■ Signs and Symptoms of Alzheimer's Disease

The signs and symptoms of NCD due to AD include a range of cognitive functions: attention, executive function, learning and memory, language, perceptual motor skills, and social cognition. These symptoms impact virtually all performance skills. Since AD is a progressive disease, the first signs can be mistaken for normal aging. Even though there are small changes in process skills with normal aging, a healthy older adult can continue to learn and problem-solve at any age. Researchers are generating new information on normal aging versus mild NCD. A person with mild NCD will have more impairment of process skills than is expected with normal aging but will not yet meet the diagnostic criteria for major NCD due to AD.

Defining the progressive stages of AD is an arbitrary process, and various researchers use different ideologies. Reisberg, a prominent researcher in the study of AD, has proposed seven stages (Reisberg & Sclan, 1992). These stages range from stage 1, in which there is no impairment, to stage 7, which is very severe decline. Most researchers use a three-stage approach (Goldman, Wise, & Brody, 2004; Samuels & Neugroschl, 2004; Shenk, 2003). The Clinical Dementia Rating (CDR) is used to measure dementia (Hughes, Berg, & Danziger, 1993). This scale defines three levels of dementia or NCD as mild, moderate, and severe.

This chapter will use the three-stage approach, which correlates with the *DSM-5*'s levels of severity for NCDs: mild, moderate, and severe. The first stage, or early stage, is a mild NCD and is what used to be referred to as mild cognitive disorder. The second or middle stage occurs at the onset of major NCD, with a moderate level of severity. The late stage is severe major NCD. It is important to remember that each person with AD is a unique individual, with unique concerns, needs, and strengths. Although such individuals do not always fit into a rigid classification system, using the three stages will give the reader general guide-lines for better understanding the problems facing the person with AD and his or her caregivers.

■ Course and Prognosis of Alzheimer's Disease

Mild Stage

For mild NCD due to AD, the early or mild stage usually lasts 2 to 3 years (Gauthier, 2002). The cognitive changes in the mild stage require com-pensatory strategies and accommodations for the individual to maintain independence. The per-son who recognizes that his or her memory is impaired may be better able to make necessary adaptations. Eventually all cognitive domains are impacted in the early or mild stage.

Complex Attention

The person takes longer to perform familiar tasks and begins making mistakes. It becomes difficult to do two things at once, such as talk while driv-ing or cook while following a recipe.

Executive Function

The person in the mild stage of AD begins to have difficulty with IADLs. Bills may be forgotten, and having automatic bill payment becomes a neces-sary strategy. Medication management may need to be monitored by a caregiver. Problems with planning, organizing, sequencing, and abstract-ing become apparent as the person begins to have difficulty in the workplace or following written directions such as a recipe (Hales & Yudofsky, 2003). For example, the person may begin to prepare a meal, become distracted, and forget to complete it; in another example, the person pre-paring food might be unable to properly sequence the steps or leave out important ingredients.

Learning and Memory

Short-term memory is significantly impaired, which makes new learning very difficult. The per-son forgets tasks, loses the thread of a conversa-tion, and misplaces things. **Long-term memory** begins to be impaired (Hales & Yudofsky, 2003). The person might be able to remember a phone number long enough to repeat it but will forget it if there is any delay in using it. **Procedural mem-ory**, such as knowing how to write, will remain intact. However, other types of memory begin to show deficits including **personal episodic memory**, which is time-related information about one's self, such as where and if one ate yesterday evening; **semantic memory**, such as remember-ing the name of a common object; and general knowledge, such as remembering the name of the highest mountain in the world.

Language.

Aphasia, an abnormal neurological condition in which language is impaired, appears in the mild stage. The person can usually maintain sentence structure, though it becomes less com-plex. Poor semantic memory leads to difficulty with word retrieval (the ability to name an object when shown a picture of it) and word list genera-tion (e.g., being able to quickly name words in a common category or beginning with the same letter). When forgetting a word, the person may substitute inappropriate words, making sentences incomprehensible. This would be an example of **paraphasia**, which means saying the wrong word, substituting a word that sounds alike, or using a word in the same category as the intended word. **Anomia** is the phenomenon in which a per-son searches in vain for a word and says "thing-amajig" or just gives up. **Circumlocution** may occur, in which the person tries to express an idea by talking around the intended word with exten-sive description and elaboration (Liu, McDowd, & Lin, 2004).

Perceptual-Motor Abilities

Visuospatial abilities decline in the mild or early stage of AD. The person starts to have difficulty with **topographical orientation**, getting lost in a familiar neighborhood or failing to recognize a familiar intersection. There may be some dis-orientation within the home, such as putting the frying pan in the freezer or the wallet in the dish-washer (Bear et al., 2001).

Social Cognition

It is not unusual to see personality changes. The family notices that the person is more rigid and irritable and less spontaneous or adventurous. Some persons with AD become suspicious, think-ing that one's things are being stolen or that his or her spouse is being unfaithful. The person may become less attuned to body language and seem inconsiderate. Depression is seen in up to 25% of people in the mild stage of AD. Depression or anxiety may lead to withdrawal from routine social activity. In some cases, delusional thinking may emerge (Kovach, 1997).

Moderate Stage

In the middle or moderate stage of AD, which can last from 2 to 10 years, there is continued decline across all neurocognitive domains. While a person in the mild stage of AD may be able to live independently, by the moderate stage there is a severe impact on function. All areas of performance skills begin to show deficits, psychiatric symptoms increase, and behavior disturbances arise.

Complex Attention

There is difficulty with maintaining attention in environments with multiple stimuli such as loud noises and bright or changing light. Attention cannot be divided between two tasks, such as walking and talking simultaneously. The ability to focus attention for a length of time will be reduced, with the need for prompts or redirection several times a minute.

Executive Function

The person in the moderate stage of AD is no longer able to problem-solve. The ability to plan, weigh consequences, consider alternative strategies, and judge outcomes is lost. The caregiver, who is now responsible for complex tasks and problem solving, may be able to guide and prompt the person with AD through some of the steps as a way to keep him or her engaged in meaningful tasks.

Learning and Memory

Recent and **remote memory** worsens. The person may think he or she is back at an earlier stage of life and become focused on a past worry, such as getting the children to school on time. The person becomes less bothered by the memory loss. There is disorientation to place and time, and in the course of decline, the person may not recognize his or her own face in the mirror, much less friends, or family members a condition known as **prosopagnosia**. New information is not retained for more than a few moments. There is difficulty organizing thoughts and thinking logically, and inability to cope with new or unexpected situations. Thinking is concrete, with no ability to take into account ideas or objects that are not present (National Institute on Aging, 2003; Shenk, 2003; Zgola, 1999).

Language

There are increased symptoms of aphasia, and the person loses fluent language. Language is limited to the concerns of the moment or reminiscing about the past. There may be diminished verbal responsiveness, or verbalizations may be impulsive and inappropriate. There is difficulty understanding simple questions or instructions. The person has trouble following a conversation and may be unable to keep track of his or her own thoughts or words (Frank, 2003). Internal speech is part of executive function and is necessary for an individual to make plans or mentally problem-solve. A person who can no longer use words effectively loses this ability of rational planning. His or her actions will become impulsive and disorganized, requiring step-by-step direction and supervision for any occupation (Zgola, 1999).

Perceptual-Motor Skills

Visuospatial abilities continue to decline. Visual inattention, which is seen in the mild stage, begins to seriously limit function in the moderate stage (Liu et al., 2004). The person gets lost in familiar environments, and is unable to become oriented if he or she moves to a new environment. Constructional skills are compromised, and the person is unable to sort out the arms and legs of garments while trying to get dressed. There is a loss of ability to judge depth and distance. The person may step highly over a mark on the ground or choose to walk around it. He or she may not be able to distinguish furniture from designs on the carpet or interpret changes in flooring. These visuospatial impairments can lead to falls. Judging direction and distance is problematic, resulting in knocking things over when trying to grasp them or grasping at thin air (Zgola, 1999).

Social Cognition

There is little or no awareness of social standards, as manifested by immodest dress or inappropriate topics of conversation. The person will not be able to consider the needs of a minor or a pet. He or she will need the caregiver to assist with community participation such as doctor appointments, shopping, and restaurant outings.

Psychiatric Symptoms

Psychiatric symptoms that emerged in the mild stage worsen. Depression and anxiety are frequently seen, and the presence of depression is associated with increased mortality. The person may lose control over his or her emotions, having outbursts of fear or anger. Visual hallucinations are not uncommon, and auditory hallucinations can also occur. Sleep is disturbed, with increased daytime napping and frequent nighttime wakefulness (Kovach, 1997).

Behavior Disturbances

Behavior disturbances increase the likelihood that the individual will need nursing home placement. It is in the moderate stage of AD that wandering and agitation become a problem (National Institute on Aging, 2003). The person paces, seemingly without a goal or destination. Pacing could be a sign of stress or anxiety, or perhaps it is the person's need for activity and exercise. Agitation could be the person's only way to respond to fear or frustration (Kovach, 1997). Loss of impulse control manifests in sloppy table manners, undressing at inappropriate times or places, and vulgar or rude language (Vickers et al., 2000). There is a loss of social propriety and **disinhibition**, a failure of the filtering system that determines which thoughts to keep to one's self and which thoughts to act upon. This inability to inhibit impulses can cause offense to others or become dangerous if the person with AD acts upon aggressive impulses (Zgola, 1999).

Severe Stage

The severe or late stage of AD can last as long as 8 or more years. At this stage, the person with AD is fully dependent on others for basic ADLs, such as bathing, dressing, and eating. Motor skills are affected, and the person eventually becomes immobile and incontinent.

Complex Attention

Attention is now measured in seconds, and the caregiver will need to give frequent but simple cues for performing simple actions such as eating or lifting an arm during dressing. Awareness of the environment is very limited. The person in the severe stage of AD eventually may only respond to pain, hunger, and fear.

Executive Function

All problem-solving and planning skills are seriously impaired, and purposeful, goal-directed occupation is lost.

Learning and Memory

There is no ability to create new memories and little or no recognition of close family members. Despite these deficits, it is still important to bring into the environment personal and meaningful objects such as mementos and family pictures.

Language

Speech is limited to one or two words, or speech and vocabulary may be totally unintelligible. Over time, speech will decline to the point where it is lost. The person no longer smiles or communicates with facial expression (Shenk, 2003). There can be instances of moaning or crying, and since these are universal sounds of distress, it is important for caregivers to explore the possible causes of discomfort. Receptive language is also seriously impaired. The person cannot process the meaning of words but may respond to a calm and soothing tone of voice or touch.

Perceptual-Motor Skills

In the severe stage of AD, if the person attempts to ambulate, he or she will be at risk for falling. Neurological symptoms develop, including **hyperreflexia**, apraxic gait, and frontal release signs (grasp and snout reflexes). Eventually, the person becomes bedbound with loss of postural control. **Paratonia** is a primitive reflex in which there is involuntary resistance in an extremity in response to a sudden passive movement. Thus, if a caregiver quickly moves the person's arm, he or she automatically resists the movement (Goldman et al., 2004). Seizures may occur, and contractures, pressure ulcers, urinary tract infections, and pneumonia may develop from immobility. There is incontinence of bladder and bowel. Appetite decreases, and eventually, the person develops **dysphagia**, or the loss of ability to chew and swallow (Kovach, 1997). The person begins to experience **agnosia**, having difficulty recognizing objects and familiar people.

Social Cognition

Social interaction is very limited. With a few words, and by taking the person's hands, a family member or caregiver may be able to capture the person's attention momentarily. Despite the loss of productive communication, the person may benefit from gentle hugs and caresses from a loved one.

Psychiatric Symptoms

The sleep cycle is very disturbed as the person spends 60% of time sleeping, including much of the daytime. Hallucinations persist for some (Kovach, 1997).

■ Course and Prognosis

The course of AD tends to be slowly progressive, with the loss of about 3 points per year on the Mini Mental State Examination (MMSE), a standard cognitive assessment instrument (Neugrosch et al., 2004). The stages outlined in the previous section of this chapter illustrate the progression of the signs and symptoms of AD. A 2004 study reported the average survival time following diagnosis of AD to be 4 to 6 years. On average, those who are newly diagnosed live approximately half as long as do people of the same age without AD. However, some people can survive as long as 20 years after the first appearance of symptoms (Alzheimer's Association, 2009; Varadarajan et al., 2000).

AD progresses until death. Death is usually a result of complications, such as infection, or the eventual inability of the individual to maintain nutrition and hydration. Despite suspected under-reporting, AD is the 6th leading cause of death in the United States (Alzheimer's Association, 2015).

■ Diagnosis of NCD

There are four primary criteria in the diagnosis of NCDs. First, there is a decline in performance in one or more of the cognitive domains. These cognitive domains include complex attention, executive function, learning and memory, language, perceptual-motor abilities, and social cognition (see Table 11.1) (American Occupational Therapy Association, 2014; American Psychiatric Association, 2013). If there is a mild decline in performance, the diagnosis will be a mild NCD; if there is a significant decline in cognition, the diagnosis will be a major NCD. The diagnostician determines that there is a decline in performance based on 1. Concern of the individual or the observation of someone who knows the individual, and 2. Cognitive impairment documented by standardized neuropsychological testing, or other quantified clinical assessment (American Psychiatric Association, 2013).

The second criterion for NCD is the finding that cognitive deficits cause some degree of impairment in occupational functioning. For a mild NCD, the cognitive deficits do not necessarily interfere with

independent living. However, the individual will begin to have difficulty with IADLs, especially those requiring executive function such as financial or medication management. The person may be able to use compensatory strategies or may begin to need some assistance. Routine ADLs remain intact. For a major NCD, the cognitive deficits interfere with independent living; the individual loses the ability to manage IADLs and will need assistance or total care for ADLs.

The third criterion specifies that delirium cannot be the only cause of the cognitive impairment. The fourth criterion rules out other disorders, such as depression or schizophrenia as the cause of the cognitive impairment (American Psychiatric Association, 2013). AD is not the only type of NCD. In fact, the diagnosis of mild or major NCD includes a specifier for each type of NCD. These specifiers include AD, frontotemporal lobar degeneration, Lewy body disease, vascular disease, TBI, substance/medication use, HIV infection, prion disease, Parkinson's disease, Huntington's disease, other medical condition, multiple etiologies, and unspecified (American Psychiatric Association, 2013).

The diagnosis is a time-consuming process, but an important one, as the thorough medical investigation may reveal a condition that can be treated. The possibility of reversible dementia will be discussed later.

The National Institutes of Health (NIH) (National Institute on Aging, 2003) has outlined the following steps in diagnosing AD:

1. A detailed patient history should include a description of how and when the symptoms developed, the patient's and family's medical condition and medical history, and an assessment of the patient's emotional state and living environment.
2. Interviewing family members or close friends, which can provide information on how behavior and personality have changed.
3. Physical and neurological examinations and laboratory tests, which help determine neurological functioning and identify possible non-AD causes of dementia.
4. A **computerized tomography** (CT) scan or a magnetic resonance imaging (MRI) test, which can reveal changes in the brain's structure and function that indicate mild or early AD.

5. Neuropsychological tests that measure memory, language skills, and other cognitive functions, which help indicate what kind of cognitive changes are occurring.

■ Medical Management
General Treatment Approach

Goldman et al. (2004) describes the following four pillars of complete dementia care:

1. Supportive care for the patient
2. Supportive care for the family and/or caregiver
3. Disease treatment
4. Symptom treatment, including cognitive, mental, and behavioral symptoms

Supportive care includes assessing the environment for aspects of safety, as well as looking at how the environment can improve function and well-being. Very early in the disease process, the person with AD needs to discuss financial and medical concerns such as wills and advance directives. It is important to determine the level of care that is needed, who will provide the care, and additional supports such as day programs. The family may need to help make decisions regarding ability to drive and work. Maintaining the person's dignity and privacy is always important. The person with AD will also need ongoing medical care and evaluation of vision and hearing.

Minati et al. (2009) summarizes a number of evidence-based interventions that may be helpful in the treatment of persons with AD. These include individual- and group-based structured activities, psychological therapy, and cognitive rehabilitation. Cognitive strategies based on implicit learning include spaced retrieval, vanishing cues, and errorless learning. However, it is important to note that this type of "learning" depends on implicit aspects of cognition not as rapidly affected by the disease; such treatments should be used only to the extent that they are therapeutic for the individual. Other cognitive interventions include cognitive stimulation, reminiscence therapies, and external memory aids. These authors assert that "person-centered therapeutic interventions" are helpful in addressing emotional issues that underlie much of the problem behavior and distress associated with AD for both the patient and caregiver (Minati, 2009).

Support for the caregiver is critical. Approximately 80% of people with dementia are cared for by their families in the community (Neugrosch et al., 2004). Caring for someone who is progressively losing memories and skills can be stressful, sad, and frightening. Caregiving can become a 24-hour-a-day job. Complicating the stress of caring for a person with AD is the tendency of caregivers to withhold the diagnosis from friends and family and the social isolation that may result from embarrassing behavior or functional decline (Neugrosch et al., 2004). For caregivers, the stress of caregiving leads to increased risk of depression, sleep disturbance, and substance abuse and can indirectly result in patient neglect (Neugrosch et al., 2004). The Alzheimer's Association can refer caregivers for support, resources, and advocacy.

Disease treatment is meant to target the etiology or cause of the progressive decline in AD. The etiology of AD is still unknown. Former President Ronald Reagan brought national attention to the disorder when, in 1994, he announced that he had been diagnosed with AD. Following his death, his widow, Nancy Reagan, publicly campaigned for increasing dementia research funds and for limiting obstacles to stem cell research. Until the causes of AD are better understood, medical management of the vascular process continues to be important not just for persons with vascular dementia but also for AD.

Symptom treatment targets cognitive decline, psychiatric symptoms (including psychosis or depression), and behavior disturbances. As the disease progressed and the symptoms become more distressing, it is imperative for the caregiver to understand the reasons for behavior changes and finds ways to support the individual with AD while keeping him or her safe. The occupational therapist has an important role in helping the caregiver to consider the individual as a whole person, to explore environmental stressors and adaptations, and to discover productive ways to perform occupations. Occupation-based symptoms management will be discussed in the next section.

Pharmacotherapy can also be useful for some symptoms. The use of medications will not stop the disease process, but relieving the associated symptoms can comfort the person with AD and improve the quality of life for both patient and caregivers. Pharmacotherapy strategies will also be discussed.

Behavioral and Environmental Management

According to Hilgeman, Burgio, and Allen (2009), the environment surrounding a person with AD should be modified so as to restore the balance between the challenges presented and the person's current level of function. By creating an appropriate level of demand, the physical environment can serve to help maintain function and simultaneously provide stimulation and comfort to the individual with AD. Environmental considerations should be made for declining cognitive function as well as sensory loss and the potential for pain and discomfort. Some specific suggestions from Hilgeman et al. (2009) include

1. Reducing the size of space and number of individuals
2. Simplifying visual and auditory stimuli
3. Providing choices/options
4. Increasing the amount of familiar and meaningful stimuli
5. Providing redundant cues in multiple modalities
6. Increasing the sensory contrast of important stimuli

An appropriate environment is perhaps one of the most effective ways to manage problem behaviors of persons with AD. Hilgeman et al. (2009) point out that aggression is often a result of too much or too little stimulation, the anticipation or experience of pain, and frustration with one's inability to perform daily tasks or effectively communicate. They suggest breaking up long periods of low or high arousal activities with sensory stimulation or relaxation, providing orienting cues, emphasizing nonverbal communication, and working to relieve immediate discomforts. Addressing other underlying factors such as pain and depression may also help ameliorate agitated behavior. Neugrosch et al. (2004) add that infections, constipation, delirium, and medication or substance intoxication may also lead to agitated behavior in persons with AD. They suggest strategies such as promoting exercise, socialization, recreation, and predictable routines. Another way to address troublesome behavior, such as agitation, is to consider the "ABCs" (Neugrosch et al., 2004; Xie et al., 2009). This refers to the antecedents, the nature of the behavior itself, and the consequences. By considering factors that frequently lead up to the behavior, changes can be made to try to avoid the issue before it begins. Some changes may involve simplifying the task, providing different cues, or offering choices. The consequences of behavior should also be considered so that uncooperative behavior, such as acting out in avoidance of a task, is not reinforced, and positive behavior is not punished or ignored.

The DICE approach is an occupation-based method of interpreting and managing symptomatic behavior for persons with major NCD (Fraker, Kales, Blazek, Kavanaugh, & Gitlin, 2014). The occupational therapist or other health professional guides the caregiver through the four steps of DICE: Describe, Investigate, Create, and Evaluate. Using the example of difficult behavior during bathing (the patient strikes out at the caregiver), the therapist first asks the caregiver to "describe" in detail the context (who, what, when, how); the social and physical environment; the perspective of the patient as much as possible; and the degree of distress felt by both caregiver and the patient. In the second step, "investigate," the therapist explores other possible factors, such as the patient's pain, medications, medical conditions, sleep, and sensory factors. The therapist also explores the caregiver's expectations and social and cultural factors. In the third step, "create," the therapist collaborates with the caregiver to create strategies to enhance communication, simplify the task, modify the environment and stimuli, and create meaningful activities for the patient. The therapist may need to educate the caregiver in how much support is needed for the patient to be successful. After the caregiver implements the strategies, the last step is "evaluate." In this essential step, the therapist and caregiver review the outcomes, determine which strategies were safe and effective, and if other strategies need exploration. In the case of a patient becoming combative during bathing, strategies such as warming the bathroom, undressing and sponge bathing only part of the body at a time, using favorite scents, and timing the bath when the patient is most relaxed are examples of strategies that may be productive.

Patients with AD may engage in a variety of problematic behaviors other than or in addition to aggression and agitation. Some examples include wandering, grabbing others, and swallowing inedible objects. A helpful guide for dealing with these behaviors based on Allen's Cognitive Disability Model and the 25 cognitive levels and modes is written by Pollard (2005) and listed as a recommended learning resource at the end of the chapter.

Pharmacotherapy

Prescription drugs are frequently used in managing symptoms such as impaired cognition, depression, delusions and hallucinations, and agitation or aggression. Medications commonly used in treating cognitive symptoms work as cholinesterase inhibitors. These include donepezil (Aricept), rivastigmine (Exelon), and galantamine (Reminyl). Inhibiting acetylcholinesterase leaves more acetylcholine in the synapse, which facilitates the activity of remaining neurons. The various cholinesterase inhibitors tend to perform equally in comparison group studies, but it is possible for individuals to respond more favorably to one drug than another (Farlow & Boustani, 2009). In a study of patients in the mild stage of AD, those given cholinesterase inhibitors were treated with less antipsychotics and less anxiolytics than those not taking cholinesterase inhibitors (Fereshtehnejad, Johnell, & Eriksdotter, 2014). These medications do not inhibit cell loss, but research does show that there is improvement in cognitive function, behavioral symptoms, and ADL (Wang et al., 2014). This improvement seen in increased function in ADLs also results in delayed placement in nursing homes (Peterson, Stevens, & Ganguli, 2001). Some studies show that treatment with cholinesterase inhibitors can restore cognition to the level seen about 6 months prior to the start of treatment (Liu et al., 2004). This means that the person may be able to again do the things he or she could do half a year ago, such as dressing with verbal prompts only. However, these treatments cannot halt the progression of AD, and cognitive decline will continue. Common side effects of cholinesterase inhibitors include nausea, vomiting, diarrhea, and loss of appetite (Farlow & Boustani, 2009).

Memantine (Namenda) is another medication used in an attempt to slow the progression of AD. It works by blocking excess glutamate, a chemical involved in memory function (National Institute on Aging, 2003). Memantine has few long-term side effects but may cause temporary confusion or sedation while the dosing is being adjusted. Memantine by itself does not enhance cognitive function (Wang et al., 2014). A combination of memantine and a cholinesterase inhibitor is the preferred treatment for moderate to severe AD (Fan & Chiu, 2014). However, as AD progresses and the person is no longer able to share meaningful interactions, medication may be discontinued (Farlow & Boustani, 2009).

At the present, pharmacological advances in the treatment of AD include large-scale clinical trials of an antihistamine drug called Dimebon (latrepirdine). This agent appears to have mitochondrial stabilization properties that promote neuronal function and inhibit cell death, leading to improved cognition in people with AD. Investigators are also exploring drug treatments that target amyloid-beta production and aggregation, but so far, success has been minimal (Massoud & Gauthier, 2010). Fan and Chiu (2014) assert that a crucial drawback in researching AD drugs is that the patients do not receive treatments early enough in the progression of NCD. For treatments to be most effective, patients, families, and/or clinicians must recognize the early signs and symptoms of AD and begin the diagnostic and treatment process.

Depression is seen in as many as 25% to 30% of persons with dementia. Depression can occur in the early stage of AD and, if untreated, can lead to earlier institutionalization and death, aside from the emotional suffering. Select serotonin reuptake inhibitors (SSRIs) are the first line of treatment for depression, followed by the use of agents with dual effects on the serotonin and norepinephrine systems (Peterson et al., 2001). Many SSRIs have anticholinergic side effects, so fluoxetine (Prozac) and sertraline (Zoloft) are usually most appropriate for individuals with dementia (Farlow & Boustani, 2009). The accumulation of research evidence suggests that antidepressants should be used only after nonpharmacologic approaches have been tried, with the exception of severe depression with suicidal symptoms (Leong, 2014).

Delusions and hallucinations can begin in the mild stage of AD but are more common in the moderate stage. Low-dose neuroleptics are sometimes used, and the atypical neuroleptics such as risperidone (Risperdal) and olanzapine (Zyprexa) are less likely to cause side effects than the typical antipsychotic medications (Peterson et al., 2001). Corbett (2014) argues that risperidone is the only neuroleptic that should be used for persons with AD, and only in cases of a preexisting psychosis or severe aggression. However, the use of these medications is controversial due to increased risk of stroke and death as well as only limited, if any, long-term improvements (Ballard, Corbett, Chitramohan, & Aarsland, 2009; Corbett, Burns, & Ballard, 2014; Kales et al., 2012; Minati et al., 2009).

Disruptive behavior such as agitation and aggression is often a sign of a medical problem. Urinary tract infections or pneumonia can create delirium with agitation or aggression. Ruling out these and other concerns, such as environmental stress or pain, is the first step in reducing problem behaviors. If the behavior is truly caused by the underlying dementia, low-dose neuroleptics, such as risperidone and olanzapine, and the antidepressant aripiprazole may be beneficial (Gallagher & Hermann, 2015). However, the use of neuroleptics in this situation may not be the best approach. Psychological interventions and caregiver training should be the first management strategies used, prior to pharmaceutical interventions (Ballard et al., 2009; Corbett et al., 2014; Madhusoodanan & Ting, 2014).

■ Impact on Occupational Performance

Mild Stage

With the progressive loss of performance skills, AD affects increasing areas of occupation and performance patterns. Although this section outlines the expected impact of AD on client factors, it is important to remember that each individual will perform differently. Someone who has always been flexible and adaptive may compensate in ways that support function; another person who is prone to anxiety or has fewer coping skills might have more significant functional losses.

In the mild stage, ADLs remain intact. The first signs of memory impairment manifest in IADLs. The person experiencing neurocognitive deficits cannot adequately or safely fulfill the responsibilities of child-rearing or caring for others. When orientation to place is impaired, mobility within the community may no longer be safe. The person easily becomes lost in a new environment. The person with mild AD will be disoriented while vacationing or traveling away from home, and sometimes, this is when family members begin to note the symptoms of AD. Financial management begins to deteriorate. The person may forget to pay a bill or may misplace it. Shopping becomes a problem when the person is disoriented, loses track of what

he or she is trying to purchase, and has difficulty making the money transactions. Compensations can include shopping only in a familiar neighborhood and using a credit or debit card.

Other IADLs may also be impacted. Meal preparation can be a problem if the person starts the task, gets distracted, and then forgets to finish preparing and even eating the meal. Health management can be a problem if the person forgets to make or keep appointments or forgets to take medication. Home management may not be a problem if there are well-established routines and no unexpected problems arise. However, routine car maintenance might be neglected, and response to problems and emergencies might be less organized.

The ability to drive is an IADL that deserves special attention. As a general rule, persons with mild stage dementia who wish to continue to drive should have their driving skills evaluated. Many states offer driving assessments through their state departments. The Family Caregiver Alliance (2002) advises families to observe for behavioral signs that the person with dementia is no longer able to drive with safety. It is possible to determine a person is no longer safe to drive when he or she:

1. Has become less coordinated
2. Has difficulty judging distance and space
3. Gets lost or feels disoriented in familiar places
4. Has difficulty engaging in multiple tasks
5. Has increased memory loss, especially for recent events
6. Is less alert to things happening around him or her
7. Has mood swings, confusion, or irritability
8. Needs prompting for personal care
9. Has difficulty processing information
10. Has difficulty with decision making and problem solving

Memory loss impacts performance in education. Learning becomes very difficult, if not impossible. Reading is problematic. The person is likely able to read but will have difficulty retaining or remembering what is read. Work is also seriously impacted. Tasks that are routine may remain intact, but poor attention will impact the ability to get work started, attend to all details, and follow the task through to completion. As job performance deteriorates, relationships with co-workers and supervisors can become strained.

Some employers make efforts to arrange work-loads and expectations in order to maintain the worker in employment as long as possible. In other cases, the person in the mild stage of AD may have to seek early or medical retirement. The person will likely need assistance in deter-mining benefits and making plans for productive retirement. Volunteer exploration and participa-tion will be difficult. New routines are difficult to establish, and the task demands, as with regular employment, may be too high for the person with memory and other cognitive impairments.

Leisure exploration will be difficult for the same reasons. Learning new tasks or routines, even for leisure, will be very difficult. The person might be able to maintain established leisure pat-terns that have little demand for problem solving. Other activities may be given up; attending the bridge club becomes stressful instead of relaxing when it is hard to remember your partner's name or what cards were just played.

The person with mild stage AD will find social participation no longer easy or enjoyable. The family begins to notice that the person avoids social contact, is rigid or irritable, and is no longer spontaneous. He or she may drop out of commu-nity and family events, or attend without actually participating. The changed behavior could be a result of depression, deteriorating language skills, or fear of embarrassment. For the same reasons, intimacy and sexual expression will be diminished.

In the mild stage, motor skills will be unaf-fected. As cognition declines, the process skills of temporal organization are impacted. It is easy to be distracted in the middle of a task and then for-get to continue, sequence, and properly terminate it. If the task is new or unfamiliar, adaptation may be too demanding. Communication and interac-tion skills are impaired as language problems develop, and the person may no longer be able to clearly articulate thoughts and needs.

Performance patterns begin to deteriorate. The person might rigidly cling to habits or routines as he or she becomes aware of, and attempts to compensate for, memory loss. Another person may begin to neglect habits and routines; the gar-bage is not taken out, or the person stops going to church. Roles begin to change: a grandmother can no longer baby-sit but needs help to go shopping; a father can no longer help his family do the taxes, even though he worked all of his life as an accountant.

Cultural and spiritual contexts remain strong, but participation begins to decline as a result of memory impairment and communication dif-ficulties. Family and friends need to provide ever-increasing support to ensure the person is included in family, cultural, and spiritual events.

Client factors that are impacted in the mild stage are the mental functions: memory, orientation, perception, higher-level cognition, mental func-tions of language, and calculation. Self-concept will be impacted as the individual fears embar-rassment or worries that his or her competence is declining.

Moderate Stage

In the moderate stage of AD, there is impairment in all areas of occupation, and the person can no longer live alone. ADLs are not always attended to, and, when attempted, performance may be poor or inadequate. The person may attempt to shower but have difficulty setting the water temperature. Showering may consist of just getting wet, with no attention to the need for soap or shampoo. If shampoo is used, regulation is poor, with too much or too little used, using it on the top of the head only or forgetting to rinse. Dressing requires decision making such as choosing attire based on weather and occasion and the sequence of don-ning each article. The person with AD might make mistakes in these decisions, as well as in under-standing the need to remove dirty clothing and replace with clean. Although the person begins misplacing eyeglasses and dentures in the mild stage, by now, these articles might be lost or even unnoticed. Toilet hygiene is no longer productive as the person may neglect to clean the body or properly refasten clothing. Eating difficulties and weight loss typically begin in the moderate stage of AD (Neugrosch et al., 2004). The sleep-wake cycle is often disturbed, and wandering in the night can create a crisis for caregivers.

IADLs are neglected or performed without proper sequence and completion. Home man-agement tasks that are repetitive, such as folding towels, can be performed after someone else has sorted, laundered, and dried them. The person is dependent in areas of community mobility, finan-cial management, and shopping. Some cleaning and cooking tasks may be done with supervision and direction. Safety is a major concern for the person in the moderate stage of AD. At first, he or she may be safe if left home alone for an hour. As the symptoms progress, there can be risk for wandering, letting a stranger in the house, or setting a fire while trying to cook.

There is a loss of ability to perform in areas of work or education. Leisure participation is limited to activities that do not require problem solving or decision making such as singing or going out with a friend or family member to church or a restaurant. In fact, friends or family are needed for any social participation as the person will have difficulty initiating or maintaining social interaction outside of his or her immediate environment.

Motor skills remain intact in the mild stage. By the moderate stage, some of these skills are affected. The decline in visuospatial skills leads to many problems. Positioning and reaching are not always effective. Poor judgment of distance, direction, and floor or ground surfaces creates fall risk. By the middle stage, all process skills are impacted. Attention is limited, and serious memory impairment compromises all aspects of knowledge, temporal organization, organizing space and objects, and adaptation.

In the mild stage, the person begins to have problems with communication and interaction skills. By the moderate stage, information exchange is limited because of memory impairment and aphasia. As a result, social interactions are affected, often becoming limited to caregivers. Communication may be driven by anxiety, and it is not unusual for the individual to perseverate, asking the same question or expressing the same worry over and over again.

Performance patterns are severely limited. The individual may attempt to engage in habits and may be successful in some such as brushing hair or teeth. Habits that require problem solving or adaptations, such as setting an alarm clock or sewing a button, will be less productive if attempted at all. While most people have established routines for workdays, weekends, and holidays, the person in the moderate stage of AD can no longer differentiate days. This loss of routine can contribute to the person's anxiety and depression. Caregivers can help by maintaining structure in the day, as well as creative use of meaningful occupations. Roles continue to be lost, and family and friends need to support the most significant roles by reminiscing and affirming the individual's importance.

Cultural contexts begin to diminish in moderate stage AD. Personal and temporal contexts may be confused, and some days, the person may believe he or she is in an earlier stage of life. Some cultural, social, and spiritual contexts may remain intact, but as the condition progresses, there is less attention given to beliefs and values that defined the individual.

Client factors of mental functions are seriously impaired. Orientation to person, place, and time is affected. Personality changes; instead of spontaneity, there is disinhibition; instead of motivation and goal direction, there is apathy or anxiety; instead of fluent verbal and nonverbal communication, there is disinterest or perseveration. There is progressive impairment in all cognitive functions. The person may have hallucinations or delusional ideas. Emotions are not well regulated, and there can be outbursts of anger, fear of an imagined threat, or crying spells that come and go suddenly.

Severe Stage

During the severe stage of AD, all areas of occupation diminish and are lost. The person is fully dependent in all ADLs and can no longer ambulate with safety. All performance skills and patterns are impaired, and eventually the person loses all functional capacity. Speech is reduced to a few words and then lost entirely. The person may moan or cry, and caregivers need to assess this as a possible response to pain, discomfort, or psychosis. There is no awareness or understanding of cultural, social, or spiritual contexts. Mental functions are completely impaired, and now there is serious impact on neuromusculoskeletal and movement-related functions. Nerve cell damage takes a toll on muscle strength and tone, and voluntary movement is limited. Once the ability to swallow is lost, the family must make the decision to provide artificial life support or allow the natural course of the illness to proceed to death.

It is important to note that individuals with AD will show a wide variance in the signs and symptoms within these stages. This is true for several reasons. An individual with a strong set of beliefs and values may maintain these ideas longer than expected; the woman who always took care and pride in her appearance will maintain grooming habits in the moderate stage; someone who has always been organized may adapt for memory loss more productively. Conversely, a formerly shy person may become very impulsive and disinhibited or become even more withdrawn.

The course of the disease is also dependent upon the extent and the areas of neuronal damage.

Non-Alzheimer's Neurocognitive Disorder

Several other types of non-Alzheimer's NCDs may be seen by occupational therapists. These types include

- Vascular NCD
- Frontotemporal NCD
- NCD with Lewy bodies
- Reversible NCD

Vascular NCD

Weiner and Lipton (2009) state that vascular NCD is second to AD as the most common type of NCD, accounting for approximately 10% to 20% of late-onset cases. However, some researchers suggest that "mixed" AD and vascular dementia may be the most common form, and in Japan, China, and Russia, vascular dementia is more common than AD. While there is a slightly greater risk of AD for women, vascular dementia is more likely to occur in men, although this gender difference becomes less prominent with age (Szoeke et al., 2009). For persons having a stroke, 20% to 30% are diagnosed with NCD within 3 months. The prevalence of vascular NCD increases from 13% at age 70 to more than 44% at age 90 (American Psychiatric Association, 2013).

Vascular NCD can be caused by large multi-infarcts, which are blockages in the large vessels of the brain. Lacunar strokes, in which the small arteries are affected, can also cause vascular NCD. Lacunar strokes affect very small areas of tissue, and people with a history of arrhythmias, or irregular heartbeat rhythms, may be especially at risk for this problem (Cohen & Eisdorfer, 2001). While factors such as hypertension, diabetes, **dyslipidemia** or abnormal lipid levels, coronary artery disease, and nicotine dependence have been known to contribute to vascular NCD, nicotine use is a completely preventable risk factor and should be a focus of clinical intervention as well as public health campaigns (Chandra & Anand, 2015).

Frontotemporal Neurocognitive Disorder

Memory/learning and perceptual-motor symptoms are less prominent in FTNCD. This form of dementia was first identified by Pick in 1906 and was known as Pick's disease (Kertesz, 2004).

Some researchers refer to this condition as Pick's complex and believe that it includes an overlapping of the following syndromes: primary progressive aphasia, corticobasal degeneration, progressive supranuclear palsy, and motor neuron disease (Kertesz, 2003). The most prominent feature of FTNCD is a change in character and social conduct. The DSM-5 specifies two types of FTNCD: behavioral variant and language variant. In behavioral variant FTNCD, there is a decline in personal hygiene and socialization. Insight is usually impaired as is social cognition. Mental rigidity and inflexibility combined with distractibility can cause the person to appear memory impaired, when, in fact, memory may yet be intact. There may be perseverative and stereotyped behavior, such as humming or hand rubbing. Utilization behavior refers to touching or grasping anything within sight and inappropriate use of objects such as trying to drink from an empty cup.

A striking feature of behavior variant FTNCD is the combination of disinhibition with apathy, although, at various stages of the disease, one or the other symptom may predominate. Disinhibited behaviors manifest as abnormal demonstration of sexual acting-out, or **hypersexuality hyperorality** (a condition created by oral insertion of objects), and utilization behavior. For the middle-aged or older person, hypersexuality may consist of verbalizations or gestures. Hyperorality can be seen in excessive overeating or in developing a limiting food preference, such as eating only milk and bananas. Some may grab food, eat from other's plates, or eat inedible objects. Another group of behaviors are sometimes referred to as "negative symptoms" because they represent a lack in behavior. These include apathy, amotivation, indifference, and flat affect. There may be striking disinterest in the affairs of the family. The person may neglect to change clothing or lack the ability to attend to any task to completion (Mosimann & McKeith, 2003). However, episodic memory is generally less impaired in comparison with AD (Xie et al., 2009).

In language variant FTNCD, speech is impaired. There are three subtypes commonly seen: **semantic variant** (impaired single word comprehension, poor object and/or person knowledge, errors in reading aloud); **agrammatica/**nonfluent variant (grammatical simplification and errors, effortful halting speech); and **logopenic** variant (impaired single word retrieval, impaired repetition of phrases and sentences).

This disorder was often mistaken for AD, as its course is progressive. Survival is usually shorter and decline is faster in FTNCD than it is in AD.

Neurocognitive Disorder with Lewy Bodies

NCDLB has often been misdiagnosed as AD or delirium or viewed as Parkinson's disease plus AD. Lewy bodies are microscopic spherical neuronal inclusion bodies within the cytoplasm of a cell. In NCDLB, Lewy bodies are found in the cortical and subcortical structures of the brain distinguishing NCDLB from Parkinson's disease, in which Lewy bodies are found in the substantia nigra (Neugrosch et al., 2004).

Just as with AD, the etiology of NCDLB is unknown. The exact mechanism through which Lewy bodies form is not clearly understood. It is thought that Lewy bodies cause neuronal degeneration and eventually lead to cell death (Bras, 2015). Examination at autopsy reveals, in addition to Lewy bodies, the presence of senile plaques. Unlike the findings of AD, there are sparse neurofibrillary tangles (Mosimann & McKeith, 2003). Familial aggregation may occur, but in most cases of NCDLB, there is no family history (American Psychiatric Association, 2013).

Reversible Neurocognitive Disorder

The idea that NCD may be reversible is a topic of debate. Most researchers today believe that reversible NCD is very uncommon (Knopman & Jankowiak, 2005). In many cases, what seemed to be a reversible NCD was simply some other cause of cognitive impairment that was misdiagnosed as NCD or dementia. Burke et al. refer to the term of reversible NCD as a misnomer and state that NCD should only be used to identify cognitive impairment in cases of irreversible degenerative brain disease (Burke, Sengoz, & Schwartz, 2000). A possible exception to this rule is in cases of substance-induced NCD. The person who begins to show signs of substance-induced NCD but is able to achieve stable abstinence prior to age 50 may show substantial and even complete recovery of neurocognitive functions (American Psychiatric Association, 2013).

It is a fact that cognitive impairment can be misdiagnosed as NCD. Having a potentially treatable impairment misidentified, and left untreated, could have drastic and dire consequences for the person's function and way of life. As a result, it is important to review what some may refer to as reversible NCD and others see as reversible cognitive impairment.

CASE STUDY 1

Mrs. L. was born in South America. She was bilingual, speaking her native Spanish as well as flawless English. In her early years, she had the luxury of maids and a cook. She was a widow before her two children were grown. At age 60, her adult daughter died, leaving Mrs. L. as the primary caregiver for her two young grandchildren. Soon after her daughter's death, Mrs. L. fled her native land for political reasons, bringing her orphaned grandchildren to live in New York. After raising them, she continued to live with her adult granddaughter, G.

Mild Stage

When Mrs. L. was 82, G. married and her new husband moved into their home. Mrs. L. had always told G. that "when you marry and no longer need me, it will be my time to die." She seemed angry at G. and showed her irritation by complaining. Nevertheless, she continued to prepare the family meals, make beds, and do some of the laundry. In spite of failing vision, she was aware of the need to dust. She continued to take impeccable care of her appearance, always setting her hair at night and never going out without wearing hose and high heels. Her social life was full, with friends and neighbors frequently visiting. She took pride in serving tea and dessert to her weekly women's support group who met at her apartment. There were times when Mrs. L. misplaced her dentures (in odd places such as in a plant pot) or forgot to use detergent when washing the dishes.

She was often anxious and needy when G. came home from work, and she became defensive and easily upset when questioned about mistakes. Her granddaughter attributed these aberrations to Mrs. L.'s increased stress as a result of the marriage.

Moderate Stage

At age 86, Mrs. L. broke her hip; her granddaughter had a new, colicky baby; and the family moved to a larger apartment in the same complex. As a result of these crises, Mrs. L. seemed to have slowed down and became more dependent on G. She began making more obvious mistakes, such as using the toilet brush to scrub the floor and neglecting to wash the dishes before putting them away. G. took over the housekeeping and cooking duties.

Mrs. L.'s hearing and sight continued to decline, and she complained about "nothing ever being right." G. got her books on tape, but Mrs. L. could not learn to operate the tape player. She continued to entertain her weekly women's group, basking in the compliments from her friends for the tasty desserts that they knew were now being made by G.

Mrs. L. became a picky eater, putting catsup on everything, including salads and fruit. She was still very particular about her appearance, but she began to need help doing her hair and became neglectful of her denture care. She could still fold laundry, make beds, and take her bath independently.

There were times when Mrs. L. became fearful of G.'s husband, accusing him of wanting to hurt her granddaughter.

At age 91, the family moved out of the apartment complex, where they had lived for many years, to a new home. Mrs. L. was no longer able to make impromptu visits to her neighbors, and her circle of friends now rarely visited. Mrs. L. was afraid to use anything in the new kitchen, especially the unfamiliar gas stove. Her appetite continued to be poor, and she was losing weight. Strategies to enable her to make her own tea and toast were unsuccessful, and she would forget to eat food left for her in the refrigerator when G. went to work.

Mrs. L. began to have incontinence of bowel and bladder, yet she would resist her granddaughter's suggestions that she needed to shower or bathe. Ironically, when Mrs. L. fell and broke her wrist, she became amenable to assistance. Insurance covered about 6 weeks of home health care, and Mrs. L. seemed to enjoy the attention.

Severe Stage

At age 92, it was clear that Mrs. L. could not be left alone. She continued to be incontinent; she couldn't lift herself from the toilet and seemed afraid to use a bedside commode. When her granddaughter came home from work, she would follow her about, repeating the same question over and over. She was not eating lunch or dinner. Her granddaughter, pregnant with her second child, was having difficulty bathing Mrs. L. On one occasion, they both ended up falling on the bathroom floor during a bathing session. In-home care proved unaffordable, and G. made the difficult decision to place Mrs. L. in a nursing home. The nursing home, known for its excellence, proved to be a positive move for Mrs. L. She regained some of her weight and seemed much less anxious. Mrs. L.'s deep-rooted social personality and gift for charming those around her made a reappearance. This served to ensure that a constant stream of staff and residents dropped by her room for brief chats. When G. and her family visited, Mrs. L. remained cool, as if to reprimand G. for sending her away.

Within a year, Mrs. L. was not always able to recognize G. when she came to visit. Sometimes, she mistook G. for her daughter. Eventually, she completely lost the ability to recognize G. Her granddaughter continued to visit with her own children, who delighted in playing word games with Mrs. L. The youngest child, himself learning to speak, would say a few words or phrases to Mrs. L., which she would mimic. This would set both children to giggling, in turn pleasing Mrs. L. to have had such an amusing effect on the children.

At age 94, Mrs. L. seemed no longer able to speak English. Her verbalizations in Spanish were limited to a few words, which were sometimes unintelligible. She was no longer able to ambulate and needed total care for feeding. Shortly after her 95th birthday, Mrs. L. died peacefully of heart failure.

Mr. B. is a 71-year-old African American who is cared for at home by his wife. Mrs. B. describes him as having been a quietly dignified person before the onset of his illness. He enjoyed spending time with his family, including his four children and other members of his extended family.

As a young college graduate in the 1960s, Mr. B. was unable to find work in his field of engineering but did get an unskilled job with the phone company. His supervisor recognized his talents and abilities, and, over time, he had a series of promotions that eventually took him to the position of personnel manager.

When Mr. B. was 60, his company was bought out and he was given an early retirement. Soon after this, he started taking classes in cabinet making and began working for an architect who was building a local church.

At age 64, Mr. B. began making errors in measurement in his work. He was aware of, and troubled, by this difficulty. He decided to cut back his hours at work. Mrs. B. noted at this time that he sometimes appeared confused. During family gatherings, he was not only quieter than his usual self, but he would actually distance himself by sitting in another room. Although he was still driving, he began misplacing things. Mrs. B. had some concerns about these behaviors but attributed them to the stress of life changes.

It was when Mr. B. was no longer able to read a ruler that Mrs. B. began to realize something was seriously wrong. At about this time, Mr. B. had an episode in which he got lost on the way to the dentist. Mrs. B. turned to her family physician for help, and an 18-month period of medical and neurological testing ensued.

At age 66, Mr. B. had a stroke. During hospitalization, the diagnosis of vascular dementia was finally made. When Mr. B. left the hospital, he was able to walk and perform his self-care activities independently.

At first, things went well at home. Both Mr. and Mrs. B. adjusted to a routine in which she would make sure that he was up, dressed, and had breakfast before she left for work. His lunch was prepared and left for him to retrieve from the refrigerator. One day, Mrs. B. came home from work and found that the stove had been left on. At this point, she realized that Mr. B. was no longer safe when left alone, and she enrolled him in a day-care program.

About 8 months later, Mrs. B. made the decision to stop working. The day program cost almost as much as her pay. It was becoming more and more difficult to help Mr. B. get dressed and out of the house every morning. In fact, Mr. B. started choosing to undress himself several times a day. He began having problems speaking and understanding what others said to him. Mrs. B. felt he was losing his personality; he wasn't able to focus on conversation or show interest, even when his grandchildren visited. He was still ambulating with help. He began having difficulty swallowing, was losing weight, and was having bladder infections. He was no longer continent of bowel or bladder.

At age 69, Mr. B. had another stroke. Despite the efforts of the rehabilitation service, he could no longer ambulate. He returned home in a wheelchair. His home did not have a ground floor bedroom, so Mrs. B. converted the living room to his bedroom. For about 1 month, his insurance provided a home health aide who would give Mr. B. a weekly bed bath. Eventually, Mrs. B. took over this responsibility, along with complete care for dressing and feeding him. Mr. B. often did not recognize Mrs. B. and no longer recognized his children.

During a recent visit to the outpatient clinic, Mrs. B. talked about the difficulty of getting through each day. "I rarely get out unless one of the family members can stay with my husband, and even then, I'm just too tired. I think about the reality that someday I may need to put him in a nursing home. I'll do it when it gets to the point where I'm no longer able to take care of him or if my health goes bad. But if that happens, I'll lose our life savings—it's not much, but enough to help pay bills with my social security check." She also related an incident that illustrated the small daily frustrations of caring for her husband: "I was feeding him lunch, and he reached for the glass of milk with his left hand. I helped place the glass in his outstretched hand, but he began raising his right hand to his mouth as if to drink. Obviously, that wasn't working, so I took the glass out of his left hand and put it in his right hand. This must have totally confused him, and he just looked at me as if to say 'what did you do that for?' I felt so helpless and so bad that I couldn't even help him."

Mr. B., who at 71 is still handsome, sits straight and tall in his wheelchair, appearing to emanate dignity and calm, faintly smiling and nodding as his wife tells their story.

RECOMMENDED LEARNING RESOURCES

Mace, N. L., & Rabins, P. V. (2012). *The 36-hour day: A family guide to caring for persons with Alzheimer's disease* (5th ed.). Baltimore, MD: Johns Hopkins University Press.

Peterson, R. (2014). *Mayo clinic on Alzheimer's disease.* New York, NY: RosettaBooks.

Pollard, D. (2005). *A cognitive link: Managing problematic bodily behavior.* Monona, WI: SelectOne Rehab.

Robinson, A., Spencer, B., & White, L. (2007). *Understanding difficult behaviors: Some practical suggestions for coping with Alzheimer's disease and related illnesses.* Ypsilanti, MI: Eastern Michigan University Alzheimer's Education Program.

The National Institute on Aging. (2015). *Caring for a person with Alzheimer's disease: Your easy-to-use guide from the national institute on aging.* Silver Spring, MD. Retrieved from www.nia.nih. gov/Alzheimers

The National Institute on Aging. (2015). *Alzheimer's disease: Unraveling the mystery.* Silver Spring, MD: Retrieved from www.nia.nih.gov/Alzheimers

REFERENCES

Alzheimer's Association. (2015). Alzheimer's disease facts and figures. *Alzheimer's and Dementia, 11*(3), 332.

American Occupational Therapy Association. (2014). *Occupational therapy practice framework: Domain & process* (3rd ed.). Bethesda, MD: Author. doi.org/10.5014/ajot.2014.682006

American Psychiatric Association. (2013). *Diagnostic and statistical manual of mental disorders* (5th ed.). Washington, DC: Author.

Ballard, C., Corbett, A., Chitramohan, R., & Aarsland, D. (2009). Management of agitation and aggression associated with Alzheimer's disease: Controversies and possible solutions. *Current Opinion in Psychiatry, 22*(6), 532–540. doi: 10.1097/YCO.0b013e32833111f9

Beacher, F., Daly, E., Simmons, A., Prasher, V., Morris, R., Robison, C., … Murphy, D.G. (2009). Alzheimer's disease and Down syndrome: An in vivo MRI study. *Psychological Medicine, 39*(4), 675–684. doi: 10.1017/S0033291708004054

Bear, M. F., Connors, B. W., & Paradiso, M. A. (2001). *Neuroscience: Exploring the brain* (2nd ed.). Baltimore, MD: Lippincott Williams & Wilkins.

Blazer, D. G., Steffens, D. C., & Busse, E. W. (2004). *The American psychiatric publishing textbook of geriatric psychiatry* (3rd ed.). Washington, DC: American Psychiatric Publishing, Inc.

Bras, J. (2015). Genetics of dementia with Lewy bodies. In S. Schneider, & J. Bras (Eds.), *Movement disorder genetics* (pp. 65–74). London: Springer.

Breitner, J. C., & Albert, M. S. (2009). *The American psychiatric publishing textbook of Alzheimer disease and other dementias.* Arlington, VA: American Psychiatric Publishing, Inc.

Burke, A., Hall, G., Yaari, R., Fleisher, A., Dougherty, J., Young, J., … Tariot, P. (2015). *Pocket reference to Alzheimer's disease management.* London: Springer.

Burke, D., Sengoz, A., & Schwartz, R. (2000). Potentially reversible cognitive impairment in patients presenting to a memory disorders clinic. *Journal of Clinical Neuroscience, 7*(2), 120–123. doi: 10.1054/ jocn.1999.0162

Chandra, M., & Anand, K. (2015). Assessment of nicotine dependence in subjects with vascular dementia. *International Journal of Research in Medical Sciences, 3*(3), 1–4. doi:10.5455/2320-6012. ijrms20150301

Jack, C., Barnes, J., Bernstein, M., Borowski, B., Barnes, J., Bernstein, J., Weiner, M. (2015). Magnetic resonance imaging in Alzheimer's disease neuroimaging initiative 2. *Alzheimer's & Dementia, 11*, 740–756. doi:10.1016/j.jalz.2015.05.00

Cohen, D., & Eisdorfer, C. (2001). *The loss of self.* New York: W.W. Norton & Co.

Coppus, A., Evenhuis, H., Verberne, G. J., Visser, F., Van Gool, P., Eikelenboom, P., & Van Duijn, C. (2006). Dementia and mortality in persons with Down syndrome. *Journal of Intellectual Disability Research, 50*(10), 768–777.

Corbett, A., Burns, A., & Ballard, C. (2014). Don't use antipsychotics routinely to treat agitation and aggression in people with dementia. *The BMJ, 349*, g6420. doi: 10.1136/bmj.g6420

DeCarli, C. (2001). The role of neuroimaging in dementia. *Clinical Geriatric Medicine, 17*(2), 255–279. doi: doi.org/10.1016/S0749-0690(05)70068-9

Family Caregiver Alliance. (2002). *Dementia & driving: Fact sheet.* Retrieved from National Center on Caregiving.

Fan, L., & Chiu, M. (2014). Combotherapy and current concepts as well as future strategies for the treatment of Alzheimer's disease. *Neuropsychiatric Disease and Treatment, 10,* 439–451. doi: 10.2147/NDT.S45143

Farlow, M. R., & Boustani, M. (2009). *The American psychiatric publishing textbook of Alzheimer's disease and other dementias.* Arlington, VA: American Psychiatric Publishing.

Fereshtehnejad, S., Johnell, K., & Eriksdotter, M. (2014). Anti-dementia drugs and co-medication among patients with Alzheimer's disease. *Drugs and Aging, 31*(3), 215–224. doi: 10.1186/s13195-014-0065-2

Fraker, J., Kales, H. C., Blazek, M., Kavanaugh, J., & Gitlin, L. N. (2014). The role of the occupational therapist in the management of neuropsychiatric symptoms of dementia in clinical settings. *Occupational Therapy in Health Care, 28*(1), 4–20. doi: 10.3109/07380577.2013.867468

Frank, C. (2003). Dementia with Lewy bodies. *Canadian Family Physician, 49*(10), 1304–1311.

Gallagher, D., & Hermann, N. (2015). Agitation and aggression in Alzheimer's disease: An update on pharmacological and psychosocial approaches to care. *Neurodegenerative Disease Management, 5*(1), 77–83. doi: 10.4081/gc.2015.5460

Gauthier, S. (2002). Advances in the pharmacotherapy of Alzheimer's disease. *Canadian Medical Association Journal, 166*(5), 616–626.

Girard, T. D., Pandharipande, P. P., & Ely, E. W. (2008). Delirium in the intensive care unit. *Critical Care, 12*(Suppl. 3), 1–9. doi: 10.1097/CCM.0b013e31829a6f1e

Goldman, L. S., Wise, T. N., & Brody, D. S. (2004). *Psychiatry for primary care physicians* (2nd ed.). Atlanta, GA: AMA Press.

Gorelick, P., Scuteri, A., Black, E., DeCarli, C., Greenberg, S.,Iadecola, C., Seshardi. (2011). Stroke: 42:2672-2713. doi10.1161/STR.ob013e3182299496,

Hales, R. E., & Yudofsky, S. C. (2003). *The American psychiatric publishing textbook of clinical psychiatry* (4th ed.). Washington, DC: American Psychiatric Publishing, Inc.

Hilgeman, M. M., Burgio, L. D., & Allen, R. S. (2009). *The American psychiatric publishing textbook of Alzheimer disease and other dementias* (4th ed.). Arlington, VA: American Psychiatric Publishing, Inc.

Hughes, C. P., Berg, L., & Danziger, W. L. (1993). A new clinical scale for the staging of dementia. *British Journal of Psychiatry, 140,* 566–572.

Kales, H. C., Kim, H. M., Zivin, K., Valenstein, M., Seyfried, L. S., Chiang, C., … Blow, F. C. (2012). Risk of mortality among individual antipsychotics in patients with dementia. *The American Journal of Psychiatry, 169,* 71–79. doi: 10.1176/appi.ajp.2011.11030347

Kanehisa, M., Limviphuvadh, V., & Tanabe, M. (2010). *Neuroproteomics.* Boca Raton, FL: CRC Press.

Karch, C., & Goate, A. (2015). Alzheimer's disease risk and mechanisms of disease pathogenesis. *Biological Psychiatry, 77,* 43–51. doi: org/10.1016/jbiopsych.2014.05.006

Kawas, C. H., & Brookmeyer, R. (2001). Aging and the public health effects of dementia. *New England Journal of Medicine, 344*(15), 1160–1161. doi: 10.1056/NEJM200104123441509

Kertesz, A. (2004). Frontotemporal dementia/Pick disease. *Archives of Neurology, 61*(6), 969–971. doi: 10.1001/archneur.61.6.969

Kertesz, A. (2003). Pick complex: An integrative approach to frontotemporal dementia: Primary progressive aphasia, corticobasal degeneration, and progressive supranuclear palsy. *Neurologist, 9*(6), 311–317. doi: 10.1097/01.nrl.0000094943.84390.cf

Knopman, D., & Jankowiak, J. (2005). Recovery from dementia: An interesting case. *Neurology, 64*(4), E18–E19.

Kovach, C. R. (1997). *Late-stage dementia care: A basic guide.* Milwaukee, WI: Taylor & Francis.

Lahiri, D. K., Zawia, N. H, Sambamurti, K., & Maloney, B. (2008). Early-life events may trigger biochemical pathways for Alzheimer's disease: The "LEARn" model. *Biogerontology, 9*(6), 375–379. doi: 10.1007/s10522-008-9162-6

Leong, C. (2014). Antidepressants for depression in patients with dementia: A review of the literature. *Consultant Pharmacist, 29*(4), 254–263. doi: 10.4140/TCP.n.2014.254

Liu, C., McDowd, J., & Lin, K. (2004). Visuospatial inattention and daily life performance in people with Alzheimer's disease. *American Journal of Occupational Therapy, 58*(2), 202–210.

Madhusoodanan, S. & Ting, M. B. (2014). Pharmacological management of behavioral symptoms associated with dementia. *World Journal of Psychiatry, 4*(4), 72–79. doi: 10.5498/wjp.v4.i4.72

Massoud, F., & Gauthier, S. (2010). Update on the pharmacological treatment of Alzheimer's disease. *Current Neuropharmacology, 8*(1), 69–80. doi: 10.2174/157015910790909520

Minati, L., Edginton, T., Bruzzone, M. G., Giaccone, G. (2009). Reviews: Current concepts in Alzheimer's disease: A multidisciplinary review. *American Journal of Alzheimer's Disease and Other Dementias, 24*(2), 95–121. doi: 0.1177/1533317508328602

Mitchell, S. L. (2015). Advanced dementia. *New England Journal of Medicine, 372*(26), 2533–2544.

Mosimann, U. P., & McKeith, I. G. (2003). Dementia with Lewy bodies-diagnosis and treatment. *Swiss Medical Weekly, 133*(9–10), 131–142. doi. org/10.7892/boris.43041

National Institute on Aging. (2003). *Alzheimer's disease: Unraveling the mystery.* Washington, DC: National Institutes of Health.

Neugrosch, J. A., Kolevzon, A. K., Samuels, S. C., & Marin, D. B. (2004). *Kaplan and Sadock's comprehensive textbook of psychiatry* (8th ed.). Philadelphia, PA: Lippincott Williams & Wilkins.

Peterson, R. C., Stevens, J. C., & Ganguli, M. (2001). Practice parameter: early detection of dementia: mild cognitive impairment (an evidence based review). *Neurology, 56*, 1133–1142. doi: 10.1212/WNL.56.9.*1133*

Pollard, D. (2005). *A cognitive link: Managing problematic bodily behavior.* Monona, WI: SelectOne Rehab.

Reed, T. T., Sultana, R., & Butterfield, D. A. (2010). *Neuroproteomics.* Boca Raton, FL: CRC Press.

Reisberg, B., & Sclan, S. G. (1992). Functional assessment staging (FAST) in Alzheimer's disease: Reliability, validity and ordinality. *International Psychogeriatric, 4*, 55–69.

Reitz, C., Tang, M. X., Schupf, N., Manly, J. J., Mayeux, R., & Luchsinger, J. A. (2010). A summary risk score for the prediction of Alzheimer's disease in elderly persons. *Archives of Neurology, 67*(7), 835–841.

Rocca, W., Mielke, M., Vemuri, P., & Miller, V. (2014). Sex and gender difference in the causes of dementia: A narrative review. *Maturitas, 79*, 196–201.

Rocchi, A., Pellegrini, S., Siciliano, G., & Murri, L. (2003). Causative and susceptibility genes for Alzheimer's disease: A review. *Brain Research Bulletin, 61*(1), 1–24.

Ryan, N., Rossor, M., & Fox, N. (2015). *Alzheimer's disease in the 100 years since Alzheimer's death. Brain: A Journal of Neurology, 134*(7), 1–6. doi: 10.1093/brain/awv316

Sadock, B. J., Sadock V. A., & Ruiz, P. (2014). *Kaplan & Sadock's synopsis of psychiatry: Behavioral sciences/clinical psychiatry* (11th ed.). Philadelphia, PA: Lippincott Williams & Wilkins.

Samuels, S. C., & Neugroschl, J. A. (2004). *Kaplan & Sadock's comprehensive textbook of psychiatry* (8th ed.). Philadelphia, PA: Lippincott Williams & Wilkins.

Schneider, R. K., & Levenson, J. L. (2008). *Psychiatry essentials for primary care.* Philadelphia, PA:The American College of Physicians.

Seitz, D. P., & van Zyl, L. T. (2006).Delirium concisely: Condition is associated with increased morbidity, mortality, and length of hospitalization. *Geriatrics, 61*(3), 18.

Shah, K., Qureshi, S. U., Johnson, M., Parikh, N., Schulz, P. E., & Kunik, M. E. (2009). Does the use of antihypertensive drugs affect the incidence or progression of dementia? A systematic review. *American Journal of Geriatric Pharmacotherapy, 7*(5), 250–261.

Shenk, D. (2003). *The forgetting.* New York: Anchor Books.

Stone, J., Johnstone, D., Mitrofanis, J., & O'Rourke, M. (2014). The mechanical cause of age-related dementia (Alzheimer's disease): The brain is destroyed by the pulse. *Journal of Alzheimer's Disease, 44*, 355–373. doi: 10.3233/JAD-141884

Varadarajan, S., Yatin, S., & Aksenova, M. (2000). Review: Alzheimer's amyloid beta-peptide associated free radical oxidative stress and neurotoxicity. *Structural Biology, 130*(2–3), 184–208.

Vickers, J. C., Dickson, T. C., & Adlard, P. A. (2000). The cause of neuronal degeneration in Alzheimer's disease. *Progress in Neurobiology, 60*(2), 139–165. doi: 10.1016/S0301-0082(99)00023-4

Wang, H., Yu, J., Tang, S., Jiang, T., Tan, C., Meng, X., Wang, C., Tan, M., & Tan, L. (2014). Efficacy and safety of cholinesterase inhibitors and Memantine in cognitive impairment in Parkinson's disease, Parkinson's disease dementia, and dementia with Lewy bodies: Systematic review with meta-analysis and trial sequential analysis. *Journal of Neurology, Neurosurgery & Psychiatry. 86*(2):135–43. doi: 10.1136/jnnp-2014-307659

Weiner, F. W., & Lipton, A. M. (Eds.). (2009). *The American psychiatric publishing textbook of Alzheimer disease and other dementias.* Arlington, VA: American Psychiatric Publishing, Inc.

Wu, J., Basha, M. R., Brock, B., Cox, D. P., Cardozo-Palaez, F., McPherson, C. A., … Zawia N. H. (2008). Alzheimer's disease (AD)-like pathology in aged monkeys after infantile exposure to environmental metal lead (Pb): Evidence for a developmental origin and environmental link for AD. *Journal of Neuroscience, 28*(1), 3–9. doi: 10.1523

Xie, S. X., Libon, D. L., Wang, X., Massimo, L., Moore, P., Vesely, L., … Grossman, M. (2009). Longitudinal patterns of semantic and episodic memory in frontotemporal lobar degeneration and Alzheimer's disease. *Journal of the International Neuropsychological Society, 15*(2), 1–9. doi: 10.1016/j.neuroimage.2010.01.041

Zgola, J. M. (1999). *Care that works: A relationship approach to persons with dementia.* Baltimore, MD: The John Hopkins University Press.

Zlomuzica, A., Dere, D., Binder, S., Silva, M., Huston, J., & Dere, E. (2015). Neuronal histamine and cognitive symptoms in Alzheimer's disease. *Neuropharmacology*, 1–11. doi: 0.1016/j.neuropharm.2015.05.007

Complex Trauma

Brandon G. Morkut and Ben J. Atchison

According to her stepgrandmother, 9-year-old Brittney was removed over a year ago from her biological mother's and stepfather's care due to neglect, subjection to chronic domestic violence, and exposure to methamphetamine. This situation resulted in her current placement with her stepgrandmother. Brittney's stepgrandmother reports Brittney's biological father, mother, grandmother, and stepfather frequently used methamphetamine. Additionally, Brittney's biological father was violent toward her mother while she was pregnant and continued the erratic episodes of violence after Brittney was born, an event her biological father failed to attend. She also stated that a year after Brittney was born, her biological father left Brittney and her mother, which resulted in Brittney's mother marrying her stepfather. Over the years, she lived with her stepfather and mother, Brittney demonstrated significantly poor school attendance due to living in multiple residences that included a motel, an apartment in which they were evicted from due to producing a filthy and unsafe living environment, a "shack in the country," and eventually a camper without running water that was infested with cockroaches. Presently, Brittney is described by her stepgrandmother as struggling academically in all areas, lacking efficient problem-solving skills, grappling to understand cause and effect, and having few friends at school. Her stepgrandmother continues to explain that Brittney visits her mother 4 hours per week at the public library and visits her stepfather in jail with her mother every other week. Furthermore, her stepgrandmother stated that Brittney has not seen or had contact with her biological father since he left her at the age of 1 year. Brittney is unaware of the fact that her biological father is in jail as a result of drug abuse and that, in addition to Brittney, he has fathered four other children.

DEFINITION AND DESCRIPTION

Prior to the 19th century, child abuse was not only acceptable but was, essentially, legally sanctioned. At that time, children did not receive equal legal status like domesticated animals with regard to protection against cruelty and/or neglect. It was not until 1962 that the term "battered child syndrome" became part of the medical terminology and not until 1976 that all of the states in the United States had adopted laws mandating the reporting of suspected child abuse.

Trauma, from the Greek word meaning "wound," was originally used in medicine for a serious physical injury, but it is more widely used now to refer to emotional shock following a stressful event or an experience that is deeply distressing. The American Heritage Dictionary defines trauma as "a serious injury or shock to the body, as from violence or an accident," which is what comes to mind when thinking of "trauma care" or a "trauma unit." This chapter is focused on the second component of this definition, which is "an emotional wound or shock that creates substantial, lasting damage to the psychological development of a person, often leading to neurosis, and an event or situation that causes great distress and disruption" (American Heritage, 2011).

In 2013, the American Psychiatric Association published the *Diagnostic and Statistical Manual of Mental Disorders 5th edition* (DSM-5) in response to an abundance of new research data and practical knowledge related to mental health disorders (American Psychiatric Association, 2013). To represent children who experienced or witnessed the traumatic event(s), the DSM-5 Task Force established posttraumatic stress disorder for children 6 years and younger under the classification of a trauma- and stressor-related disorder (American Psychiatric Association, 2013). Posttraumatic stress disorder (PTSD) was originally created and published in the DSM-III in 1980 in response to the large number of Vietnam veterans returning home with psychiatric problems. Until the publication of the DSM-5, PTSD was the only trauma-related diagnosis used for both children and adults (van der Kolk, 2005).

The main attributes used to describe PTSD for children 6 years and younger include experiencing, witnessing, or learning about death, violence, or injury, especially toward a caregiver, one or more times. As a result of the trauma experience,

children may encounter intrusive thoughts, avoidance, or negative emotional reactions to reminders of the traumatic event in conjunction with physiological dysregulation, as demonstrated by disturbance in sleep, hypervigilance, concentration difficulties, and angry outbursts (American Psychiatric Association, 2013). Unfortunately, there continues to be a population of children who continually experience a dark and unsafe world as a result of chronic exposure to interpersonal violence, neglect, abuse (e.g., physical, emotional, or sexual), and maltreatment, in addition to a caregiver who repeatedly fails to provide protection or is unavailable during times of extreme stress. As a result, these children often receive a cluster of diagnoses to identify their complex behaviors and negative emotional reactions, which can impair their ability to successfully participate in age-appropriate daily activities (e.g., school, play, self-care, toilet training, etc.) and to develop positive peer relationships. Frequent inaccurate disorders include bipolar disorder, attention deficit/hyperactivity disorder (ADHD), anxiety disorders, oppositional defiance disorder (ODD), conduct disorder, obsessive-compulsive disorder (OCD), and sensory processing disorder (SPD). Furthermore, the impact of receiving multiple mental health diagnoses most often leads to interventions focusing on behavioral control. This can limit a clinician's ability to provide effective research-based interventions as reflected by addressing symptoms based on a single etiology (e.g., complex trauma).

In 2009, the Consensus Proposed Criteria for **Developmental Trauma Disorder** (DTD) was established by the National Child Traumatic Stress Network (NCTSN)-affiliated Task Force led by Bessel A. van der Kolk, MD, and Robert S. Pynoos, MD (van der Kolk, 2009, 2014). The cornerstone of the Task Force was to develop proposed criteria that reflect the true reality and outcomes in children exposed to chronic interpersonal trauma experience. The authors of the Task Force hoped that this new set of criteria would lead to the acceptance of the diagnosis of DTD in the publication of the revision of DSM-5. This more complete and holistic set of criteria would result in a more comprehensive approach to intervention so that children would receive the proper care to improve their quality of life and ability to appropriately react to daily experiences (van der Kolk et al., 2009). Extensive review of empirical literature, surveys of NCTSN clinicians, discussions with clinical experts, and preliminary analysis of data representing thousands of children in various clinical and child service system settings (e.g., state child welfare systems, juvenile detention centers, and inpatient psychiatric settings) allowed the NCTSN Task Force to construct a proposed set of criteria for DTD, which contained the most clinically significant symptoms displayed by children following complex trauma. DTD symptoms include affective and physiological dysregulation, attentional and behavioral dysregulation, and self- and relational dysregulation (van der Kolk, 2014). Furthermore, to meet the criteria for DTD exposure, the child must have experienced or witnessed multiple adverse events over a minimum period of 1 year that begins in early childhood or adolescent, in conjunction with chronic exposure to interpersonal violence and significant interruptions of protective caregiving, which may include exposure to severe and repeated emotional abuse (van der Kolk, 2005, 2014). Unfortunately, several months after submitting their proposal for DTD, it was rejected by the DSM subcommittee with consensus that no new diagnosis was required to fill a "missing diagnostic niche" and "The notion that early childhood adverse experiences lead to substantial developmental disruptions is more clinical intuition than a research-based fact" (van der Kolk, 2014, p. 16).

Clinicians, including occupational therapists, who treat children with a history of chronic trauma, have increasingly called for a diagnosis that more adequately addresses the multiple domains of concern that result from developmentally adverse interpersonal trauma because the multitude of signs and symptoms cannot be accurately described by current diagnoses. As of the date of the publication of this chapter, the term *complex trauma* most accurately describes and represents children and adolescent subjected to repetitive adverse experiences. As defined by experts in the field of childhood trauma, complex traumas "describe both a constellation of causal risk factors involving repeated interpersonal trauma by caregivers early in life; and the resulting dysregulation that occurs across a range of areas including emotional, behavioral, interpersonal, physiological, and cognitive functioning" (Greeson et al., 2011, p. 93). Therefore, this chapter will focus on the complex trauma because this is the condition most relevant to occupational therapy practice.

ETIOLOGY

Complex trauma can be the result of multiple exposure to traumatic events, maltreatment, or polyvictimization beginning in early childhood or adolescent, occurring within the context of unpredictable, uncontrollable, and violent environments in conjunction with inconsistent or absent protective caregiving. The abuse, whether it is physical, sexual, or emotional, and neglect a child experiences from a caregiver are often **transgenerational**, that is, the caregiver's actions are based on his or her own previous parenting experiences (Perry, 2001). The most deadly form of child trauma is caused by neglect, as death can occur from accidents that occur in the absence of supervision or during abandonment. Failure to seek necessary medical attention in cases of injury, illness, or a life-threatening medical condition places a child at risk for death as well. Fatal injuries are caused by a variety of traumatic actions including severe head trauma, such as violently shaking an infant or small child; forceful punching of the fist to the abdomen, chest, or head; scalding; intentional drowning; suffocation; poisoning; and starvation.

Multiple risk factors related to complex trauma have been identified (Center for Disease Control and Prevention, 2015; World Health Organization, 2014):

- Parental risk factors include young or single parents, those who did not graduate from high school, and those who either were abused themselves as children or endured a severely dysfunctional home life. Difficulty providing quality care to a large number of dependent children can also increase the risk of abuse.
- Adults with psychiatric disorders such as depression and bipolar disorder are more likely to abuse children.
- A common theme when interviewing abusive individuals is their unrealistic expectations of infant or child development. Often, they expect maturation of developmental milestones significantly beyond the age of the child. This is especially true for toilet training expectations.
- The perpetrator's childhood: Approximately 80% of offenders were themselves abused as children.
- Substance abuse: Children in alcohol-abusing families are nearly four times more likely to

be mistreated, almost five times more likely to be physically neglected, and 10 times more likely to be emotionally neglected than children in non–alcohol-abusing families.

- Family support systems: Other factors include the disintegration of the nuclear family and violence between other family members and, in addition, the loss of child-rearing support from the extended family members.

- Children at higher risk for abuse include infants who are felt to be "overly fussy," as well as children with congenital anomalies, chronic/recurrent conditions, and children with chronic diseases as well as children with learning disabilities, speech/language disorders, and intellectual disability.

- Specific "trigger" events that occur just before many fatal parental assaults on infants and young children include an infant's inconsolable crying, feeding difficulties, a toddler's failed toilet training, and exaggerated parental perceptions of acts of "disobedience" by the child.

- Family income strongly correlates to incidence rates. Children from families with annual incomes below $15,000 per year are more than 25 times more likely than are children from families with annual income above $30,000 to be harmed or endangered by abuse or neglect. Poverty clearly predisposes a person to child abuse. However, it must be recognized that all data available can only be based on reported cases. It is very likely that trauma exposure exists among other classes as well, but those families are often protected by position and wealth and thus their cases do not necessarily become part of a community's child protective services system.

- Parents' or caregivers' characteristics that may increase child maltreatment include difficulty bonding with their newborn, involvement in criminal activity, and inability to provide quality nurturing to their child.

- Multiple nonbiological, transient caregivers living in the home.

- Neglect and medical neglect are most often attributed to female caretakers, while sexual abuse is most often associated with male offenders.

- Younger children are at risk: If the child is unwanted, 67% of abused children are <1 year old, and 80% are <3 years

- Adopted and foster children are at higher risk.

INCIDENCE AND PREVALENCE

Child maltreatment most often occurs within the home (Perry, 1997) and an estimated 91.6% of maltreated children are victimized by one or both parents (US Department of Health & Human Service, 2016). Bruce Perry, MD, PhD, best describes infants and children raised in violent and erratic settings as "incubated in terror" (Perry, 1997, p. 2). Data collected during the 2014 financial fiscal year and analyzed by the National Child Abuse and Neglect Data System (NCANDS) indicate that an estimated 702,000 victims experienced child abuse and neglect. Child victims were similar for both boys (48.9%) and girls (50.7%). Three-quarters (75%) of maltreated children were victims of neglect, while 17% of the children experienced physical abuse and 8.3% were victims of sexual abuse. Approximately 75% of sexual abuse is inflicted upon girls. Girls also are more likely to suffer from sexual abuse, emotional abuse, and neglect. Boys, on the other hand, are more likely to experience physical trauma (other than sexual abuse). Data from the *Child Maltreatment 2014* report (US Department of Health & Human Service, 2016) also indicate more than one-half (54.1%) of perpetrators were women and 44.8% were men. In addition, mothers (40.7%) were the most frequent perpetrator of maltreatment in relation to 20.5% of fathers. With regard to age of perpetrator, 83.2% of perpetrators were between the ages of 18 and 44 years in conjunction with ages 25 through 34 years representing the highest group of perpetrators.

Unfortunately, an estimated 1,580 children nationally died from abuse and neglect during the 2014 financial fiscal year. Children <1 year old were the most vulnerable to maltreatment, and almost three-quarters (70.7%) of all child fatalities were younger than 3 years old. Boys had a higher child fatality rate than did girls, and 79.3% of child fatalities involved at least one parent. Further, 2014 child maltreatment data indicate that 72.3% of child fatalities were due to neglect, and 41.3% of child deaths were the result of physical abuse. Retrospectively, 1.1% of the child fatalities were caused by emotional and sexual abuse (US Department of Health & Human Service, 2016).

SIGNS AND SYMPTOMS

Complex trauma is composed of seven domains of impairment observed in children subjected to reoccurring trauma exposure. Those domains include attachment, biology, affect regulation, dissociation, behavioral regulation, cognition, and self-concept (Cook et al., 2007).

Attachment

The most significant signs of exposure to interpersonal trauma are maladaptive behaviors related to the disruption of attachment. The type of relationship between a child and caregiver influences the response to present and future emotional and physical experiences. A normal child-caregiver relationship develops into a secure attachment in about 55% to 65% of the general population (Cook, Blaustein, Spinazzola, & van der Kolk, 2003). In a secure attachment, the caregiver responds to stressful situations by providing the child a safe environment and a sense of protection. This in turn influences the child's ability to appropriately regulate affect and behavior. Over 80% of children who experience chronic trauma demonstrate insecure attachment patterns (Cook et al., 2003). Repeated exposure to unpredictable and uncontrollable stressful environments, in conjunction with erratic, hostile, rejecting, or abusive caregiving, is a precursor to an insecure child-caregiver attachment (Cook et al., 2007). Insecure attachment and associated signs can be subcategorized into three typologies: avoidant, ambivalent, and disorganized.

Avoidant attachment develops as a result of persistent caregiver rejection and failure to provide basic emotional and physical support to his or her child. These children often become skilled at distancing their emotions in conjunction with avoiding the establishment of meaningful relationships with peers and adults. Children with ambivalent attachment experience a range of predictable patterns of detachment and neglect to excessive intrusiveness from their parents. Disorganized attachment develops when children are traumatized by repeated exposure to uncontrollable and unpredictable stress, for example, physical or sexual abuse, in conjunction with the consistent absence of a nurturing, reliable, and protective caregiver. Children who demonstrate difficulty organizing an adaptive response to daily experiences, due to childhood trauma, display significant challenges regulating their emotions. In addition, they experience problems in managing stress and developing empathy (Cook et al., 2007).

It has been hypothesized that disorganized attachment interferes with efficient neurodevelopmental connections between the right and left hemispheres of the orbital prefrontal cortex, which is responsible for regulating emotions, conscious decision-making, and social behavior (Cook et al., 2003). Other brain structures associated with the development of attachment that can be affected by complex trauma include the amygdala, hippocampus, hypothalamic-pituitary-adrenal (HPA) axis, and the neurotransmitters oxytocin, dopamine, and norepinephrine, which impact, respectively, on threat detection, new memory and learning, response to threat detection, and release of hormones critical for healthy emotional states that are critical for affective development (Henry, Sloane, & Black-Pond, 2007). Attachment dysfunction leads to intense preoccupation with the safety of the caregiver or other loved ones and difficulty tolerating reunion with them after separation. Other outcomes that emerge due to poor attachment include the following (Cook et al., 2003):

- Problems with personal boundaries
- Chronic feelings of distrust and suspicion
- Social isolation
- Establishing and maintain healthy relationships thought life
- Difficulty attuning to other people's emotional states and perspective taking

Biology

As a result of being in a state of chronic fear and stress, the child's brain alters its typical bottom-up organization (i.e., brainstem, midbrain, limbic structure, and cerebral cortex) and redirects neural systems to support repeated survival-based reactions or "flight, fight, or freeze" to stressful experiences. Due to repeated activation of the HPA axis, which controls stress responses, traumatized children can habitually be in a continuous hyperarousal state (Gaskill & Perry, 2014; Perry, 2001). Other brain structures impacted by maltreatment include the thalamus, which is vital for sensory and motor signal relay and the regulation of consciousness and sleep. The thalamus plays a role in controlling the motor systems of the brain, which are responsible for voluntary bodily movement and coordination and the corpus callosum, the structure connecting the two cerebral hemispheres (Gaskill & Perry, 2014). In a study of 900 children with a history of maltreatment, caregiver-generated survey data of sensory processing indicated difficulty with sensory modulation. It has been postulated that sensory modulation disorder is a result of difficulty in the brain's ability to filter and inhibit extraneous environmental stimuli (Bialer & Miller, 2011). Survey data indicated 53.1% of the sample population demonstrating signs associated with difficulty filtering auditory sensations, 51.7% displaying sensory-seeking responses, and 23.8%demonstrating patterns of sensory overresponsivity to tactile input (Atchison, 2007).

■ Affect Regulation

A common deficit observed in children with complex trauma histories is their inability to distinguish and interpret internal states of arousal in conjunction with difficulty accurately identifying emotions, for example, mad, happy, and sad, in self and others (Cook et al., 2003). Impaired affect regulation is the result of exposure to inconsistent displays of affect and behavior (e.g., a cheerful expression combined with rejecting behavior) or to inconsistent responses to display of emotion (e.g., infant distress is united inconsistently with rejection, anger, nurturance, or detachment) (Cook et al., 2007). **Alexithymia**, or the impaired capacity to describe emotions or bodily states, is a persistent sign of affect dysregulation. This includes difficulty describing internal states and communicating basic needs such as hunger or elimination, as well as expressing emotions, wishes, and desires (Sayar, Kosfe, Grabe, & Topbas, 2005; Way, Yelsema, Van Meter, Hyter, & Black-Pond, 2007). Due to difficulty with identifying, interpreting, and regulating emotions, traumatized children may avoid emotional situations including positive experiences, display dissociation, or chronic emotional "numbing" and develop maladaptive coping strategies (Cook et al., 2007).

■ Dissociation

Dissociation is a predominate attribute in children exposed to complex trauma. Essentially, dissociation is a loss in the ability to process and integrate information and experiences. As a result, conscious awareness fails to respond to physical sensations, disconnection between thought and emotion is facilitated, and involuntary repetitive behavior may emerge (Brand & Lanius, 2014). As described by Putnam (1997), dissociation serves three primary functions during exposure to overwhelming trauma, which is evident by a

protective "freeze" response, suppression of painful emotions and memories, and detachment from one's self. Unfortunately, a child who habitually dissociates as a coping strategy can intensify difficulties with self-concept, behavior management, and affect regulation (Cook et al., 2007).

■ Behavioral Regulation

Traumatized children often demonstrate difficulty regulating their behavior to participate in age-appropriate daily activities. It is important to note that traumatized children's maladaptive behavior patterns are reflections of their difficulty adapting to significant stress (Cook et al., 2003). Maladaptive behaviors include difficulty with arousal regulation and modulation, which is demonstrated by the lack of and recovery from extreme affective states such as fear, anger, and shame that emerge from chronic trauma exposure. These affective states may be manifested by prolonged and extreme emotional tantrums on one side of the spectrum to catatonic-like immobilization. Disorders of bodily functions may occur including disturbances in sleeping, eating, and elimination (Egger, Costello, Erkanli, & Angold, 1999; Glod, Teicher, Hartman, & Harakal, 1997; Noll, Trickett, Susman, & Putnam, 2006). Furthermore, the alteration of affective states may lead to misperception of risk, combined with poor impulse control and difficulty understanding consequences of negative behaviors. When experiencing a sense of threat, maladaptive attempts at self-soothing may include head banging, body rocking, and compulsive masturbation (Ford et al., 2000). Self-harm among chronically traumatized children and adolescents has been described in the literature. These include dangerous actions such as setting fires, sexual promiscuity, and actions of self-harm such as cutting, picking, and burning one skin and other self-mutilation actions (Brown, Houck, Hadley, & Lescano, 2005).

■ Cognition

Exposure to maltreatment can be associated with impairment in cognitive function, which can be identified by late infancy. By early childhood, maltreated children may display less cognitive flexibility and problem-solving skills, which can affect their future academic growth and performance (Cook et al., 2003; Egeland, Sroufe, & Erickson, 1983).

Further attributes related to cognitive dysfunction as a result of complex trauma include the following (Cook et al., 2003, 2005):

- Delayed language development
- Problems with object constancy
- Difficulties with sustained attention to task to complete a task
- Visual perceptual problems
- Difficulty understanding complex visual-spatial patterns
- Lack of persistent curiosity

■ Self-Concept

The sense of feeling worthy and belonging and being accepted and the perception of being capable of engaging and completing novel and challenging tasks are frequent deficients in complexly traumatized children (Ferrer & Fugate, 2003). The early caregiver relationship significantly influences the development of an unblemished sense of self. These factors include a responsive caretaker to the child's needs and a caretaker who offers quality and frequent touch and eye contact. In childhood, the development of a healthy self-concept is facilitated by the child being able to safely explore and interact successfully within his or her environment, ask questions without feeling they are an annoyance, and engage in make-believe play (Ferrer & Fugate, 2003). Common symptoms associated with an impaired self-concept identified in traumatized children consist of feeling unsuccessful, powerless, helpless, incompetent, and unlovable (Cook et al., 2003). As a result of a lack of reoccurring positive experiences to develop a healthy self-concept beginning in early infancy through adolescent by adulthood, these children can endure a substantial degree of self-blame (Liem & Boudewyn, 1999).

COURSE AND PROGNOSIS

Complex trauma is marked by observable alterations in behavior across multiple domains with prognosis directly related to the extent of exposure, the application of appropriate interventions, and **resiliency** factors. Signs and symptoms and associated impairments are characterized by progressive deterioration with episodic signs of symptom severity in childhood and adolescence, as well as persistent challenges across the lifespan in many cases as evident by the Adverse Childhood Experiences (ACE) study. The ACE study examined 17,337 middle-class multiethnic Kaiser Permanente health care insurance members by means of a general medical questionnaire that included 10 questions related to potential adverse experiences, that is, witness to parental violence, household dysfunction, neglect, and abuse (Felitti & Anda, 2010). Results identified that the number of adverse experiences in the first 18 years of life increased the probability to develop cancer, heart disease, diabetes, liver disease, and stroke. Elevated ACE scores were also associated with depression, alcoholism, drug use, obesity, cigarette smoking, sexual promiscuity, and domestic violence (van der Kolk, 2005). To analyze adult death rates, a 14-year follow-up was initiated, and data indicated that participants with an ACE score of 6 or higher exhibited a shorter lifespan of almost 20 years compared to participants with ACE score 0 (Felitti & Anda, 2010). The multiple consequences that emerge as a result of chronic trauma and impact on the course are detailed in a seminal white paper by the NCTSN Complex Trauma Task Force titled Complex Trauma in Children and Adolescents (Cook et al., 2003). Two major considerations for course and prognosis are directly related to the extent of neurobiologic damage and resiliency factors.

■ Neurobiologic

The impact of chronic trauma on brain development has been reported in the literature with the primary benefit of these studies being a better understanding of the scope of the problems associated with trauma exposure as well as informing clinicians about the intervention approaches necessary to improve the prognosis for healing and recovery. Ito, Teicher, Glod, and Harper (1993) reported that children exposed to chronic trauma had left hemisphere EEG abnormalities in anterior, temporal, and parietal areas. Taylor et al. (2006) found decreased amygdala activation among children who experienced detached emotional engagement from parents. In a task requiring identification of emotions, Taylor also found a significant positive correlation between the activation of the amygdala and right ventrolateral prefrontal cortex, a finding that indicates reduced inhibition of the amygdala.

Curtis and Cicchetti (2007) found that maltreated children categorized as nonresilient had decreased left hemisphere activation when compared to resilient maltreated children and decreased left parietal activity compared to non-maltreated children. Neuroendocrine changes have been documented in the aftermath of childhood interpersonal trauma.

Bevans, Cerbone, and Overstreet (2008) found that exposure to childhood trauma was related to alterations in diurnal cortisol variation. Cortisol, a steroid hormone, is released in response to stress and acts to restore homeostasis. However, prolonged cortisol secretion results in significant physiological changes including immunological and neurological changes.

Cicchetti and Rogosch (2001) found that maltreated children with internalizing problems and coexisting internalizing and externalizing problems had elevated cortisol compared to non-maltreated children. Neuroimaging studies have indicated reduced growth of the hippocampus and limbic abnormalities as well as diminished growth in the left hemisphere and compromised function of the corpus callosum, the structure that allows for efficient interhemispheric connectivity (Teicher, 2000). Henry et al. (2007) summarized brain structures affected as a result of chronic trauma, which are illustrated in Table 12.1.

Recognition of the brain behavior connection linking trauma and neurodevelopmental function is critical to occupational therapists working with this population so that appropriate intervention is provided to improve the prognosis for healing and engagement and participation in occupations.

■ Resiliency Factors

Human resiliency refers to the ability of an individual to recover from adverse or traumatic events in a manner that is adaptive and nonpathologic. While the risks of pathologic responses are indeed great among children who have experienced trauma, there is the potential to gain competence across a variety of domains if provided with the necessary intervention, including those that address both internal and external factors (Cherry & Galea, 2015; Masten, 2014). Resilience is most threatened by the loss of organic and relational protective systems, which occur in response to traumatic events. The extent of brain damage and associated cognitive, perceptual, and self-regulatory dysfunction, along with severely compromised caregiver relationships, are key factors that compromise resilience (Teicher, Anderson,

& Polcari, 2002). In addition, loss of motivation to seek out interpersonal relationships, to interact with one's environment, and to learn and to develop new skills greatly inhibits recovery. However, supportive relationships, family connections, and cognitive resources help protect one and serve as "inoculations against adversity" (Kagan, 2004). Several factors have been found to be the most critical for promoting resilience, including (a) positive attachment and connections to emotionally supportive and competent adults within a child's family or community, (b) development of cognitive and self-regulation abilities, (c) positive beliefs about oneself, and (d) motivation to act effectively in one's environment (Luthar, Cichetti, & Becker, 2000; Masten, 2014; Wyman, Sandler, Wolchik, & Nelson, 2000).

MEDICAL MANAGEMENT

Due to the impact of chronic **polyvictimization**, or multiple types of trauma, the child may demonstrate signs of comorbid psychiatric disorders. These common mental health disorders include posttraumatic stress disorder, depression, attention deficit/hyperactivity disorder, oppositional defiant disorder, anxiety disorders, bipolar disorder, dissociative disorders, and personality disorders. Traditional medical management of trauma will include psychopharmacological intervention, which, in best practice, is prescribed as an adjunct to psychosocial treatment modalities. Medication should only be used in conjunction with trauma-specific treatment and not in the absence of it. In a survey sample representing 1,699 children, ages infancy through 18 who were exposed to chronic trauma, it was determined that most trauma intervention occurs in an outpatient setting with varied treatment modalities (Pynoos et al., 2008). The frequency of intervention modalities identified is as follows:

• Weekly psychotherapy (78%)
• Self-management/coaching (62%)
• Family therapy (56%)
• Play therapy (55%)
• Expressive therapies (41%)
• Pharmacotherapy (27%)
• Community outreach (25%)

Traditional models of intervention are typically provided by either a social worker or a psychologist;

TABLE 12.1 Impact of Complex Trauma on Specific Brain Areas

Area	Function
	ATTACHMENT
Neurotransmitters	Enables communication of different areas of brain structures
HPA axis (hypothalamic-pituitary-adrenal)	Allows response to perceived threats
Axis	"fight/flight/freeze" response
Amygdala	Primary role is threat detection-initiates the "fight/flight/fright freeze" response; connected to many other brain structures
Hippocampus	New memory and learning
Corpus callosum	Connects cerebral hemispheres to smoothly integrate functions; emotional regulation
Fusiform face area (FFA)	Facial recognition; especially important for infant recognition of caregiver
	AFFECT REGULATION
Locus caeruleus	Located in the brainstem—arousal and alertness
Thalamus	"Relay station" screening and distribution of sensory input to other brain areas
Striatum	Reward center of brain
Orbitofrontal cortex (OFC)	Regulation of emotion, decision-making, social behavior
	INFORMATION PROCESSING
Amygdala and hippocampus	New memory formation
Anterior cingulated	Associated with conflict mentoring, resolution, and executive function
Orbitofrontal cortex	Conscious decision-making

however, there are existing models of assessment and intervention that are grounded in interdisciplinary and transdisciplinary approaches, which include several professional disciplines on a team including occupational therapy (Hyter, Atchison, Henry, Sloane, & Black-Pond, 2001; Koomar, 2009; Richardson et al., 2015).

IMPACT ON OCCUPATIONAL PERFORMANCE

Occupational performance areas are significantly compromised as a result of complex trauma, Evidence of compromised client factors has been determined including those related to motor and praxis skills, sensory-perceptual skills, emotional regulation skills, cognitive skills, and communication and social skills, which impact on all areas of occupation (Richardson et al., 2015; Richardson, Henry, Sloane & Black-Pond, 2008; Atchison, 2007; Pynoos et al., 2008). In addition, the physical context in which the trauma occurs can greatly impact the child's ability to engage in an activity in the same or similar location, due to overwhelming reminders or "trauma triggers" of the event (Petrenchik, 2015).

■ Personal Activities of Daily Living (PADL)

Bathing

As a result of physiological manifestations of stress, regulations of bodily functions are compromised leading to difficulties in PADL. Stress responses are especially impacted by children with a history of sexual abuse while being bathed as well as being physically abused by immersion in hot or cold water.

Toileting

Encopresis, or the act of passing feces in inappropriate places such as in clothing or other places, is known to occur more frequently among children who have experienced sexual abuse, although it is not a specific indicator of child abuse. Enuresis, or the repeated voiding of urine in the clothing and in inappropriate places, often accompanies encopresis among traumatized children. Whether intentional or not, it is essentially an expression of the child's only mechanism of control in the midst of complete submission to the perpetrators of abuse.

Feeding and Eating

There are many relational factors between a primary caregiver and a child with regard to nutritional intake, beginning in the initial attachment process in infancy. A negative nurturing relationship with an infant including lack of attunement, irritability, depression, and other maternal problems will result in significant maladaptive, disorganized responses. These include difficulty with oral mechanisms such as suckling, sucking, swallowing and breathing, rhythm, food refusal, and overactive response to certain smells and tastes. Toddlers will often present with severe dental decay, or "bottle rot," a condition resulting from persistently being bottle fed with high concentrates of sugar while dental development is taking place. Children exposed to chronic trauma are at a higher risk for developing an eating disorder as they grow older. In a home where physical or sexual abuse is taking place, the child may turn to an eating disorder to gain a sense of control. Similar to the psychodynamics associated with encopresis and enuresis, they are able to control their food intake or their weight. Children who are compulsive eaters or those who hoard and hide food are usually using food to help them deal with feelings of anger, sadness, hurt, loneliness, abandonment, fear, and pain.

Personal Hygiene and Grooming

Complex trauma often results in children who lack the attention needed to provide proper hygiene and grooming, which often comes to the attention of school personnel and may facilitate a referral to child protective services. This may be the result of incompetent parents who lack the intellectual requirements to facilitate a child's awareness of healthy grooming or willful neglect of one, but not all, children among a set of siblings.

Sexual Activity

Reactions to chronic sexual abuse include significant dysfunction in sexual activity including hypersexuality, which is often demonstrated by a preoccupation with sexual organs of self, parents, and others expressed in drawings and in language. Children with a history of molestation are seven times more likely to become drug/alcohol dependent (Pynoos et al., 2008). In a study on the effects of sexual abuse of 938 adolescents admitted to residential, therapeutic communities for the treatment of substance abuse and related disorders, 64% of the girls and 24% of the boys reported histories of sexual abuse (Hawke, Jainchill, & DeLeon, 2000).

■ Instrumental Activities of Daily Living (IADLs)

Childhood maltreatment has a significant impact on IADLs. A common occurrence among a group of siblings in an abusive and neglectful environment is for one child, usually the oldest, to take on the role of a parent, referred to as **parentification** as there is an absence of an adult care provider willing or able to provide care for others. Oftentimes, neglected children are exposed to dangerous in-home situations such as fire hazards, firearms, and insect and animal infestation from parents operating methamphetamine labs. Parents might become physically or mentally unable to care for a child. Other times, alcohol or drug abuse may seriously impair judgment and the ability to keep a child safe.

■ Rest and Sleep

Exposure to trauma often results in substantial difficulty with rest and sleep patterns as the child often exhibits hypervigilance and overactive. Multiple exposures to violence and trauma result in autonomic and endocrine hyperarousal, which are observed overreactions to stimuli. This may include being easily startled and craving high-risk, stimulating, or dangerous activity, all of which impair the balance of play, work, and rest. The NCTSN clinician survey (Pynoos et al., 2008) found that 73% of children with complex trauma histories experienced sleep disturbances, a finding that has been supported by additional studies (Egger et al., 1999; Glod et al., 1997; Noll et al., 2006). While not a common occurrence, victims of chronic abuse may experience "sleep terrors," which are also called "night terrors." In a typical episode, an individual will sit up in bed and begin to scream or shout, which may include kicking and thrashing. The child may say or shout nonsensible exclamations with an intense fearful expression with eyes wide open and heart racing. In addition, the child may sweat, breathe heavily, and be very tense. Evidence further indicates increased bed-wetting among complexly traumatized children (Petrenchik, 2015, cited in Humphreys et al., 2009).

■ Education

In a study that included a sample of 9,336 children receiving trauma intervention across the United States, 41% had academic problems including behavior problems in school settings, including preschool programs (Pynoos et al., 2008). Academic functioning is a significant area of developmental competence beginning with preschool to higher education. In addition to intellectual abilities, success is significantly tied to a child's ability to regulate internal events or experience and to effectively interact with peers and teachers. By preschool, trauma-exposed children demonstrate problems in both of these areas as demonstrated by poor frustration tolerance, a higher incidence of anger and noncompliance, and significantly higher dependency on others for support (Cook et al., 2005; Egeland et al., 1983; Vondra, Barnett, & Chichetti, 1990). In elementary school, children are more likely to avoid challenging tasks, and thus are overly reliance on teachers' guidance and feedback (Shonk & Cicchetti, 2001). Complexly traumatized children may further demonstrate negative attention-seeking behaviors, poor attendance, and incomplete homework assignments (Petrenchik, 2015). By middle school and high school, they are more likely to be considered having a lack of motivation and learning below average, and there is a higher incidence of disciplinary referrals and suspensions (Eckenrode, Laird, & Doris, 1993). Developmental delays and emotional/behavioral dysregulation, learning disabilities, and intellectual impairment that cannot be accounted for by neurological or other factors that are experienced by children exposed to trauma can profoundly affect their school performance (Cook et al., 2005). A cycle is often created whereby a student's lack of success in school reduces his or her self-esteem and increases a lethargic response that is often perceived by adults as laziness or willful disobedience. A variety of school intervention programs, with a focus on creating trauma-informed or trauma-sensitive classrooms, have been utilized and are described in the literature as a means of addressing these students' needs (Atchison, 2011; Macy, Macy, Gross, & Brighton, 2003; Stein et al., 2003). The key components of a trauma-sensitive classroom that emerge from descriptions of intervention programs for children exposed to chronic trauma include

- Establishing and maintaining a safe classroom
- Predictability
- Acquiring affective regulation skills through positive adult interactions
- Considering the classroom's level of sensory input (i.e., bright-colored posters, objects hanging and moving from the ceiling, noise volume, and rich-stimulating scents).
- Assistance in making meaning of students' experiences

Unfortunately, there exists a paucity of awareness in most school systems regarding the need for classroom-based intervention that addresses the child as the victim of chronic abuse. The child, because of the many challenges he or she has in response to trauma experiences, acts out and behaves in ways that are interpreted as willful and thus being labeled as oppositional defiant or other diagnoses that lay blame solely on the child, leading to continuous conflicts with school personnel. The lack of appropriate intervention leads to academic underperformance, nonattendance, disciplinary problems, a high dropout rate, and failure to complete diplomas, which ultimately leads to poor success in vocational pursuits.

■ Work

Persons exposed to reoccurring early childhood trauma typically show disinterest in work, with ill-defined employment interests and poor employment-seeking skills or vocational interests. Acquisition of job performance skills, due to the lack of antecedent skills that typically emerge from home as well as academic environment, leads to the inability to get or keep jobs. Persistent conflict with coworkers or supervisors is also a significant barrier to successful work performance. Other factors, which influence low work performance and employment, include impaired emotional regulation during stressful situations and an absence of self-awareness as noted by a lack of appropriate hygiene and social skills (Petrenchik, 2015).

■ Play and Leisure

The lack of acquisition in the components of interpersonal competence, poor self-concept, difficulty with social communication, sensory processing disorders, and intellectual impairment have a significant impact on play exploration, constructive play, and symbolic play. Typical early childhood behavior among those exposed to complex trauma will often reflect traumatic events, which may include sexual acting out or violent play with dolls, seemingly disorganized and nonpurposeful interaction with items that may indicate a reenactment of events. Persistent themes may be noted as the child is essentially reliving the event in an attempt to control or gain mastery over fears that continue to create fear or that overwhelm the child. The child may be easily triggered by environmental stimuli, including other children and adults, which result in rage and physical aggression during play sessions with other children or alone (Petrenchik, 2015). As the child transitions to adolescence and adulthood, the pursuit of leisure interests is compromised due to these maladaptive play behaviors.

■ Social Participation

In a sample of 9,336 children with a history of trauma who were receiving intervention across the United States, 48% were reported to have had difficulty with social engagement within the home and in the community (Pynoos et al., 2008). Within peer groups, there is a significant degree of isolation, deviant affiliations, persistent physical or emotional conflict, avoidance/passivity, involvement in violence or unsafe acts, and age-inappropriate affiliations or style of interaction. Family interaction is marked by interpersonal conflict, avoidance/passivity, running away, detachment and surrogate replacements, attempts to physically or emotionally hurt family members, or nonfulfillment of responsibilities within the family. Many individuals with complex trauma histories are at high risk for dysfunctional social participation within their communities. This includes a high incidence of arrests and recidivism, detention, convictions, incarceration, violation of probation or other court orders, increasingly severe offenses, crimes against other persons, and disregard or contempt for the law and conventional moral standards (Pynoos et al., 2008). In addition, any inappropriate, avoiding, or aggressive behaviors as a result of poor mental health can greatly impact the child's ability to develop and maintain healthy peer relationships (Petrenchik, 2015).

CASE STUDY 1

Meghan is a 6-year-5-month-old girl who has been living with her stepgrandmother and infant stepbrother for over a year as a foster placement. Primary concerns for Meghan include her emotional outburst, which often results in Meghan throwing objects and breaking toys. In addition, Meghan has been displaying highly sexualized behaviors toward her stepbrother. Meghan was removed from her biological father and stepmother due to chronic neglect, physical and sexual abuse, and exposure to drugs and domestic violence. On one occasion, Meghan once was forced to put her soiled pants on her head, then in her mouth, and eventually forced to swallow some of her own feces. The stepgrandmother noted that Meghan does not have any contact with her biological mother. Meghan's father was attending weekly visits with her and then suddenly stopped showing up. Meghan frequently states she misses her father, and the stepgrandmother noted that Meghan was making good progress until her father stopped attending visits. The stepgrandmother did not have any information related to Meghan's prenatal care, development, and medical history but stated her biological mother and father both had a history of drug and alcohol abuse. Currently, Meghan does not take medication or display signs of fine and gross motor challenges. However, Meghan is struggling academically as indicated by her inability to read and write her name, follow multi-step directions, and problem-solve efficiently. Her difficulty with sustained attention has also been observed.

Meghan demonstrates irregular sleep patterns causing her to wake in the middle of the night, which occasionally results in her kicking her bed-room walls and dismantling her room. Meghan has verbally expressed aggression by telling her stepgrandmother that she was going to shoot people and stab her stepbrother. She lacks the awareness of "stranger danger" and continues to display sexualized behaviors as evident by talking to her dolls in a sexual manner and has removed the diaper from her stepbrother and proceeded to touch him inappropriately.

CASE STUDY 2

David is an 11-year-9-month-old adolescent male residing with his adoptive mother, her fiancé, and adoptive 4-year-old sister. At 2 years old, David was placed with his adoptive mother as a foster placement and then adopted by her 1 year later at the age of 3 years. Prior to being adopted, David resided in five different foster homes. The adoptive mother's concerns for David include aggression and lack of remorse as evident by David threatening to suffocate his 4-year-old sister with a pillow a few days prior to the start of the new school year. The incident resulted in a 5-day inpatient stay at a mental health facility followed by outpatient appointments at Community Mental Health. Currently, David wears a hat due to trichotillomania, a compulsive disorder in which a person constantly pulls out his or her hair. His other diagnoses include fetal alcohol syndrome (FAS) and obsessive-compulsive disorder (COD).

David was born 2 months premature and removed from his biological mother at birth as a result of testing positive for cocaine in his system. It is unknown who David's father is as his biological mother reportedly has had frequent multiple sex partners. David last visited his biological mother at her house when he was 7 years of age in the company of his adoptive mother. The visit was brief as a result of excessive use of alcohol by individuals in the home, including his biological mother.

David's adoptive mother reports that he is a good reader and speller and enjoys puzzles and drawing. His drawings are frequently similar to that of an elementary child. David's adopted mother further states that he has a first grade math competency level and demonstrates a limited understanding of cause and effect and difficulty with time orientation. His recent full scale IQ score was 68. His problem-solving skills are limited to simple challenges. David is suspected of having some sensory processing challenges, specifically in regard to sounds as noted by his aggressive response toward individuals making noise he perceives as threatening and irritating. When David is upset, he yells, slams doors, and attacks his sister and mother. David is easily frustrated and does not process his emotions well. His adoptive mother states she has rarely seen him cry. David does laugh and smile at times but most often presents with a flat affect.

RECOMMENDED LEARNING RESOURCES

American Professional Society on the Abuse of Children (APSAC)
350 Poplar Avenue
CHO 3B-3406
Elmhurst , IL 60126
877-402-7722
www.apsac.org

The Annie E. Casey Foundation
701 St. Paul Street
Baltimore, MD 21202

The Child Trauma Academy
5161 San Felipe, Suite 320
Houston, TX 77056
866-943-9779
www.childtrauma.org

The Doris Duke Charitable Foundation
650 Fifth Avenue, 19th Floor
New York , NY 10019
212-974-7000
www.ddcf.org

National Children's Traumatic Stress Network
Center for Mental Health Services
Substance Abuse and Mental Health Services Administration

Department of Health and Human Services
5600 Fishers Lane
Parklawn Building, Room 17C-26
Rockville, MD 20857
www.nctsn.org

The National Institute for Trauma and Loss in Children
42855 Garfield Road
Suite 111
Clinton Township, MI 48038
www.starrtraining.org/contact-tlc

REFERENCES

American Heritage Dictionary, 5th ed (2011). *Houghton Mifflin Harcourt Trade.*

American Occupational Therapy Association. (2014). Occupational therapy practice framework: Domain and process (3rd ed). *American Journal of Occupational Therapy, 68*(Suppl. 1), S1–S48. Retrieved from http://dx.doi.org/10.5014/ajot.2014.682006

American Psychiatric Association. (2013). *Diagnostic and statistical manual of mental disorders* (5th ed.). Arlington, VA: American Psychiatric Association.

Atchison, B. (2011). Creating trauma informed classroom: The school intervention project. National Child Traumatic Stress Network Webinar Series. Retrieved from www.http://learn.nctsn.org/ on February 12, 2011.

Atchison, B. (2007). Sensory modulation disorders among children with a history of trauma: A frame of reference for speech pathologists. *Language, Speech, and Hearing Services in Schools, 38,* 109–116. doi: 10.1044/0161-1461(2007/011)

Bevans, K., Cerbone, A., & Overstreet, S. (2008). Relations between recurrent trauma exposure and recent life stress and salivary cortisol among children. *Development and Psychopathology, 20*(1), 257–272. doi: 10.1017/S0954579408000126

Bialer, D. S., & Miller, L. J. (2011). *No longer a secret: Unique common sense strategies for children with sensory or motor challenges.* Arlington, TX: Future Horizons.

Brand, B., & Lanius, R. (2014). Chronic complex dissociative disorders and borderline personality disorder: Disorders of emotion dysregulation. *Borderline Personality Disorders and Emotional Dysregulation, 1,* 13. doi: 10.11186/2051-6673-1-13

Brown, L. K., Houck, C. D., Hadley, W. S., & Lescano, C. M. (2005). Self-cutting and sexual risk among adolescents in intensive psychiatric treatment. *Psychiatric Services, 56*(2), 216–218. doi: 10.1176/appi.ps.56.2.216

Center for Disease Control and Prevention. (2015). *Child maltreatment: Risk and protective factors.* Retrieved from http://www.cdc.gov/violenceprevention/childmaltreatment/riskprotectivefactors on January 25, 2016.

Cherry, K., & Galea, S. (2015). Resilience after trauma. In D. Ajdukovic, et al. (Eds.), *Resiliency: Enhancing coping with crisis and terrorism* (pp. 35–40). Fairfax, VA: IOS Press.

Cook, A., Spinazzola, J., Ford, J., Lanktree, C., Blaustein, M., & Sprague, C. (2007). Complex trauma in children and adolescents. *Focal Point, 21*(1), 4–8. doi: 10.4236/health.2013.52040

Cook, A., Spinazzola, J., Ford, J., Lanktree, C., Blaustein, M., Cloitre, M., ... van der Kolk, B.. (2005, May). Complex trauma in children and adolescents. *Psychiatric Annals, 35*(5), 390–398. doi: 10.3402/ejpt.v2i0.5622

Cook, A., Blaustein, M., Spinazzola, J., & van der Kolk, B. (Eds.) (2003). *Complex trauma in children and adolescents.* Los Angeles, CA: National Child Traumatic Stress Network. Retrieved from http://www.NCTSNet.org

Curtis, W. J., & Cicchetti, D. (2007). Emotion and resilience: A multilevel investigation of hemispheric electroencephalogram asymmetry and emotion regulation in maltreated and nonmaltreated children. *Development and Psychopathology, 19*(3), 811–840. doi: 10.1017/S0954579407000405

Eckenrode, J., Laird, M., & Doris, J. (1993). School performance and disciplinary problems among abused and neglected children. *Developmental Psychology, 29,* 53–62.

Egeland, B., Sroufe, A., & Erickson, M. (1983). The developmental consequence of different patterns of maltreatment. *Child Abuse and Neglect, 7,* 459–469.

Egger, H. L., Costello, E. J., Erkanli, A., & Angold, A. (1999). Somatic complaints and psychopathology in children and adolescents: Stomach aches, musculoskeletal pains, and headaches. *Journal of the American Academy of Child and Adolescent Psychiatry, 38*(7), 852–860.

Felitti, V. J., & Anda, R. F. (2010). The relationship of adverse childhood experiences to adult medical disease, psychiatric disorders and sexual behavior: Implications for healthcare. In R. A. Lanius, E. Veremetten, & C. Pain (Eds.), *The impact of early life trauma on health and disease. The hidden epidemic* (pp. 77–87). New York: Cambridge University Press.

Ferrer, M., & Fugate, A. (2003). *Helping your school-age child develop a healthy self-concept.* Retrieved from https://edis.ifas.ufl.edu/fy570, on February 8, 2016.

Ford, J. D., Racusin, R., Ellis, C., Daviss, W. B., Reiser, J., Fleischer, A., & Thomas, J. (2000). Child maltreatment, other trauma exposure, and posttraumatic symptomatology among children with oppositional defiant and attention deficit hyperactivity disorders. *Child Maltreatment, 5,* 205–217. doi: 10.4236/health.2013.52040

Gaskill, R. L., & Perry, B. D. (2014). Child sexual abuse, traumatic experiences and their effect on the developing brain. In P. Goodyear-Brown (Ed.), *Handbook of child sexual abuse: Identification, assessment and treatment* (pp. 29–49). New York: Wiley, 2012.

Glod, C. A., Teicher, M. H., Hartman, C. R., & Harakal, T. (1997). Increased nocturnal activity and impaired sleep maintenance in abused children. *Journal of the American Academy of Child and Adolescent Psychiatry, 36*(9), 1236–1243.

Greeson, J. K. P., Ake, G. S., Howard, M. L., Briggs, E. C., Ko, S. J., Pynoos, R. S., … Fairbank, J. A., (2011). Complex trauma and mental health in children and adolescents placed in foster care: Findings from the national child traumatic stress network. *Child Welfare, 90*(6), 91–108.

Hawke, J., Jainchill, N., & DeLeon, G. (2000). School professionals' attributions of blame for child sexual abuse. *Journal of Child and Adolescent Substance Abuse, 9*(3), 35–47.

Henry, J., Sloane, M., & Black-Pond, C. (2007). Neurobiology and neurodevelopmental impact of childhood traumatic stress and prenatal alcohol exposure. *Language, Speech, and Hearing Services in Schools, 38,* 99–108.

Humphreys, C., Lowe, P., & Williams, S. (2009). Sleep disruption and domestic violence: Exploring the interconnections between mothers and children.

Child and Family Social Work, 14, 6–14. doi: 10.1111/j.1365-2206.2008.00575.x

Hyter, Y., Atchison, B., Henry, J., Sloane, M., & Black-Pond, C. (2001). A response to traumatized children: Developing a best practice model. *Occupational Therapy in Health Care, 15*(3), 113–140.

Ito, Y., Teicher, M. H., Glod, C. A., & Harper, D. (1993). Increased prevalence of electrophysiological abnormalities in children with psychological, physical, and sexual abuse. *Journal of Neuropsychiatry and Clinical Neurosciences, 5*(4), 401–408.

Kagan, R. (2004). *Rebuilding attachment with traumatized children: Healing from losses, violence, abuse and neglect.* New York. NY: Haworth Press.

Koomar, J. A. (2009, December). Trauma- and attachment-informed sensory integration assessment and intervention. *Sensory Integration Special Interest Section Quarterly, 32*(4), 1–4.

Liem, J. H., & Boudewyn, A. C. (1999). Contextualizing the effects of childhood sexual abuse on adult self and social functioning: An attachment theory perspective. *Child Abuse and Neglect, 23,* 1141–1157.

Luthar, S. S., Cicchetti, D., & Becker, B. (2000). The construct of resilience: A critical evaluation and guidelines for future work. *Child Development, 71,* 543–562.

Macy, R. D., Macy, D. J., Gross, S. I., & Brighton, P. (2003) Healing in familiar settings: Support for children and youth in the classroom and community. *New Directions for Youth Development, 98,* 51–79.

Masten, A. S. (2014). Promoting the capacity for peace in early childhood: Perspectives from research on resilience in children and families. In J. F. Leckman, C. Panter-Brick, & R. Salah (Eds.), *Pathways to peace: The transformative power of families and child development* (pp. 251–271). Cambridge MA: MIT Press.

Maten, A., & Coatsworth, J. (1998). The development of competence in favorable and unfavorable environments: Lessons from research of successful children. *American Psychologist, 53,* 205–220.

Noll, J. G., Trickett, P. K., Susman, E. J., & Putnam, F. W. (2006). Sleep disturbances and childhood sexual abuse. *Journal of Pediatric Psychology, 31*(5), 469–480.

Perry, B.D. (2001). Bonding and attachment in maltreated children: Consequences of emotional neglect in childhood. The Child Trauma Academy. Retrieved from http://www.childtrauma.org/images/stories/Articles/attcar4_03_v2_r.pdf, on October 18, 2015.

Perry, B. D. (1997). Incubated in terror: Neurodevelopmental factors in the 'cycle of violence.' *Child Trauma Academy Press*, 1–24. Retrieved from https://childtrauma.org/wpcontent/uploads/2013/11/Incubated_In_Terror.pdf

Petrenchik, T. (2015, April). Developmental trauma and the brain: Understanding and working with children on the arousal regulation continuum. *Workshop presented at the American Occupational Therapy Association Annual Conference & Expo*, Nashville, TN. Retrieved from https://www.aota.org/-/media/Corporate/Files/Practice/Children/SchoolMHToolkit/childhood-trauma.pdf

Putnam, F. W. (1997). *Dissociation in children and adolescents: A developmental perspective*. New York: Guilford Press.

Pynoos, R., Fairbank, J. A., Briggs-King, E. C., Steinberg, A., Layne, C., Stolbach, B., & Ostrowski, S. (2008). Trauma exposure, adverse experiences, and diverse symptom profiles in a national sample of traumatized children. Paper presented at the 24th Annual Meeting of the International Society for Traumatic Stress Studies, Chicago, IL, November 15, 2008.

Richardson, M., Black-Pond, C., Sloane, M, Atchison, B., Hyter, Y, & Henry, J. (2015). Neurodevelopmental impact of child maltreatment. Mental health issues of child maltreatment. In P. Clements, S. Soraya, & E. Gibbins (Eds.), *Mental health issues of child maltreatment*. St. Louis, MO: STM Learning, Inc.

Richardson, M., Henry, J., Black-Pond, C., & Sloane, M. (2008). Multiple types of maltreatment: Behavioral and developmental impact on children in the child welfare system. *Journal of Child and Adolescent Trauma, 1*, 1–14. doi: 10.1080/19361520802505735

Sayar, K., Kose, K., Grabe, H., & Topbas, M. (2005). Alexithymia and dissociative tendencies in an adolescent sample from Eastern Turkey. *Psychiatry and Clinical Neurosciences, 59*(2), 127–134. doi: 10.1111/j.1440-1819.2005.01346

Shonk, S. M., & Cicchetti, D. (2001). Maltreatment, competency deficits, and risk for academic and behavioral maladjustment. *Developmental Psychology, 37*, 3–17.

Spinazzola, J., Ford, J. D., Zucker, M., van der Kolk, B. A., Silva, S., Smith, S. F., & Blaustein, M. (2005). Survey evaluates complex trauma exposure, outcome, and intervention among children and adolescents. *Psychiatric Annals, 35*(5), 433–439.

Stein, B. D., Jaycox, L. H., Kataoka, S. H., Wong, M., Tu, W., Elliott, M. N., & Fink, A. (2003). A mental health intervention for schoolchildren exposed to violence. *Journal of the American Medical Association, 290*, 603–611.

Teicher, M. H., Andersen, S. L., & Polcari, A. (2002). Developmental neurobiology of childhood stress and trauma. *Psychiatric Clinics of North America, 25*(Special Issue: Recent advances in the study of biological alterations in post-traumatic stress disorder), 397–426.

Taylor, S., Eisenberger, N., Saxbe, D., Lehman, B., & Liberman, M. (2006). Neural responses to emotional stimuli are associated with childhood family stress. *Biological Psychiatry, 60*, 296–301.

Teicher, M. D. (2000). Wounds that time won't heal: The neurobiology of child abuse. *Cerebrum: The Dana Forum on Brain Science, 2*(4), 50–67.

U.S. Department of Health and Human Services, Administration for Children and Families, Administration on Children, Youth and Families, Children's Bureau. (2016). *Child Maltreatment 2014*. Retrieved from http://www.acf.hhs.gov/programs/cb/research-data-technology/statistics-research/child-maltreatment

van der Kolk, B. A. (2014). *The body keeps the score. Brain, mind, and body in the healing of trauma*. New York: Penguin Random House.

van der Kolk, B. A., Pynoos, R., Cicchetti, M., Cloitre, M., D'Andrea, W., Ford, J., … Teicher, M. (2009). Proposal to include a developmental trauma disorder diagnosis for children and adolescents in DSM-V. *National Children's Traumatic Stress Network*. Retrieved from http://www.traumacenter.org/announcements/DTD_papers_Oct_09.pdf

van der Kolk, B. A. (2005). Developmental trauma disorder: Toward a rational diagnosis for children with complex trauma histories. *Psychiatric Annals, 35*(5), 2–8.

Vondra, J. I., Barnett, D., & Cicchetti, D. (1990). Self-concept, motivation, and competence among preschoolers from maltreating and comparison families. *Child Abuse and Neglect, 14*, 525–540.

Way, I., Yelsma, P., Van Meter, A, & Black-Pond, C. (2007). Understanding alexithymia and language skills in children: Implications for assessment and intervention. *Language, Speech and Hearing Services in Schools, 38*, 128–139.

World Health Organization. (2014). *Child maltreatment*. Retrieved from http://www.who.int/mediacentre/factsheets/fs150/en/, on February 7, 2016.

Werner, A. A., & Smith A. E. (1992). *High risk children from birth to adulthood*. Ithaca, NY: Cornell University Press.

Wyman, P. A., Sandler, I., Wolchik, S., & Nelson, K. (2000). Resilience as cumulative competence promotion and stress protection: Theory and intervention. In D. Cicchetti & J. Rappaport (Eds.), *The promotion of wellness in children and adolescents* (pp. 133–184). Washington, DC: Child Welfare League of America.

13 Obsessive-Compulsive and Related Disorders

Cynthia A. Grapczynski

KEY TERMS

Obsessive-compulsive disorder
Body dysmorphic disorder
Hair-pulling disorder
Skin-picking disorder
Hoarding disorder
Obsessions
Compulsions
Repetitive behaviors
Trichotillomania
Excoriation

Betsy, a 23-year-old on-again–off-again student, waited impatiently for the occupational therapist to contact her. Betsy has been admitted to an outpatient mental health facility to begin treatment for her obsessive-compulsive disorder (OCD). Betsy's OCD began when she was about 12 years old, coming on quite suddenly and quickly becoming debilitating. Betsy's OCD is related to contamination issues, and she cannot touch anything that she has not cleaned herself, including food, and she showers four to five times a day, with intermittent hand washing between showers. As a result, Betsy's appearance is disheveled; her hair is dry and flyaway; her hands and face are dry and scaly with some spots reddened and some bleeding. She wears the same clothes all the time because these are the only clothes she believes have been decontaminated appropriately. Because she will only eat food she has cleaned and prepared for herself, Betsy is very thin; she is also very tired from the compulsive ritualistic behaviors that take up so much of her time. Betsy completed high school under great duress, with many absences due to her compulsions. She has attempted college, but her compulsive behaviors were so demanding that she has had to drop out.

The occupational therapist is a member of the team that will be treating Betsy for OCD with cognitive-behavioral therapy and exposure response therapy. Attempts have been made before to treat Betsy, but she has been unable to complete the program. This is her third attempt, and she is hoping to be able to be successful this time. The occupational therapist is supposed to work with Betsy on relaxation therapy, mindfulness, and energy conservation, of which Betsy is skeptical. Betsy believes that her thoughts are out of her control and the anxiety she experiences because of her obsessions is so profound that she does not believe there is any hope for her to ever find relief. She believes that no one understands the extent of her suffering, and she is often short-tempered with family and others. Betsy has very few friends for this reason and the fact that her hand washing is disruptive to any social activities in which she might engage.

DESCRIPTION AND DEFINITIONS

Obsessive-compulsive disorder (OCD) is the primary disorder identified in the *Diagnostic and Statistical Manual of Mental Disorders, 5th Edition* [*DSM-5*] (American Psychological Association [APA], 2013) category of Obsessive-Compulsive and Related Disorders (OCRDs). The *DSM-5* has made changes in the description and the classification of OCD, one of which is that OCD is now leading the new diagnostic category of OCRDs. A second significant change is that the *DSM-5* does not require that people recognize the senselessness or excesses of their obsessions and compulsions. However, it does allow a way to distinguish degree of insight or lack thereof in OCD, through the use of specifiers, which may help to improve differential diagnoses (Abramowitz & Jacoby, 2014). These changes also reflect more precisely clinical symptoms and distinguish severity among symptoms (Schieber, Kollei, de Zwaan, & Martin, 2015; Snorrason, Stein, & Woods, 2013).

OCRDs include all disorders marked by obsessive thoughts and/or repetitive behaviors, including OCD, and five other related disorders. The related disorders included in the OCRD category include (a) **body dysmorphic disorder** (BDD), (b) **hoarding disorder**, (c) **hair-pulling disorder**, (d) **skin-picking disorder**, and (e) other specified and OCRDs (APA, 2013). The related disorders are included due to similarities of symptoms and characteristics. These include the following: (a) some empirical evidence that supports inclusion; (b) the primary symptom of all these disorders is repetitive behaviors; (c) all have similar age of onset, comorbidity patterns, and family loading; (d) all share brain circuitry and neurotransmitter abnormalities; and (e) all have overlapping treatment response profiles (Abramowitz & Jacoby, 2014; Schieber et al., 2015). Each of these OCRDs will be discussed individually.

■ Obsessive-Compulsive Disorder

OCD is a common, heterogeneous, neuropsychiatric disorder that is experienced by both adults and children (Grant, 2014; National Alliance on Mental Illness [NAMI], 2013). The hallmark of this disorder is the presence of obsessions and/or compulsions that cause anxiety and interfere with daily functioning and relationships (NAMI, 2013). **Obsessions** consist of persistent, unwanted, intrusive thoughts that can only be resolved, mostly, but not always, by **compulsions**, which are irrational excessive behaviors or mental acts repeated again and again. These repetitive behaviors are expected to resist or somehow control or banish obsessive thoughts to prevent feared consequences (Abramowitz & Jacoby, 2014; Bokor & Anderson, 2014; Jukel, Siebers, Kienast, & Mavrogiorgou, 2014; NAMI, 2013). These obsessions and/or compulsions must be upsetting, create problems in the completion of daily life activities, and last at least 1 hour every day to meet the *DSM-5* criteria.

■ Body Dysmorphic Disorder

BDD presents as a severe preoccupation with a perceived defect in physical appearance that results in distress and serious social or occupational functioning impairment (Schieber et al., 2015; Veale & Bewley, 2015). Although the perceived flaw may be a normal variation, or appear slight to the objective observer, it nevertheless causes "…enormous shame or interference in a person's life" (Veale & Bewley, 2015, p. 2278). Additionally, BDD can result in bodily harm, due to overexercise and unnecessary surgeries (NAMI, 2013).

The obsession with the physical aspect causes **repetitive behaviors** or mental acts such as mirror checking, rumination, and camouflaging, to hide or distract from the perceived defect, which, on average, occur 3 to 8 hours per day (Phillips, 2014). While BDD is considered a significant psychiatric diagnosis, it is seldom seen in the mental health clinic unless there is co-occurring depression, inability to leave the home, or risk of suicide (Veale & Bewley, 2015). According to Pavan et al. (2008), the individual with BDD focuses emotionally charged attention on a specific part of the body. This body part is so despised or disgusting to the individual that this focus can interfere with relationships and social functioning, damage the self-esteem, and severely impact quality of life (Buhlmann, Teachman, Gerbershagen, Kikul, & Rief, 2008; Marques et al., 2011). Comorbidities include OCD, depression (80% lifetime), substance abuse, and suicidal ideation, to name the most common (Pavan et al., 2008).

■ Hoarding Disorder

Hoarding disorder (HD) is a condition that impedes the ability of an individual to discard apparently unnecessary possessions, value notwithstanding, and creates clutter that interferes with the safe use of the living space (Nordsletten & Mataix-Cols, 2014; Saxena et al., 2011). Extreme distress is created by the idea of throwing anything away, and can make the living space unhealthy (NAMI, 2013; Saxena et al., 2011). The accumulation of articles is often disorganized, substantially compromising intended use of living space, keeping individuals from sleeping in their bed, sitting in the living room, or cooking in the kitchen (Nordsletten & Mataix-Cols, 2014; Saxena et al., 2011).

Individuals with this condition often have poor insight and are not open to seeking help due to the distress caused by the thought of discarding anything, despite serious social and financial distress (Mataix-Cols, 2014; NAMI, 2013). HD can be associated with OCD, but more often is found to appear independently. Individuals with HD show higher levels of disability related to work and relationships (Saxena et al., 2011). Older individuals with HD frequently have worse general health and more medical problems of a chronic nature as well (Nordsletten & Mataix-Cols, 2014; Saxena et al., 2011).

■ Hair-Pulling Disorder

Hair-pulling disorder (HPD), also known as **trichotillomania**, is a disorder in which individuals engage in repeatedly pulling out their hair, resulting in significant hair loss or thinning of the hair (Ricketts, Brandt, & Woods, 2012). This hair pulling is self-induced and recurrent and is a result of an "increasing sense of tension" before the pulling is begun (Jacob, 2013, p. 162). Hair can be pulled out with the thumb and forefinger, or it can be scratched or rubbed out, or various implements can be used such as tweezers, pencils, and hairbrushes—even needles in some extreme cases (Jacob, 2013).

HPD creates significant psychosocial impairment and may create physical problems associated with eating the hair that can be dangerous (NAMI, 2013; Tung, Flessner, Grant, & Keuthen, 2015). Medical complications can occur, such as infection, permanent hair loss, and gastrointestinal obstruction in the event that the hair is ingested and hairballs are formed. Psychosocial domains are also affected including self-esteem, body image, emotions, and social functioning (Jacob, 2013; Ricketts et al., 2012). The disorder

is recognized as one that has a significant stigma attached because it is both visible to others and is perceived to be a disorder that can be controlled by the individual (Ricketts et al., 2012).

■ Skin-Picking Disorder

Skin-picking disorder (SPD), also known as **excoriation**, is the presence of recurrent skin picking resulting in noticeable skin lesions. Individuals with this disorder pick at their skin relentlessly, to the extent that it may use up several hours during the day. People with this disorder can be seen to have open wounds on their bodies, with myriad scabs, scars, and tissue damage from previous picking (Craig-Muller & Reichenberg, 2015; Grant et al., 2012).

SPD, left untreated, can lead to other dermatologic problems, including infection and even the need for amputation. Triggers to skin picking can include stress, anxiety, boredom, anger, and/or a perception of a blemish by the individual (Craig-Muller & Reichenberg, 2015). SPD often co-occurs with related disorders such as BDD and hair-pulling disorder, and many individuals with SPD are found to have other lifelong psychiatric disorders as well (Odlaug, Hampshire, Chamberlain, & Grant, 2015).

ETIOLOGY

The etiology of the OCRDs is unclear and complex in all types of these disorders. There do appear to be genetic, neurobiological, and sociocultural factors that work together in the development of these disorders; however, each disorder has a unique combination of factors identified (NAMI, 2013; Pavan et al., 2008; Saxena et al., 2011).

■ Obsessive-Compulsive Disorder

The etiology of OCD is unknown, and there is no way to tell which symptoms or specific elements of OCD will predict later development of the condition (Jukel et al., 2014). There is some information to indicate that genetics may play a part in this illness, to the extent that if a parent or sibling has the condition, there is a 25% chance that an individual will develop it as well (NAMI, 2013). Additionally, there are indicators that brain activity in several different areas of the OCD brain is abnormal due to a unique response to serotonin. A single gene has not been isolated, but rather genes that may affect serotonin, glutamate, and dopamine appear to be involved (Bokor & Anderson, 2014).

OCD can also occur in the wake of physical or physiological damages to the body. For example, a stroke affecting the basal ganglia, caudate, and posterior frontal lobes, or a serious traumatic injury (accident or experience of violence), and occasionally pregnancy can bring on symptoms of OCD. Psychosocial trauma, particularly related to posttraumatic stress disorder (PTSD), can bring on OCD that includes a high rate of self-injurious behavior, panic disorder, and compulsive buying (Bokor & Anderson, 2014). Pediatric autoimmune neuropsychiatric disorder associated with streptococcus (PANDAS) can also be related to the onset or the exacerbation of OCD symptoms in children, along with a variety of other symptoms such as separation anxiety and mood disorders. Occasionally, exposure to GABHS, a type of streptococcus bacteria that causes Sydenham chorea, another neurobiological disorder of childhood, can result in symptoms of OCD, along with irregular involuntary movements seen in choreic conditions (Bokor & Anderson, 2014). Any of these insults to the system can cause hyperactivity in the orbitofrontal cortex, anterior cingulate gyrus, thalamus, and striatum, leading to OCD (Seibell, Hamblin, & Hollander, 2015).

Body Dysmorphic Disorder

The cause of BDD is unknown. Research, although inconsistent, indicates that these individuals may have abnormalities in visual processing, executive functioning, and difficulty recognizing emotional facial expressions. These abnormalities result in the individual actually seeing things differently from others (Phillips, 2014). Specifically, there appears to be impairment in the brain circuitry at the frontostriatal and temporoparietal-occipital areas, which are related to how facial images and emotional information are processed (Pavan et al., 2008). These abnormalities indicate less effective connections in various areas of the brain leading to poor insight about the source or reality of BDD (Phillips, 2014).

Additionally, in the sociocultural realm, individuals with BDD appear to have unhealthy attitudes associated with physical appearance and maladaptive beliefs about the importance of appearance.

Many of these attitudes and beliefs appear to be based on past teasing or childhood neglect/abuse (Buhlmann et al., 2008; Phillips, 2014). All of these elements, when taken together, suggest a multifactorial causation and complex clinical picture in BDD (NAMI, 2013; Phillips, 2014).

Hoarding Disorder

The cause of HD appears to be genetic, without specific genes identified for about 50% of compulsive hoarding; however, it is still considered to have a familial component (Gilliam & Tolin, 2010). Research is inconsistent when considering specific genes that predispose individuals to hoarding. One common factor seen in HD is high rates of traumatic events and/or abuse in childhood, sometimes reported by those individuals diagnosed at a later age, that appears to precede onset, but this has not been empirically identified as a definitive cause of HD (Mataix-Cols, 2014).

The presence of other disorders such as brain lesions, autism spectrum disorders, and dementia can present with symptoms of HD. Research, however, indicates no specific relationship to these other disorders. HD appears to be independent of these and other obsessive-compulsive disorders, with more global impairment noted in HD and an overall poorer response to treatment than these other disorders (Gilliam & Tolin, 2010; Nordsletten & Mataix-Cols, 2014; Saxena et al., 2011).

Hair-Pulling Disorder

The cause of HPD is not known; however, research in the last 10 years suggests both biological and behavioral factors are involved, with a relationship to certain abnormalities in the brain including alteration in frontostriatal thalamic pathways. These abnormalities are similar to those found in SPD and OCD; however, there appear to be other areas of the brain that are involved in HPD (Roos, Fouche, Stein, & Lochner, 2015).

Behavioral theorists suggest a strong influence from sociocultural issues may also be part of the etiology of HPD. Issues related to family conflicts, stress, or depression may result in HPD as a learned response that ultimately develops into a habit (Jacob, 2013). The relationship of HPD to SPD may be quite strong, as SPD is frequently a co-occurring disorder in approximately 38% of those with HPD (Grant et al., 2012; Ricketts et al., 2012).

Skin-Picking Disorder

SPD's etiological information is scarcer than that found in the other OCRDs, but also does suggest an underlying neurological dysfunction. Specifically, recent imaging studies showed "…abnormalities in white matter tracts, involving top down motor generation and suppression…" (Snorrason et al., 2013, p. 406). This white matter is close to the anterior cingulate cortices, and the abnormalities seen are quite similar to those found in hair-pulling disorder (Odlaug et al., 2015).

A recent functional imaging study conducted with individuals having skin-picking disorder showed "…significant underactivation in distributed neural circuitry including the bilateral dorsal striatum, bilateral anterior cingulate, and right frontal regions" of the brain (Odlaug et al., 2015, p. 5). These results suggest that SPD is associated with both structural and functional abnormalities in the areas of the brain related to the development of habits, monitoring action, and control of inhibitory processes (Odlaug et al., 2015).

INCIDENCE AND PREVALENCE

Obsessive-Compulsive Disorder

OCD occurs in roughly 1% to 2% of the US population. Similar rates are noted in the United Kingdom, Canada, Puerto Rico, German, Korea, and New Zealand, but Taiwan has a slightly lower prevalence (Soomro, 2012). However, a recent study of OCD in Singapore (Subramaniam, Abdin, Vaingankar, & Chong, 2012) showed a lifetime prevalence of 3.0% and a 1-year prevalence of 1.1%. In Singapore, being younger and being divorced or separated had a higher association with OCD than did others in the study.

Males appear to be more often affected in childhood, but women are more often affected in adulthood (Seibell & Hollander, 2014). According to Seibell (2015), OCD is "…one of the top 20 causes of illness-related disability worldwide for individuals between the ages of 18 and 44 years" (p. 290). Seibell et al. (2015) noted that many individuals with OCD endure their condition in silence, as individuals average 9 years in treatment before the appropriate therapeutic treatment can be obtained.

Risk factors for OCD include a family history of the condition, being single, and being in a higher socioeconomic category. Additionally, individuals who have anxiety, depression, alcohol/substance abuse, and eating disorders may have an underlying OCD. More than 2% of the US population is expected to develop OCD in their lifetimes (Johnson & Blair-West, 2013; NAMI, 2013).

Body Dysmorphic Disorder

BDD is considered a fairly common disorder in the general population. In the United States, prevalence was found to be approximately 2.4%; in Germany, prevalence was recently found to be 1.7% to 1.8% (Marques et al., 2011; Schieber et al., 2015). These rates for BDD are higher than those for either anorexia nervosa or schizophrenia and occur equally in both sexes (Veale & Bewley, 2015). According to Phillips (2014), BDD rates for suicidal ideation, suicidal attempts, and completed suicides are comparatively high, but treatment research on this disorder is significantly behind that for similarly common and serious disorders.

BDD is frequently comorbid with a major depressive disorder, poor insight, social phobia, and information processing differences. BDD can be misdiagnosed as an eating disorder if the body preoccupation relates to weight, as the mean age of onset is 16.4 years, and a number of studies indicate that BDD is common among students, both male and female. Research has indicated that many individuals report sensitivity related to their appearance throughout their lives, with up to 80% experiencing depressive disorders and 78% experiencing suicidal ideation (Pavan et al., 2008; Phillips, 2014; Veale & Bewley, 2015).

Hoarding Disorder

Reports of prevalence of hoarding disorder (HD) varied widely in previous publications, as clinically significant compulsive hoarding is identified as quite common. The most recent research indicated a population prevalence of 1.3% to 1.5% in the United States (Nordsletten et al., 2013). Comorbidities of HD include anxiety disorder (~75%) and attention deficit hyperactivity disorder, along with a greater number of chronic medical conditions. The majority of people with HD report for treatment in their 50s despite the fact that symptoms may appear decades earlier (Mataix-Cols, 2014; Saxena et al., 2011).

Risk factors related to HD appear to include having a family member with the same disorder, stressful and/or traumatic life events, and environmental influences. There is not adequate research to support the popular idea that material deprivation in childhood creates a predisposition to developing hoarding disorder (Mataix-Cols, 2014).

■ Hair-Pulling Disorder

Hair-pulling disorder (HPD) is a severely under-researched and poorly understood condition, and prevalence has not been established in the pediatric population, although the condition appears between the ages of 7 and 14 (Harrison & Franklin, 2012; Kaplan, 2012). The condition is more common in women than in men, with a total lifetime prevalence of 0.6% to 3.4% and a 1-year prevalence of 1% to 2%, especially among college-age individuals (Harrison & Franklin, 2012; Jacob, 2013; Kaplan, 2012; Rogers et al., 2014). HPD is seen comorbidly in up to 60% of reported cases, most often with depression, generalized anxiety, and OCD. A recent study revealed that severity of depression was a major predictor of life disability in HPD, along with avoidance and emotional distress (Tung et al., 2015). Only 5% of individuals with HPD report any relationship to posttraumatic stress disorder (Kaplan, 2012).

■ Skin-Picking Disorder

Skin-picking disorder has only recently been recognized as an independent syndrome, and research on prevalence has been limited. Past prevalence reports estimated SPD to range from 1.4% to 1.5%, with the age of onset usually between 30 and 40 years of age (Craig-Muller & Reichenberg, 2015; Odlaug et al., 2015). A recent study by Monzani et al. (2012) looked at prevalence of SPD among a sample of 2,518 twins in the United Kingdom and established prevalence with empirically derived cutoffs. Results indicated that SPD was a "...relatively prevalent problem, particularly among women..." (p. 605), with a prevalence of 1.2% among the twins, who were all female.

Among those with SPD, there is a higher rate of the presence of other grooming disorders. A comorbidity of BDD is pronounced in SPD, with research estimates between 32% and 44.9% (Grant et al., 2012).

Signs and Symptoms

■ Obsessive-Compulsive Disorder

The primary symptoms of OCD include intrusive, irrational thoughts or impulses that occur repeatedly, known as obsessions, and repetitive acts that briefly relieve the stress associated with obsessive thoughts, known as compulsions. These obsessive thoughts cause great anxiety in the affected individual, and the repetitive acts, some of which are ritualistic, are attempts to reduce the anxiety by neutralizing the obsessive thought (Abramowitz & Jacoby, 2014). The obsessive/compulsive cycle can be vicious, generally lasting more than 1 hour, intensifying the disease process and significantly interfering with daily life processes (NAMI, 2013; Seibell & Hollander, 2014).

Leonard and Reimann (2012) point out that it is important to listen carefully to patients for potential compulsions that may not be as rule driven, prolonged, or repetitive. Some mental acts or subtle behaviors may be completed in response to an obsessive thought of which the patient is unaware. Furthermore, according to Johnson and Blair-West (2013), "any recurrent anxiety-provoking thoughts that are seen as intrusive and involuntary, and are recognized as exaggerated, excessive, or against the person's own belief system should be reviewed as possible OCD symptoms" (p. 607).

Symptoms of OCD begin in childhood, teen, and young adult years and include common categories or dimensions. These include (a) contamination, related to washing and cleaning rituals; (b) symmetry, related to ordering and positioning rituals; (c) counting, related to the need to complete a behavior a specific number of times; (d) harm, related to the fear of hurting others; and (e) forbidden thoughts/images/scrupulosity, related to sex, violence, and religion (Johnson & Blair-West, 2013; Seibell & Hollander, 2014). Also, while OCD appears similar across cultures, the culture may have an influence on the content of obsessions and compulsions. For example, studies show more aggressive and religious obsessions in the Middle East and Brazil (Grant, 2014). Individuals with OCD may also show deficits in executive functioning, motor function impulsivity, and cognitive flexibility.

■ Body Dysmorphic Disorder

The primary symptom of BDD is a highly emotionally charged focus on a particular part of the body, where an individual identifies one or more perceived flaws that are described as "ugly," "hideous," and/or otherwise intolerable (Pavan et al., 2008; Phillips, 2014). Preoccupation with the offending body part lasts for 3 to 8 hours per day and results in repetitive behaviors such as constant mirror checking, excessive grooming, reassurance seeking, and camouflaging of the defect. Furthermore, the exaggerated preoccupation with the defect produces a disproportionate emotional reaction that is akin to shame. Individuals with BDD also report a pervasive sense of inadequacy about their bodies, and the anxiety produced with social encounters can be debilitating, inhibiting social life and occupational activities, such as school or work (Buhlmann et al., 2008; Veale & Bewley, 2015). Self-esteem is noted to be seriously eroded, as well (Phillips, 2014).

While the repetitive behaviors seen in BDD are similar to those found with OCD, there are differences to note. For example, some compulsions in BDD can consist of mental acts, such as comparing oneself with others. In the use of camouflage, the affected individual will check and recheck the camouflage (e.g., makeup, hair, clothing) to ensure it is still hiding the defect. Additionally, there is evidence that individuals with BDD have maladaptive beliefs about the importance of appearance in life, and self-referential thinking, along with accessory symptoms such as reference ideas and abnormal tactile sensations (Pavan et al., 2008; Rieke & Anderson, 2009).

■ Hoarding Disorder

Hoarding is exemplified by an obsessional fear of losing items of significance that may become important at a later time, along with a disproportionate emotional attachment to possessions (Saxena et al., 2011). Symptoms include the urge to save things, difficulty discarding things, excessive acquisition, disorganization of items with no cohesive theme, and clutter to the point that activities of daily living are impaired. Function is significantly impaired as well, and there is emotional distress tied both to difficulties with function and with the idea of discarding any possessions (Mataix-Cols, 2014; Nordsletten & Mataix-Cols, 2014; Saxena et al., 2011). Additional symptoms noted include deficits in attention, decision making, and categorization (Gilliam & Tolin, 2010).

Symptoms occur early in life and generally increase in severity over time. Poor insight among those with HD further interferes with the individual's ability to see the seriousness of the situation. Symptoms that appear later in life are often related to other medical, neuropsychiatric, or neurodegenerative diseases (Mataix-Cols, 2014).

■ Hair-Pulling Disorder

The primary symptom of hair-pulling disorder (HPD), also called trichotillomania, is the self-induced removal of hair on the body. The primary areas chosen for pulling include the scalp, the eyebrows, and eyelashes. Hair pulling can be implemented with a variety of tools, from the thumb and forefinger to use of tweezers and even needles to dig out hair (Jacob, 2013; Tung et al., 2015). Episodes can occur while the individual is relaxed, known as automatic HP, or stressed, known as focused HP, but the common denominator is that the individual experiences an increasing sense of tension prior to actually pulling out the hair (Jacob, 2013). Recent research indicated a complex relationship to exist between the severity of HPD, degree of depression, and functional impairment (Tung et al., 2015). HPD most commonly affects women, with onset usually in adolescence (Ricketts et al., 2012).

■ Skin-Picking Disorder

Individuals with skin-picking disorder (SPD), also known as excoriation, spend a significant amount of their time, on a daily basis, picking at their skin. Many such individuals report that picking takes up several hours each day, sometimes causing them to be late for, or miss, school, work, or social engagements (Grant et al., 2012; Jacob, 2013). Skin picking in SPD has been shown to be repetitive to the point of creating skin lesions and tissue damage that ultimately causes emotional distress and functional impairment in social, occupational, and daily living activities. SPD can lead to complicated dermatologic conditions, scarring, infection, and need for amputation in severe cases (Craig-Muller & Reichenberg, 2015; Grant et al., 2012).

Factors that may trigger the urge to pick include stress, anxiety, boredom, fatigue, and anger. Sometimes, the feel or look of the skin may trigger picking, and emotional regulation or reactivity has been shown to predict picking activity (Grant et al., 2012).

COURSE AND PROGNOSIS

■ Obsessive-Compulsive Disorder

OCD is responsible for significant suffering, impairment, and debilitation and is the 4th most common mental illness in the United States

(Seibell et al., 2015). OCD is often chronic and has a significant impact on social and occupational functioning, often starting in early childhood or adolescence. Fifty percent of patients report their first behavioral changes, such as anxiety or a lack of self-trust, appearing before the age of 20. Later onset is associated with increased feelings of responsibility and exact attention to details, along with a need for order and cleanliness, difficulty with decision making, and often a later diagnosis of depression (Jukel et al., 2014).

A serious problem with the disorder is that of misdiagnosis, related to the shame produced by the illness, and lack of recognition. OCD is often comorbid with other psychiatric diagnoses such as schizophrenia, Tourette's syndrome, post-traumatic stress disorder, generalized anxiety disorder, and some neurological disorders, making diagnosis complex (Bokor & Anderson, 2014). Many patients go for up to 9 to 10 years before the condition is correctly diagnosed, with an average of 17 years elapsing before appropriate treatment is initiated (Seibell et al., 2015; Subramaniam et al., 2012).

Unless OCD is treated, the course of the illness is chronic, although symptoms can wax and wane. However, remission rates are low (20%) without treatment, and occupational and social impairment is the norm (Jukel et al., 2014; Seibell et al., 2015). The course of the illness with treatment has been shown to be shorter in duration and to have higher rates of symptom remission (up to 40%) and an enhanced quality of life (Jukel et al., 2014; Wheaton, Schwartz, Pascucci, & Simpson, 2015).

OCD can also have an episodic course, appearing during the initial years of the disease; however, the chronic course is more common after that. Over time, almost half of individuals with OCD experience some symptom improvement. Research indicates that approximately 24% of individuals experience a partial remission after about 2 years. In children, however, "…the rate of persistent, full OCD was 41%…with greater persistence, related to earlier onset, longer duration and a history of inpatient treatment" (Soomro, 2012, p. 3). A case report by Sinha, Bakhla, Patnaik, and Chaudhury (2014) described a seasonal course of OCD, with symptoms appearing in October and resolving themselves by April or May. The patient did experience an increase in severity of symptoms over time and was treated

with a combination of exposure response prevention therapy (ERP) and phototherapy. This combined 14-day therapy resulted in "…complete remission of OCD symptoms" (p. 161).

■ Body Dysmorphic Disorder

BDD is a serious mental health disorder, but seldom seen clinically unless there is a comorbid disorder of depression, anxiety, or risk of suicide (Veale & Bewley, 2015). Despite this fact, individuals with BDD are substantial consumers of healthcare resources, but are seldom satisfied with their experiences. The reason for this dissatisfaction, according to Pavan et al. (2008), is because these individuals usually present themselves to dermatologists and plastic surgeons to resolve their perceived physical deficits, often associated with distaste, decreased social functioning, and psychological discomfort. Without appropriate treatment, however, BDD is a chronic malady that is "…associated with markedly poor functioning and quality of life and with high rates of suicidality" (Phillips, Menard, Quinn, Didie, & Stout, 2012, p. 1109). Some researchers, however, report that individuals with BDD, whether treated or not, show little to no difference in quality of life or functional disability (Marques et al., 2011).

Despite the commonality of BDD (1.7% to 2.4% nationwide), little is known about the course of the illness or any predictors of the course. A recent prospective naturalistic study of BDD's course and predictors over 4 years, by Phillips et al. (2012), revealed significant information about the course of BDD and its predictors. The results indicated, over 4 years, with 88% receiving mental health treatment at some time during the follow-up period: (a) Both partial remission and no remission of BDD symptoms were more frequent than full remission; (b) more severe BDD symptoms at intake predicted a lower chance of remission; (c) BDD comorbid with a major depressive disorder, personality disorder, or delusional BDD beliefs did not predict greater chronicity of BDD; and (d) even with remission, a majority of these individuals relapsed.

■ Hoarding Disorder

Hoarding disorder (HD) symptoms appear in childhood and adolescence with 60% reporting symptoms by age 12 and 80% reporting symptoms by age 18 (Gilliam & Tolin, 2010).

The course of hoarding disorder appears to be chronic, with a high likelihood of comorbid mental and physical healthcare problems, as it occurs more often with depression, social anxiety, and generalized anxiety than with other conditions (Gilliam & Tolin, 2010; Nordsletten et al., 2013; Saxena et al., 2011). Compulsive hoarding is associated with significant problems with social, familial, and work-oriented activities, with the more severe hoarding associated with lower overall income. Quality of life in HD, including safety, daily activities, family contact, and general life satisfaction in one study, was shown to be significantly lower than that in individuals with OCD (Saxena et al., 2011).

A recent study Nordsletten et al. (2013) indicated that individuals with HD were likely to be older and unmarried as well as impaired enough by a physical or mental health condition that they could claim disability benefits. Mataix-Cols (2014) indicated that untreated HD is chronic and becomes progressively worse over time, with interference in daily functioning occurring at about mid-20s and clinical significance occurring by the mid-30s. The majority of individuals with HD appear for treatment in their mid-50s (Nordsletten & Mataix-Cols, 2014).

■ Hair-Pulling Disorder

The course of hair-pulling disorder (HPD) is complicated by whether the hair pulling is automatic and high focused, or low focused, as well as whether or not there are other body-focused repetitive behaviors present (Tung et al., 2015). Those individuals with HPD that is high focused appear to have greater depression and stress, as do high automatic pullers (Flessner et al., 2008).

According to Tung et al. (2015), the severity of any depression in the HPD population was a strong predictor of significant social disability, though many of the individuals in this study were not formally diagnosed with depression. Additional predictors of work and social disability included interference or avoidance of activities by individuals with HPD, along with distress caused by HPD leading to impairment in social and leisure activities, family life, and home responsibilities. Intensity of hair pulling also influences perceptions of those individuals with HPD (Ricketts et al., 2012).

■ Skin-Picking Disorder

Like most of the OCRDs, SPD has a chronic course, which worsens with time, and is difficult to manage. The disorder may fluctuate depending on the stress level, but continues for many decades and is consistently present (Snorrason et al., 2013). Individuals with SPD pick at their skin daily, sometimes for several hours, causing damage to the skin, infection, and sometimes even disfigurement (Grant et al., 2012; Monzani et al., 2012; Snorrason et al., 2013). It is also considered a stigmatizing disorder (Ricketts et al., 2012).

SPD is often comorbid with other psychiatric disorders and causes distress as well as functional disability, particularly in the case of skin ulcerations and infections, which are common (Monzani et al., 2012). Contributing to the chronicity of the disorder is the lack of awareness of SPD and therefore lack of appropriate treatment. Fewer than 20% of individuals with SPD report seeking treatment. Most people with SPD report other family members having some kind of grooming disorder, as well (Craig-Muller & Reichenberg, 2015; Grant et al., 2012; Monzani et al., 2012).

DIAGNOSIS

■ Obsessive-Compulsive Disorder

The diagnosis of OCD is generally made when an individual reports the presence of repetitive thoughts and actions to neutralize those thoughts, occurring repeatedly throughout the day and taking up 5 to 8 hours of time daily. Diagnosis of OCD can be made if either obsessions or compulsions are present, despite recommendations from the field to require both for an OCD diagnosis, to improve diagnostic accuracy and treatment (Leonard & Reimann, 2012).

There is a specifier related to degree of insight for the individual with OCD that allows for differentiation between OCD and other psychotic disorders, as well as to distinguish degree of severity of OCD. This specifier separates those who have good insight and recognize their fears as not real, from those individuals who have poor insight and believe their obsessions may be real, and those with no insight, who are considered to have a delusional belief that their fears are very real

(Abramowitz & Jacoby, 2014). Abramowitz and Jacoby (2014) also note a tic-related specifier that helps to distinguish a combination of OCD with tics, which is characterized by a physical problem that is relieved by the motoric tic response. However, diagnosis may be difficult due to shame on the part of the patient, the stigma associated with diagnosis of a mental disorder, and misdiagnosis by the health care provider (Seibell et al., 2015).

A key assessment used for identifying obsessive-compulsive behaviors is the Yale-Brown obsessive-compulsive scale (YBOCS). The YBOCS is a 10-item semistructured questionnaire designed to measure the severity of OCD symptoms. Both obsessions and compulsions are measured, looking at five different parameters: (a) time, (b) interference, (c) distress, (d) resistance, and (e) control. This measure has been shown to be reliable and valid in a number of research studies (Conelea, Schmidt, Leonard, Riemann, & Cahill, 2012).

Other rating scales used include the National Institute of Mental Health General Obsessive-Compulsive Scale, the Maudsley Obsessive-Compulsive Inventory, and the Leyton Obsessional Inventory. Other mental illness scales are also available but are not specific to OCD (Bokor & Anderson, 2014). Furthermore, according to Bokor and Anderson (2014), obsessions and compulsions must consume a minimum of 1 hour per day, must not be a response to another medication or to substance abuse, and must not be due to any other psychiatric disorders.

Body Dysmorphic Disorder

Key diagnostic criteria for BDD to meet *DSM-5* criteria include three factors: (a) significant preoccupation with a perceived physical defect for at least 1 hour per day; (b) the defect must cause the individual substantial distress, interfering with daily life, including social and occupational areas of function; and (c) repetitive behaviors or mental acts like rumination must be present (Pavan et al., 2008; Phillips, 2014).

The diagnosis of BDD may not be easy to make, as many individuals with this disorder may not discuss the degree of their concerns unless they are asked directly. Veale and Bewley (2015) note that diagnosis requires a careful review of an individual's history, particularly the degree of preoccupation with the body, how much it interferes with daily life, level of distress associated with the preoccupation, and whether the individual avoids certain activities because of body preoccupation. It is also suggested that the clinician observe carefully for attempts to camouflage body parts with clothing or makeup (Pavan et al., 2008; Phillips, 2014).

There are two specifiers that need to be considered in the diagnosis of BDD. These include muscle dysmorphia and insight regarding BDD beliefs. The muscle dysmorphia specifier identifies individuals who believe their body builds are too small or lack adequate muscle development, despite a normal or very muscular appearance. This belief could persist in the presence of other non–muscle-focused preoccupations as well. The insight specifier addresses the level of insight an individual has related to BDD beliefs. This specifier has three levels: (a) with good or fair insight, (b) with poor insight, and (c) with absent insight/delusional beliefs and contributes to distinguishing degrees of severity (Phillips, 2014; Schieber et al., 2015).

Hoarding Disorder

Key diagnostic criteria for HD include (a) persistent difficulty discarding possessions, (b) marked distress associated with discarding possessions, (c) congestive clutter that impedes normal use of living spaces and compromises their intended use, (d) significant distress or impairment at the suggestion of discarding, (e) symptoms that are not attributable to other conditions, and (f) symptoms not attributable to other relevant psychiatric conditions (DSM-5, 2013). The attachment that these individuals have to their possessions is attributed to potential value or usefulness, sentiment, and a desire not to create waste (Gilliam & Tolin, 2010; Mataix-Cols, 2014).

Additional information that can be useful in making the diagnosis of HD includes observations made by the clinician or by reliable family members about the condition of the home of individuals suspected of having HD. These observations can demonstrate floor to ceiling stacks of newspapers, books, mail, etc., that allow only a small path to be travelled within the living space; possessions piled on beds, seating areas, tables, and even kitchen appliances; and no apparent organization to the collections. Reports from family members may indicate that they themselves, or others, have intervened to help individuals discard possessions. These reports, along with photographs, may be helpful, as well (Nordsletten & Mataix-Cols, 2014). Additionally, it is important for the clinician to differentiate HD from normal collecting. One particularly important differentiation is the characteristic disorganization and clutter associated with HD, along with very little relationship seen among the myriad possessions (Mataix-Cols, 2014).

There are two specifiers that exist for HD, excessive acquisition and insight. Neither of these is required for the diagnosis, but they help to identify specific areas of concern for the clinician. Excessive acquisition refers to the continued accumulation of possessions that are unnecessary or for which there is no space. The insight specifier is the same as noted in other of the OCRDs: (a) good or fair insight, (b) poor insight, or (c) no insight/delusional (Mataix-Cols, 2014).

◼ Hair-Pulling Disorder

Key diagnostic criteria for HPD in the *DSM-5* include (a) recurrent pulling out of one's own hair leading to noticeable hair loss, (b) repeated attempts to decrease or stop pulling, (c) the disturbance is not better accounted for by another mental disorder and is not due to a general medical (e.g., dermatological) condition, and (d) the disturbance causes clinically significant distress or impairment in social, occupational, or other important areas of functioning (APA, 2013). A diagnosis of hair-pulling disorder requires individuals meet all four criteria.

While the *DSM-5* has attempted to recategorize hair-pulling disorder, the requirement for meeting all four criteria has come under review, based on the idea of a dimensional framework, which would put diagnostic criteria on a spectrum or continuum. Using a dimension framework, researchers have argued that it would be easier to predict relapses by showing systematic variances along a continuum (Houghton et al., 2015).

There are several assessments that can be used for diagnosis including the National Institute on Mental Health Trichotillomania Severity Scale, which has adequate psychometrics, and the Clinical Global Impression Severity Scale, which has good psychometrics. The latter assessment is often used to measure treatment outcomes (Houghton et al., 2015).

◼ Skin-Picking Disorder

Key criteria for SPD include (a) the presence of skin lesions, (b) clinically significant distress or functional impairment, and (c) repeated attempts to stop or decrease picking (Snorrason et al., 2013). It is important when considering SPD that the clinician looks closely to distinguish SPD from other disorders such as primary pruritic skin disorders systematic conditions related to chronic, generalized pruritus, and other psychocutaneous syndromes, such as depression, anxiety, and/or delusional infestation (Craig-Muller & Reichenberg, 2015). It can also be misdiagnosed as OCD or BDD (Grant et al., 2012). Skin picking is also found to coexist many times with other grooming disorders, and lesions may vary from several to several hundred, depending on severity. Fingernails are used to create most lesions. Some individuals, however, report using tools to pick, such as knives, tweezers, pins, and needles (Grant et al., 2012).

It is important to note that skin damage and infections are quite common. Some individuals could experience disfigurement caused by picking, making SPD a significant mental health problem (Snorrason et al., 2013). Therefore, it is imperative that clinicians ask "problem-specific questions," including personal and family history, general acuity of the problem, frequency of picking, time spent picking, awareness of picking, body parts involved, when picking occurs, attempts to resist picking, and degree of distress evoked by picking (Craig-Muller & Reichenberg, 2015).

The Skin-Picking Impact Scale (SPIS) developed by Keuthen et al. (2001) has shown good psychometrics and has been used effectively in the diagnosis of SPD (Craig-Muller & Reichenberg, 2015). Recently, a short version of the SPIS, called the SPIS-S, has been developed and appears to be more effective with individuals whose picking extends beyond the face (Snorrason et al., Olafsson 2013).

MEDICAL/SURGICAL MANAGEMENT

◼ Obsessive-Compulsive Disorder

Research has shown that the neurobiology of OCD is complex, making medical management complex, as well. The orbitofrontal cortex, anterior cingulate gyrus, and caudate nucleus of the brain are all involved in OCD. Furthermore, abnormalities in neurotransmitters like serotonin, dopamine, and glutamate are also apparent contributors to OCD. The most effective treatment for OCD is a combination of cognitive-behavioral therapy (CBT), exposure response prevention (ERP) therapy, and pharmacotherapy (Bokor & Anderson, 2014; NAMI, 2013).

CBT is a type of psychotherapy that addresses dysfunctional emotions, maladaptive behaviors, cognitive processes, and differentiation of rational and irrational thinking. ERP encourages the individual to confront images that provoke anxiety and then conscious opt to NOT implement a compulsive behavior. This combination of CBT and ERP has had the most long-term success in the treatment of OCD (Seibell & Hollander, 2014). Individuals in treatment must adhere closely to instructions to ensure that learning occurs. Any kind of avoidance or subtle distraction may weaken the outcome (Grant, 2014).

When the CBT/ERP combination is not enough, selective serotonin reuptake inhibitors (SSRIs) are also used (Bokor & Anderson, 2014). The compounds with FDA approval include paroxetine, sertraline, fluoxetine, fluvoxamine, and clomipramine (Bokor & Anderson, 2014; Seibell & Hollander, 2014). There are additional combination strategies that may be used for adults with comorbid depression or other mental illness. Adaptations of all of these treatment methods must occur if they are to be used in children and adolescents (Franklin & Foa, 2011). Psychoeducation, reduction of psychosocial stress, and guided self-help are strategies that can be used in the treatment of children with OCD, along with CBT, behavioral therapy, and SSRIs (Ferren, Palmes, & Kaplan, 2013; Thomsen, 2013).

Neuromodulation is being researched for OCD based on a deeper understanding of brain circuitry in some psychiatric conditions. The need for neuromodulation is due to individual OCD resistance to the usual treatment at a level of approximately 40% to 60%. Neuromodulation is preferable to more invasive methods, such as surgery, and includes transcranial magnetic stimulation, which modulates cortical and subcortical function to increase or decrease cortical excitability. These treatments are considered experimental because the pathophysiology of OCD remains unclear (Pallanti, Marras, & Grassi, 2015; Pittenger, 2015).

■ Body Dysmorphic Disorder

While BDD is related to OCD, it is less responsive to ERP, and this approach is unlikely to be successful. What is suggested includes some basic strategies such as motivational interviewing, focus on patients' functional impairment, and discouraging patients from seeking cosmetic dermatological, dental, or surgical treatment (Phillips, 2014). Cognitive-behavioral therapy (CBT) that is specific to BDD, following a protocol that lasts over 6 to 24 sessions, is the recommended treatment (National Institute for Health and Clinical Excellence, 2005). According to Veale and Bewley (2015), this plan is based on several randomized controlled trials, demonstrating that CBT is "...more effective in improving severity of body dysmorphic disorder, based on blinded assessment by clinicians" (p. 2280). The aim of treatment is to decrease preoccupation with the body to reduce self-focused attention and to address faulty beliefs and assumptions. This process includes self-monitoring of thoughts and behaviors. Some individuals may be helped by SSRIs over a 3-month period used in addition to the focused CBT (Pavan et al., 2008).

■ Hoarding Disorder

Management of this condition is best done through a multifaceted psychological approach based on CBT, blending motivational enhancement techniques, and goal setting with behavioral modification and skills training (NAMI, 2013; Nordsletten & Mataix-Cols, 2014). CBT for HD uses a variety of strategies to address motivational issues; information processing deficits; beliefs about, and attachment to, possessions; and behavioral avoidance (Gilliam & Tolin, 2010).

According to Gilliam and Tolin (2010), when using the CBT for HD strategies, it is imperative that goal setting is addressed at the outset of treatment to ensure that the individuals can identify personally relevant reasons to make changes in their hoarding behaviors. Simultaneous with CBT, the individual must begin the sorting and discarding process, which requires extensive therapist involvement asking challenging questions and employing behavioral experiments to help address barriers to treatment. More research is needed on both psychological treatment and pharmacological treatment, particularly due to the high cost of medications (NAMI, 2013). A lot of uncertainties remain relative to hoarding in children and adolescents, family-centered intervention, and the value of pharmacologic treatments (Mataix-Cols, 2014).

■ Hair-Pulling and Skin-Picking Disorders

HPD and SPD are combined here because recent neuroimaging research has shown substantial similarities between the two disorders, particularly in the frontostriatal circuitry of the brain, and the medical management, therefore, is similar. The areas of the brain involved appear to be related to stimulus-response habit formation. There are, however, some distinct differences in brain structures between HPD and SPD, including differences in brain volume and cortical thickness (Roos, Grant, Fouche, Stein, & Lochner, 2015).

Habit reversal training (HRT) and cognitive-behavioral therapy (CBT) used singly and in combination have been successful in treating both HPD and SPD (Rogers et al., 2014). However, there is a gap between implementation of treatment and documentation of efficacy. One of the problems is that there are not many competent providers of HPD/SPD treatment, as evidenced by the "…lack of providers in 12 states and only 1 provider for another 14 states" (Keuthen, Tung, Reese, Raikes, Lee, & Mansueto, 2015, p. 11). Another significant issue is that various racial and ethnic groups respond differently to treatment, especially to web-based, self-help programs (Falkenstein, Rogers, Malloy, & Haaga, 2015).

The TLC Foundation for Body-Focused Repetitive Disorders, formerly known as the Trichotillomania Learning Center, endorses a behavioral treatment approach that includes HRT along with CBT, and medications (TLC Foundation, 2016). This combination of behavioral therapy and medication has been shown to be more effective than either HRT or CBT alone. Habit reversal training (HRT) is a behavioral treatment approach developed in the 1970s and has been found to be useful in treating HPD and SPD over the short term, but is less effective long term (Golomb et al., 2011). HRT includes awareness training, competing response training, contingency management, relaxation training, and generalization training. HRT used in combination with CBT and medications that affect serotonin and/or glutamate production in the brain has been shown to be effective for HPD and SPD as well. Other treatment strategies are being explored (Jacob, 2013; Rogers et al., 2014).

IMPACT ON OCCUPATIONAL PERFORMANCE

Because the OCRDs relate directly to functional behaviors, each of them has a significant impact on client factors and occupational performance. Client factors as defined by the *Occupational Therapy Practice Framework, 3rd Edition* (AOTA, 2014) include "…capacities, characteristics, or beliefs that reside with the person…" (p. 57). Client factors include (a) values, beliefs, and spirituality, (b) body functions, and (c) body structures. These factors can affect and be affected by performance skills, through influence on motivation and individual perceptions of value as well as through physical and physiological perceptions of the world. This section of the chapter will address client factors and discuss how the OCRDs impact each factor and ultimately impact occupational performance.

■ Values, Beliefs, and Spirituality

This category of client factors relates to cultural beliefs and values, what is held as true by an individual, and the way that individuals express meaning and purpose and connectedness in their lives. As can be seen from the descriptions of the OCRDs, this category of client factors is affected heavily. In OCD, for example, beliefs about what is safe (contamination), what is orderly (sequencing), what is repugnant (unacceptable behaviors like harming a friend), and what is moral (sexual and religious beliefs) affect social encounters, how one maintains a home, how one carries out ADLs, and how one relates to others (Bokor & Anderson, 2014; Saxena et al., 2011). In BDD, beliefs about one's attractiveness or its importance can interfere with both social and work activities. These beliefs can also have an impact on style and type of clothing or attire identified as appropriate. In HD, beliefs about what is valuable and what one can or cannot do without become important, along with an individual's sense of power over one's own behaviors (Gilliam & Tolin, 2010). In HPD and SPD, issues related to honesty with self, as well as issues of power, are present (Snorrason et al., 2013). In all of the OCRDs, issues related to the expression of meaning and purpose and connected to the world and to others are a strong presence, which the public does not understand or accept. Furthermore, the media tends to create and reinforce faulty conceptualizations of mental illness (Fennel & Boyd, 2014).

■ Body Functions

All of the OCRDs affect body functions, including mental functions, both specific and global, volunteer activities, play, leisure, and social participation.

Mental Functions

Each of the OCRDs has a unique neurobiology that affects a different area of the brain and therefore impacts mental functions slightly differently. So, for example, all of the OCRDs affect higher level cognition, such as judgment, concept formation, metacognition, cognitive flexibility, insight, attention, and awareness (Abramowitz & Jacoby, 2014; Mataix-Cols, 2014; Phillips, 2014). So, for example, research in HD has shown cognition deficits in judgment, cognitive flexibility, and insight (Grant, 2014; Phillips, 2014; Tung et al., 2015). Concentration and attention are very involved in OCD, along with perceptions, thoughts, global, and other mental functions. Depending on the severity of the OCRD, one's state of awareness and alertness may be affected, along with temperament and personality and energy level.

Sensory Functions

Sensory functions have also been researched in OCD, to examine how individuals process sensory input. According to Rieke and Anderson (2009), adults with OCD have greater sensory sensitivity and sensation avoiding than do other adults. This includes difficulty ignoring stimuli and responding readily. This difficulty suggests that adults with OCD have less efficient sensory processing patterns, which may be linked to neurocognitive processes. Also, because clinicians do not know what the individual with BDD actually sees, "...abnormalities in visual processing" are suggested, according to Phillips (2014, p. 326).

Skin and Related Functions

Individuals with HPD and SPD may have limited understanding of the protective nature of skin and hair, if they are unaware of their behavior (Rogers et al., 2014). Even with awareness, because these two disorders may be comorbid with BDD or another mental illness, the ability to interpret and act on that knowledge may be impaired, as well (Phillips, 2014; Snorrason et al., 2013).

■ Body Structures

In this category, all of the OCRDs have a relationship to the structure of the nervous system, as discussed earlier in the chapter. The research demonstrating brain abnormalities and neurotransmitter differences is testament to this connection and to the importance of understanding the stigma, the shame, the suffering, and the disability that creates the devastation of mental illness (Pallanti et al., 2015; Pittenger, 2015, Seibell, 2015).

The impact of OCRDs on occupational performance can be profound, depending on the severity of symptoms, the client factors involved, and the duration of the illness. In terms of performance skills, such things as positioning and transporting objects may be problematic for someone with a hoarding disorder. Process skills are much more involved, related to ability to attend, heed, make choices, initiate, sequence, and organize activities, any and all of which may be impaired, as in someone who is preoccupied with skin picking or some other body concerns. Social interaction skills are seriously eroded in all of the OCRDs, as indicated earlier in the chapter, including the ability to engage in social interactions.

Performance patterns in terms of habits, routines, rituals, and roles may all be seriously impaired, as the OCRDs related directly to these categories. For example, rituals may be overstressed, while routines may be erratic due to interference from obsessive thoughts or compulsive actions. The ability to perform in a particular role may also be impaired, as in attempting to play in the mud with a child when a contamination obsession is present, or attempting to prepare a meal for family when the kitchen is cluttered with things that don't belong there, but for which there is no other space.

It is evident that client factors, performance skills, and performance patterns can all be affected by the presence of OCRDs and can significantly impact one's ability to live comfortably in one's own home or even in one's own skin. Being cognizant of the many complexities involved in living a functional life is important in dealing with individuals having OCRD.

CASE STUDY 1

Eileen is 28-year-old interior designer. She has worked in her field for about 6 years, but she has had seven jobs in that length of time. Eileen has always been very conscious of her appearance, although she has never been happy with it. From the time she was little, Eileen has been aware of what she believes is a serious flaw in her appearance. When she turned 13, this flaw became more of an issue for her because she suddenly became interested in boys and she was sure no one would be interested in her because of this flaw. Eileen has tried numerous ways to conceal the flaw, but is never satisfied with the result.

The flaw is located on her left ear. At the top of the ear where it would normally curl, for about one-half inch along the curled edge, Eileen's ear is flat. When she was little, it was easy to cover with her hair, but she would never let her mother put her hair in pigtails or braids or a ponytail that others girls wore. If her mother was insistent, Eileen would wear earmuffs all day until she could take out the braids or pigtails. If anyone noticed it or asked about it, she said she had "cold ears."

As Eileen has gotten older and wanted to try different hairstyles, she has become acutely aware of this defect, to the point that she spends hours every day focused on it. Getting through high school was very difficult for Eileen, because she was so self-conscious about her appearance. She refused to present in class and used to sit with her face downcast, her head resting in her hand, and her hand covering her ear. She did not date in high school because she was so self-conscious that she was unable to make eye contact with anyone who spoke to her, which earned her a reputation as a snob. Eileen developed one good friend in high school, Kate. Kate was willing to listen to Eileen's concerns and would sympathize to a degree. However, once Kate went to college, she changed, and told Eileen that she had a "problem" and needed help to deal with it. This event prompted devastation in Eileen, and she cried for weeks, expressing feelings of worthlessness. Eileen and Kate have not spoken since that time. While Eileen was studying for her interior design career, she arranged all her classes for later in the day, so she would have plenty of time to work on covering up her flawed ear.

Since getting her design credential, Eileen has had numerous jobs. The reason is that she usually quits or loses the job because she is unable to keep her appointments in a timely fashion and often has difficulty focusing on client conversations and desires due to her preoccupation with her ear flaw. It typically takes Eileen 3 hours to prepare for work. Every morning when she is getting ready for work, she spends most of her time fussing with her hair to cover the flawed part of her ear and then moving around the room, as she might do if she was working at a client's home, to see if the flaw is revealed. If she does find that certain movements display the ear, then Eileen attempts to control her movements more closely, resulting in stilted and awkward movements that actually draw more attention to her than usual. During the workday, Eileen is so obsessed with her hair and her ear, that she frequently checks herself in store windows, the car mirror, and in the bathroom. Many days, she wears a hat to cover her flaw and then has to spend time rearranging or adjusting it. These behaviors have resulted in client requests for another designer and have cost her the job in several cases. The loss of her last job resulted in another significant episode of depression.

As a result of her obsession with her ear flaw and her inability to work or concentrate on anything else, Eileen has no social life. She does not have the money to live independently, so she lives at home with her widowed mother, a teacher. Eileen's mother has tried numerous strategies to help Eileen address her concerns, even agreeing to take her to a plastic surgeon, particularly following Eileen's most recent depressive episode. The surgery proposed by the physician, however, was so expensive that Eileen could not afford it, and since she is over age, she is no longer covered by her mother's insurance. The physician did recommend a psychiatric consult, based on Eileen's depression, which her mother thought would be a good idea. This encounter has convinced Eileen that her preoccupation with her ear flaw may actually be abnormal and that perhaps she should think about seeing a psychiatrist, especially since she has already experienced two depressive episodes. Eileen has agreed to think about it, primarily because she is so unhappy and has found herself recently thinking about suicide.

CASE STUDY 2

Jerry is a disabled veteran of the Gulf War. He is 52 years old and comes from a large family with seven siblings, all of whom live in the same area where Jerry lives. Jerry has never married, and when he returned from the Gulf War with a disability, he was invited to live with his sister and her family. Recently, Jerry was asked to leave his sister's home because he had accumulated so much stuff that he had filled up his own space and had begun to encroach on the family space. It was decided that Jerry needed his own place. Because Jerry is disabled, he is unable to work, but he does receive disability and a small military pension, enabling him to live independently in a subsidized housing environment. His apartment is one bedroom, with a living/dining area, bathroom, and kitchenette. It is about 550 square feet.

According to Jerry's sister, he has always been a "collector" of sorts, not of anything particular, but rather of odds and ends that appealed to him, or that had some sentimental value. He has saved a lot of his papers and grade school report cards, along with a great deal of his high school memorabilia. He has saved similar memorabilia from the activities of his many nieces and nephews, special events that he has attended, posters, correspondence, newspaper and magazine articles he has found interesting, and so on. When he was younger, his collectibles could be contained in several boxes in his room, or in his closet, and his mother would periodically suggest that he get rid of some stuff. He never did, but he would just compress his stuff so it fit into fewer boxes.

Since Jerry has been back home after his military experience and several months in the hospital because of his injury, his collecting has become excessive, notes his sister. She states that she had to ask him to move because his room was filled with boxes and also loose papers he had saved—cards, articles, more correspondence, and souvenirs from his recent volunteer work with the Boys and Girls Club. She objected when she could not get into the room to run the vacuum, and he agreed to move some things to the family garage. But that became impossible as well, said his sister, so she asked him to move.

Jerry's other siblings refuse to go to his house because there is no place to sit in the living/dining room area or the kitchenette. There is a small stove, but that is covered with magazines and unopened mail and is currently not usable. Jerry generally does not cook anyway, preferring to eat directly from the refrigerator, in which he keeps ready-to-eat foods such as yogurt, cheese and crackers, some fruit, and other things he can eat from the carton. He likes to order Chinese food once every couple of weeks if he can. The tabletop is covered with mail and magazine articles, while newspapers are stacked 6 to 7 ft high all through the house. Even in the bedroom, part of the bed, along with the floor, the dresser tops, and one chair, is covered with both boxes and loose papers. It is difficult to get into the bathroom, but there is a slender path to the toilet and sink. The bathtub/shower is full of boxes of memorabilia.

Outside of his volunteer work, Jerry has few interests and he does not socialize much. He has never been comfortable in social situations, preferring his own company or the company of family. Jerry is good with children, which allows him to continue his work with the Boys and Girls Club. He does visit his siblings for family gatherings, but it is difficult for him to get around because of his disability. So his interests are focused inside the house including reading, watching television, maintaining correspondence with old military buddies, and looking at pictures and other stuff from the children of his family members.

The family has suggested both cleaning up Jerry's apartment and even helping him to do it, but he has refused any assistance, saying that he would be afraid they would discard something that was really important to him or that he might need later. The family has also suggested that his hoarding may be a mental health problem, but Jerry doesn't see it that way. He has, however, been seeing a counselor for a recent episode of depression, and his collecting/hoarding behavior was broached in that meeting. Jerry agreed to let the counselor visit him in his apartment, but he is uncertain if he will be able to do anything to change the living environment or lifestyle with which he is comfortable.

LEARNING RESOURCES

Adam, D. (2015). *The man who couldn't stop: OCD and the true story of a life lost in thought.* New York, NY: Sarah Crichton Books.

Goodman, W. K. (Ed.). (2014). *OCRD: An issue of psychiatric clinics of North America.* Philadelphia, PA: Elsevier.

Grant, J. E., & Chamberlain, S. R. (2014). *Clinical guide to obsessive–compulsive and related disorders.* Oxford, UK: Oxford University Press.

Grant, J. E., Stein, D. J., Woods, D. N., & Keuthen, N. J. (2012). *Trichotillomania, skin picking, and other body-focused repetitive behaviors.* Arlington, VA: American Psychiatric Publishing.

Grayson, J. (2014). *Freedom for obsessive–compulsive disorder.* New York: Berkley Publishing Group.

Hershfield, J., & Corby, T. (2013). *The mindfulness workbook for OCD: A guide to overcoming obsessions and compulsions using mindfulness and cognitive behavioral therapy.* Oakland, CA: New Harbinger Books.

International OCD Foundation. *PO Box 961029,* Boston, MA: (617) 973-5801. https://iocd.org

Lak, C. W. (Ed.). (2015). *Obsessive–compulsive disorder: Etiology, phenomenology and treatment.* Fareham, UK: Onus Books.

Stein, D. J., & Fineburg, N. (Eds.). (2015). *Obsessive–compulsive and related disorders.* (2nd ed.). Oxford, UK: Oxford University Press.

Storch, E. A., & Lewin, A. B. (Eds.). (2015). *Clinical handbook of OCRD: A case-based approach to treating pediatric and adult populations.* Springer Trichotillomania Learning Center. 207 McPherson St, #H, Santa Cruz, CA, 95060: (831) 457-1004. www.trich.org.

Yadin, E., & Foa, E. B. (2012). *Treating your OCD with exposure and response (ritual) preventive therapy: Workbook* (2nd ed.). Oxford, UK: Oxford University Press.

REFERENCES

Abramowitz, J. S., & Jacoby, R. J. (2014). Obsessive–compulsive disorder in the *DSM-5. Clinical Psychology Science and Practice, 21*(3), 221–235. doi: 10.1111/cpsp.12076

American Occupational Therapy Association. (2014). Occupational therapy practice framework: Domain and process (3rd ed.). *American Journal of Occupational Therapy, 68*(Suppl.1), S1–S48. doi: 10.5014/ajot.2014.682006

American Psychological Association. (2013). *Diagnostic and statistical manual of mental disorders* (5th ed.). Arlington, VA: APA. doi: 10.1176/appi.books.9780890425596

Buhlmann, U., Teachman, B. A., Gerbershagen, A., Kikul, J., & Rief, W. (2008). Implicit and explicit self-esteem and attractiveness beliefs among individuals with body dysmorphic disorder. *Cognitive Therapy and Research, 32*(2), 213–225. doi:10.1007/s10608-006-9095-9

Bokor, G., & Anderson, P. D. (2014). Obsessive–compulsive disorder. *Journal of Pharmacy Practice, 27*(2), 116–130. doi: 10.1177/0897190014521996

Conelea, C. A., Schmidt, E. R., Leonard, R. C., Riemann, B. C., & Cahill, S. (2012). The Children's Yale-Brown Obsessive Compulsive Scale: Clinician versus self-report format in adolescents in a residential treatment facility. *Journal of Obsessive-Compulsive and Related Disorders, 1*(2), 69–72.

Craig-Muller, S. A., & Reichenberg, J. S. (2015). The other itch that rashes: A clinical and therapeutic approach to pruritus and skin picking disorders. *Current Allergy and Asthma Report, 15*(6). doi: 10.1007/s11882-015-0532-2

Falkenstein, M., Rogers, K., Mally, E. J., & Haaga, D. A. F. (2015). Race/Ethnicity and treatment outcome in a randomized controlled trial for trichotillomania. *Journal of Clinical Psychology, 71*(7), 641–652.

Fennel, D., & Boyd, M. (2014). Obsessive–compulsive disorder in the media. *Deviant Behavior, 35*(9), 669–686. doi: 10.1080/01639625.2013.872526

Ferren, T., Palmes, G. K., & Kaplan, S. G. (2013). Psychopharmacologic treatment of refractory pediatric obsessive compulsive disorder. *Journal of Child and Adolescent Psychopharmacology, 23*(7), 509–512. doi: 10.1089/cap.2013.0025

Flessner, C. A., Conelea, C. A., Woods, D. W., Franklin, M. E., Keuthen, N. J., & Cashin, S. E. (2008). Styles of pulling in trichotillomania: Exploring differences in symptom severity, phenomenology, and functional impact. *Behavior Research and Therapy, 46*(3), 345–357. doi: 10.1016/j.brat.2007.12.009

Franklin, M. E., & Foa, E. B. (2011). Treatment of obsessive–compulsive disorder. *Annual Review of Clinical Psychology, 7*(1), 229–243. doi:10.1146/annurev-clinpsy-032210-104533

Gilliam, C. M., & Tolin, D. F. (2010). Compulsive hoarding. *Bulletin of the Menninger Clinic, 74*(2), 93–121. doi: 10.1521/bumc.2010.74.2.93

Golomb, R., Franklin, M. E., Grant, J. E., Keuthen, N. J., Mansueto, C. S., Mouton-Odum, S., … Woods, D. (2011). *Treatment guidelines for trichotillomania and skin picking and other body-focused repetitive behaviors.* Santa Cruz, CA: Trichotillomania Learning Center.

Grant, J. E. (2014). Obsessive–compulsive disorder. *New England Journal of Medicine, 37*(7), 646–653. doi: 10.1056/NEJMcp1402176

Grant, J. E., Odlaug, B. L., Chamberlain, S. R., Keuthen, N. J., Lochner, C., & Stein, D. J. (2012). Skin picking disorder. *American Journal of Psychiatry, 169*(11), 1143–1149. doi: 10.1176/appi.ajp.2012.12040508

Harrison, J. P., & Franklin, M. E. (2012). Pediatric Trichotillomania. *Current Psychiatry Reports, 14*(2), 188–196.

Houghton, D. C., Balsis, S. Stein, D. J., Compton, S. N., Twohig, M. P., Saunders, S. M., … Woods, D. W. (2015). Examining *DSM* criteria for trichotillomania in a dimensional framework: Implications for *DSM-5* and diagnostic practice. *Comprehensive Psychiatry, 60*, 9–16. doi: 10.1016/j.comppsych.2015.04.011

Jacob, A. P. (2013). Trichotillomania. *Nursing Journal of India, civ* (4), 162–164. Retrieved from http://search.proquest.com.exproxy.gvsu.edu/docview/1536920197?accountid=39473

Johnson, C., & Blair-West, S. (2013). Obsessive–compulsive disorder: The role of the GP. *Australian Family Physician, 42*(9), 606–609. Retrieved from http://search.proquest.com/ezproxy.gvsu.edu/docview/1470780489?accountid=39473

Jukel, G., Siebers, F., Kienast, T., & Mavrogiorgou, P. (2014). Early recognition of obsessive–compulsive disorder. *Journal of Nervous and Mental Disease, 202*(12), 889–891. doi: 10.1097/NMD.0000000000000220

Kaplan, A. (2012). Update on trichotillomania. *Psychiatric times, 29*(8), 19. Retrieved from http://search.proquest.com/ezproxy.gvsu.edu/docview/1038452269?accountid=39473

Keuthen, N. J., Tung, E., Reese, H. E., Raikes, J., Lee, L, & Mansueto, C. S. (2015). Getting the word out: Cognitive-behavioral therapy for trichotillomania (hair-pulling disorder) and excoriation (skin-picking) disorder. *Annals of Clinical Psychiatry, 27*(1), 10–15.

Keuthen, N. J., Deckersbach, T., Wilhelm, S., Engelhard, I., Forker, A., O'Sullivan, R. L., … Baer, L. (2001). The skin picking impact scale (SPIS): Scale development and psychometric analyses.

Psychosomatics, 42(5), 397–403. doi: 10.1176/appi.psy.42.5.397

Leonard, R. C., & Rieman, B. C. (2012). The co-occurrence of obsessions and compulsions in OCD. *Journal of Obsessive–Compulsive and Related Disorders, 1*(3), 211–215. doi: 10.1016/j-jocrd.2012.06.002

Mataix-Cols, D. (2014). Hoarding disorder. *New England Journal of Medicine, 370*(21), 2023–2030. doi: 10.1056/NEJMcp1313051

Marques, L., LeBlanc, N., Robinaugh, M. A., Weingarden, B. S., Keshaviah, A., & Wilhelm, S. (2011). Correlates of quality of life and functional disability in individuals with body dysmorphic disorder. *Psychosomatics, 52*(3), 245–254. doi: 10.1016/j.psym.2010.12.015

Monzani, B., Rijsdijk, F., Cherkas, L., Harris, J., Keuthen, N., & Mataix-Cols, D. (2012). Prevalence and heritability of skin picking in an adult community sample: A twin study. *American Journal of Medical Genetics Part B, 159B*(5), 605–610. doi: 10.1002/ajmg.b.32067

National Alliance on Mental Illness. (2013). Obsessive–compulsive disorder. *National Alliance on Mental Illness.* Retrieved from www.nami.org/Learn-More/Mental-Health-Conditions/Obsessive-Compulsive-Disorder

National Institute for Health and Clinical Excellence. (2005). Obsessive compulsive disorder: Core interventions in the treatment of obsessive–compulsive disorder and body dysmorphic disorder: CG31. Retrieved from www.nice.org.uk/guidance/cg31

Nordsletten, A. E., & Mataix-Cols, D. (2014). Ask the experts: Hoarding disorder. *Neuropsychiatry, 4*(1), 17–21. doi: 10.2217/npy.13.83

Nordsletten, A. E., Reichenberg, A., Hatch, S. L., Fernandez de la Cruz, L., Pertusa, A., Hotoph, M., & Mataix-Cols, D. (2013). Epidemiology of hoarding disorder. *The British Journal of Psychiatry, 203*(6), 445–452. doi: 10.1192/bjp.bp.113.130195

Odlaug, B. L., Hampshire, A., Chamberlain, S. R., & Grant, J. E. (2015). Abnormal brain activation in excoriation (skin-picking disorder): Evidence from an executive planning fMRI study. *The British Journal of Psychiatry, 208*, 168–174. doi: 10.1192/bjp.bp.114.155192

Pallanti, S., Marras, A., & Grassi, G. (2015). Outcomes with neuromodulation in obsessive–compulsive disorder. *Psychiatric Annals, 45*(6), 316–320. doi:10.3928/00485713-20150602-07

Pavan, C., Simonato, P., Marini, M., Mazzoleni, F., Pavan, L., & Vindigni, V. (2008). Psychopathologic aspects of body dysmorphic disorder: A literature review. *Aesthetic Plastic Surgery, 32*(3), 473–484. doi: 10.1007/s00266-008-9113-2

Phillips, K. A. (2014). Body dysmorphic disorder: Common, severe and in need of treatment.

Psychotherapy and Psychosomatics, *83*(6), 325–329. doi: 10.1159/000366035

Phillips, K. A., Menard, W., Quinn, E., Didie, E. R., & Stout, R. L. (2012). A 4-year prospective observational follow-up study of course and predictors of course in body dysmorphic disorder. *Psychological Medicine*, *43*(05), 1109–1117. doi: 10.1017/S0033291712001730

Pittenger, C. (2015). Glutamate modulators in the treatment of obsessive–compulsive disorder. *Psychiatric Annals*, *45*(6), 308–315. doi: 10.3928/00485713-20150602-06

Ricketts, E. J., Brandt, B. C., & Woods, D. W. (2012). The effects of severity and causal explanation on social perceptions of hair loss. *Journal of Obsessive–Compulsive and Related Disorders*, *1*(4), 336–343. doi: 10.1016/j.jocrd.2012.07.007

Rieke, E. F., & Anderson, D. (2009). Adolescent/adult sensory profile and obsessive–compulsive disorder. *American Journal of Occupational Therapy*, *62*(2), 138–145. doi: 10.5014/ajot.63.2.138

Rogers, K., Banis, M., Falkenstein, M. J., Malloy, E. J., McDonough, L., Nelson, S.O., … Haaga, D. A. F. (2014). Stepped care in the treatment of trichotillomania. *Journal of Counseling and Clinical Psychology*, *82*(2), 361–367. doi: 10.1037/a0035744

Roos, A., Fouche, J.-P., Stein, D. J., & Lochner, C. (2015). White matter integrity in hair-pulling disorder (trichotillomania). *Psychiatry Research: Neuroimaging*, *211*(3), 246–250. doi: 10.1016/j.pscychresns.2012.08.005

Saxena, S., Ayers, C. R., Maidment, K. M., Vapnik, T., Wetherell, J. L., & Bystritsky, A. (2011). Quality of life and functional impairment in compulsive hoarding. *Journal of Psychiatric Research*, *45*(4), 475–480. doi: 10.1016/j.jpsychires.2010.08.007

Schieber, K., Kollei, I., de Zwaan, M., & Martin, A. (2015). Classification of body dysmorphic disorder—What is the advantage of the new DSM-5 criteria? *Journal of Psychosomatic Research*, *78*(3), 223–227. doi: 10.1016/j.jpsychores.2015.01.002

Seibell, P. J. (2015). Guest Editorial: Obsessive–compulsive disorder. *Psychiatric Annals*, *45*(6), 290–291. doi: 10.3928/00485713-20150602-03

Seibell, P. J., Hamblin, R. J., & Hollander, E. (2015). Obsessive–compulsive disorder: Overview and standard treatment strategies. *Psychiatric Annals*, *45*(6), 297–302. doi: 10.3928/00485713-20150602-04

Seibell, P. J., & Hollander, E. (2014). Management of obsessive–compulsive disorder. *F1000Prime Reports*, *6*: 68. doi: 10.12703/P6-68

Sinha, P., Bakhla, A. K., Patnaik, A. K., & Chaudhury, S. (2014). Seasonal obsessive–compulsive disorder. *Industrial Psychiatry Journal*, *23*(2), 160–162. doi: 10.4103/0972-6748.151701

Snorrason, I., Olafsson, R. P., Flessner, C. A., Keuthen, N. J., Franklin, M. E., & Woods, D. W. (2013). The SPIS: Factor, structure, validity and development of a shorter version. *Scandinavian Journal of Psychology*, *54*(4), 344–348. doi: 10.1111/sjop.12057

Snorrason, I., Stein, D. J., & Woods, D. W. (2013). Classification of excoriation (skin-picking) disorder: Current status and future directions. *Acta Psychiatrica Scandinavica*, *128*(5), 406–407. doi: 10.1111/acps.12153

Soomro, G. M., (2012). Obsessive–compulsive disorder. *British Medical Journal*, *2012*: 1004. Published online January 18, 2012. Retrieved from www.ncbi.nlm.nih.gov/pmc/articles/PMC3285220/?report=reader

Subramaniam, M., Abdin, E., Vaingankar, J. A., & Chong, S. A. (2012). Obsessive–compulsive disorder: Prevalence, correlates, help-seeking and quality of life in multiracial Asian population. *Social Psychiatry Psychiatric Epidemiology*, *47*(12), 2035–2043. doi:10.1007/s00127-012-0507-8

The TLC Foundation for Body-Focused Repetitive Behaviors. (2016). *Expert Consensus Treatment Guidelines*. Santa Cruz, CA: Author.

Thomsen, P. H. (2013). Obsessive–compulsive disorders. *European Child and Adolescent Psychiatry*, *22*(S1), 23–28. doi: 10.1007/s00787-012-0357-7

Tung, E. S., Flessner, C. A., Grant, J. E., & Keuthen, N. J. (2015). Predictors of life disability in trichotillomania. *Comprehensive Psychiatry*, *56*, 239–244. doi: 10.1016/j.comppsych.2014.09.018

Veale, D., & Bewley, A. (2015). Body dysmorphic disorder. *British Medical Journal*, *350*(9), h2278. doi: 10.1136/bmj.h2278

Wheaton, M. G., Schwartz, M. R., Pascucci, O., & Simpson, H. B. (2015). Cognitive-behavior therapy outcomes for obsessive–compulsive disorder: Exposure and response prevention. *Psychiatric Annals*, *45*(6), 303–307. doi: 10.3928/00485713-20150602-05

CHAPTER 14

Somatic Symptoms and Related Disorders

Michael J. Urban

Mr. Smith is a 30-year-old man who works at a local construction company. While at work one day, he was helping to move some 8 foot 2 × 4 pieces of lumber, which was a normal job function. After moving 50 boards, he noticed his back was sore and he started to have difficulty with getting in and out of his truck or going to stand from sitting in a chair. Mr. Smith the next day called out of work to rest his back. After 2 days of no resolve, he went to see his doctor as instructed by his supervisor and was diagnosed initially with a lumbar strain needing therapy.

After completing 4 weeks of the physical therapy for his back and being out of work, Mr. Smith was referred to an occupational therapist for work hardening as his body had become deconditioned. His pain was still reported to be at an 8/10 constantly with difficulty with any kind of bending or performing transitions from a seated or supine surface. The report for transition from physical therapy showed all the therapeutic exercises to stretch his back and modalities that were used. The occupational therapist started to conduct the evaluation that comprised a full check of Mr. Smith's full body active range of motion (AROM), passive range of motion (PROM), strength, sensation, hobbies, leisure pursuits, interests, work classification, job description, ability to complete his activities of daily living (ADLs) and instrumental activities of daily living (IADLs), and current cognitive status, which included memory and risk of depression. The evaluation also reviewed his current physical capacity and mechanics to complete basic lifting, pushing, pulling, carrying, and functional positional and mobility ability. Each client factor, performance pattern, and performance skill noted to be a weakness was identified in relation to the impact on his ability to complete his basic daily needs and work functions.

Testing noted that Mr. Smith clinically and objectively demonstrated signs consistent with depression and several inconsistencies and self-limiting behaviors. He was noted to have a 10% loss of full forward trunk flexion and poor body mechanics and posturing for daily habitual routines. With functional testing, Mr. Smith often reported having 10/10 pain and reported he could not lift the 10-lb box from the table to carry to another table. The occupational profile noted that Mr. Smith enjoyed spending time with his 4-month-old son since his injury and his injury has allowed his wife to return to work earlier to a higher paying job. When showing pictures of him carrying his son to the occupational therapist, he disclosed that his son weighed 21 lb.

DESCRIPTION AND DEFINITIONS

Somatosensory sensation can be viewed as subjective and objective in its own right as we all perceive pain differently. **Pain** is a physical suffering or discomfort caused by illness or injury (American Psychiatric Association, 2013). It is a reaction to some kind of physical, biological, or emotional trauma that disrupts the harmony of our everyday life.

Somatic symptom disorder is a disorder where the physical symptoms cannot be fully explained by a general medical condition, another mental disorder, or the effects of a substance. They could be the result of a factitious or a malingering disorder. **Malingering** is the intentional production of false or grossly exaggerated physical or psychological problems (American Psychiatric Association, 2013). Despite the unknown origins, they are noted to cause significant impairments to everyday engagement in social occupational performance and all areas of daily living. **Occupational performance** is an act accomplishing a selected action (The American Occupational

Therapy Association, 2014). The *Diagnostic and Statistical Manual of Mental Disorders 5th Edition* (DSM-5) uses the term somatic symptom and related disorders as a broad classification grouping a variety of disorders. Changes were made to the classifications from DSM-IV to DSM-5 to consolidate similar conditions into one classification cluster (see Table 14.1).

When medical providers think about a somatic disorder, they view it as chronic pain without a known cause (American Psychiatric Association, 2013). **Chronic pain** is pain that causes clinically significant distress or impairment in social, occupational, or other important areas of functioning for a duration >6 months (American Psychiatric Association, 2013). As occupational therapy practitioners, we must think about the areas of daily functioning that have been impaired. Individuals in this classification often display an increased attention to their bodily sensations with the attributions of those sensations expressed negatively. These two cognitive components foster the individual learning the help-seeking behaviors associated with the sick role that are only reinforced through attention

TABLE 14.1 Somatic Symptom Disorder and Related Disorders

DSM-5 Classifications Compared to DSM-IV	
DSM-IV	DSM-5
Somatization disorder	Somatic symptom disorder
Undifferentiated somatoform disorder	Illness anxiety disorder
Conversion disorder	Conversion disorder
Pain disorder	Psychological factors affecting a medical condition
Hypochondriasis	Factitious disorder
Somatoform dysmorphic disorder and somatoform disorder NOS	Other specific and nonspecific somatic symptom disorders

TABLE 14.2 Most Common Symptoms Reported with Somatic Disorders

Abdominal pain	Amnesia
Back pain	Bloating
Chest pain	Chronic pain
Diarrhea	Difficulty swallowing
Dizziness	Headaches
Impotence	Joint pain
Nausea and sometimes vomiting	Pain during intercourse
Pain during urination	Painful menstruation
Pain in the legs or arms	Palpitations
Paralysis or muscle weakness	Sexual inactivity
Shortness of breath	Vision changes

and/or sympathy. The level of distress caused by the fixation developing or even acquiring a serious illness or debilitating impairment preoccupies the individual into severe forms of self-limiting and habit-forming behaviors. Table 14.2 compiles the most common symptoms reported by an individual with no medical root cause noted.

ETIOLOGY

There is no known cause for somatic sensory and related disorders, as the physical complaints cannot be fully explained by a medical condition or substance abuse. These disorders are neither testable nor physically or medically identifiable and thus are difficult to treat by medical professionals (Crane et al., 2012). Due to the unknown origin, physicians report this classification of disorders as difficult to identify and treat properly (Crane et al., 2012; de Waal, Arnold, Eekhof, & van Hemert, 2004; Voigt et al., 2012). The impact on a client can result in the loss of physical, social, and occupational performance. Most clients diagnosed with a form of somatic-related disorder typically have a history or an associated diagnosis of depression and/or anxiety, which could exacerbate the condition (Crane et al., 2012; de Waal et al., 2004). **Depression** is a lack of interest or pleasure in daily activities for more than a 2-week period and represents a change from previous functioning (American Psychiatric Association, 2013).

INCIDENCE AND PREVALENCE

There is no difference in prevalence by gender, age, or ethnicity (Crane et al., 2012). For people with somatoform disorders, costs are two times higher than those with other medical conditions in the United States (Crane et al., 2012). Some literature does suggest that somatoform symptoms and related disorders are the third most common psychiatric condition behind depression and anxiety (Crane et al., 2012; de Waal et al., 2004; Douzenis & Seretis, 2013; Neng & Weck, 2013). Current literature cannot accurately document the incidence and prevalence rates due to the difficulty with properly diagnosing the disorders due to their unknown origin and the recent changes from DSM-IV to DSM-5, which increased the identification of individuals who are psychologically impaired (Voigt et al., 2013).

SIGNS AND SYMPTOMS

Complaints of pain that cause significant distress and disability with daily occupations are abundant in all areas of health care practice. The correlation between chronic pain and psychiatric disorders is well known but hard to treat due to the subjectivity in nature of the complaints (American Psychiatric Association, 2013; Crane et al., 2012; de Waal et al., 2004; Dimsdale et al., 2013; Douzenis & Seretis, 2013). A key characteristic stems around the excessive fixation or concern the client has about physical symptoms or health (Crane et al., 2012; de Waal et al., 2004; McCabe et al., 2009; Neng & Weck, 2013). Somatic symptom disorder, illness anxiety disorder, conversion disorder, and psychological factors affecting other medical conditions all derive from this overall notion but with slight variations (Arnold, de Waal, Eekhof, & van Hemert, 2006; Bener, Al-Kazaz, Ftouni, Al-Harthy, & Dafeeah, 2013; de Waal et al., 2004; Dimsdale et al., 2013; Katz, Rosenbloom, & Fashler, 2015). These characteristics prominently appear in a medical setting rather than a mental health care setting.

SOMATIC SYMPTOM DISORDER

Clients with somatic symptom disorder may present with one or multiple complaints of muscle and joint pains, low back pain, tension headaches, chronic fatigue, non–cardiac-related chest pain, palpitations, nonulcer dyspepsia, irritable bowel, dizziness, and insomnia (American Psychiatric Association, 2013; Bener et al., 2013; Crane et al., 2012; de Waal et al., 2004; Kroenke, Spitzer, deGruy, & Swindle, 1998). Clients also are noted to have a higher medical history that includes depression, irritable bowel syndrome, fibromyalgia, chronic pain, posttraumatic stress disorder, antisocial personality disorder, and a history of sexual or physical abuse. Due to the physical fixation, this classification can be difficult to identify and can greatly impact a client's overall occupational performance with daily tasks.

■ Illness Anxiety Disorder

Clients diagnosed with **hypochondriasis** have been reclassified as **illness anxiety disorder** under the DSM-5 (American Psychiatric Association, 2013). Hypochondriasis is a preoccupation with fears of having or the idea that one has a serious disease based upon the person's misinterpretation of bodily symptoms (American Psychiatric Association, 2013). A key characteristic factor is the preoccupation of having or acquiring a serious illness. Clients in this cluster have a high anxiety about health leading to excessive or maladaptive health behaviors, such as repeatedly checking their bodies for signs of illness or avoiding the doctor altogether. Clients in this classification tend not to be relieved by negative test results, and the reassurance of negative findings from doctors does not decrease the client's anxiety.

■ Conversion Disorder

Conversion disorder is often referred to as functional neurological symptom disorder or psychogenic (American Psychiatric Association, 2013; Arnold et al., 2006; Crane et al., 2012; Dimsdale et al., 2013; Katz et al., 2015). A client with conversion disorder is characterized by one or more symptoms related to a motor or sensory impairment when all medical testing is considered normal or the symptoms reported are inconsistent in nature. Typical motor symptoms are tremors, **dystonic movements**, gait abnormalities, abnormal limb posturing, and weakness or paralysis. Dystonic movement is a neurological movement disorder in which sustained muscle contractions cause twisting and repetitive movements or abnormal postures (American Psychiatric Association, 2013). Sensory symptoms include altered, reduced, or an absence of hearing, visual, or skin sensation. Other symptoms can include reduced or absence of speech volume, sensation of a lump in the throat, and altered articulation. Examples of loss of motor function could present with a client who is unable to abduct the shoulder greater than 40 degrees when tested but then can use the same arm to scratch the back of the head, which uses approximately 85 to 95 degrees of shoulder abduction.

■ Psychological Factors Affecting Other Medical Conditions

Psychological factors affecting other medical conditions are noted to be behavioral or psychological factors that can exacerbate or have an influence on the pathophysiology of the medical condition (American Psychiatric Association, 2013). Characteristics associated in this classification include poor adherence to medical recommendations, coping styles, patterns of interpersonal interactions, psychological distress, and other maladaptive behaviors that impact denial of a medical condition. Examples of these factors can include chronic occupational stress leading to increased risk for hypotension to conditions with a clear medical etiology impacted by the psychological factors such as knowingly ignoring the signs of a heart attack. This classification helps to clarify the impact that lifestyle, personality, or occupational stressors have on a medical condition. In this classification, individuals can choose to ignore or continue to engage in the factors that have a negative impact on their overall general well-being and health. If the behaviors or psychological components are deemed to stem from the medical condition, a more appropriate diagnosis and classification will be provided. Simple examples of this disorder classification would be the impact of a chronic stressful lifestyle on irritable bowel syndrome.

■ Factitious Disorders

The last defined classification for somatic symptoms and related disorders is **factitious disorders** (American Psychiatric Association, 2013). Factitious disorders are falsifications of an illness for oneself or others. In this classification, the individual reports various symptoms to obtain a diagnosis from a doctor, often to gain attention. In some cases, the individual is able to convince the doctor to perform surgery to the extent of loss of limb as an act of mutilation. Factitious on others differs from factitious on self in that the caregiver will project false reports of symptoms on behalf of someone in his or her care such as a child or elder. The end result can be unnecessary medical procedures including surgery. Individuals with a type of factitious disorders use to be diagnosed with **Munchausen's syndrome** (factitious on self) or **Munchausen's syndrome by proxy** (factitious on others) (Ferrara et al., 2014). Munchausen's syndrome was named after Karl Friedrich Hieronymus Von Munchausen, a German cavalry officer who was known for exaggerating his adventures to attract attention. People who exaggerate their symptoms do so not for financial gain but for increased sympathy (American Psychiatric Association, 2013; Ferrara et al., 2014). Munchausen's syndrome by proxy is the exaggerating of an illness, typically upon a child, to gain sympathy for the caregiver (American Psychiatric Association, 2013; Ferrara et al., 2014).

Individuals with factitious disorder could go to extremes to alter medical test results to help support their subjective complaints. Examples of this could include placing blood in their urine sample and physical self-harm. The differential diagnosis for factitious and all related disorders is challenging for health care professionals due to there being little to no evidence of the individual deceiving the doctor into believing that the symptoms are real despite the lack of medical documentation to support claims (Ferrara et al., 2014). Occupational therapy practitioners

as part of an interdisciplinary medical team need to be cognizant of any inconsistencies noted during functional tasks. Early return to functioning and appropriate diagnosis and medical treatment is essential to help minimize the development of such disorders mentioned related to somatic symptoms (Clark, Bair, Buckenmaier, Gironda, & Walker, 2007; Ferrara et al., 2014).

COURSE AND PROGNOSIS

Somatic symptoms and related disorders can occur across the life span in different variations and frequencies. The nature of and pattern of somatic complaints can be part of the normal aging process expected with the course of maturation. Examples of this would include older adults with some health issues having an increased worry over various symptoms than a younger individual or healthier peer. In children, examples of normal progression for somatic complaints are noted with common recurrent abdominal pain, fatigue, or headaches but without any worry of fixation of the somatic complaints (American Psychiatric Association, 2013).

Illness anxiety disorders are noted to have an unclear development and course but are noted to be rarer in children than adults (American Psychiatric Association, 2013; Bener et al., 2013). One explanation for this difference in children versus an adult is the increase in anxiety symptoms as people age, with the most common anxiety fixating on memory loss (American Psychiatric Association, 2013; Bener et al., 2013). Conversion disorders tend to have increased onset of nonepileptic attacks in the 30s, while motor symptom onset peaks in the 40s (American Psychiatric Association, 2013). Factitious disorders are noted to have an onset in early adulthood after a hospitalization, which are often lifelong in nature (American Psychiatric Association, 2013; Ferrara et al., 2014).

Because of the psychological complexity involved, somatic symptoms and related disorders often result in a poor prognosis (Simms, Prisciandaro, Krueger, & Goldberg, 2012). Due to the complexity and severity noted with each disorder, the ability to provide proper medical treatment often is limited. Medical treatment is further complicated by the individual's tendency to not remain constant with one health care provider long enough to receive a proper diagnosis (Crane et al.,

2012; de Waal et al., 2004; Simms et al., 2012). To be successful in treating an individual, the health care provider needs to be knowledgeable and tactful in the approach to diagnosing and treating the disorders (Arnold et al., 2006; de Waal et al., 2004; Simms et al., 2012). If the individual feels the provider does not believe his or her reported symptoms or if the provider accuses the individual of making up the symptoms, the patient-provider rapport will be destroyed, thus yielding a poor prognosis over the long term (Crane et al., 2012; de Waal et al., 2004; McCabe et al., 2009; Neng & Weck, 2013).

Since the prognosis and duration is relatively unknown, the occupational therapy practitioner needs to be able to build a strong rapport with all individuals to allow for proper assessments of impairments of occupational performance. The ability to train an individual in how to adapt to the changes in his or her medical conditions can help redesign daily occupational performance patterns to compensate for any perceived impaired client factors. Through the use of compensatory techniques and a complete occupational profile, occupational therapy practitioner can help to remediate the impact of any perceived impairments. Thus, the outcomes of impaired occupational performance are more likely to improve while helping the individual and the medical team with proper medical management of the condition.

DIAGNOSIS

Individuals with somatic symptom disorder typically have one or more somatic symptoms that are distressing or have a significant impact on daily functioning. Pain is the most common and specific form, but symptoms can range from specific complaints of pain to complaints of general fatigue (de Waal et al., 2004). The nature of the complaint can sometimes represent normal bodily functions and does not have to necessarily indicate severe pathology. Diagnosis is made based on the three criteria in the DSM-5 being met with the intensity from mild to severe corresponding to the number of symptoms reported in the second criterion (see Table 14.3).

Somatic symptoms are assessed based on psychological responses such as the client's emotions, thinking, and behavior of the symptoms. Diagnosing a client's symptom as unexplained is no longer an accepted practice as it was in the past because often symptoms need to be further examined (American Psychiatric Association, 2013; Dimsdale et al., 2013; Katz et al., 2015; Voigt et al., 2013). Client's suffering from somatic symptoms may feel that professionals are not viewing their complaints seriously and will report lower satisfaction levels with their medical care (American Psychiatric Association, 2013). To diagnose somatic symptoms and related disorders, the physicians cannot discredit the seriousness of the root cause as psychological and thus need to concurrently rule out all root physiological causes. Once all physical systems of possible alignment are ruled out, the physician will initiate a psychiatric treatment approach, which would require referral to appropriate services and pharmacological treatment. Table 14.3 details the DSM-5 diagnostic criteria the physician uses to properly diagnose a patient with a type of somatic symptom disorder.

TABLE 14.3 DSM V Diagnostic Criteria

A. One or more distressing symptoms that result in significant daily life disruptions

B. Excessive thoughts, feelings, or behaviors related to the somatic symptoms of associated health concerns as manifested by at least one of the following:

1. Disproportionate and persistent thoughts about the seriousness of one's symptoms
2. Persistently high levels of anxiety about health or symptoms
3. Excessive time and energy focused on these symptoms or health concerns

C. Any one somatic symptom may not be continuously present, but a persistent state of being symptomatic is noted greater than 6 months.

From American Psychiatric Association. (2013). *Diagnostic and Statistical Manual of Mental Disorders* (5th ed.). Washington, DC: Author.

MEDICAL/SURGICAL MANAGEMENT

Medical management for somatic symptom disorder can include treating the somatic symptoms, reducing the health-related anxieties and preoccupations with health concerns, and modifying or substituting the maladaptive illness behaviors. The nature of the subjective complaints may not be clearly associated with a physical cause but more of a learned sick role psychologically manifested. To help determine if pain is related to a form of somatic sensory disorders, the medical providers need to look holistically at the patient to see if the subjective complaints and reports of physical impairments with daily tasks increase with emotional distress and psychological disturbances (Katz et al., 2015). The danger in jumping straight to dismissing the patient's complaints and diagnosing a mental condition can destroy the medical rapport between the provider and the patient. The recognition and early diagnosis of mental health conditions is considered essential in the proper management to help medical providers to not improperly diagnose a patient with a form of somatic symptom disorder (Bener et al., 2013).

The clinical association between somatic symptom disorders and other mental health conditions is high. An example of comorbidities associated with somatic symptom disorders is anxiety, stress, and depression (American Psychiatric Association, 2013; Bener et al., 2013; Katz et al., 2015; Wolfe, Walitt, Katz, & Häuser, 2014). It has been noted that psychological disorders increase with age with the peak age group typically to be males aged 45 to 54 years old (Bener et al., 2013; Douzenis & Seretis, 2013; Katz et al., 2015). The lack of clear methods on how to assess each criterion for somatic symptom disorders often leads the medical providers to rely on their clinical judgment to properly diagnose patients, thus impacting effective medical management by providers (Bener et al., 2013; Katz et al., 2015; Knaster, Karlsson, Estlander, & Kalso, 2012; Kroenke et al., 1998).

Medical diagnosis and management is essential for positive outcomes. **Cognitive-based therapy** (CBT) has been noted as an effective means to treat patients with various forms of somatic symptom disorders (Arnold et al., 2006; Pfingsten, Hildebrandt, Leibing, Franz, & Saur,

1997; Riebel, Egloff, & Witthöft, 2013). CBT is a multimodal approach to treatment, which includes a focus on at least three of the following: relaxation, stress management, goal setting/contracting, self-monitoring, self-talking, assertiveness training, modeling, imagery, pacing, and/or family training as interventions that can be delivered as individual or group sessions (Arnold et al., 2006; Chang & Compton, 2013; Pfingsten et al., 1997; Riebel et al., 2013). CBT as an occupational therapy technique would focus on stress management, activity regulation, emotional awareness, cognitive restructuring, and improving interpersonal communication (Arnold et al., 2006; Chang & Compton, 2013; Pfingsten et al., 1997; Raine et al., 2015; Willmuth & Callahan, 2002). The goals for CBT are to focus on the reduction of physiological arousal through relaxation techniques, promote engagement in pleasurable and meaningful occupations, increase self-awareness of emotions associated with the somatic complaints, modify dysfunctional beliefs, and enhance communication of thoughts and emotions associated with symptoms.

In moderate to severe cases, psychiatric consultation should be included to allow for proper differential diagnosis of other mental health conditions that may be influencing the somatic complaints. Medications used to treat somatic symptom disorder focus on the comorbidities of symptoms such as depression and anxiety with the prescription of tricyclic antidepressants, serotonin reuptake inhibitors, serotonin-noradrenaline reuptake inhibitors, antipsychotics, and general analgesics if warranted. Selective serotonin reuptake inhibitors (SSRIs) and serotonin-noradrenaline reuptake inhibitors (SNRIs) are the first line of treatment for patients with predominant pain symptoms and may also include anticonvulsants such as gabapentin or pregabalin. These medications are used to block or limit serotonin reuptake, thus blocking the stimulation of nerves for pain, depression, and anxiety. Common brand names are noted in Table 14.4.

Occupational therapy in the treatment of somatic symptoms and related disorders is critical and essential to help promote the well-being and engagement with daily occupations. The Practice Framework 3rd Edition (The American Occupational Therapy Association, 2014) views pain as generalized or localized sensations that can be signaling potential or actual damage to

TABLE 14.4	Common Brand Medication Names for Somatic Symptoms and Related Disorders
Generic Name	**Brand Name**
citalopram	Celexa
escitalopram	Lexapro
fluoxetine	Prozac
paroxetine	Paxil
sertraline	Zoloft

bodily structures. The role of occupational therapy as part of an interdisciplinary team to help treat patients with reports of various pain syndromes is vital given our skill set of analyzing the impact of somatic symptoms on client factors and occupational performance.

IMPACT ON OCCUPATIONAL PERFORMANCE

The American Occupational Therapy Association (AOTA) defines occupational performance as the skills observed while clients engage and move within their environment to complete their daily occupations (The American Occupational Therapy Association, 2014). To best understand the impact of somatic symptoms and related disorders on occupational performance, one must have an understanding of the impact of pain syndromes and the perception of pain on client factors, which influence performance. When we think of pain, it is easy to understand the cause and impact on the client if it is associated with an acute injury or surgical procedure, but after the bodily structures heal and the presence of pain still remains, the perplexity related to the chronic pain is unclear.

The occupational therapy practitioner is skillfully trained to analyze the client through a different lens related to how the client must meet the demands of the tasks to properly engage in the task. When looking at the client with reports of chronic pain, the first thing an occupational therapy practitioner must review is the client's medical history to have an understanding of what root etiology there was leading up to the current state. The review of the medical chart helps the practitioner to identify possible chronic conditions that may have permanently altered the basic bodily functions, such as a herniated disc with nerve root

impingement that is leading to structural integrity issues with the functions of the joints, bones, and nerves of spine. In this situation, even with surgery, the length of nerve root impingement, severity of the injury, and the surgical versus nonsurgical medical treatment will start to paint a clearer picture of what functional limitations a client may have when attempting to engage in his or her daily occupations.

Regardless of surgical intervention or not, a person with reports of chronic pain due to a herniated disc could present with decreased joint alignment, altered sensations, and muscular impairment (strength, tone, reflexes, mass, etc.) along the impinged nerve root distribution. Due to pain and changes with soft tissue integrity from the injury, the client may learn various maladaptive methods to engage in daily occupations to the fullest potential. Using a full functional assessment of the client, the occupational therapy practitioner is able to analyze how the clients move and participate in their daily occupational demands. Through early identification of maladaptive posturing and body mechanics, the practitioner is able to help the client reduce the impairments through remedial and compensatory techniques. It is imperative to assess the client's perception of his or her physical impairments related to occupational performance.

The traditional medical model uses medications and surgical interventions to try to correct soft tissue abnormalities and may overlook the mental component of pain. Some models use health psychologists as part of the interdisciplinary team to address this component. Occupational therapy uses a holistic approach through a functional lens to assess and treat the client. The client's perception of perceived disability related to pain has an impact on the overall occupational performance. The modification and correction of abnormal postures during the engagement in occupations can reduce the strain on compromised joint integrity and soft tissue, thus breaking the negative cycle for pain. When thinking of pain and the impact on occupational performance, the occupational therapy practitioner needs to understand and articulate the impact of the perception of pain, physical impairments, and mental integrity in relation to occupational performance.

A visualization of the client factors that can impact occupational performance is represented by the symbol for the Olympics (see Fig. 14.1). Each ring represents a different factor that can increase a client's pain including stress, anxiety, depression, poor sleep, poor body mechanics/posture, and muscle tension/weakness related to the client's impairments. As one component in the client's life starts to spin more out of control, such as stress or poor body mechanics, it causes the rest of the components to spin faster, thus leading to an increased perception of pain and disability.

The components and their connectedness to one another when associated with occupational performance can help the medical team provide the best treatment strategies to help the client achieve his or her optimal occupational performance. Occupational therapy plays a vital role in identifying the impacted client factors and performance patterns that are leading to an altered perception by the client related to occupational performance. Explaining to the client how to safely engage to his or her fullest limits related to impaired joint and muscular systems can help

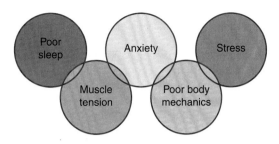

Figure 14.1 Factors that increase a client's pain.

decrease the stress and anxiety often expressed and noted through self-limiting behaviors due to a fear of increased pain while engaging in daily occupations. The ability for the client to learn how to control one factor in the Olympic ring example can help to eventually slow the negative impact of the other rings that are impacted.

Through the use of meaningful and purposeful occupations, a client can become lost in the task and work within his or her limits to safely complete daily occupations that were perceived to be unmanageable. Opportunities for this can be promoted though the occupational therapy session in various settings to include work hardening/return-to-work programs, outpatient clinics, subacute clinics, and pediatric settings. To understand the role of occupational therapy in various settings, we will examine 2 clients and how their perception of pain and disability related to somatic symptoms and related disorders may present in a pediatric and an adult case.

CASE STUDY

Ben is a 10-year-old boy who was in an accident and sustained a fracture with mild medial and ulnar nerve involvement to his dominant right radius and ulna while playing on the school playground. He was casted for 4 to 6 weeks after being set with internal fixation to protect the nerves and soft tissue. Ben has poor pain tolerance and favored his right upper extremity by not using it while casted leading to increased joint stiffness and atrophy in the right hand. He was referred to occupational therapy after the school teacher noted that he could not use a utensil for

school tasks after the cast was removed and he was asking for help to don his coat.

The occupational therapist reviewed the medical history provided by the orthopedist and observed Ben in the classroom. He has no restriction, and the orthopedist has encouraged him and his family to actively use his right hand. His parents, however, sympathized with his reports of pain, thus promoting him to not use his arm to complete his work for school if his arm hurt. Ben was observed to not cross or transfer any objects past midline to use his right upper extremity. He was noted to hold his right upper extremity in severe shoulder protraction with elevation leading to tightness in the upper trapezius and pectoralis major and minor, which also lead to shoulder impingement from the abnormal posturing. The changes in his body mechanics due to an abnormal posturing of his dominant upper extremity lead to increased anterior shoulder pain and tenderness over the anterior bursae.

As a result, Ben was noted to have decreased active and passive range of motion (ROM), impaired strength across the right upper extremity equal to 50% loss of full active ROM. Due to the ongoing pain and the perception that if he used his right upper extremity he would hurt himself again,

Ben is at risk for developing complex regional pain syndrome. Ben also reported that he liked to have others write and type papers for him and to not have to do any house chores. When asked to play with a building block set using his right hand, he started to cry as he expressed an increase in pain in his hand. Ben's family reported that he used to love to play with his 1-year-old puppy but now could not hold him due to his injury. The occupational therapist noted in the evaluation that when Ben was engaged and completely distracted during functional testing, he had full passive ROM and 75% of full active ROM in all the joints of the right upper extremity.

CASE STUDY 2

Sara is a 36-year-old female veteran who presented to her primary care physician with complaints and signs of increased muscle twitching and decrease motor coordination in all four extremities. Sara, who just retired from the military, denies any injury or trauma while in the service to have led to the cause of these problems. Preliminary testing does not support a general organic cause due to pathology. Sarah is referred to neurology for further testing for which the doctor states clinically the symptoms present like the early onset of amyotrophic lateral sclerosis (ALS), but medical testing and electromyography (EMG) studies do not support the diagnosis. Throughout testing, Sara starts to display an increase in symptoms for which the neurologist noted and starts to ask her about her feelings about all of the testing and results. Sara reports that the added medical appointments for testing have increased her stress and anxiety over having ALS. The neurologist refers Sara to a psychologist to help her with the added stress and to rule out the possibility of symptoms stemming from a psychological component.

Sara is angered by the referral but still attends the appointment for the psychologist. Testing now notes a positive screen for depression and anxiety along with Sara reporting that she was a victim of an assault upon leaving the service. The

stress, anxiety, and fear of being a victim have left her unable to work, properly care for personal hygiene, or take care of her home. The psychologist has a close working relationship with the therapy department and refers Sara to occupational therapy for assistance with reengagement into daily functional tasks. The occupational therapist upon evaluation notes generalized poor personal hygiene, impaired accommodation to various settings, a hyperactive startle reflex, 5/5 strength and full active ROM in all extremities, slowed mental processing, and reduced self-awareness. The medical record was reviewed, and the therapist notes through the medical chart and semistructured interview that the symptoms increased with stress and appeared to have manifested after the trauma of an assault. Sara is working with the psychologist on the psychological impact of the assault, but the physical manifestations have precluded her from being able to perform self-care. Due to the muscle twitching impacting her gross and fine motor coordination, she is a fall risk during bathing and dressing. Her impaired gross and fine motor coordination also leads to frequent dropping of items and precludes the use of utensils for self-feeding. Sara would love to be able to bathe and dress again within a reasonable amount of time.

LEARNING RESOURCES

Somatic Symptom Disorders YouTube Video
https://www.youtube.com/watch?v=h5eHWYJTlsE

Somatic Symptom Disorders Summary and Screening Tool
http://www.aafp.org/afp/2007/1101/p1333.html

Treatment of Functional Impairment in Severe Somatoform Pain Disorder Article
http://jpepsy.oxfordjournals.org/content/26/7/429.full

Conversion Disorder
https://www.nlm.nih.gov/medlineplus/ency/article/000954.htm

Conversion Disorder CBS This Morning YouTube Clip
https://www.youtube.com/watch?v=gbQK8ucIcAw

Danielle's Journey with Conversion Disorder YouTube
https://www.youtube.com/watch?v=6xhypWbI0bk

REFERENCES

American Psychiatric Association. (2013). *Diagnostic and Statistical Manual of Mental Disorders* (5th Ed.). Washington, DC: Author

Arnold, I. A., de Waal, M. W. M., Eekhof, J. A. H., & van Hemert, A. M. (2006). Somatoform disorder in primary care: Course and the need for cognitive-behavioral treatment. *Psychosomatics*, *47*(6), 498–503. Retrieved from http://doi.org/10.1176/appi.psy.47.6.498

Bener, A., Al-Kazaz, M., Ftouni, D., Al-Harthy, M., & Dafeeah, E. E. (2013). Diagnostic overlap of depressive, anxiety, stress and somatoform disorders in primary care. *Asia-Pacific Psychiatry : Official Journal of the Pacific Rim College of Psychiatrists*, *5*(1), E29–E38. Retrieved from http://doi.org/10.1111/j.1758-5872.2012.00215.x

Chang, Y.-P., & Compton, P. (2013). Management of chronic pain with chronic opioid therapy in patients with substance use disorders. *Addiction Science & Clinical Practice*, *8*(1), 21. Retrieved from http://doi.org/10.1186/1940-0640-8-21

Clark, M. E., Bair, M. J., Buckenmaier, C. C., Gironda, R. J., & Walker, R. L. (2007). Pain and combat injuries in soldiers returning from Operations Enduring Freedom and Iraqi Freedom: implications for research and practice. *Journal of Rehabilitation Research and Development*, *44*(2), 179–194. Retrieved from http://doi.org/10.1682/JRRD.2006.05.0057

Crane, D. R., Morton, L. B., Fawcett, D., Moore, A., Larson, J., & Sandberg, J. (2012). Somatoform disorder: Treatment utilization and cost by mental health professions. *Contemporary Family Therapy*, *34*(3), 322–333. Retrieved from http://doi.org/10.1007/s10591-012-9182-x

De Waal, M. W. M., Arnold, I. A., Eekhof, J. A. H., & van Hemert, A. M. (2004). Somatoform disorders in general practice: Prevalence, functional impairment and comorbidity with anxiety and depressive disorders. *The British Journal of Psychiatry: The Journal of Mental Science*, *184*, 470–476. Retrieved from http://doi.org/10.1192/bjp.184.6.470

Dimsdale, J. E., Creed, F., Escobar, J., Sharpe, M., Wulsin, L., Barsky, A., … Levenson, J. (2013). Somatic symptom disorder: An important change in DSM. *Journal of Psychosomatic Research*, *75*(3), 223–228. Retrieved from http://doi.org/10.1016/j.jpsychores.2013.06.033

Douzenis, A., & Seretis, D. (2013). Descriptive and predictive validity of somatic attributions in patients with somatoform disorders: A systematic review of quantitative research. *Journal of Psychosomatic Research*, *75*(3), 199–210. Retrieved from http://doi.org/10.1016/j.jpsychores.2013.05.005

Ferrara, P., Vitelli, O., Romani, J., Bottaro, G., Ianniello, F., Fabrizio, G., … Gatto, A. (2014). The thin line between Munchausen syndrome and Munchausen syndrome by proxy. *Journal of Psychological Abnormalities in Children*, *3*(2), 2–3. Retrieved from http://doi.org/10.4172/2329-9525.1000115

Katz, J., Rosenbloom, B. N., & Fashler, S. (2015). Chronic pain, psychopathology, and DSM-5 somatic symptom disorder. *Canadian Journal of Psychiatry*, *60*(4), 160–167.

Knaster, P., Karlsson, H., Estlander, A. M., & Kalso, E. (2012). Psychiatric disorders as assessed with SCID in chronic pain patients: The anxiety disorders precede the onset of pain. *General Hospital Psychiatry*, *34*(1), 46–52. Retrieved from http://doi.org/10.1016/j.genhosppsych.2011.09.004

Kroenke, K., Spitzer, R. L., deGruy, F. V., & Swindle, R. (1998). A symptom checklist to screen for somatoform disorders in primary care. *Psychosomatics*, *39*(3), 263–272. Retrieved from http://doi.org/10.1016/S0033-3182(98)71343-X

McCabe, C., Cohen, H., Hall, J., Lewis, J., Rodham, K., & Harris, N. (2009). Somatosensory conflicts in Complex Regional Pain Syndrome Type 1 and Fibromyalgia Syndrome. *Rheumatic Manifestations of Other Diseases, 11*, 461–465. Retrieved from http://doi.org/10.1007/s11926-009-0067-4

Neng, J. M. B., & Weck, F. (2013). Attribution of somatic symptoms in hypochondriasis. *Clinical Psychology and Psychotherapy, 124*, 116–124. Retrieved from: http://doi.org/10.1002/cpp.1871

Pfingsten, M., Hildebrandt, J., Leibing, E., Franz, C., & Saur, P. (1997). Effectiveness of a multimodal treatment program for chronic low-back pain. *Pain, 73*(1), 77–85. Retrieved from http://doi.org/S0304395997000833 [pii]

Raine, R., Raine, R., Haines, A., Haines, A., Sensky, T., Sensky, T., … Black, N. (2015). Systematic review of mental health interventions for patients with common somatic symptoms: can research evidence from secondary care be extrapolated to primary care? *British Medical Journal, 325*(7372), 1082.

Riebel, K., Egloff, B., & Witthöft, M. (2013). Modifying the implicit illness-related self-concept in patients with somatoform disorders may reduce somatic symptoms. *International Journal of Behavioral Medicine, 21*, 861–868. Retrieved from http://doi.org/10.1007/s12529-013-9362-6

Simms, L. J., Prisciandaro, J. J., Krueger, R. F., & Goldberg, D. P. (2012). The structure of depression, anxiety and somatic symptoms in primary care. *Psychological Medicine, 29*(6), 997–1003. Retrieved from http://doi.org/10.1016/j.biotechadv.2011.08.021.Secreted

The American Occupational Therapy Association. (2014). Occupational therapy practice framework: Domain & process (3rd ed.). *American Journal of Occupational Therapy, 68*(Suppl. 1), S1–S48. Retrieved from http://doi.org/doi:10.5014/ajot.2014.682006

Voigt, K., Wollburg, E., Weinmann, N., Herzog, A., Meyer, B., Langs, G., & Löwe, B. (2012). Predictive validity and clinical utility of DSM-5 somatic symptom disorder—Comparison with DSM-IV somatoform disorders and additional criteria for consideration. *Journal of Psychosomatic Research, 73*(5), 345–350. Retrieved from http://doi.org/10.1016/j.jpsychores.2012.08.020

Voigt, K., Wollburg, E., Weinmann, N., Herzog, A., Meyer, B., Langs, G., & Löwe, B. (2013). Predictive validity and clinical utility of DSM-5 somatic symptom disorder: Prospective 1-year follow-up study. *Journal of Psychosomatic Research, 75*(4), 358–361. Retrieved from http://doi.org/10.1016/j.jpsychores.2013.08.017

Willmuth, M. E., & Callahan, C. D. (2002). Cognitive rehabilitation. *Journal of Head Trauma Rehabilitation, 17*(6), 575–577. Retrieved from http://doi.org/10.1097/00001199-200212000-00009

Wolfe, F., Walitt, B. T., Katz, R. S., & Häuser, W. (2014). Symptoms, the nature of fibromyalgia, and diagnostic and statistical manual 5 (DSM-5) defined mental illness in patients with rheumatoid arthritis and fibromyalgia. *PLoS ONE, 9*(2). Retrieved from http://doi.org/10.1371/journal.pone.0088740

15 Feeding and Eating Disorders

KEY TERMS

Anorexia nervosa
Avoidant/restrictive
 food intake disorder
Bulimia nervosa
Cognitive-behavioral
 therapy
Eating disorder
Family-based therapy
Feeding disorder
Pica
Rumination

Amy Wagenfeld and Linda M. Olson

Lucy was admitted to 4C, the inpatient psychiatric unit at her regional hospital. At admission, Lucy is 5'6" tall and weighs 90 lb. This is Lucy's second day in the unit, and her occupational therapist (OT) has just arrived for her initial interview. Lucy is frantic. She does not want to be on the unit; she wants to go for a long run. She is not allowed beyond the end of the hallway, which she has estimated to be 50 yards long. If she briskly walks back and forth for 2 hours, she might actually burn off some calories. But so far, whenever she starts to walk, a nurse gently guides her back to her room. Good thing the OT has arrived; maybe he will help her figure out ways to get exercise, because that is what matters right now.

With intense societal pressure to be thin and social media perpetuating this trend, so-called celebrity "role models" often succumb to the pressure and place excessive personal value on thinness and weight control. The domino effect is that achieving extreme thinness can become a goal for those who idolize celebrity role models. Negatively comparing oneself with the societal "ideal" can lead to a distorted self-image (Treasure, Claudino, & Zucker, 2010) and, for too many, eating disorders. This chapter discusses six **feeding and eating disorders**: how they are diagnosed and classified and their prevalence and clinical presentations. Evidence-based research on the causality and intervention of feeding and eating disorders will be explored. The impact of feeding and eating disorders on occupational performance will be discussed throughout the chapter as well as in the case studies at the conclusion of the chapter.

DESCRIPTION AND DEFINITION

Activities that contribute to health and occupational performance include eating a balanced diet, engaging in meaningful leisure pursuits, exercising in moderation, and participating in fulfilling social relationships. Food restricting or purging behaviors "prevent clients from engaging in activities that contribute to health" (Costa, 2009, p. 13). Many people experience internal conflict with regard to eating at some point in their lives, but not to the point at which it threatens good health and occupational performance. According to the *DSM-5* (American Psychiatric Association [APA], 2013), feeding and eating disorders include **anorexia nervosa**, **bulimia nervosa**, **binge eating**, **pica**, **rumination**, and **avoidant/restrictive food intake disorder**. Eating disorders (particularly anorexia nervosa, bulimia nervosa, and binge eating disorder) are among the most common health concerns in young people, particularly female adolescents and young women (Treasure et al., 2010), but to a lesser extent, men are also impacted (Grave, 2011). Most adults seeking treatment for eating disorders are in their 20s or 30s, having dealt with their issues for on average 8 years (Murphy, Straebler, Basden, Cooper, & Fairburn, 2012). Eating disorders are understood to arise from a combination of behavioral, biological, emotional, psychological, interpersonal, and social factors (Costa, 2009). While each of the feeding and eating disorders has different clinical presentations, these six disorders feature severe disturbances in eating behavior that clinically impede an individual's life. Life-threatening effects of eating disorders can be electrolyte imbalance, cardiac arrhythmias, and intercurrent infarction (Treasure et al., 2010). Anxiety, low self-esteem, obsessional thoughts and actions, feelings of low self-worth, and perfectionism are classic characteristics associated with eating disorders. Hypotension and bradycardia, constipation, GI issues, and long-term estrogen deficiency are common side effects of anorexia nervosa (Grave, 2011). Other serious long-term effects of anorexia nervosa and bulimia nervosa include reproductive issues, osteopenia and osteoporosis, impaired brain growth, and dental health.

On a more systemic level, eating disorders can threaten to take over the entire family system; the family becomes consumed by it and has limited community engagement. Mealtimes become war zones. For children and adolescents with eating disorders, constant prompting to eat can lead to created dependency (Clark & Nayar, 2012).

■ Anorexia Nervosa

Anorexia nervosa is described as the oldest recorded eating disorder, with accounts of it dating back to the 19th century. Anorexia nervosa presents as a profound refusal to maintain a normal body weight at 85% of expected weight, excessive concern with and distorted body image, and failure to recognize that there is a problem (Quiles-Cestari & Pessa Ribeiro, 2012; Trudeau, 2016, in press). It is a relentless pursuit of thinness through diet and exercise with an accompanying intense and unremitting fear of gaining weight or becoming fat, despite being extremely thin (Treasure et al., 2010; Walsh, 2011). Food is always on the minds of those with anorexia nervosa. For example, a person might obsess about the number of calories, the fat content, or how many minutes of exercise it will take to burn off a desperately desired cookie.

■ Bulimia Nervosa

Bulimia nervosa features episodic and recurring binge eating and purging of food to avoid weight gain. Behaviors such as self-induced vomiting, misuse of laxatives, diuretics, enemas, or other medications to avoid weight gain are hallmarks of bulimia nervosa (Treasure et al., 2010; Trudeau, in press; Walsh, 2011). Fasting or excessive exercise to compensate for high caloric intake is common in individuals with bulimia nervosa as well as anorexia nervosa. Like anorexia nervosa, a distorted perception of body image (shape and weight) is common for individuals with bulimia nervosa.

■ Binge Eating Disorder

Binge eating disorder was first described in the medical literature in 1952 (Walsh, 2011). Binge eating disorder is a condition in which there are both recurrent episodes of excessive eating within a discrete period of time and a perceived sense of lack of control over the eating. Most individuals with binge eating disorder tend to be "overweight, obese, and middle-aged" (Walsh, 2011, p. 526). The difference between binge eating disorder and bulimia nervosa is that individuals with binge eating disorder do not engage in compensatory behaviors like purging or misuse of laxative and diet pills. A transition from restrictive eating to binge eating is common, but going from binge eating to severely restricted eating is less so (Treasure et al., 2010).

■ Pica

Pica is a dangerous form of self-injurious behavior. It is described as a perverted appetite for nonnutritive, nonfood substances such as clay, soil, laundry starch, hair, chalk, crayons, and ashes (Aparna, Austin, & Mattews, 2012; Tabers, 2013). The word pica is derived from the Latin for magpie, a species of bird that eats whatever it finds (Aparna et al., 2012). Pica can lead to death or life-threatening consequences due to choking or intestinal obstruction and may require surgery to remove inedible objects (Williams & McAdam, 2012). It can also lead to poisoning, burns, and parasitic infections and cause significant harm to dental and digestive structures.

■ Rumination

Rumination is the nonpurposeful regurgitation of recently ingested food from the stomach to the mouth, where it is either rechewed, reswallowed, or expelled (Eckern, Stevens, & Mitchell, 1999; Mousa, Montgomery, & Alioto, 2014). It has been recognized in the medical literature for over 100 years (Eckern et al., 1999). Regurgitation typically happens during or immediately following a feeding. The sensation associated with the regurgitation is felt as pressure, the need to belch, nausea, pain, or discomfort (Mousa et al., 2014). Individuals with rumination typically describe the process as being effortless with no gagging or retching (Mousa et al., 2014). Those with rumination understand that the food is undigested yet report that it tastes normal. Lacking social conventionality, rumination is often a very secretive behavior (Eckern et al., 1999). It is not life threatening but can have medical and psychological ramifications for the individual and family.

■ Avoidant/Restrictive Food Intake Disorder

Avoidant/restrictive food intake disorder is a new diagnostic category in the *DSM-5* (APA, 2013). It replaces and extends the category of Feeding Disorder of Infancy or Early Childhood in the *DSM-IV*. The reason for the change was to expand the category to make the disorder applicable across the life span and to make the diagnostic criteria more explicit (APA, 2013). While typically seen in children and adolescents, avoidant/restrictive food intake disorder can also be diagnosed in adults (Bryant-Waugh & Kreipe, 2012). Avoidant/restrictive food intake disorder may present in a variety of ways; some individuals eat only a very narrow range of foods, while others restrict food intake in response to emotional crises, unpleasant experiences, or untoward feelings (Bryant-Waugh & Kreipe, 2012). Food avoidance is not driven by cognitive misperceptions about weight or body shape, nor is it the result of lack of availability of food or a culturally sanctioned practice (Bryant-Waugh & Kreipe, 2012; Katzman, Stevens, & Norris, 2014). Those with avoidant/restrictive food intake disorder are more likely to have a coexisting medical condition such as autism spectrum disorder, attention deficit hyperactivity disorder, anxiety disorder, and obsessive-compulsive disorder than individuals with anorexia nervosa or bulimia nervosa (Bryant-Waugh & Kreipe, 2012; Fisher et al., 2014). It has been suggested that there are five types of food refusal. They include

- Learning dependent food refusal
- Medical complications–related food refusal
- Selective food refusal
- Fear-based food refusal
- Appetite awareness and autonomy-based food refusal (Dovey and colleagues as cited in Kreipe & Palomaki, 2012)

An individual with avoidant/restrictive food intake disorder is dependent on enteral feeding and/or oral nutritional supplements and may demonstrate notable interference with psychosocial function (Bryant-Waugh & Kreipe, 2012; Norris & Stevens, 2014).

ETIOLOGY

The heritable characteristics of eating disorders are strong. Twin and family studies show the incidence rates to be between 50% and 83% (Treasure et al., 2010). Research also indicates that eating disorders represent a complex interaction of physiological, genetic, psychological, social-emotional, and cognitive factors. There is a strong link between coexisting mental health conditions such as depression and anxiety, borderline personality disorder, affective disorder, substance abuse (the latter two more closely associated with bulimia nervosa) (Treasure et al., 2010), and eating disorders. Further, there is a relationship between general adversity (abuse, neglect) and increased risk of developing an eating disorder (Treasure et al., 2010). Parallels are also noted between eating disorders and addictions; both have associated tendencies such as compulsive behaviors, diminished self-control, and engagement in repetitive behaviors despite knowing the negative consequences (Costa, 2009).

For some individuals with bulimia nervosa and binge eating disorder, overeating may be considered a form of self-regulation (Gardiner & Brown, 2010). An explanation for this behavior is that when people are under stress, eating helps to balance the body's biochemistry; serotonin levels increase and cortisol decreases (Gardiner & Brown, 2010). From a sensory regulation perspective, people who are hyporesponsive to sensory input (tactile and proprioceptive) may be drawn to consuming large amounts of highly textured and flavored foods (or nonnutritive substances) in an effort to modulate (Gardiner & Brown, 2010). This potential causation of eating disorders could apply to individuals with bulimia nervosa, binge eating disorder, and pica. Although there are similarities, there are also etiological characteristics specific to each eating disorder. A description of etiology specific to each eating and feeding disorder follows.

The cause of anorexia nervosa is multifactorial and includes genetics, sociocultural, familial, and individual factors and/or experiencing an adverse event, personality, and psychological vulnerability (Quiles-Cestari & Pessa Ribeiro, 2012). Like anorexia nervosa, the cause of bulimia nervosa is most likely multifactorial and includes sociocultural, familial, and individual characteristics as well as psychological factors (Frank, 2015).

One suggested cause of binge eating disorder may be a genetic mutation of the melanocortin 4 receptor gene, which makes a protein that stimulates hunger (Branson et al., 2003). A mutation in this gene may lead to reduced protein production so that the body (inaccurately) feels excessive hunger (Branson et al., 2003). Like anorexia nervosa and bulimia nervosa, binge eating disorder may also have psychological roots, for example, negative emotions, loneliness, and anger (Zeek, Stelzer, Linster, Joos, & Hartmann, 2011).

The practice of pica has been reported as far back as 1800 BCE in regions of the Far and Middle East (n.a., 2011). Since the time of Hippocrates, it has been proposed that pica is a symptom of anemia, but it has never been proven (Aparna et al., 2012). The question remains as to whether iron deficiency is a cause or effect of pica (Aparna et al., 2012). No further etiology for pica has been reported in the medical or psychological literature.

The cause of rumination is not understood. Rumination is commonly believed to be behavioral, that is, a learned disorder that allows for voluntary relaxation of the diaphragm that leads to belching and regurgitation of food (Talley, 2011).

Although not for certain, avoidant/restrictive food intake disorder may be caused by mechanical oral motor factors such as low tone or coordination, tactile defensiveness, previous history of choking, and/or a conditioned response to gastrointestinal issues that preclude food intake (Kreipe & Palomaki, 2012). These issues combined with an individual's medical history and, for children, caregiver response to these issues and subsequent learned behaviors may exacerbate avoidant/restrictive food intake disorder (Kreipe & Palomaki, 2012).

INCIDENCE AND PREVALENCE

It is estimated that up to 24 million people of all ages and genders have anorexia, bulimia, or binge eating disorder in the United States with the highest incidence rate of anorexia nervosa and bulimia nervosa occurring between the age of 10 and 19 years (Renfrew Center Foundation for Eating Disorders, 2003). With only 35% of people with anorexia, bulimia, or binge eating disorder receiving specialized treatment (Noordenbox, 2002), the incidence rate for these three eating disorders cannot be considered absolute. More specific information on incidence and prevalence by diagnosis follows.

■ Anorexia Nervosa

Anorexia nervosa was previously thought to impact only young Caucasian women with upper socioeconomic status. It actually affects both men and women of all ages, races, and ethnicities across the world (Costa, 2009), but mostly younger Caucasian women. The prevalence rate is reported at a range between 0.3% and

1% (Hoek, 2007; Renfrew Center Foundation for Eating Disorders, 2003). Comorbidity is the rule rather than the exception, with anxiety and depression the most common. It has been estimated that one-fifth of people with attention deficit hyperactivity disorder (ADHD) and autism spectrum disorder have anorexia nervosa (Treasure et al., 2010).

■ Bulimia Nervosa

A 12-month prevalence of bulimia nervosa among young females is reported at 1% to 1.5% (APA, 2013; Hay & Claudino, 2010; Hoek, 2007). Prevalence is highest among young adults since it peaks in older adolescence and early adulthood. There is approximately a "10:1 ratio of females versus males" (APA, 2013, p. 347). Like anorexia nervosa, comorbid psychological conditions such as anxiety and depression may also be present in individuals with bulimia nervosa.

■ Binge Eating Disorder

The 12-month prevalence of binge eating disorder in the United States adult population is 1.6% female and 0.8% male. It is more prevalent among individuals seeking weight loss treatment than in the general population and is equally as prevalent among white females as ethnic minorities (APA, 2013, p. 351).

■ Pica

Pica has been observed in people across all cultures and age groups (Aparna et al., 2012). In the United States, it appears to be more common among individuals living in the Southeast. Considered by some to be a learned behavior, it is more frequently noted in individuals with autism spectrum disorder, Prader-Willi syndrome, and psychological conditions such as stress and anxiety (APA, 2013; n.a., 2011). It is difficult to determine the prevalence rate because people are reluctant to admit to engaging in pica and the definitions of pica vary (Blinder, 2008) because of varied cultural practices.

■ Rumination

Originally, it was thought that rumination occurred only in intellectually impaired children or adults, but recent research suggests that healthy individuals with no cognitive challenges can also be diagnosed with rumination syndrome (Mousa et al., 2014). To that end, there have been no systematic incidence studies on rumination in humans (Talley, 2011).

■ Avoidant/Restrictive Food Intake Disorder

There has been limited study of the prevalence of avoidant/resistant food intake disorder (Nicely, Lane-Loney, Masciulli, Hollenbeak, & Ornstein, 2014). Studies have noted rates range from 1.4% to 5% for youth and adolescents treated at eating disorder facilities (Fisher et al., 2014; Norris et al., 2013; Ornstein et al., 2013). Being a new category in the *DSM-5* (APA, 2013), future prevalence study has been recommended.

SIGNS AND SYMPTOMS

There are a number of signs and symptoms common among the six eating and feeding disorders. They are presented below in Table 15.1.

COURSE AND PROGNOSIS

Although eating disorders have the highest mortality rate of any mental disorder, like diagnostic rates, the mortality rate of eating disorders varies depending on studies and reports (Crow et al., 2009). Part of the reason why there is a large variance in the reported number of deaths caused by eating disorders is that those with an eating disorder may ultimately die of heart failure, organ failure, malnutrition, or suicide. Often, the medical complications of death are reported instead of the eating disorder that compromised a person's health.

The complex nature and frequency of relapse of anorexia nervosa make its prognosis the bleakest among eating and feeding disorders (Miller & Golden, 2010). Over 20% of individuals with anorexia nervosa continue to present with the condition at long-term follow-up. Vomiting and purgative abuse have been shown to lead to the worst prognosis, while excessive exercise and dieting does not necessarily portend poor prognosis (Steinhausen, 2008). It has been found that the outcome for adolescent onset is more positive than for adult onset (Steinhausen, Boyadjieva, Griogoroiu-Serbanescu, & Neumarker, 2003). For younger individuals, a positive parent-child relationship has protective qualities to diminish poor outcomes for both anorexia nervosa and bulimia nervosa

TABLE **15.1**	Signs and Symptoms Associated with Feeding and Eating Disorders	
Characteristics	**Symptoms**	**Specific Feeding and Eating Disorders**
Behaviors		
Restrictive behaviors		
	Cutting back on food consumption	Anorexia nervosa, bulimia nervosa, avoidant/resistant food intake disorder
	Strict rules about eating (when, where, caloric intake)	Anorexia nervosa, bulimia nervosa, avoidant/resistant food intake disorder
	Long-term fasting (>8 hours)	Anorexia nervosa, bulimia nervosa
	Ritualized behaviors (shopping, preparation, consumption, cutting food into tiny pieces, ingesting hot food, ritualized order of eating)	Anorexia nervosa, bulimia nervosa, avoidant/resistant food intake disorder
	Little variety in foods	Anorexia nervosa, bulimia nervosa, avoidant/resistant food intake disorder
	Avoiding social eating	Anorexia nervosa, bulimia nervosa, binge eating disorder, pica, rumination, avoidant/resistant food intake disorder
	Social competitiveness (who can eat less)	Anorexia nervosa, bulimia nervosa
	Self-mutilation	Anorexia nervosa, bulimia nervosa, pica, avoidant/resistant food intake disorder
Binge eating		
	Eating excessive amount of food in discrete amount of time based on situation (objective)	Bulimia nervosa, binge eating disorder
	Food intake not excessive in light of context but determined to be large by individual (subjective)	Anorexia nervosa, bulimia nervosa
	Eating quickly	Bulimia nervosa, binge eating disorder
	Eating until uncomfortably full	Bulimia nervosa, binge eating disorder
	Eating in isolation because of feeling embarrassed	Anorexia nervosa, bulimia nervosa, binge eating disorder, pica, rumination
	Eating large amounts when not hungry	Binge eating disorder
	Shame and self-disgust from eating	Anorexia nervosa, bulimia nervosa, binge eating disorder
Fixations		
	Obsessive fascination with recipes and reading cookbooks	Anorexia nervosa, bulimia nervosa
	Increased use of spices, salt, and gum chewing	Anorexia nervosa, bulimia nervosa
	Intensive, unrelenting, compulsive	Anorexia nervosa, bulimia nervosa, binge eating disorder, pica, rumination, avoidant/resistant food intake disorder

TABLE 15.1 *Continued*

Characteristics	Symptoms	Specific Feeding and Eating Disorders
Purgative behavior		
	Misuse of diet pills, diuretics, laxatives	Anorexia nervosa, bulimia nervosa
	Excessive exercise	Anorexia nervosa, bulimia nervosa
	Self-induced vomiting or spitting	Bulimia nervosa, rumination
Fluid intake		
	Limited (<1 quart per day)	Anorexia nervosa
	Excessive (>1.5 quarts per day)	Bulimia nervosa
	Increased tea and coffee consumption	Anorexia nervosa
Body checking		
	Repeated weighing	Anorexia nervosa, bulimia nervosa, binge eating disorder
	Pinching or measuring body parts	Anorexia nervosa, bulimia nervosa
	Repeated checking of protrusion of body bones (i.e., hips)	Anorexia nervosa, bulimia nervosa
	Obsessive checking that clothes fit	Anorexia nervosa, bulimia nervosa
	Mirror gazing	Anorexia nervosa, bulimia nervosa
	Comparing self with others	Anorexia nervosa, bulimia nervosa, binge eating disorder
Body avoidance		
	Refusing to weigh self	Bulimia nervosa, binge eating disorder
	Refusing to look at self in mirror	Anorexia nervosa, bulimia nervosa, binge eating disorder
	Wearing bulky clothes	Anorexia nervosa
	Self-mutilation	Anorexia nervosa, bulimia nervosa, pica
	Refusing to touch self	Anorexia nervosa
Psychopathology		
	Anxiety	Anorexia nervosa, bulimia nervosa, binge eating disorder, rumination, avoidant/resistant food intake disorder
	Depression	Anorexia nervosa, bulimia nervosa, binge eating disorder, rumination
	Body image disturbance	Anorexia nervosa, bulimia nervosa
	Preoccupation with body weight and shape	Anorexia nervosa, bulimia nervosa
	Overevaluation of shape and weight to determine self-worth	Anorexia nervosa, bulimia nervosa
	Minimizing or denying symptom severity	Anorexia nervosa, bulimia nervosa

(Continued)

TABLE 15.1 *Continued*

Characteristics	Symptoms	Specific Feeding and Eating Disorders
	Disturbance in way body is experienced	Anorexia nervosa, bulimia nervosa
	Intense fear of weight gain, despite being significantly underweight	Anorexia nervosa, bulimia nervosa
	Impaired concentration	Anorexia nervosa, bulimia nervosa
	Emotionally labile	Anorexia nervosa, bulimia nervosa
	Irritation	Anorexia nervosa, bulimia nervosa, avoidant/resistant food intake disorder
	Apathy	Anorexia nervosa, bulimia nervosa
	Personality changes	Anorexia nervosa, bulimia nervosa
	Poor insight and judgment	Anorexia nervosa, bulimia nervosa, binge eating disorder
	Social withdrawal	Anorexia nervosa, bulimia nervosa, binge eating disorder, pica, rumination, avoidant/resistant food intake disorder
	Decreased libido	Anorexia nervosa, bulimia nervosa
Physical	Weight loss or failure of growth, e.g., disruption of menses	Anorexia nervosa, bulimia nervosa, rumination, avoidant/resistant food intake disorder
	Reductions in waking erections (men)	Anorexia nervosa, bulimia nervosa
	Reduced libido	Anorexia nervosa, bulimia nervosa
	Hair loss	Anorexia nervosa, bulimia nervosa
	Nail biting	Anorexia nervosa, bulimia nervosa, pica
	Sensitivity to cold	Anorexia nervosa, bulimia nervosa
	Weakness and fatigue	Anorexia nervosa, bulimia nervosa, pica, avoidant/resistant food intake disorder
	Low blood pressure	Anorexia nervosa, bulimia nervosa
	Bradycardia	Anorexia nervosa, bulimia nervosa
	Diminished bone density	Anorexia nervosa, bulimia nervosa
	Osteoporosis	Anorexia nervosa, bulimia nervosa
	Muscle loss	Anorexia nervosa, bulimia nervosa
	Dehydration	Anorexia nervosa, bulimia nervosa
	Syncope	Anorexia nervosa, bulimia nervosa
	Dry skin	Anorexia nervosa, bulimia nervosa
	Lanugo (downy body hair)	Anorexia nervosa, bulimia nervosa
	Electrolyte imbalance	Bulimia nervosa, rumination
	Gastric issues	Anorexia nervosa, bulimia nervosa, binge eating disorder, rumination, avoidant/resistant food intake disorder
	Esophageal inflammation and rupture	Bulimia nervosa, rumination, pica

TABLE 15.1 Continued

Characteristics	Symptoms	Specific Feeding and Eating Disorders
	Tooth decay	Bulimia nervosa, rumination, pica
	Pancreatitis	Bulimia nervosa, binge eating disorder
	Ulcers	Bulimia nervosa
	Irregular bowel movements	Anorexia nervosa, bulimia nervosa, pica, rumination, avoidant/resistant food intake disorder
Cognitive perceptual		
	Poor concentration	Anorexia nervosa, bulimia nervosa
	Denies hunger or fatigue	Anorexia nervosa, bulimia nervosa
	Preoccupation with diet and exercise	Anorexia nervosa, bulimia nervosa
	Calorie counting	Anorexia nervosa, bulimia nervosa
	Loss of memory	Anorexia nervosa, bulimia nervosa
	Poor concentration	Anorexia nervosa, bulimia nervosa

From Eckern et al. (1999), Gardiner and Brown (2010), Grave (2011), Mousa et al. (2014), and Treasure et al. (2010).

(Steiner & Martine, 2012). (Herzog et al., 1999) and colleagues' longitudinal study of 246 patients with anorexia nervosa and bulimia found that 74% of individuals with bulimia nervosa achieved a full recovery compared to 33% of those with anorexia nervosa. Partial recovery occurred in 99% of individuals with bulimia nervosa and 83% of those with anorexia nervosa. Relapse rate was found to be approximately 33% for both anorexia nervosa and bulimia nervosa (2003). Recovery from anorexia nervosa becomes more difficult the longer it persists, yet the opposite is true for bulimia nervosa (Treasure, Claudino, & Zucker, 2010). Coexisting obsessive-compulsive characteristics add to the chronicity of both anorexia nervosa and bulimia nervosa (Steiner & Martine, 2012). The prognosis for binge eating disorder is more favorable than for bulimia nervosa. The remission rate is >50% (National Association of Anorexia Nervosa and Associated Disorders, 2015).

Pica may stop spontaneously after several months or require dopamine-regulating medication to control the behaviors (National Library of Medicine [NLM], 2015a). It tends to be more persistent and leads to poorer prognosis in individuals with developmental disabilities than the general population. Rumination may also stop spontaneously or require psychotherapy or aversive conditioning (NLM, 2015a). Like pica,

for individuals with developmental and intellectual disabilities, the prognosis for rumination tends to be poorer than for the general population (NLM, 2015b). The prognosis for individuals with avoidant/resistant food intake has not been reported in the literature, but early treatment is very important. Left untreated, it may lead to anorexia nervosa or bulimia nervosa (Sheppard Pratt Center for Eating Disorders, 2015).

Until clients are ready to make behavioral changes, they will not recover from an eating disorder. Recovery also depends on hope, healing, empowerment, and connection (Clark & Nayar, 2012). Recovery from an eating disorder has been described as "when individuals with a history of an eating disorder appear indistinguishable from healthy controls" (Bardone-Cone et al., 2009, p. 3). From an occupational therapy perspective, recovery is dependent upon achieving a balance between work, leisure, and self-care (Crist, Davis, & Coffin, 2000).

DIAGNOSIS

■ Anorexia Nervosa

The diagnostic criteria for anorexia nervosa include "restriction of caloric intake relative to body requirements that leads to significantly low body weight in relationship to age, sex, developmental trajectory, and physical health status" (APA, 2013, p. 339). Suicide rate is high for individuals with anorexia and is reported at 12 per 100,000 annually (APA, 2013). The ICD-9-CM (International Statistical Classification of Diseases and Related Health Problems) code for anorexia nervosa is 307.1. The ICD-10-CM codes vary based on subtype; restricting type is F50.01 and binge eating/purging type is F50.02.

■ Bulimia Nervosa

Bulimia nervosa is diagnosed when an individual engages in binge eating and compensatory purging behaviors at least one time per week for 3 months and does not occur exclusively during episodes of anorexia nervosa (APA, 2013). Eating occurs within a discrete amount of time (e.g., 1 hour). Food intake is significantly larger than what would be typically expected, and the individual experiences a sense of loss of control of the eating (APA, 2013). Compensatory behaviors occur such as vomiting, misuse of laxative and diuretics, fasting, and/or excessive exercise (APA, 2013). Unlike those with anorexia nervosa, individuals with bulimia nervosa tend to be of normal weight or slightly overweight (Frank, 2015). An individual with bulimia nervosa presents with self-evaluation that is "overly influenced by body shape and weight" (APA, 2013, p. 345). The ICD-9-CM code for bulimia nervosa is 307.51 and the ICD-10-CM code is F50.2.

■ Binge Eating Disorder

Binge eating disorder refers to recurring episodes of eating quickly, with loss of control, and ingesting significantly more food in a discrete period of time (e.g., 1 hour) than most people would eat under similar circumstances regardless of hunger or satiety. It is associated with marked distress and occurs, on average, at least once a week over 3 months (APA, 2013). Binge eating disorder is not associated with inappropriate compensatory behaviors, nor does it occur exclusively during the course of anorexia nervosa or bulimia nervosa (APA, 2013, p. 351). The ICD-9-Cm code is 307.51, and the ICD-10-CM code is F50.8.

■ Pica

To be diagnosed with pica, the individual must have engaged in eating nonfood items for at least 1 month (APA, 2013; Aparna et al., 2012). The ICD-9-CM code for pica is 307.52, and the ICD-10-CM codes for childhood pica are F98.3 and F50.8 for adults.

■ Rumination

Rumination is diagnosed via the Rome III criteria, which includes symptoms such as regurgitation and rechewing or expulsion of food, with no retching for at least 1 month, with onset at least 6 months prior to diagnosis. While most often diagnosed in children with intellectual disabilities, adult cases in the general population have been documented. Rumination does not occur exclusively within the context of anorexia nervosa, bulimia nervosa, binge eating disorder, or avoidant/restrictive food intake disorder (APA, 2013; Mousa et al., 2014). The ICD-9-CM code for rumination is 307.53, and the ICD-10-CM code is F98.21.

■ Avoidant/Restrictive Food Intake Disorder

Nutritional insufficiency and weight loss resulting from excluding specific food groups or inadequate vitamin or mineral intake must occur for a diagnosis of avoidant/restrictive food intake disorder (Bryant-Waugh & Kreipe, 2012). There are no validated assessments to diagnose avoidant/restrictive food intake disorder. Assessment is typically via interview with the client (or family if child is young), weight and height measurement, and assessment of clinical intake. An avoidant/restrictive food intake disorder cannot be associated with an individual's self-perception of his/her body weight or shape, associated with a concurrent medical condition such as food allergy or intolerance, or better explained by psychiatric conditions such as schizophrenia, in which an individual might have delusions about the safety of his or her food (Bryant-Waugh & Kreipe, 2012; Norris & Stevens, 2014, p. 445), cultural practices, or with the presence of another eating disorder (APA, 2013). The ICD-9-CM code for avoidant/restrictive food intake disorder is 307.59 and the ICD-10-CM code is F50.8.

MEDICAL/SURGICAL MANAGEMENT

Interpersonal challenges tend to worsen self-esteem. These challenges can be the catalyst to engage in atypical eating behaviors as a maladaptive way to gain self-control (Murphy et al., 2012). Fully manifesting eating disorders tend to occur in the context of or are amplified by traumatic interpersonal events (Murphy et al., 2012).

Psychological therapies are the typical means for managing eating disorders. Self-help groups and family interventions are the main types of therapy intervention for individuals with eating disorders (Gardiner & Brown, 2010). **Cognitive-behavioral therapy** (CBT) is the most common psychological intervention for adults and **family-based therapy** (FBT) for children, youth, and adolescents (Kosmerly, Waller, & Robinson, 2015; Treasure et al., 2010). Both are evidence-based treatment approaches for individuals with eating disorders. These highly structured interventions have been shown to be more effective than less structured psychological treatment approaches. If psychotherapy services are not available or are ineffective, the next treatment option for those with eating disorders (anorexia nervosa or bulimia nervosa) may be the use of medications such as antidepressants or mood stabilizers (Treasure et al., 2010). In the case of rumination, a muscle relaxant such as baclofen may be used to "reduce regurgitation and belching… and decrease how often the lower esophageal sphincter relaxes" (Mousa et al., 2014, p. 4). For some eating disorders, particularly pica, applied behavioral analysis treatment techniques are often the preferred treatment method.

When there is a concern regarding an individual's physical or emotional safety, especially in individuals with anorexia nervosa, inpatient hospitalization may be required. The goal of this hospitalization would be to reestablish a safe nutritional status and address emotional issues.

Typical treatment for avoidant/restrictive food intake disorder includes psychological or behavioral interventions, nutritional counseling, and medical monitoring (Katzman & Stevens, 2014). Avoidant/restrictive food intake disorder can be managed clinically using food or drink supplements high in calories and fat or via enteric feeding (Bryant-Waugh & Kreipe, 2012).

IMPACT ON OCCUPATIONAL PERFORMANCE

The effect of an eating disorder negatively influences occupational performance. Behaviors are obsessive and maladaptive. Eating disorders globally impact a person's ability and drive to perform adaptive occupations (Clark & Nayar, 2012). While loss of occupational role is a key area of concern for all individuals with eating disorders, anorexia nervosa, in particular, can literally consume a person and lead to a singular focus on food to the exclusion of all else in daily life (Trudeau, 2016). Diminished engagement in purposeful occupation is noted and accompanied by unreasonably high self-expectations. It is not uncommon for an individual with an eating disorder to lose sight of what is (was) fun and important for him or her. Personal causation is at issue. Isolation is common. Roles that are lost may include friend, spouse, parent, worker, and hobbyist (Quiles-Cestari & Pessa Ribeiro, 2012). This loss leads to a dearth of interpersonal connections and even, due to the obsessive inward nature of the disorders, lack of empathy for others.

A client-centered approach to occupational therapy intervention for individuals with eating and feeding disorders entails finding meaning and purpose in life. It can also focus on self-esteem because it is a critical contributor to recovery from eating disorders and an important part of the treatment process (Karpowicz, Skerseter, & Nevonen, 2009). Engagement in social and community activity bolsters self-esteem. Intervention can be directed at increasing socialization, a life function often lost when an individual is entrenched in an eating disorder (Clark & Nayar, 2012). Motivational interviews may help a client with an eating disorder prepare to authentically engage in making adaptive behavioral changes. Occupational therapy can focus on enhancing self-efficacy and self-concept, identifying role deficits, and identifying positive role models (Gardiner & Brown, 2010). For instance, with anorexia nervosa and bulimia nervosa, exercise may become the focal point of a client's life—all day, every day. The occupational therapy practitioner must become skilled at understanding the client's desire and motivation to engage in an activity and the activity demands and associated contraindications. Striking a balance between autonomy and safety is paramount. Too much high-intensity activity will perpetuate undesired behaviors and weight loss. An occupational therapy practitioner needs to be aware of this persistent drive and work with the individual to reevaluate the value of such behavior. It becomes, in essence, helping the client find balance between engaging in moderate exercise and engagement in other meaningful work and leisure activities. This entails client-centered intervention to engage in meaningful active recreation that stops before becoming excessive, to increase socialization, to set limits, and to reduce anxiety and depression (Gardiner & Brown, 2010).

CONCLUSION

To varying extents, all aspects of daily life are negatively impacted by an eating disorder. Meal preparation, grocery and clothes shopping, interpersonal relationships, work, and leisure all suffer. An important role that occupational therapy practitioners can perform when working with clients with eating disorders is to help them organize their lives in order to find a workable balance between engaging in daily skills that they need to do in order to achieve a sense of personal fulfillment (Costa, 2009). Eating disorders are serious mental health conditions that warrant careful and sensitive client-centered treatment from an interdisciplinary team of health practitioners.

CASE STUDY 1

Lucy is a 38-year-old manager of a local bank in a midsized town in the Pacific Northwest. Lucy works about 50 hours a week, where she supervises 10 employees, and is responsible for employee training and customer service. Lucy has been married to Zachary, an elementary school music teacher, for 15 years. They have three children, ages 12, 6, and 2, all conceived via in vitro fertilization. They try to share household tasks, but due to Lucy's long work hours, Zachary ends up doing almost all of it, including child care. Lucy used to love to cook, garden, run, do Zumba, hike, bike, and swim. Girls' night at the local dinner theatre was also something Lucy looked forward to every month. Now, she spends her time being in motion: walking, pacing, and marching in place when she is at work, home, the grocery store, and everywhere. She goes to the gym 6 days a week before work, where she does strength training and cardio workouts. Before bed, she does 100 sit-ups and 50 push-ups as well as prepares lunches for everyone for the next day. Her favorite lunch is two cups of raw chopped chard and a whole sliced cucumber. Sometimes, she also brings celery sticks. She used to pack some carrots, but decided that while they were tasty, she really did not need to eat them. She is thirsty, but doesn't like to drink much because it makes her stomach seem huge when she looks down.

Lucy's story actually begins when she was 12 years old. Lucy is the oldest child in a family with six children. Life was very hectic at home, and there was often a lot of strife between Lucy's parents and siblings. She was always an overachiever, always seeking to be the best at everything she did, from playing the viola and softball to being on student council and having the most friends. Lucy sought out praise and approval and was loath to make a mistake, much less be chastised for it. No matter what she achieved, it never seemed to be enough.

The summer after seventh grade, Lucy's aunt and uncle invited her to come to Nova Scotia to babysit their four children while they rehearsed for a musical theatre troupe. The hours were long and the responsibility intense for a 12-year-old girl. She had wrestled with whether to accept the job or not. It was a chance to go someplace she had never been, but going would mean a summer away from friends and her routines, which were important to her. And she was getting intense pressure from her parents to say yes, which ultimately, being the good girl, she agreed to go. Once she arrived in Nova Scotia, she realized that she was in over her head. Her aunt and uncle were absent for much of the day and night. The children were hard to take care of, on top of making meals and trying to keep the summer cottage clean and tidy. There was no time for Lucy to do what she wanted to do, except for an occasional day off, when she hiked five miles each way into town to look at shop windows as she longed to be home with her family and back into her routine.

While in Nova Scotia, Lucy began to experience a great deal of comfort in restricting what she ate and found that it gave her an incredible high. Finally, she could control something in what had become a very chaotic life. She tried to convey how she felt to her mom, but was dismissed and told to stay the course and honor her commitment; after all, she was a good girl and needed to remember that. By the end of the summer, Lucy went from being a healthy 85-lb girl who had her first period 3 months before the Nova Scotia trip to a 63-lb waif, whose period ultimately stopped for 3 years. When her parents and siblings came to pick her up for their end of the summer vacation, her parents were horrified, but they had no idea what to do. So, they did nothing. Lucy continued to bask in the glory of being in charge of her weight and loved how she could go for a day without eating and exercise seemingly nonstop. She was in full control of herself, but also felt very out of control at the same time, which was confusing. Over the years, Lucy would cycle through times when she could allow herself to eat, and then, following another traumatic life event or when she felt her busy life spinning out of control, the cycle would begin again.

CASE STUDY 2

Milo is 4 years old and was diagnosed with autism spectrum disorder (ASD) when he was 3 years old. He lives in Vermont with his mother and two older sisters. Both sisters are typically developing and attend the local elementary school. Milo's cousin Jonas also has ASD. Milo was verbal until age two, when he began to lose his speech. Although Milo's Mom (Candice) was puzzled, she attributed Milo's loss of speech to having two older sisters who spoke for him. Although his motor skills developed normally, there was a certain quality to them that Candice at times thought were just not right, but again, she shrugged it off by telling herself that Milo was his own person and was just developing according to "his" plan. And didn't boys usually develop more slowly than girls? At least it seemed that way with what Candice had experienced with her daughters. When first enrolled in preschool at age 2 years 6 months, his teachers immediately identified that things were not "right" with Milo. He did not talk, avoided interacting with his peers, walked only on his toes, and preferred to twirl his fingers and, at every chance he could, to eat dirt and rocks. Outside play was scary for the teachers; one needed to be by Milo's side at every minute to make certain that Milo was not putting dirt or rocks in his mouth. They did not know how to stop this behavior and were very concerned that Milo would get sick or, worse, to even choke on something or eat something poisonous and die. When the lead teacher called Candice in for a conference, the classroom teaching staff expressed their concerns about Milo's behaviors and strongly recommended that Milo get evaluated to determine what might be causing these behaviors. Reluctantly, Candice agreed. It took her several months to process that Milo might have a condition, so time went by and no evaluation was done. When she was ready, Candice made an appointment with her pediatrician, and after extensive testing, Milo was diagnosed, at age 3, with ASD and pica.

CASE STUDY 3

It is just another typical Friday night for 28-year-old Treena. After a long day of working as a front desk clerk at a hotel, she heads to the grocery store. She tells herself that this time it will be different. No more buying three gallons of mint chocolate chip ice cream; instead, she is going to buy a large platter of preprepared fruits and eat them while doing what she does every Friday night: watching reruns of a fashion show in which the hosts help women learn to dress to their best potential for their body type. She longs to have a friend to join her, but it seems like they are all busy with their own lives and their own families. No one wants to hang out with her. It is the story of her life, it seems.

At the store, Treena heads to the produce aisle and, after a lot of deliberation, selects a platter of fruit that comes with a pint of fruit dip. This, she thinks, will be the start of a new me. But since she was already at the store, it was logical to pick up a few more things that were on sale, including frozen pancakes and her favorite brand of peanut butter. As she was passing through the frozen food aisle, she saw the ice cream and decided to buy it, but promised herself that she could portion control and not eat a full gallon while watching a 60-minute episode of the fashion show. Besides, she was going to eat her fruit. And that would be enough. Once home, she puts away her groceries and jumps into the shower, noticing that the waistband of her pants had made a deep impression on her stomach, maybe deeper than ever. After comfortably settling onto the couch with the television remote in hand, she began to think about the ice cream. "No, fruit first," Treena told herself. So she ate the platter of fruit, dipping pieces of fruit in the caramel dip and then swirling each piece in the peanut butter she had picked up on sale. Then, despite being full, she opened the mint chocolate chip ice cream and had a taste, then another, and then, by the time the fashion television show had ended, the fruit was gone, the container of dip was empty, half of the peanut butter had been eaten, and there was one spoonful left of ice cream. So she ate it. And then she cried. "Was this any way to live?" she asked herself.

RECOMMENDED LEARNING RESOURCES

National Eating Disorders Association
http://www.nationaleatingdisorders.org/resource-links
Center for Eating Disorders
http://www.center4ed.org/resources.asp

National Association of Anorexia Nervosa and Associated Disorders
http://www.anad.org/resources/
Academy for Eating Disorders
http://www.aedweb.org/

REFERENCES

American Psychiatric Association. (2013). *Diagnostic and statistical manual of mental disorders* (5th ed.). Arlington, VA. doi:10.1176/appi.books.9780890423349

Aparna, P. V., Austin, R. D., & Mattews, P. (2012). Pica. *Indian Journal of Dental Research, 23*(3), 426–427.

Bardone-Cone, A. M., Harney, M. B., Maldonado, C. R., Lawson, M. A., Robinson, D. B., Smoth, R., & Tosh, A. (2009). Defining recovery from an eating disorder: Conceptualization, validation, and examination of psychosocial functioning and psychiatric comorbidity. *Behaviour, Research and Therapy Journal, 48*(3), 194–202. Retrieved from http://www.ncbi.nlm.nih.gov/pmc/articles/PMC2829357/pdf/nihms-161878.pdf. doi:10.1016/j.brat.2009.11.001

Blinder, B. J. (2008, May 1). An update on pica: Prevalence, contributing causes, and treatment. *Psychiatric Times*. Retrieved from http://www.psychiatrictimes.com/eating-disorders/update-pica-prevalence-contributing-causes-and-treatment

Branson R., Potoczna N., Kral, J. G., Lentes, K.-U., Hoehe, M. R., & Horber, F. F. (2003). Binge eating as a major phenotype of melanocortin 4 receptor gene mutations. *New England Journal of Medicine, 348*(12), 1096–2003.

Bryant-Waugh, R., & Kreipe, R. E. (2012). Avoidant/restrictive food intake disorder in DSM-5. *Psychiatric Annals, 42*(11), 402–405.

Clark, M., & Nayar, S. (2012). Recovery from eating disorders: A role for occupational therapy. *New Zealand Journal of Occupational Therapy, 59*(1), 13–17.

Costa, D. M. (2009). Eating disorders: Occupational therapy's role. *OT Practice*, 13–16.

Crist, P. H., Davis, C. G., & Coffin, P. S. (2000). The effects of employment and mental health status on the balance of work, play/leisure, self-care, and rest. *Occupational Therapy in Mental Health, 15*(1), 27–42.

Crow, S. J., Peterson, C. B., Swanson, S. A., Raymond, N. C., Specker, S., Eckert, E. D., & Mitchell, J. E. (2009). Increased mortality in bulimia nervosa and other eating disorders. *American Journal of Psychiatry, 166*, 1342–1346.

Eckern, M., Stevens, W., & Mitchell, J. (1999). The relationship between rumination and eating disorders. *International Journal of Eating Disorders, 26*(4), 414–419.

Fisher, M. M., Rosen, D. S., Ornstein, R. M., Mammel, K. A., Katzman, D. K., Rome, E. S., et al. (2014). Characteristics of avoidant/restrictive food intake disorder in children and adolescents:

A "new disorder" in DSM-5. *Journal of Adolescent Health, 55*, 49–52.

Frank, K. W. G. (2015). What causes eating disorders and what do they cause? *Biological Psychiatry, 77*(7), 602–603.

Gardiner, C., & Brown, N. (2010). Is there a role for occupational therapy within a specialist child and adolescent mental health eating disorder service? *British Journal of Occupational Therapy, 73*(1), 38–41. doi: 10.4276/030802210X12629548272745.

Grave, R. D. (2011). Eating disorders: Progress and challenges. *European Journal of Internal Medicine, 22*, 153–160.

Hay, P. J., & Claudino, A. C. (2010). Bulimia nervosa. *BMJ Clinical Evidence Review Update 7*, 1009.

Herzog, D. B., Dorer, D. J., Keel, P. K., Selwyn, S. E., Ekeblad, E. R., et al. (1999). Recovery and relapse in anorexia and bulimia nervosa: A 7.5-year follow-up study. *Journal of the American Academy of Child and Adolescent Psychiatry, 38*(7), 829–837.

Hoek, H. W. (2007). Incidence, prevalence and mortality of anorexia and other eating disorders. *Current Opinion in Psychiatry, 19*(4), 389–394.

Karpowicz, E., Skerseter, I., & Nevonen, L. (2009). Self-esteem in patients treated for anorexia nervosa. *International Journal of Mental Health Nursing, 18*, 318–325.

Katzman, D. K., Stevens, K., & Norris, M. (2014). Redefining feeding and eating disorders: What is avoidant/restrictive food intake disorder? *Paediatrics and Child Health, 19*(8), 445–446.

Kosmerly, S., Waller, G., & Robinson, A. L. (2015). Clinician adherence to guidelines in the delivery of family based therapy for eating disorders. *International Journal of Eating Disorders, 48*(2), 223–229.

Kreipe, R. E., & Palomaki, A. (2012). Beyond picky eating: Avoidant/restrictive food intake disorder. *Current Psychiatric Reports, 14*, 421–431.

Miller, C. A. & Golden, N. H. (2010). An introduction to eating disorders: Clinical presentation, epidemiology, and prognosis. *Clinical Nutrition in Practice, 25*(2), 110–115.

Mousa, H. M., Montgomery, M., & Alioto, A. (2014). Adolescent rumination syndrome. *Current Gastroenterology Reports, 16*(398), 1–6. doi: 10.1007/s11894-014-0398-9

Murphy, R., Straebler, S., Basden, S., Cooper, Z., & Fairburn, C. G. (2012). Interpersonal psychotherapy for eating disorders. *Clinical Psychology & Psychotherapy, 19*, 150–158.

National Association of Anorexia Nervosa and Associated Disorders. (2015). *Binge eating disorder*. Retrieved from http://www.anad.org/get-information/about-eating-disorders/binge-eating-disorder/

National Library of Medicine. (2015a). *Pica*. Retrieved from http://www.nlm.nih.gov/medlineplus/ency/article/001538.htm

National Library of Medicine. (2015b). *Rumination*. Retrieved from http://www.nlm.nih.gov/medlineplus/ency/article/001539.htm

Nicely, T. A., Lane-Loney, S. A., Masciulli, E., Hollenbeak, C. S., & Ornstein, R. M. (2014). Prevalence and characteristics of avoidant/resistant food intake disorder of a cohort of young patients in day treatment for eating disorders. *International Journal of Eating Disorders, 2*, 21. Retrieved from http://www.jeatdisord.com/content/2/1/2

Noordenbox, G. (2002). Characteristics and treatment of patients with chronic eating disorders. *International Journal of Eating Disorders, 10*, 15–29.

Norris, M. L., Robinson, A., Obeid, N., Harrison, M. Spettigue, W., et al. (2013). Exploring avoidant/resistant food intake disorder in eating disordered patients: A descriptive study. *International Journal of Eating Disorders, 47*(5), 495–499.

Ornstein, R. M., Rosen, D. S., Mammel, K. A., Callahan, S. T., Forman, S., et al. (2013). Distribution of eating disorders in children and adolescents using the proposed DSM-5 criteria for feeding and eating disorders. *Journal of Adolescent Health, 53*(2), 303–305.

Pica. (2011). *Dental abstracts. 56*(3), 160–161.

Quiles-Cestari, L. M., & Pessa Ribeiro, R. P. (2012). The occupational roles of women with anorexia nervosa. *Revista Latino-Americana de Enfermagem, 20*(2), 235–242.

Sheppard Pratt Center for Eating Disorders. (2015). *Avoidant/resistant food intake disorder*. Retrieved from http://eatingdisorder.org/eating-disorder-information/eating-disorder-information/arfid/

Steiner, H., & Martine, F. F. (2012). *Fast facts: Eating disorders—Course and prognosis*. Abingdon: Health Press Limited. Retrieved from http://search.proquest.com/docview/1174305129?accountid=15099

Steinhausen, H. C. (2008). Outcomes of eating disorders. *Child and Adolescent Psychiatric Clinics of North America, 18*, 225–242. doi:10.1016/j.chc.2008.07.013

Steinhausen, H. C., Boyadjieva, S., Griogoroiu-Serbanescu, M., & Neumarker, K. J. (2003). The outcome of adolescent eating disorders: Findings from an international collaborative study. *European Child & Adolescent Psychiatry, 12*(Suppl. 1), 91–I98.

Taber's Cyclopedic Medical Dictionary. (2013). *Pica*. Philadelphia, PA: FA Davis.

Talley, N. J. (2011). Rumination syndrome. *Gastroenterology & Hepatology, 7*(2), 117–118.

The Renfrew Center Foundation for Eating Disorders. (2003), *Eating disorders 101 guide: A summary of issues, statistics and resources*. Retrieved from www.renfrew.org

Treasure, J., Claudino, A. M., & Zucker, N. (2010). Eating disorders. *The Lancet, 375*, 583–593.

Trudeau, S. (2016). Psychological conditions. In A. Wagenfeld (Ed.), *Foundations of theory and practice for the occupational therapy assistant* (pp. 391–403). Baltimore, MD: Wolters Kluwer, Lippincott, Williams & Wilkins.

Walsh, T. (2011). The importance of eating behavior in eating disorders. *Physiology & Behavior, 104*, 525–259.

Williams, D. E., & McAdam, D. (2012). Assessment, behavioral treatment, and prevention of pica: Clinical guidelines and recommendations for practitioners. *Research in Developmental Disabilities, 33*, 2050–2057.

Zeek, A., Stelzer, N., Linster, H. W., Joos, A., & Hartmann, A. (2011). Emotion and eating in binge eating disorder and obesity. *European Eating Disorders Review, 19*(5), 426–437.

16

Substance-Related and Addictive Disorders

Addiction
Co-occurring disorders
Cravings
Delirium tremens
Fetal alcohol syndrome
Intoxication disorder
Impaired control
Pharmacological criteria
Risky use
Social impairment
Substance abuse
Substance/medication-
    induced disorders
Substance-related
    disorders
Substance use disorder
Tolerance
Withdrawal
Withdrawal disorder

Emily Raphael-Greenfield

Laura, an 80-year-old Caucasian woman, is being seen daily by an occupational therapist (OT) in a subacute facility. She has broken her hip and successfully undergone hip replacement surgery. Before her fall, she was living by herself in a four-bedroom house where she and her husband raised their children. Her husband passed away 10 years ago, and none of her three children live nearby. The OT has observed that Laura keeps to herself in the subacute rehabilitation facility and never has any visitors. The therapist encourages Laura to describe her daily life prior to her accident and gently probes for details surrounding her fall. Laura is hesitant to discuss how she used to spend her days and the fall, but she liked the therapist and admitted to her that she was very lonely and was having a hard time living by herself and taking care of her house. When asked if she had any friends, she shook her head and said that she used to but not anymore. She told the therapist that she had worked as an accountant for 30 years while also raising her children. She used to see her children and grandchildren often, but she said, "My family is angry with me." When asked why, the client shook her head and said sadly, "I spoiled things."

The therapist knew that the client was not depressed because she had been screened with a depression scale, but she had never been screened for alcohol use, which is linked with falls and other orthopedic injuries. The therapist decided to administer the CAGE Questionnaire, which is a standardized screening tool for alcohol use disorders that can be administered by any health care provider (Silver, 2015). She asked Laura the following four questions:

1. Have you ever thought you should **C**ut down on your drinking? Although Laura was upset by the question, she began to describe how she and her husband were social drinkers and occasionally

shared a bottle of wine with friends. Since his death, she had begun to drink alone. She described herself as a late-onset drinker who had lost her tolerance for alcohol. She had tried to stop her drinking but had failed. (Yes.)

2. Have people **A**nnoyed you by criticizing your drinking? Laura stated with great embarrassment that her children were critical of her drinking, and for the last 3 years, they had refused to allow her to see her grandchildren whom she adored. She was extremely annoyed with them. (Yes.)

3. Have you ever felt bad or **G**uilty about your drinking? Laura felt that she has really messed up her life, especially by spoiling her relationship with her family. (Yes.)

4. Have you ever had a drink first thing in the morning to steady your nerves or to get rid of a hangover (**E**ye opener)? Laura started to cry and said that the morning she fell and broke her hip, she had started the day with a drink. (Yes.)

The therapist totaled her score, which was a four, which is considered clinically significant. The OT reported her findings to the medical team, which included a psychologist who considered a diagnosis of alcohol use disorder for Laura. Because Laura was in a subacute rehab facility, she was in a controlled environment where alcohol was prohibited, which was going to help her remain abstinent in the short run. Her therapist also knew that building a trusting relationship with Laura was going to help her patient face and overcome her substance use problem in the long term. Another part of Laura's plan consisted of collaborating with her to design a discharge plan, which included not only continuing outpatient physical rehabilitation but also setting her up in a day program that treated substance use problems, locating self-help services such as Alcoholics Anonymous (AA), and reinvolving her family in her life to help her recover from this late-onset alcohol use disorder.

DESCRIPTION AND DEFINITIONS

Substance-related disorders and addiction are widespread phenomena that affect all sectors of a population and OT specialty areas on a national and global basis (AOTA, 2014). Because OTs are likely to encounter clients with addiction in all treatment settings, a background in signs and symptoms as well as familiarity with medical interventions will enable our profession to make a unique contribution to improving our clients' occupational performance (Thompson, 2007).

DSM-5 changed the classification system of substance-related disorders from that used in DSM-IV-TR. DSM-5 has retained the two main categories of substance-related disorders—substance use disorders and substance-induced disorders—but dropped the terminology of substance dependence and **substance abuse**. Substance abuse usually is defined as the state that occurs when the use of the substance leads to failure in carrying out a variety of occupational roles, interpersonal and legal problems, and risky behaviors (APA, 2000). DSM-5's newer system of classification for all classes of substances is based on the pattern of use and its associated behavioral and psychological factors. The three types of disorder listed in the DSM-5 for all substance classes are Use disorders, Intoxication disorders, and Withdrawal disorders (APA, 2013).

Clients are now described as having substance use problems, which are further categorized into two phases: intoxication and withdrawal. **Substance use disorder** refers to irreversible brain circuit changes in severe disorders and repeated behavioral relapses and strong cravings in the presence of substance-related stimuli (APA, 2013). **Intoxication disorder** refers to the short-term symptoms associated with current use of the substance, including the problematic behaviors and psychological changes. **Withdrawal disorder** describes the symptoms that occur immediately and for a longer period after a client who has been heavily using a substance stops ingesting. These withdrawal symptoms also cause suffering and problematic functioning (APA, 2013).

There are 10 classes of drugs that are encompassed by the DSM-5 **substance-related disorders:** alcohol; caffeine; cannabis; hallucinogens; inhalants; opioids; sedatives, hypnotics, and anxiolytics; stimulants; tobacco; and other substances and nonsubstance (gambling). DSM-5 describes diagnostic criteria and specifiers for each drug class. The classes are presented alphabetically (see Table 16.1). All drugs that are taken in excess activate the neurons in the brain's reward system to release the chemical dopamine at higher levels than do naturally occurring stimuli (NIDA, 2015b). This reaction is so intense that normal activities are ignored. The drugs produce a pleasurable feeling state, which is referred to as a "high."

Rather than stimulating the reward system in the brain through adaptive behavior, drugs of abuse directly trigger the reward circuits (APA, 2013). Gambling is included because it also activates the brain's reward system and produces similar behavioral patterns (Bonder, 2015). When a person is diagnosed with a substance use disorder and other psychiatric conditions, this is referred to as **co-occurring disorders** (CODs) (Moyers, 2011).

Substance use is defined as the consumption of the substance by any of the following means: orally, smoking, inhaling, or intravenously. Substance use produces long-term physiological, cognitive, and behavioral symptoms in contrast with the immediate effects of intoxication. Clients are diagnosed with substance use disorders when they exhibit disturbed patterns of behavior after ingesting a substance. DSM-5 criteria for diagnosing substance use disorders are organized into four categories: impaired control, social impairment, risky use, and pharmacological criteria (APA, 2013).

Impaired control (APA, 2013) is defined as taking larger amounts than intended over time, many unsuccessful attempts to reduce use and also a persistent desire to decrease or discontinue, and one's daily activities revolve around obtaining the substance and/or recovering from its use. **Cravings** are the desire for the drug that precludes thinking of anything else and are associated with specific reward pathways in the brain and occur

---

TABLE 16.1 Substance-Related Disorders

Substance Use Disorders (10 Classes of Drugs)

1. Alcohol
2. Caffeine
3. Cannabis
4. Hallucinogens
5. Inhalants
6. Opioids
7. Sedatives, hypnotics, and anxiolytics
8. Stimulants
9. Tobacco
10. Other substances and nonsubstance (gambling)

From American Psychiatric Association (APA). (2013). Substance-related and addictive disorders. In *Diagnostic and statistical manual of mental disorders* (5th ed.). Author. doi: 10.1176/appi.books.9780890425596.249120

more likely in an environmental context of previous use. Cravings are documented by asking the client if there was a time when he or she could not think of anything else other than getting the substance. Cravings are viewed as a signal of an impending relapse (APA, 2013). **Social impairment** (APA, 2013) is defined as persistent substance use associated with the inability to carry out key occupational roles, serious social and interpersonal problems, and withdrawal from leisure and other family activities. **Risky use** (APA, 2013) is defined as consuming the substances even when it is physically hazardous and despite knowing that the substance use is causing persistent physical, legal, and/or psychological difficulties. **Pharmacological criteria** (APA, 2013) are defined as tolerance and withdrawal. **Tolerance** is defined as requiring increased amounts of the substance in order to get the desired effect or a significantly reduced effect when usual dosage is consumed; tolerance is difficult to determine by history alone and is established by laboratory tests. **Withdrawal** is defined as a syndrome that occurs when blood or tissue concentrations decline in a person who has used heavily, which makes him or her more likely to consume again to relieve symptoms. For most classes of substances, a past history of withdrawal is associated with a more severe clinical picture. When a person is experiencing both the symptoms of tolerance and withdrawal, he or she is described as having an **addiction**.

Substance-induced disorders include intoxication, withdrawal, and other substance/medication-induced mental disorders, including substance-induced psychotic disorder, substance-induced depressive disorder, substance-induced bipolar disorder, substance-induced anxiety disorder, substance-induced OCD and related disorders, substance-induced sleep problems, substance-induced sexual dysfunction, substance-induced delirium, and substance-induced dementia (see Table 16.2). According to the DSM-5, these types of substance-induced disorders are usually reversible, but severe, temporary, brief states and related to the ingestion of a specific substance; conditions usually disappear within 1 month or so of cessation of acute withdrawal, severe intoxication, or use of the medication. All of the 10 classes of substances that produce substance use disorders can produce the substance/medication-induced mental disorders, but these disorders can also be caused by many other medications commonly used in medical practice (APA, 2013) (see Table 16.3). Common characteristics of these types of substance-/medication-induced disorders include appearance of clinically significant symptoms of a relevant mental disorder that occur within 1 month of a substance intoxication or withdrawal or taking a medication, capability of the substance/medication to produce a mental disorder, and presence of significant problems in several areas of occupational functioning (APA, 2013).

Intoxication disorders usually consist of changes in perception, wakefulness, attention, thinking, judgment, psychomotor behavior, and interpersonal behavior. The type of intoxication sought determines the route of administration. The most intense intoxication is produced by rapid and efficient absorption into the bloodstream intravenously, smoking, or intranasal "snorting." These three methods of administration

TABLE 16.2 Substance-Induced Disorders

Drugs	Actions During Intoxication	Actions During Withdrawal
Sedating drugs (sedatives, hypnotics, anxiolytics, alcohol)	Depressive disorder Sleep disorders Sexual disorders	Anxiety disorder
Stimulating drugs (amphetamines, cocaine)	Psychotic disorder Anxiety disorder Sleep disorders Sexual disorders	Depressive disorder

From American Psychiatric Association (APA). (2013). Substance-related and addictive disorders. In *Diagnostic and statistical manual of mental disorders* (5th ed.). Author. doi: 10.1176/appi.books.9780890425596.249120

TABLE 16.3 Medication-Induced Disorders

Medications	Mental disorders
Anesthetics, antihistamines, antihypertensive, other medications and toxins	Neurocognitive disorders
Anticholinergic, cardiovascular, steroid drugs, stimulant-like and depressant-like prescription or over-the-counter drugs	Psychotic disorders
Steroids, antihypertensive, disulfiram, prescription or over-the-counter depressant or stimulant-like substances	Depressive disorders, anxiety disorders, sleep disorders, sexual dysfunctions

From American Psychiatric Association (APA). (2013). Substance-related and addictive disorders. In *Diagnostic and statistical manual of mental disorders* (5th ed.). Author. doi: 10.1176/appi.books.9780890425596.249120

are more likely to lead to an escalating pattern of withdrawal. Short-acting substances, rather than longer acting ones, have a higher potential for the development of withdrawal (APA, 2013).

Withdrawal disorders occur after a person who has used a substance for a long period stops ingesting the substance. Withdrawal disorders are described by specific behavioral, psychological, and physical symptoms that can last hours, days, and weeks and can cause significant distress and occupational dysfunction. When a substance such as heroin, which has prolonged, uncomfortable withdrawal symptoms, is used, it may make treatment of the disorder more challenging (Bonder, 2015).

Medications or substances can cause serious central nervous system (CNS) side effects, such as dystonic reactions, confusion, and dizziness, but the side effects disappear once the medication or substance is eliminated from the body. The criteria for diagnosing substance/medication-induced mental disorders involve gathering descriptions of symptoms, a history of substance/medication use, a mental status exam, and lab findings (APA, 2013).

OTs need to be aware of the medications that can cause CNS side effects because the cognitive, behavioral, and physical symptoms that they cause may occur in any acute, rehabilitation, and community practice site (Bonder, 2015). One example is medication-induced movement disorders, such as dystonia, akathisia, and tardive dyskinesia. All of these movement disorders are caused by the use of typical antipsychotic medications, and their appearance can further stigmatize clients. The movement disorders are usually controlled by rebalancing medication regimens.

Dystonia is defined as prolonged muscle contractions. Akathisia is defined as restlessness and fidgeting. Tardive dyskinesia is defined as involuntary athetoid and choreiform movements of the tongue, face, and limbs.

ETIOLOGY

There are five factors that help to explain the causes and origins of substance-related disorders: biological and genetic, temperament, psychological explanations, sociocultural factors, and age (Fig. 16.1). The neurological pathways that are implicated in all substance use disorders are the mesolimbic dopamine reward pathway and the prefrontal cortex (Bonder, 2015). The reward pathway is changed by substance use, which causes unrestrained cravings (Gutman, 2006). The reward response is changed so that "go" signals are enhanced and "stop" signals are inhibited. The prefrontal cortex controls decision making, which becomes impaired with substance use (Clay, Allen & Parran, 2008) (see Fig. 16.2).

The genetic factors underlying the etiology of alcohol disorders are more thoroughly understood and researched than any of the other substances (Sells, Stoffel & Plach, 2011). In early 20th century America, the cause of alcohol disorders was considered to be a moral failing. It is now considered to be a disease (Bonder, 2015). There is no single gene but rather a variety of genes that are thought to make a person vulnerable to developing alcoholism (NIAAA, 2005a). Based on biological relative and adoptive parent studies with

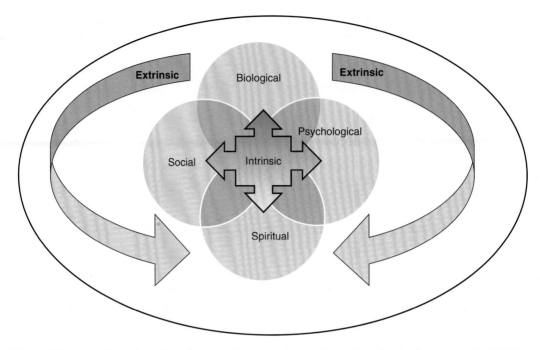

Figure 16.1 Intrinsic and extrinsic factors affecting etiology. (From Rundio, A., & Lorman, B.. (2015). *Core curriculum of addictions nursing* (3rd ed.). Philadelphia, PA: Lippincott Williams & Wilkins.)

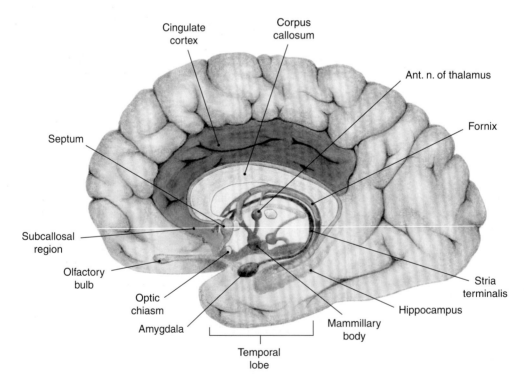

Figure 16.2 The anatomical brain. (From Herron, A., & Brennan, T. K.. (2015). *The ASAM essentials of addiction medicine* (2nd ed.). Philadelphia, PA: Lippincott Williams & Wilkins.)

twins, it is thought to be a combination of genetic predisposition triggered by environmental issues. The onset of familial alcoholism is earlier, and its prognosis is poorer than patterns of nonfamilial alcoholism. Women diagnosed with alcohol use disorders have a later onset, drink smaller amounts, and progress more rapidly with the disease (Bonder, 2015). The genetic factors linked to drug disorders are more complex, but genes are considered important in explaining the level of risky behavior associated with these disorders (Sells et al., 2011).

The development of substance use disorders in adulthood is associated with childhood and adolescent "difficult" temperaments (NIAAA, 2005a). Youth with self-regulation problems, which translate into behavioral problems in the classroom and the community, may self-medicate with alcohol, drugs, and illicit use of medications. Research on adults with sensory modulation disorders demonstrated that a majority used CNS depressant substances, including alcohol, sedatives, hypnotics, and anxiolytics, while 15% to 18% used stimulants or a combination of both (Quadling, Maree, Mountjoy, Bosch, & Kotkin, 1999).

Psychological theories that explain the etiology of substance use include theories of behaviorism and cognitive behavior (NIAAA, 2005a). Classical conditioning explains how drinking and drug use become linked to person, location, and time of day. Operant conditioning explains how substance use becomes paired with stressors as triggers and perceived calm after use. These theories explain how the user discounts negative consequences because they occur later and are not connected with the positive effects of using. There is also research with children that reveals the power of modeling where young users learn their alcohol use behaviors from observing and imitating what others are doing in real life and in the media (NIAAA, 2005a).

Sociocultural influences on the etiology of alcohol and drug use include the relationship between alcohol and drug use and family, peer, and social relationships. It is not clear if this relationship is causal or just associative. The influence of family has been researched, for example, if a child grows up in a family where substance use adversely impacts family functioning, the child is at greater risk for developing substance use problems. There is a link between adolescents who have early adverse experiences such as parental divorce, parental drinking, a parental psychiatric disorder, or sexual abuse and adolescents trying to cope by using substances (Monti et al., 2005). Economic and sociological explanations rather than neurochemical explanations have also been posited for the high rates of usage among inner-city minority populations by neuroscientist Hart (2013) who has studied how the availability of cheap illicit substances and absence of healthier alternative occupations and racist law enforcement in low-resource neighborhoods explain addiction patterns rather than the hard wiring of brains.

Researchers have found protective factors such as supportive extended family members, a child's calm temperament, or positive family rituals can interrupt the cycle (NIAAA, 2005a). The influence of peers is profound during mid to late adolescence when it is most likely that alcohol and drugs are tried for the first time, due to greater independence, need for peer approval, availability of substances, and greater tolerance, for example, on college campuses. Adolescents report that they use more substances because they are bored and have positive associations with intoxication. They also believe that substances foster increased sociability and reduce anxiety (NIAAA, 2005a). There is a strong link in women between histories of sexual and physical abuse and alcohol use disorders (Maniglio, 2011). If women use alcohol excessively during pregnancy, there is a greater risk for **fetal alcohol syndrome**, a condition in which the infant exhibits CNS damage and retardation (Jones & Streissguth, 2010). Alcohol is often used to self-medicate symptoms of other psychiatric disorders, which results in dual diagnosis or co-occurring disorders.

There are two age groups that deserve special attention in terms of etiology: college age students and older adults. Excessive drinking on campuses is now reported to be at epidemic proportions, particularly among males, ages 18 to 25, even though drinking among college-bound students is lower than that among their non–college-bound peers because of the pressure to achieve. College campuses have traditionally been considered safe places to drink and use substances, but there are numerous negative consequences associated with this permissive environment, including serious injuries, death, sexual harassment and assault, problems for roommates and friends, destruction of property, academic problems, anxiety, and depression (National Center on Addiction and Substance Abuse, 2007). Because of their use of alcohol in combination with prescription and over-the-counter medications, older adults also present with particular difficulties. While the majority of older adults do not drink or use drugs at all or only in moderation, research has shown that in adults over 60, 15% of men and 12% of women drank more than the recommended guidelines (Adams, Barry & Fleming, 1996).

INCIDENCE AND PREVALENCE

Prevalence is the percentage of persons within a particular population who have a specific disease or illness at a given time. Incidence is the percentage or rate of new cases within a population during a particular time period (Center for Substance Abuse Treatment, 2007). The prevalence of Americans aged 12 or older, who reported being current alcohol drinkers, was 52.2%, which was similar to the rate in 2012 (52.1%). Nearly one-quarter or 22.9% of persons aged 12 or older in 2013 were described as binge alcohol users in the 30 days prior to the survey. Binge drinking is defined as five or more drinks on the same occasion. The rate in 2013 was similar in 2012 (23.0%). Heavy drinking, which is defined as five or more drinks on each of 5 days, was reported by 6.3% of the population aged 12 or older, which was similar to the rate of heavy drinking in 2012 or 6.5% (SAMHSA, 2014).

An estimated 24.6 million Americans aged 12 or older in 2013 used an illicit drug during the month prior to the survey, which represents 9.4% of the population aged 12 or older, according to the National Survey on Drug Use and Health (NSDUH) (Fig.16.3). Illicit drugs include marijuana, cocaine, heroin, hallucinogens, inhalants, psychotherapeutics, or the nonmedical use of prescription medications (SAMHSA, 2014). The most commonly used illicit drug was marijuana, which was used by 19.8 million users over the last month, representing 80.6% of illicit drug users (Fig.16.4).

Young adults, aged 18 to 25, used illicit drugs at the highest rate (21.5%) in 2013, after that youths aged 12 to 17 (8.8%), and then adults aged 26 or older (7.3%). This represents a decrease from 2012 in the number and percentage of current illicit drug users among youths aged 12 to 17 from 2.4 million (9.5%) in 2012 to 2.2 million

Percentage who used any illicit drug in last 12 months

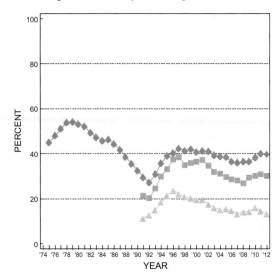

Figure 16.3 Percentage using any illicit drug. (From Ries, R. K., Fiellin, D. A., Miller, S. C., & Saitz, R. (2014). *The ASAM principles of addiction medicine* (5th ed.). Philadelphia, PA: Lippincott Williams & Wilkins.)

(8.8%) in 2013 (SAMHSA, 2014; National Center on Addiction and Substance Abuse, 2011).

The prevalence of alcohol and illicit drug use is higher among males than females. In 2013, 57.1% of males aged 12 or older were current drinkers compared to females (47.5%). Among youths aged 12 to 17, however, the percentage of

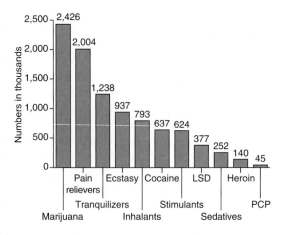

Figure 16.4 Prevalence of different drugs. (From Ries, R. K., Fiellin, D. A., Miller, S. C., & Saitz, R. (2014). *The ASAM principles of addiction medicine* (5th ed.). Philadelphia, PA: Lippincott Williams & Wilkins.)

males and females who were current drinkers was 11.2% and 11.9%, respectively. The incidence for both male and female youths was lower than those of 2012 (12.6% and 13.2%, respectively). In the young adult group, ages 18 to 25, 62.3% of males and 56.9% of females were reported to be current drinkers in 2013. In this same age group in 2013, 44.4% of males and 31.4% of females reported binge drinking in 2013. The rate of binge drinking for females aged 18 to 25 decreased from the incidence reported in 2012 (33.2%), while binge drinking among males in this age group remained the same. Among persons aged 26 or older, an estimated 62.2% of males and 50.1% of females reported current drinking in 2013, but in this age group, the rate of binge drinking for males was approximately twice the rate for females (30.7% vs. 14.7%) (SAMHSA, 2014).

The prevalence of alcohol use among pregnant women aged 15 to 44 in 2012–2013 included an annual average of 9.4% reporting current alcohol use, 2.3% reporting binge drinking, and 0.4% reporting heavy drinking. Alcohol use during the second and third trimesters in 2012–2013 was reportedly lower than during the first trimester (5.0% and 4.4% vs. 19.0%) (SAMHSA, 2014).

Among persons aged 12 or older in 2013, the prevalence of current illicit drug use was 3.1% in Asians, 8.8% in Hispanics, 9.5% in Whites, 10.5% in Blacks, 12.3% in American Indians or Alaska Natives, 14.0% in Native Hawaiians or other Pacific Islanders, and 17.4% in persons reporting two or more races. Between 2002 and 2013, the incidence of current illicit drug use increased from 8.5% to 9.5% for whites, and among blacks, the rate increased from 2004 (8.7%) to 2013 (10.5%) (SAMHSA, 2014).

Prevalence of substance use is also explained by biological, genetic, and socioeconomic factors. Epidemiological research has demonstrated differences in metabolism and absorption rates of alcohol in different ethnic groups (Wall, Luczak, & Hiller-Sturmhofel, 2016). For example, Asians have the lowest risk of alcohol use disorders, while Whites experience the highest risk. Hispanics have higher rates and Asians have lower rates of heavy drinking patterns. Hispanics and Blacks compared to Whites and Asians are more likely to experience health and social problems from drinking. Access to health care, preventive services, and alternatives to drug use are less available and underfunded for lower socioeconomic groups in

this society (Hart, 2013). Hart also emphasizes that only about 10% to 15% of substance users, whether they use alcohol, prescription medications, or illicit drugs, become addicted and 75% of substance users do not develop these serious dysfunctional patterns. Underserved minorities face more discrimination, stronger legal consequences, and increased incarceration when they use drugs recreationally than do the Caucasian youth population. There are also fewer resources for healthy living and treatment in inner cities and rural areas, which makes advanced states of substance-related disorders harder to treat in these areas (Sells et al., 2011).

The prevalence of adult US citizens with a COD is approximately five million (Center for Substance Abuse Treatment, 2007). Studies of clients in mental health settings found that 20% to 50% had a lifetime co-occurring substance use disorder, while other studies of individuals in substance abuse treatment found that 73% had co-occurring mental health disorders during their lifetimes. The majority of these mental health disorders are described as depressive, bipolar, posttraumatic stress, and personality disorders. Clients diagnosed with more than one mental health disorder are not uncommon (Center for Substance Abuse Treatment, 2007).

SIGNS AND SYMPTOMS

■ Alcohol

Alcohol is a CNS depressant that causes a brief period of intoxication followed by slowing of cardiac and respiratory responses over time. Overdose and death can occur from a single episode when there is a very high level of intake, for example, during fraternity hazing (Bonder, 2015). The signs and symptoms are organized into alcohol use disorders, alcohol intoxication disorders, and alcohol withdrawal disorders within DSM-5 (see Table 16.4). Alcohol use disorders have the following signs and symptoms: within a 12-month period, the use of alcohol leads to significant psychological distress and problems in functioning, including increased tolerance and cravings; a great deal of time spent acquiring, using, and recovering from alcohol consumption; unsuccessful efforts to decrease or stop its use; inability to carry out important occupational roles; serious problems with interpersonal functioning and

TABLE 16.4 Substance Use Disorders

Drug Class	Use D/O	Signs and Symptoms for Classes		Withdrawal D/O
		Intoxication D/O		
1. Alcohol	Within a 12-mo period significant psychological distress and problems in functioning, increased tolerance and cravings	Hypersexual or aggressive behavior, mood lability, impaired judgment, slurred speech, incoordination, unsteady gait, nystagmus, impaired attention, memory, stupor or coma		Autonomic hyperactivity, hand tremors, insomnia, vomiting, transient visual, tactile or hallucinations, psychomotor agitation, generalized tonic-clonic seizures, anxiety, irritability, tachycardia, DTs
2. Caffeine	N/A	Restlessness, nervousness, insomnia, flushed face, diuresis, gastrointestinal disturbance, muscle twitching, disorganized thinking or speech, cardiac rhythm changes, excessive energy, psychomotor retardation		Headache, difficulty concentrating, fatigue, depressed mood, and flu-like symptoms
3. Cannabis	Experience tolerance and withdrawal when not using, avolition, lack of concern for future, paranoia, depression, aggression and hostility, emotional lability	Induces euphoria and relaxation, perceptual and cognitive distortions, poor concentration, conjunctival irritation, increased appetite, dry mouth, tachycardia		(Lasts12 h–30 d) Irritability, anger, anxiety, sleep difficulties, decreased appetite, restlessness, depressed mood, flu-like symptoms, anorexia, sweating, nausea, vomiting, diarrhea
4. Hallucinogens Phencyclidine (PCP) LSD, Peyote, Ecstasy, K2	Severe behavioral, psychological, and legal effects (violence, psychosis, hospitalization), cravings and tolerance, disruptions in occupational role functioning	Phencyclidine (PCP) – low dose: intoxication, unsteady gait, slurred speech; high dose: seizure, coma, paranoia, psychosis, suicidal and aggressive behavior; nystagmus, hypertension, tachycardia, lowered response to pain, ataxia, dysarthria, muscle rigidity		K2 withdrawal can be acute and require hospitalization. Agitation, cravings, sweating, nausea, tremors, hypertension, tachycardia, headaches

Substance		Effects	Withdrawal
	Use is continued despite risks and hazards.	Ecstasy—increases body temperature during physical exertion, leading to hyperthermia and excessive water consumption	Sleep disturbance, nausea, tremors, and irritability, all lasting several days
	Cravings and tolerance, disruptions in occupational role functioning	K2—tachycardia, hypertension, heart attacks, nausea and vomiting, electrolyte abnormalities, seizures, syncope (fainting), inadvertent overdose because of unregulated higher substance concentration	
	Use is continued despite risks and hazards.		
5. Inhalants Many ordinary substances, which are toxic, can be abused with significant medical/psychological effects.	Cravings and tolerance, disruptions in occupational role functioning	Increase in dopamine production increases cravings and drug consumption. Immediate high that lasts up to 15 min. Pleasurable experiences and grandiosity reported. High-risk behaviors including crime, disinhibition, dizziness, nystagmus, incoordination, slurred speech, unsteady gait, lethargy, depressed reflexes, psychomotor retardation, muscle weakness, blurred vision, coma	
	Use is continued despite risks and hazards.		
	Depression, suicide, impaired memory and learning		
6. Opioids (stimulants) Heroin, and the following medicinal drugs, which are used without supervision and/or obtained illicitly: analgesics, anesthetics, cough suppressants, methadone, Vicodin, OxyContin	Cravings and tolerance, disruptions in occupational role functioning	When not used for pain management, blissful euphoria, itchiness, nausea and vomiting; drowsiness, lethargy, cognitive changes including impaired memory and attention, hallucinations, pupil constriction, slower speech, drooling, apathy, coma, inadvertent overdose because unregulated higher substance concentration	Can last 7–10 d—increased tolerance and habituation, flu-like symptoms, sneezing, lower back pain, tactile hallucinations (ants), anorexia, depression, muscle aches, nausea/vomiting, rhinorrhea (runny nose), pupil dilation, yawning, diarrhea, fever, watery eyes, tremors, panic, cramps, insomnia
	Use is continued despite risks and hazards.		Withdrawal symptoms can be so severe and life-threatening that users continue to use.
	Depression, suicide, impaired memory and learning		

(Continued)

TABLE 16.4 Continued

Drug Class	Use D/O	Signs and Symptoms for Classes	
		Intoxication D/O	Withdrawal D/O
7. Sedatives, hypnotics, and anxiolytics Benzodiazepines (Valium, Librium, Xanax, Ativan, Halcion, Klonopin, Dalmane, Restoril)	Even though prescribed for chronic conditions, such as anxiety and insomnia, but drugs build tolerance that creates potential for substance use disorder, including slowed respiration and drowsiness Efforts to control its use are unsuccessful even when user knows they should stop. Use interferes with occupational role functioning. Cravings occur and use is continued despite risks and hazards.	Less common than other substance-induced intoxication. Eventual overdose is possible as tolerance builds and larger amounts consumed. Suppression of respiration, slurred speech, incoordination, unsteady gait, nystagmus, impaired cognition, stupor, or coma	Anxiety attacks, lethargy, fatigue or insomnia, depersonalization, emotional lability, memory problems, seizures, and withdrawal delirium
8. Stimulants Cocaine and methamphetamine are always used illicitly. Amphetamines, bath salts		Cocaine: Tachycardia, pupillary dilation, elevated or lowered blood pressure, sweating or chills, nausea/vomiting, weight loss, psychomotor agitation or retardation, muscle weakness, impaired respiration, chest pain or arrhythmias, confusion, seizures, and coma Methamphetamine—cardiac complications, diaphoresis, dental grinding, pulmonary problems, increased energy, attention, curiosity, interest in surroundings, hypersexuality; decreased anxiety, motor dysfunction, psychosis, cognitive impairment, loss of brain tissue	Cocaine: No physical withdrawal but psychological symptoms can last a number of months: apathy, extreme fatigue, increased appetite, hypersomnia, disorientation, depression, strong cravings Methamphetamine (can last for a year or more)—hospitalization required to manage psychosis, depression, suicidal ideation, irritability, hypersomnia, increased appetite, cravings, aggression, paranoia, anxiety

9. Tobacco Nicotine is a stimulant.	Physically addicting and habituating. Habits become linked with daily activities. Associated with many pleasant social effects.	Not considered intoxicating but can be toxic if consumed in large amounts	Irritability, anger, anxiety, decreased concentration, increased appetite, restlessness, depression, insomnia, symptoms can last for months after stopping.
10. Other substances and nonsubstances Gambling	Persistent gambling despite its causing distress and dysfunction, attempts to hide the problem, unsuccessful attempts to control the behavior, spending and borrowing of larger amounts of money, negative impacts relationships and occupational roles		

From American Psychiatric Association (APA). (2013). Substance-related and addictive disorders. In *Diagnostic and statistical manual of mental disorders* (5th ed.). Author. doi: 10.1176/appi.books.9780890425596.249120

relationships; leisure and recreational activities not developed or given up; and continued use despite its physical and legal risks and its negative effect on the body and mind (APA, 2013). The signs and symptoms for alcohol intoxication include recent consumption of alcohol followed by inappropriate sexual or aggressive behavior, mood lability, impaired judgment, slurred speech, incoordination, unsteady gait, nystagmus or involuntary eye movement, impaired attention or memory, or stupor or coma. The signs and symptoms of alcohol withdrawal include stopping consumption of alcohol after a prolonged and heavy use, and within several hours or days of cessation, a person experiences autonomic hyperactivity or sweating and increased pulse rate; hand tremors; insomnia; nausea or vomiting; transient visual, tactile, or auditory hallucinations; psychomotor agitation; anxiety; or generalized tonic-clonic seizures (loss of consciousness, stiffness of muscles, and jerking movements) (APA, 2013). Mild degrees of withdrawal symptoms are common and are usually managed in the community without medical interventions. In approximately 5% of people with chronic alcohol use disorders who terminate their drinking, the condition of **delirium tremens (DTs)** develops, which consists of seizures, hallucinations, and severe tremors, which can lead to death. Alcohol withdrawal can produce life-threatening symptoms such as DTs, and the protocol is currently to admit these patients with moderate and severe withdrawal

symptoms to the hospital (Elliott, Geyer, Lionetti & Doty, 2012).

Alcohol use has been analyzed by the amount of substances consumed by males and females (NIAAA, 2010) (see Table 16.5). The amount of alcohol consumed has also been standardized by NIAAA and defined as one unit or standard drink. One standard drink consists of 0.5 to 0.6 fluid ounces or 1.2 tablespoons of absolute ethanol (see Table 16.6).

The vast and changing numbers of abused drugs make its classification more complex than that of alcohol use. Rather than being categorized by amounts and patterns of consumption, drug use is categorized by classes of drugs and whether they are prescription or nonprescription drugs (Sells et al., 2011). Classifications of drugs also change as new drugs are created and their trends of usage shift. In the late 1970s, the United States experienced a peak in drug use that was followed by a national decline in the 1980s. After an increase in the 1990s, the use has been relatively stable for the last two decades. While Ecstasy, considered a club drug, reached its popularity in the 1990s, it was surpassed by oxycodone, a painkiller, in the last decade (SAMHSA, 2014). Figure 16.5 shows a comparison of drug use worldwide.

■ Caffeine

Caffeine is the most commonly consumed mind-altering substance globally. OTs are rarely involved in the treatment of this disorder, except

TABLE 16.5 Drinking Types by Gender

Type of Drinker	Low risk	At risk
Male drinker (younger than 65)	No more than 4 drinks/d No more than 14 drinks/week	5 drinks or more per day 15 drinks or more per week Harmful side effects: Injuries, coronary heart disease and other health problems, alcohol use disorders
Female drinker	No more than 3 drinks/d No more than 7 drinks/week	4 drinks or more per day 8 drinks or more per week Harmful side effects: Injuries, birth defects, fetal alcohol syndrome, coronary heart disease and other health problems, alcohol use disorders

From National Institute on Alcohol Abuse and Alcoholism (NIAAA). (2010). *Rethinking drinking: Alcohol and your health.* Bethesda, MD: Author. Retrieved from http://rethinkingdrinking.niaaa.nih.gov/ NIH Publication No. 13–3770 on June 27, 2015

TABLE **16.6** A Standard Drink	
A Standard Drink	
One Standard Unit or Standard Drink 0.5 or 0.6 absolute ethanol	Different Drink Equivalents 12 oz of beer or wine cooler 8–9 oz of malt liquor 5 oz of table wine 3–4 oz of fortified wine (port, sherry) 2–3 oz of cordial, liqueur, aperitif 1.5 oz of spirits (whiskey, gin, vodka)

Adapted from National Institute on Alcohol Abuse and Alcoholism. (n.d.). *"What is a standard drink?"* Retrieved from http://pubs.niaaa.nih.gov/publications/Practitioner/pocketguide/pocket_guide2.htm on August 21, 2015.

to assist clients to find alternative activities that produce desired positive outcomes. For example, an OT may help a client learn how to socialize without drinking coffee if a client is experiencing negative side effects. Although research is beginning to document its health benefits, there are still people who experience adverse reactions and cannot stop using it, as with other addictive substances (Higdon & Frei, 2006; Juliano & Roland, 2004). There is no caffeine use disorder because that would include an inordinate number of people. The signs and symptoms for caffeine intoxication include restlessness, nervousness, excitement, insomnia, flushed face, diuresis, gastrointestinal disturbance, muscle twitching, disorganized thinking or speech, cardiac rhythm changes, excessive energy, and psychomotor retardation (APA, 2013).

The symptoms of caffeine withdrawal must take place within 24 hours of the last caffeine intake and include headache, difficulty concentrating, fatigue, depressed mood, and flu-like symptoms. The signs and symptoms of caffeine intoxication disorder and caffeine withdrawal disorder are summarized in Table 16.4.

■ Cannabis

The most commonly used illicit drug, cannabis (Fig. 16.6), also called weed, pot, ganja, and a large number of other slang terms, is made from the shredded leaves and flowers of *Cannabis sativa*, which is a hemp plant (SAMHSA, 2014). In 2013, marijuana was used by 81% of current illicit drug users and the only drug used by 64.7% of them. A number of states are legalizing

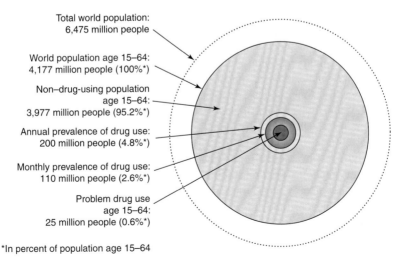

Total world population:
6,475 million people

World population age 15–64:
4,177 million people (100%*)

Non–drug-using population
age 15–64:
3,977 million people (95.2%*)

Annual prevalence of drug use:
200 million people (4.8%*)

Monthly prevalence of drug use:
110 million people (2.6%*)

Problem drug use
age 15–64:
25 million people (0.6%*)

*In percent of population age 15–64

Figure 16.5 Comparison of drug use worldwide. (From Ries, R. K., Fiellin, D. A., Miller, S. C., & Saitz, R. (2014). *The ASAM principles of addiction medicine* (5th ed.). Philadelphia, PA: Lippincott Williams & Wilkins.)

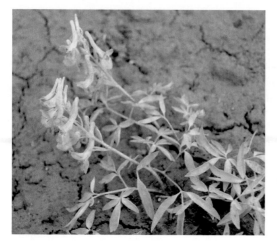

Figure 16.6 Picture of marijuana plant. (From Ries, R. K., Fiellin, D. A., Miller, S. C., & Saitz, R. (2014). *The ASAM principles of addiction medicine* (5th ed.). Philadelphia, PA: Lippincott Williams & Wilkins.)

marijuana for medicinal and recreational purposes, which means that its use is gaining greater acceptance in American society. Its therapeutic benefits, as well as its adverse health effects, are still being researched. It is smoked in the form of rolled cigarette joints, water pipes, and marijuana cigars, brewed in tea, mixed into foods when dispensed for medicinal purposes, and served as concentrated resins. The mind-altering or psychoactive chemical in cannabis is delta-9-tetrahydrocannabinol (THC). THC is similar to cannabinoid neurotransmitters that occur in the body and activate the following areas of the brain: hippocampus and orbitofrontal cortex, which are responsible for forming new memories and learning complex new tasks; the cerebellum and the basal ganglia, which regulate balance, posture, coordination, and reaction time; and the body's dopamine reward system, which contributes to the pleasurable "high" sought by recreational users (NIDA, 2015b).

Pleasant experiences with cannabis are not universal. Instead of euphoria and relaxation, some users experience anxiety, fear, distrust, panic, hallucinations, delusions, and a loss of a sense of personal identity (NIDA, 2015b). These adverse reactions often occur when an excessive amount is taken, the user is inexperienced, or the potency is high. Over the past three decades, the potency of marijuana is increasing, rising from 3.7% in the 1990s to 9.6% in 2013. These

levels have been established from THC content in confiscated cannabis samples (NIDA, 2015b). There is some research that demonstrates a link between cannabis use and psychotic disorders such as schizophrenia if there is a preexisting genetic vulnerability. There are also studies that show marijuana use can exacerbate symptoms in people who have already been diagnosed with schizophrenia (Radhakrishnan, Wilkinson, & D'Souza, 2014). Because cannabis use impairs judgment, motor coordination, and reaction time, research has established a connection between its use and problems with driving accidents, including fatal ones (NIDA, 2015b). There is also evidence that marijuana can be addictive; about 9% of people who use it cannot stop using it even though it interferes with many occupational roles and areas. There is also growing evidence that marijuana use during development can cause permanent adverse changes in the brain, which has implications for its use during pregnancy on the developing fetus and during adolescence when there is a potential loss of IQ on intelligence tests and the development of learning problems (NIDA, 2015b). The physical effects of cannabis use include breathing problems and increased heart rate (NIDA, 2015a). The signs and symptoms of cannabis use disorder, cannabis intoxication disorder, and cannabis withdrawal disorder are summarized in Table 16.4.

■ Hallucinogens

Hallucinogens are taken by the user to escape. These drugs are found in plants and mushroom and have been used in religious ceremonies for centuries. Their chemical structure is similar to neurotransmitters such as acetylcholine and serotonin (NIDA, 2014b). Some of the general effects of this class include hallucinations, depersonalization/derealization, distortions of time and perception, mood swings, elevated body temperatures, and seizures. Lysergic acid diethylamide (LSD) is one of the most powerful hallucinogens and was discovered in 1938. LSD is not considered to be an addictive drug because although it produces tolerance, it usually does not result in compulsive drug-seeking behavior. Unlike most other drugs and because there is so much variation in their composition, hallucinogens have an unpredictable and therefore dangerous effect on individuals. The fact that this class of drugs is produced in laboratories and is readily available contributes to its variability. Although PCP developed a bad reputation as a street drug in the 1960s due to its adverse reactions during intoxication (violence and suicidality), people still abuse it because it causes intense feelings of strength, power, invulnerability, and numbing of the mind (NIDA, 2014b).

More recently, the hallucinogen or synthetic cannabinoid, K2, which is marketed as fake marijuana, potpourri, or herbal high, has been gaining in popularity because users believe it is natural and safer than other drugs. It is, however, not natural and has been created in laboratories and never meant for human ingestion. It is sold cheaply in small colorful packages with comical characters, meant to appeal to youth, and is easily available in tobacco and smoke shops. K2 contains a mixture of herbs that have been laced with psychoactive chemicals. While the Federal Government has classified some of the synthetic cannabinoids as illegal to sell, laboratories quickly change the formula to avoid these banned substances and sell them as potpourri, labeled as not meant for consumption. Standard urine toxicology tests cannot detect K2. It is thought to stay in the body for prolonged periods of time and to have a similar chemical structure as carcinogens, which are cancer-causing substances (NIDA, 2012a).

The risk of overdose with K2 is high because the amount of psychoactive agents varies within each batch. The length of its effect varies from 30 minutes to 2 hours. It causes the following signs and symptoms, including euphoria and relaxation, perceptual and sensory distortions, hallucinations, poor concentration, drowsiness, confusion and agitation, difficulty forming thoughts, loss of motivation, no concern for the future, emotional lability, aggression, depression, anxiety, paranoia, headaches, tachycardia, hypertension, heart attacks, nausea and vomiting, electrolyte abnormalities, seizures, and syncope (fainting) (NIDA, 2012a). Withdrawal can take 6 hours or longer and may require hospitalization. The signs and symptoms of hallucinogen use disorder, hallucinogen intoxication disorder, and hallucinogen withdrawal disorder are summarized in Table 16.4.

Hallucinogens have the potential for long-term cognitive damage. Although most people experiment with this class of drugs and are deterred from further use by the negative consequences after a few times, other people use them heavily for a longer period of time and develop hallucinogen persisting perception disorder. Diagnostic criteria include persistent perceptual changes, sometimes described as flashbacks, memory loss, depression, loss of speech, thinking problems, weight loss, and liver malfunction (APA, 2013).

■ Inhalants

Inhalants are chemical vapors or gases that when inhaled cause psychoactive effects. These include a broad range of volatile solvents and gas products (e.g., airplane glue, paint thinner, nail polish remover), aerosols (e.g., hairspray), anesthetics (e.g., nitrous oxide), and nitrites (e.g., poppers, room odorizers). Inhalants are abused by inhaling either through the nose or through the open mouth (SAMSHA, 2003). Because of their easy availability due to the difficulty of restriction of use of legal, inexpensive, everyday substances, inhalants have become popular with teens. Because the inhalants are so readily available, many young people do not consider them harmful or understand their negative consequences. While teens more frequently inhale glue and lighter fluid, adults inhale nitrous oxide and room odorizers. Lifetime prevalence by gender and race is higher for Caucasian males (8.9%) and females (9.8%) than for Black males (5%) and females (6.8%) (SAMSHA, 2003). People who abuse inhalants seek treatment in emergency rooms rather than treatment in hospitals. Signs of inhalant use include redness or sores around the mouth or nose, chemical breath odor, dizzy appearance, excess salivation, and unexplainable collection of inhalable substances. Even with first use, lethal and debilitating effects can occur including sudden death, cardiac effects, coma, seizures, brain damage, and lead poisoning (SAMSHA, 2003). With longer term use, there is evidence of neurological damage causing decreased concentration, memory impairment, and learning difficulties, but the research has not established if these changes are transitory or long term (SAMSHA, 2003). The signs and symptoms of inhalant use disorder, inhalant intoxication disorder, and inhalant withdrawal disorder are summarized in Table 16.4.

■ Opioids

Opioids include narcotics, which were developed to block or reduce pain and produce drowsiness for legitimate medical procedures. Users of nonprescribed opioids seek withdrawal and relaxation, and they typically have a low tolerance for pain, anxiety, and stimulus thresholds. There are illicit opioids, such as heroin, and other substances that are prescription drugs prescribed for cough suppressants or for relief of pain or sensation (analgesics and anesthetics) that are used for nonmedical purposes (Bonder, 2015). Most people begin with using prescriptions for controlling pain but change to nonprescription use or heroin because of lower costs and lack of availability of prescribed medication (Rabin, 2014). Although heroin use is less frequent than that of the prescription medications, it has extremely serious health and addictive consequences. Heroin is an opioid made from morphine extracted from the poppy plant. Heroin can be consumed by injection, snorting or sniffing, or smoked. These three methods rapidly deliver the drug to the brain, which results in changes in the brain and addiction whereby uncontrollable cravings occur heedless of consequences. The opioid binds with opioid receptors in the brain and body, which are involved in the perception of pain and reward, as well as in the brainstem, which is responsible for controlling blood pressure, arousal, and respiration (NIDA, 2014d). Overdose with heroin often results from the suppression of breathing, which results in hypoxia in the brain (loss of oxygen) that can have serious psychological and neurological effects. Research has demonstrated destruction of the brain's white matter after heroin use, which may impair decision making, emotional regulation, and ability to manage stress (NIDA, 2014a, 2014d). There are a number of serious health problems caused by heroin use, including fatal overdose, pneumonia, irreversible damage to vital organs (lungs, liver, kidney, brain), spontaneous abortion, HIV, hepatitis, collapsed veins, heart lining and valve infections, abscesses, constipation, stomach cramps, and liver or kidney disease (NIDA, 2014d). The signs and symptoms of opioid use disorder, opioid intoxication disorder, and opioid withdrawal disorder are summarized in Table 16.4.

CNS Depressants

Sedatives, hypnotics, and anxiolytics are drugs that decrease activity in the brain and are therefore termed CNS depressants (NIDA, 2014e). CNS depressants are used as medications to treat anxiety and sleep disorders. These medications include benzodiazepines (Valium, Xanax, Halcion, Restoril, and ProSom), which are used for short- but not long-term treatment of anxiety or sleep because of their risk for developing tolerance and addiction. This class also includes nonbenzodiazepine sleep medications (Ambien, Lunesta, and Sonata), which are thought to have fewer side effects and less risk of developing addiction than do the benzodiazepines. The last class of CNS depressants is the barbiturates (Mebaral, Luminal Sodium, and Nembutal), which are used in surgery, have a higher risk of overdose, and therefore are not used for sleep or anxiety problems (NIDA, 2014e). The CNS depressants increase the neurotransmitter gamma-aminobutyric acid (GABA) neural activity, which has an inhibitory effect on the brain, resulting in a drowsy or a calming effect.

There are two patterns of developing substance use disorders with this class of drugs. First, the drugs are prescribed for a specific purpose and the person develops tolerance and cravings over time, or second, the person obtains the drugs illegally and they are not used in a prescribed fashion (Bonder, 2015). When a person stops taking CNS depressants, the body can experience a rebound effect, including seizures. While withdrawal from benzodiazepines is not life threatening, it can be with barbiturates. Stopping CNS depressants and combining CNS depressants with other medications should be closely monitored (NIDA, 2014e). The signs and symptoms of sedatives, hypnotics, and anxiolytics use disorder; sedatives, hypnotics, and anxiolytics intoxication disorder; and sedatives, hypnotics, and anxiolytics withdrawal disorder are summarized in Table 16.4.

Stimulants

Stimulants involved in substance use disorders consist of amphetamines and cocaine (NIDA, 2013). Amphetamines can be prescribed for the treatment of ADHD; methamphetamine and cocaine are never prescribed and always used illicitly (Bonder, 2015). Cocaine is an addictive stimulant derived from the coca plant. In a powdered form, it is either inhaled through the nose (snorted) or mixed with water and injected. Crack is the crystallized form of cocaine that is heated to form vapors that are smoked. Injecting or smoking cocaine produces a more intense, but shorter-lasting, sensation than does snorting. To extend the length of the high, people often binge, taking bigger doses over a short period of time (NIDA, 2013). Cocaine increases the level of dopamine in the synapses in the brain, which amplifies its effects, causing the "high." The other bodily systems affected by cocaine include blood vessels, body temperature, gastrointestinal problems, strokes, heart attacks, death, and risk for contracting HIV through risky sexual behavior. Snorting leads to loss of a sense of smell, nosebleeds, swallowing problems, and runny nose. Injecting cocaine can lead to increased risk for contracting HIV, hepatitis C, and other blood-borne illnesses. Cocaine binging can lead to severe paranoia. When combined with other drugs or alcohol (polydrug use), cocaine poses a high risk for a serious overdose (NIDA, 2013). The signs and symptoms of stimulant use disorder, stimulant intoxication disorder, and stimulant withdrawal disorder are summarized in Table 16.4.

■ Tobacco

Tobacco is a stimulant and causes one in every five deaths in the United States, serious illnesses attributable to smoking for 16 million Americans, and the deaths of 41,000 nonsmokers from second-hand smoke each year (NIDA, 2014c). Nicotine is the stimulant, which is smoked, chewed, or inhaled. Nicotine stimulates the adrenal gland, which releases the hormone epinephrine. This stimulates the CNS, increasing respiration, blood pressure, and heart rate. Nicotine also stimulates the production of dopamine. Cigarette smoking, which is a mixture of many chemicals that are carcinogenic, causes 90% of lung cancer cases in the United States (NIDA, 2014c). Other medical complications include oral cancers, emphysema, heart disease, leukemia, cataracts, and pneumonia. On average, people who are smokers shorten their lifespan by 10 years. Smoking by pregnant women and maternal smoking is associated with increased risks of miscarriage, stillborn, premature infants, and learning and behavioral problems in older children (NIDA, 2014c). If a person quits smoking, there are immediate positive health consequences, including reduced risk of heart disease, cancer, and stroke. The signs and symptoms of tobacco use disorder and tobacco withdrawal disorder are summarized in Table 16.4. There is no category of tobacco intoxication disorder (APA, 2013).

■ Gambling

Gambling, a non–substance-related disorder, shares many of the same criteria as do substance-related disorders even though it does not involve ingestion of a substance. The signs and symptoms include impulsivity, unsuccessful attempts to cut down, preoccupation with spending time gambling, a return to gambling even after significant losses, attempts to conceal a gambling habit from others, negative impacts on relationships and job functioning, and persistent participation in gambling despite financial risks (APA, 2013). The signs and symptoms of gambling use disorder are summarized in Table 16.4.

COURSE AND PROGNOSIS

■ Alcohol

Although it is thought to be an intractable condition, only a small percentage of longtime chronic users will experience serious psychological and physical problems including liver damage, cognitive impairment, peripheral neuropathy, cardiomyopathy, stroke, sleep disorders, pancreatitis, cancer, injuries, drowning, homicide, suicide, fatal falls and/or burns, domestic violence, sexual assaults, motor vehicle crashes, depression, homelessness, unemployment, social isolation and loss of contact with family, and incarceration. Those who use both alcohol and drugs have a poorer outcome (Bonder, 2015; NIAAA, 2010). Unsafe use of alcohol and drugs is associated with increased levels of violence and conflict, and the presence of conflict increases the risky consumption of alcohol and drugs (World Health Organization, 2008).

Most people with this disorder have a more auspicious prognosis and improve (see Fig. 16.7). They may benefit from four types of evidence-based treatments, including brief interventions, cognitive-behavioral therapy, motivation interviewing, and 12-step programs (Stoffel & Moyers, 2004). Prognostic factors include cultural attitudes toward drinking, availability and price of alcohol, stress levels and impaired ways of coping with stress, heavy peer pressure regarding substance use, and cognitive distortions, which exaggerate the positive effects of alcohol (APA, 2013; see Fig. 16.8).

In adolescents, alcohol use disorder is often comorbid with conduct disorder. Ninety percent of individuals develop alcohol use disorder before the age of 40. The 10% of older adults who become chronic users develop more severe intoxication with lower levels of consumption and develop other medical complications (APA, 2013; Adams et al., 1996). Fetal alcohol spectrum

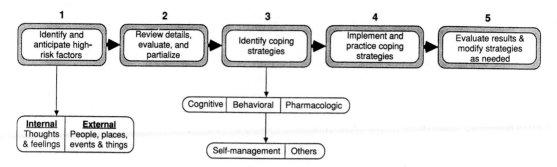

Figure 16.7 Managing addiction. (From Lowinson, J. H., Ruiz, P., Millman, R. B., & Langrod, J. G. (2004). *Substance abuse.* Philadelphia, PA: Lippincott Williams & Wilkins.)

disorders (FASDs) are the physical, mental, behavioral, and learning disorders that occur in an individual whose mother consumed alcohol during pregnancy. It occurs in approximately 1% of the live birth population in the United States (SAMSHA, 2007). Alcohol damages the developing fetus more than do other substances that are used illicitly. FASDs are the most preventable cause of developmental disabilities in children.

Most individuals with FASD do not have the facial features associated with this illness (short palpebral fissures, indistinct philtrum, and thin upper lip). The extent of the disorder depends on when and how much alcohol the mother consumed during the pregnancy. The behavioral outcomes can include poor judgment and impulsivity, depression, and substance and alcohol abuse (SAMSHA, 2007).

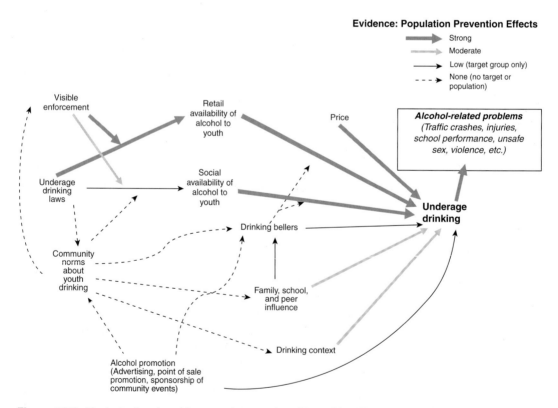

Figure 16.8 Alcohol-related problems and prevention. (From Ries, R. K., Fiellin, D. A., Miller, S. C., & Saitz, R. (2014). *The ASAM principles of addiction medicine* (5th ed.). Philadelphia, PA: Lippincott Williams & Wilkins.)

■ Caffeine

Because the half-life of caffeine is approximately 4 to 6 hours, the symptoms of caffeine intoxication and withdrawal are short-lived and do not present with long-term consequences. There are several exceptions to this benign description of its course: if a person consumes more than 5 grams of caffeine at one time, he or she will require immediate medical attention; older adults grow more sensitive to the intense effects of caffeine and complain about increased sleeplessness and restlessness; children and adolescents with low body weight may be at increased risk for caffeine intoxication, especially if they are consuming caffeine drinks, such as soft drinks and energy drinks (APA, 2013).

■ Cannabis

The development of cannabis use disorder most commonly occurs during adolescence and early adulthood. Early onset of use of cannabis before the age of 15 is considered a serious risk factor for future externalizing and internalizing mental health disorders, including depression and conduct disorders (APA, 2013). In adolescence, the onset of the disorder is usually gradual. Cannabis, along with tobacco and alcohol, are generally the first substances tried by adolescents with cannabis used more often than alcohol because its behavioral and cognitive consequences are considered less harmful. This may explain the rapid transition from cannabis use to cannabis use disorder. While milder cases of cannabis use disorder among teenagers arouse disapproval by peers, parents, and school staff, severe cases result in more solitary and daily consumption that is hidden from others leading to mood, energy level, and appetite changes and serious impairment in school functioning, including drop in grades, truancy, loss of interest in previous activities, and deficits in prosocial behaviors. Adults diagnosed with cannabis use disorder involve patterns of daily consumption, medical and psychosocial problems, and unsuccessful attempts to stop using (Volkow et al., 2014; APA, 2013; Cousijn et al., 2012; D'Souza, Sewell, & Ranganathan, 2009).

■ Hallucinogens

When phencyclidine (PCP) is the primary drug used among those admitted to substance use treatment settings, the patients are younger, have lower educational levels, and tend to be from the two coastal regions of the United States (APA, 2013). The continual use of PCP is associated with high risk of injuries from fights, falls, and other accidents as well as suicide; psychosis; intense rage; deficits in memory, language, and cognition; neurological and cardiovascular toxicities; intracranial hemorrhage; and, rarely, cardiac arrest (APA, 2013). Early-onset Ecstasy users are more likely to be polydrug users than those who begin using this hallucinogen later (APA, 2013). With other hallucinogens, the course is usually associated with experimentation, limited use, and high rates of recovery (APA, 2013).

■ Inhalants

Inhalant use generally declines after adolescence and diminishes in early adulthood (APA, 2013). While 10% of American children 13 to 17 years old report the use of inhalants one time, <0.5% of the same age group progress to inhalant use disorder and exhibit multiple mental health problems, including personality disorders and suicidal ideation and attempts (APA, 2013).

■ Opioids

Most problems associated with opioid use disorder are reported in late adolescence and early adulthood. The typical course of use of opioids persists for many years, punctuated by periods of remission. Successful treatment and abstinence is often followed by relapse. While 20% to 30% of opioid users achieve long-term abstinence, the mortality rates for long-term users may be as high as 2% per year (see Fig.16.9). Increasing age is associated with decreased prevalence due to early mortality rates and a diminution of symptoms after age 40. Ninety percent of Vietnam veterans were successfully treated for opioid use disorder after deployment, but these veterans also developed alcohol use and amphetamine use disorders and suicidality (APA, 2013).

■ CNS Depressants

Use of sedatives, hypnotics, and anxiolytics generally begins in adolescence and early adulthood when some individuals use these types of substances to achieve a "high" (APA, 2013). There are two courses that sedative, hypnotic, and anxiolytic use disorders generally follow. The most common course is where individuals who are often using other substances such as alcohol,

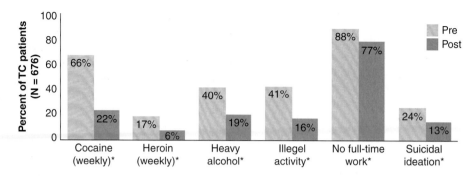

Figure 16.9 Evidence of improvement with treatment. (From Ries, R. K., Fiellin, D. A., Miller, S. C., & Saitz, R. (2014). *The ASAM principles of addiction medicine* (5th ed.). Philadelphia, PA: Lippincott Williams & Wilkins.)

opioids, and stimulants escalate occasional use of these substances especially in social situations like parties until they meet criteria for diagnosis. In this situation, there are long-term cognitive and interpersonal difficulties as well as severe withdrawal symptoms. A less common course is where individuals in their 40s who have been prescribed sedatives, hypnotics, or anxiolytics by a medical provider for anxiety, insomnia, or somatic complaints experience tolerance and self-administer higher doses until they meet criteria for diagnosis. These individuals will often seek prescriptions from several providers. As individuals age, the use of sedatives, hypnotics, and anxiolytics poses greater risks, both in terms of motor coordination and cognitive deficits and the metabolism of substances. Individuals with neurocognitive disorders such as dementia are more likely to experience intoxication and toxic side effects at lower dosages (APA, 2013).

Stimulants

Stimulant use disorders are more common in young people ages 12 to 25 than in those over 26 years old (APA, 2013). Methamphetamines are often prescribed to control weight gain, treat attention deficit disorder, and improve school, work, or athletic performance. Some individuals will begin by using medications prescribed for others. Patterns of use can be daily or episodic. In addition, there are binges where individuals consume these substances for hours and days until their supply is depleted. When amphetamine-type stimulants are taken orally and cocaine is administered

intranasally, there is a more gradual course established over months and years compared to stimulant smoking and intravenous use, which results in a rapid progression to a severe stimulant use disorder. As people use more stimulants, there is a decrease in pleasure and increase in dysphoria (APA, 2013).

Tobacco

Most adolescents in the United States experiment with tobacco, and by age 20, 20% of them become daily users (APA, 2013). It is rare for people over 21 to initiate smoking. The symptoms of tobacco use disorder appear quickly after tobacco is consumed. About 80% of individuals with this disorder attempt to stop, but 60% resume and only 5% achieve abstinence. Most people do not achieve abstinence until after age 30 (APA, 2013).

Gambling

Gambling use disorders develop gradually over many years and at earlier ages in males compared to females (APA, 2013). Females with gambling use disorder are more likely than males to have comorbid depressive, bipolar, and anxiety disorders and to seek treatment. Most individuals with this disorder report problems with one to two different types of gambling but with more trouble with one type than the other. The frequency and the amount of money involved do not determine the severity of the gambling use disorder. Some people can gamble large amounts of money once a month and not have a gambling use disorder, while others who wager small amounts on a daily basis meet criteria for this disorder. Gambling can increase in response to stress, depression, substance use, or abstinence. The course may follow periods of heavy gambling and serious problems, total abstinence, and sometimes nonproblematic gambling, which may lead to a false sense of invulnerability (APA, 2013).

DIAGNOSIS

Substance-related disorders are divided into substance use disorders and substance-induced disorders. The diagnosis of substance use disorders is based on an atypical configuration of behavior that stems from the use of a substance. Criteria A described in DSM-5 pinpoint the four types of behavior necessary in order to make a substance use diagnosis: impaired control, social impairment, risky use, and pharmacological criteria. Two examples that cause significant distress or impaired functioning must be present within a 12-month period (APA, 2013). These key characteristics were defined and explained earlier in the chapter. Pharmacological criteria include not only behaviors associated with tolerance but also physiological changes that are detected by laboratory tests, for example, high blood levels of the substance occurring with little evidence of intoxication. Withdrawal is also diagnosed with a combination of history and laboratory tests. The physiological signs of withdrawal are easily measured for the following substances, alcohol, opioids and sedatives, hypnotics, and anxiolytics, whereas the laboratory detection of withdrawal for the stimulants, tobacco, and cannabis is less obvious. The behavioral and physiological signs of withdrawal from PCP, other hallucinogens, and inhalants are not detectable (APA, 2013). DSM-5 also includes a number of specifiers to diagnose these disorders with greater precision. These specifiers consist of severity of use (mild, moderate, severe), level of remission (early, sustained, maintenance, controlled environment), use of more than one substance at a time, presence of other mental disorders, and presence or absence of perceptual disturbances (APA, 2013).

The criteria for diagnosing substance-induced disorders are divided separately into the characteristics for intoxication and for withdrawal, which are included within the descriptions of the 10 classes of substances in DSM-5. Intoxication is diagnosed based on the following criteria.

Criterion A describes a reversible substance-specific syndrome caused by the ingestion of the substance. Criterion B specifies the behavioral and psychological changes that occur with intoxication. Criterion D specifies that the signs and symptoms are not attributable to another medical or psychiatric condition. Withdrawal is diagnosed based on the following criteria. Criterion A identifies the key behavioral, psychological, physiological, and cognitive characteristics that result from the cessation or reduction in heavy use of a substance. Criterion B highlights the key functional areas of distress and impairment that occur as a result of withdrawal. Criterion D specifies that the signs and symptoms are not attributable to another medical or psychiatric condition (APA, 2013).

MEDICAL/SURGICAL MANAGEMENT

Evidence-based intervention strongly suggests the combined use of medications and psychosocial support (Fig. 16.10) for the most effective treatment of substance-related disorders (Stoffel & Moyers, 2004). Medications are primarily used for the following substance-related disorders: alcohol, opioid, and tobacco. There is often a pattern where the use of medications for these disorders competes with the use of the abused substance to block or diminish its effect (Paxos & Dugan, 2015).

■ Alcohol

The four FDA-approved medications for alcohol-related disorders are acamprosate (Campral), disulfiram (Antabuse), oral naltrexone (ReVia), and extended-release injection naltrexone (Vivitrol), but only a small percentage of US residents take these medications (SAMSHA, 2010). They are prescribed to enable a client to be abstinent, not as a means to taper the withdrawal from alcohol. The abrupt cessation of alcohol ingestion by a client who has been a heavy user can have very serious health consequences, including seizures and neurological injury.

Acamprosate is given to clients who are seeking complete abstinence and are currently not using to help decrease cravings and reduce other uncomfortable symptoms, including insomnia, restlessness, and mood changes, which might cause a relapse (NIAAA, 2005b). It requires the client to take 2 to 3 pills a day for an extended period. The side effects are generally mild, except

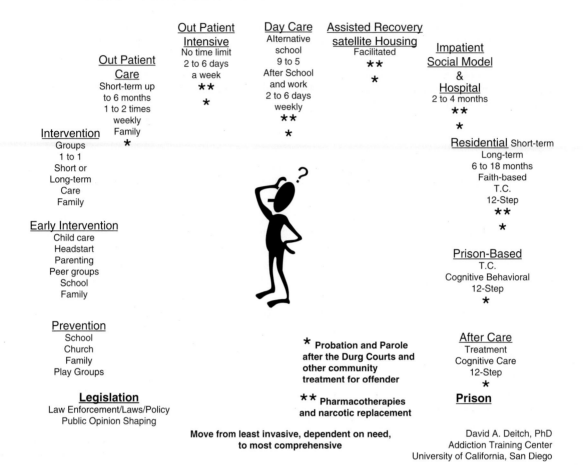

Figure 16.10 Continuum of Care Model. (From Lowinson, J. H., Ruiz, P., Millman, R. B., & Langrod, J. G. (2004). *Substance abuse.* Philadelphia, PA: Lippincott Williams & Wilkins.)

when a person first starts taking this medication, at which time there can be acute side effects, including diarrhea, nausea, anxiety, and depression, which may entail suicidal ideation or attempts that must be closely monitored (SAMHSA, 2010; Paxos & Dugan, 2015). Since it does not interfere with opioids, acamprosate is appropriate for clients who are receiving opioid maintenance therapy or taking opioids. There is also no interaction with other medications. Clients with severe kidney problems should not take this medication. Otherwise, it is a safe medication with no overdose risk and no potential for abuse and can be continued even if a person relapses and requires detoxification (SAMSHA, 2010).

Naltrexone can be taken orally or by injection. It works as an opioid antagonist (blocker) that reduces the positive effects and cravings of alcohol and is effective in individuals who have a history of opioid use but are now abstinent. It has not

been found effective in individuals using other illicit substances and should not be taken by those currently using illegal opioids or on methadone maintenance therapy (SAMHSA, 2010; Sells et al., 2011). Pills are taken orally once daily. Side effects of oral naltrexone are mild, usually subside over time, and include nausea, vomiting, headache, dizziness, fatigue, and drowsiness. Extended-release injectable naltrexone is provided once monthly. It is recommended for those who are motivated to maintain abstinence, have problems adhering to treatment regimens, and have the means to pay for its high costs. The most prominent and bothersome side effect of the injectable form is painful skin reactions at the site of the injection, which require immediate medical attention (SAMHSA, 2010).

Disulfiram has been used to treat alcohol use disorders for over 60 years. It reduces the desire to use alcohol by adversely impacting the user's metabolism and other bodily systems (Sells et al., 2011). If a person consumes alcohol while taking disulfiram, he or she will experience a toxic reaction even if the alcohol is prepared in food. The person can become sweaty, have difficulty breathing, and experience blurred vision, head and neck throbbing, confusion, vertigo or syncope, nausea, flushing, tachycardia, and restlessness. Severe reactions include life-threatening cardiac and respiratory problems, such as heart attacks, seizures, and death (SAMHSA, 2010). The reaction varies from moderate to severe in individuals, typically occurs 10 to 30 minutes after alcohol intake, and can last up to 2 weeks. Individuals taking disulfiram should carry a medical alert card indicating that they are taking it and providing emergency procedures to follow in case of a severe reaction. The drug is considered most effective if a person is trying to be abstinent or in risky drinking situations (NIAAA, 2005b). It is taken as a tablet once daily. Side effects are generally mild and usually disappear after 2 weeks and include drowsiness, a metallic taste, dermatitis, headache, and impotence (SAMHSA, 2010). There are two new promising medications for alcohol use disorders, but they are still in clinical trials, topiramate and baclofen (Sells et al., 2011).

Opioids

Medications used to treat opioid use disorders include methadone (Dolophine), a combination of buprenorphine and naloxone (Suboxone), buprenorphine (Butrans), and naloxone (Narcan). Methadone is a synthetic, long-lasting opioid, which has been used in the treatment of opioid addiction for more than 40 years. Methadone mimics the actions of opioids by binding to opiate receptors to prevent cravings and reduce the chances of relapse. This medication is controversial because it is also addictive, but it does not lead to overdose, infections, and death (Sells et al., 2011). It is usually dispensed as a premixed, colored liquid and distributed only at clinics and treatment facilities to minimize its abuse. Methadone prescriptions increased by 700% between 1998 and 2006 (Center for Substance Abuse Treatment, 2009). When methadone is used properly, it is considered very safe. Typical side effects include faintness, dizziness, nausea, vomiting, perspiring, and drowsiness. Adverse events can occur when an individual is simultaneously abusing other substances, such as benzodiazepines, other opioids,

cocaine, or alcohol, or there are interactions with other medications. Because methadone is long-lasting and is slowly released into the bloodstream from the liver and other tissues, toxicity or poisoning can occur if a patient takes methadone faster than the body can metabolize it or if the dose is increased too quickly (Center for Substance Abuse Treatment, 2009). Twelve months is considered the minimum treatment for methadone maintenance (NIDA, 2012b). The combination of buprenorphine and naloxone is also used to treat opiate addiction. Buprenorphine binds to opiate receptors to prevent highs and withdrawal symptoms, and naloxone is an opiate receptor antagonist, which blocks the opiate from binding to its receptor. Sublingual pills, which are used as tablets under the tongue, are used as maintenance therapy. Typical side effects from this combination include headache and other pain, diarrhea, rhinitis, sleeplessness, and liver damage, which must be closely monitored (Paxos & Dugan, 2015).

Tobacco

The prescription medications, varenicline (Chantix) and bupropion (Wellbutrin), are used for the treatment of tobacco addiction as well as nicotine replacement therapy (NRT) (patches, gum, lozenges, and nasal spray). Varenicline is the most recently approved medication for smoking cessation. It acts as a partial agonist/antagonist at nicotine receptors in the brain, which means that it partially stimulates the nicotine receptor but not enough to release dopamine so the person does not get pleasurable effects and decreases cravings (NIDA, 2012b). Typical side effects include nausea, constipation, flatulence, vomiting, abnormal and/or strange dreams, sleep disturbances, significant mood changes, and allergic reactions (Paxos & Dugan, 2015). Bupropion was discovered to decrease tobacco craving in patients who were depressed (NIDA, 2012b). Its most prominent side effects include dry mouth, nausea, stomach and headaches, light-headedness, ringing in the ears, decreased interest in sex, weight loss, skin rash, and sore throat. NRT provides low levels of nicotine, which prevent withdrawal symptoms that make it difficult for people to quit. Using more than one of the replacement therapies in combination has been found to be more effective (NIDA, 2012b). The patches, which are applied once a day, provide consistent levels throughout the day, while gum, lozenges, nasal spray, and inhalers deliver sporadic dosages. It is important to follow NRT protocols for maximal effect, for example, the gum must be chewed until the perception of a prickly taste and then placed in the cheek until the nicotine is absorbed. Side effects of NRT include unusual oral tastes, and if a person has a heart problem, he or she must use only low doses (Paxos & Dugan, 2015).

IMPACT ON OCCUPATIONAL PERFORMANCE

The severity level of use of the 10 classes of substances determines their impact on occupational performance. Individuals with mild use disorders probably can participate in most or all occupations. Individuals diagnosed with severe use disorders will face barriers in most or all areas of occupation. This section will summarize the common difficulties faced by users of all substances at the severe level in each occupation as well as highlight particular difficulties that accompany specific classes of substances.

■ ADLs

The primary areas of ADLs impacted by severe levels of all substance use disorders are hygiene, grooming, time management, and sexual activity (Carifio, 2014; Sells et al., 2011). The avolition characteristic of cannabis users can express itself as a decreased interest or disregard for grooming or personal hygiene. There may also be inappropriate choices of clothing for the weather or occasion. Sexual activity may be impacted and expressed as risky behavior or lowering of sexual drive or interest. Stimulant users believe they have the capacity to outperform other people in ADLs when in actuality their performance is poor (Martin, Bliven, & Boisvert, 2008).

■ IADLs

The primary IADLS impacted include communication management, driving and community mobility, health management and maintenance, medication management, financial management, and home establishment and management (Sells et al., 2011). Acute intoxication involving motor skills and reflexes can interfere with driving cars, riding bicycles, taking public transportation, and operating machinery. Doctors and clinics may be avoided to get around drug testing, and medication compliance activities may be abandoned. Complex financial and home management activities may be abandoned due to cognitive impairments and a focus on substance obtaining and using. The user's ability to provide care for others or supervise others is often compromised. Safety awareness is negatively impacted by lack of awareness of the environment. Stimulant users believe they have the capacity to outperform other people in IADLs when in actuality their performance is poor. Individuals who are using substances illicitly will often become involved in theft, prostitution, or drug dealing in order to obtain drugs or money for substances (Hoppes, Bryce, & Peloquin, 2013; Stoffel & Moyers, 2001).

■ Rest and Sleep

All three areas of this occupation (rest, sleep preparation, and sleep participation) are adversely impacted by a disrupted sleep-wake cycle, poor orientation to time, and impaired sequencing skills, which characterize most of the classes of substance use (Sells et al., 2011). Strange nightmares and insomnia often characterize this area of occupation.

■ Education and Work

Both education and work are negatively impacted by higher rates of truancy and absenteeism, tardiness, accidents, poor performance, lack of volition, and the inability to follow through with commitments. Dropping out of school and job loss and turnover often result from substance use disorders, which lead to numerous negative consequences, including financial difficulties, unstructured days that perpetuate poor self-esteem, and, in some cases, incarceration (Gutman, 2006; Hoppes et al., 2013). Employment opportunities may not be pursued due to fear of failing drug testing. Cannabis use is identified with motivational syndrome, which can affect advancement in education and work arenas.

■ Play and Leisure

Substance use disorders that develop in early adolescence interrupt typical developmental milestones in play exploration and the acquisition of leisure activities, which can aid in stress management and patterns of healthy living in adulthood. The primary focus of substance users becomes obtaining the drug and getting high. Money spent on the seeking and consuming substances is no longer available for play and leisure participation. When individuals stop using substances, they often are at a loss for how to structure their days and manage their time. When intoxicated or in withdrawal, individuals often experience anhedonia or engage in risky behaviors such as driving recklessly or participating in unprotected sexual activity (Heuchemer & Staffan, 2006; Knis-Matthews, 2003).

■ Social Participation

The inability to regulate emotions and poor orientation to person, place, time, self, and others as well as poor ADLs and IADLs often lead to impaired relationships and roles with family, friends, co-workers, peers, and community. Family members especially become angry with the users because their aberrant behavior violates trust and negatively impacts the entire family structure. For example, parents who are heavy users cannot carry out their roles (Knis-Matthews, 2003). Individuals with substance use disorders will often self-isolate because of embarrassment, fear of failing, lack of hope, slurred speech, dysphoric or apathetic mood, inability to understand what someone else says, lowered frustration, and poor judgment. During intoxication, users can become either more social or more withdrawn, while during withdrawal, mood and physiological difficulties can negatively impact social participation (Boisvert, Martin, Grosek, Clarie, 2008; Gutman, 2006; Hoppes et al., 2013; Sells et al., 2011).

Case Study 1

Case Illustration

Adolescent with Stimulant or Opioid Disorder

Donald is an 18-year-old African American adolescent male who is living in a homeless shelter in a medium-sized northeastern city. He grew up with his mother who had been addicted to heroin when he was younger, but she is now involved in a methadone maintenance program. He never knew his father. His grandmother has been a stabilizing influence in his life, and he maintains contact with her. Donald was diagnosed with ADHD in elementary school and was placed in special education classes. At age 10, he was prescribed the stimulant Adderall, an amphetamine, but living in shelters made follow-up by a psychiatrist difficult. He would get Adderall from other kids at his high school before exams and when papers were due. Donald was athletic and played on the varsity basketball team in high school. He liked to socialize with friends, and when he attended parties, he joined the crowd and smoked cannabis. He liked the relaxation that came with marijuana and began to use it on a daily basis. Since moving into the shelter, he has been experimenting with smoking K2, a hallucinogen, which he likes because it is sold as potpourri and as a natural substance and is very cheap. He can purchase it at a local tobacco store and not have to worry about getting arrested when making purchases of illicit drugs from dealers on the street. He also believes that the K2 is safer because it is sold in a package, whereas the marijuana sold on the street is unregulated and can sometimes contain toxic substances.

Donald's views about K2 changed drastically after the last time he tried it. He experienced very severe symptoms for more than an hour, including hallucinations, tachycardia, nausea and vomiting, and syncope. He was taken to the emergency room of the local hospital by the shelter staff. When he sobered up from this episode, an OTR who worked in the ER approached him about his problems with polysubstance use. She asked him what his daily schedule looked like and what his short- and long-term goals were. He said he had been a B student in school and enjoyed playing basketball and that he wanted to attend college. The OTR asked him what steps he was taking to achieve his goal. Donald said, "None, and I think I need some help." He called his grandmother and spoke to her and his mother, both of whom advised him to enroll in an inpatient program for substance use treatment. They also suggested that he try attending Narcotics Anonymous Meetings, which would provide him with daily support once he was discharged. Each of them promised to be there for him during this rough stretch. They also expressed their strong belief in him and his ability to recover from these substance-related problems.

Adult with Disabilities— Sedatives, Hypnotics, and Anxiolytics

Jose is a 50-year-old Hispanic man who has been deaf since birth. He lives by himself in an apartment in a large city in the southwestern United States. His family consists of his sister and elderly parents who live nearby. He uses sign language and reads lips in order to communicate. He was enrolled in special education in elementary and secondary school while growing up. For college, he moved away from the Southwest and attended Gallaudet University for the Deaf in Washington, DC, where he majored in political science. He loved his college experience and thrived in the deaf community. He formed lifelong friendships at Gallaudet. After graduation, he was able to obtain a job in the federal government, in the Department of Education. He worked in Washington, D.C., for 25 years, successfully supporting himself. His leisure interests included swimming and advocacy work for the deaf community. When he was in his 40s, his elderly parents became ill and he decided to return to the Southwest to help his sister care for them.

Jose did not anticipate that he would have difficulty finding a new job. The arduous job search depleted his savings and left him feeling extremely anxious and vulnerable. He consulted with his internist about his symptoms, which included insomnia and intense feelings of self-doubt and agitation during job interviews. The internist referred him to a psychiatrist who prescribed Restoril for improving his sleep and Xanax to be used when he became symptomatic before an interview. The sedative and anxiolytic medications relieved his symptoms, but he found that he needed to take more Xanax at other times besides job interviews. Whenever he was in a new situation or meeting people for the first time, he felt he performed better if he took some Xanax, which he began to self-administer in higher doses. His original psychiatrist would not prescribe additional anxiolytic medication unless Jose started therapy. Jose was not eager to be in therapy but agreed to see a therapist who knew how to communicate with people who are deaf. His sister searched the city for someone with these qualifications and could not find either a therapist or a treatment program that had expertise in working with clients who are deaf or any clients who abused substances and had a physical or sensory disability. In the meantime, Jose went to several other providers who gave him prescriptions for the sedative and anxiolytic medications.

After several years of this course, Jose noticed that he was experiencing difficulty with motor coordination, cognitive deficits, and the metabolism of the substances. His sister was especially concerned because when Jose stopped using, he experienced increased anxiety attacks, lethargy, and emotional lability. She decided to contact an old friend of Jose's from Gallaudet who was a psychiatrist, Dr. Powers. When Dr. Powers heard what was going on with her old friend, she made arrangements that he be admitted immediately to a local detox center because she was very concerned about the likelihood of seizures that can accompany sedative, hypnotic, and anxiolytic withdrawal disorders. She reassured Jose's sister that they would work together to find Jose a therapist and substance use recovery program that were specifically trained to work with clients who are deaf and living with disabilities.

ACKNOWLEDGMENTS

Kathryn Reynolds, OTS, Marcy Schlissel, OTS, Allison Schubert, OTS, and Zachary Schluger, OTS

RECOMMENDED LEARNING RESOURCES

https://medicine.wright.edu/citar/sardi

This is the SARDI Program (Substance Abuse Resources & Disability Issues). It is on the Web site of the Wright State University's Boonshoft School of Medicine. Its purpose is to improve the quality of life for people living with physical disabilities who face behavioral problems. Through participatory research, it has produced several unique programs: HIV services for people who are minorities and have physical disabilities; Deaf Off Drugs that targets the deaf community; programs for formerly incarcerated individuals who also have HIV; tobacco education and cessation programs for people with disabilities; and research resources for professionals working with people with disabilities who also have substance-related disorders.

http://www.smartrecovery.org/meetings/olschedule.htm

The SMART Program (Self Management and Recovery Training) is a free nonprofit supported outpatient treatment based on Ellis' Rational-Emotive-Behavioral Therapy. This is a form of cognitive-behavioral therapy that teaches skills for recovery. It is a form of self-help but based on scientific research rather than dependency on faith; it has been called non–12-step rehab. It includes weekly meetings, individual therapy, and the use of medications to treat substance use disorders.

Alcoholics Anonymous Online Intergroup

http://aa-intergroup.org/index.php

Online resources for the self-help approach advocated by Alcoholics Anonymous (AA), including online chat rooms, immediate assistance, a global and local directory of meetings, upcoming conferences, and AA literature.

Narcotics Anonymous Chat and Online Meetings for Drug Addicts

http://www.12stepforums.net/na

An online group with immediate 24-hour/7 days a week access for all people with drug use disorders to find support and fellowship.

Baylor College of Medicine Center for Research on Women with Disabilities

http://www.bcm.edu/crowd

Online site for the Center for Research on Women with Disabilities (CROWD) whose mission is to advance the quality of life of women with disabilities by developing and disseminating information. It is a consortium of local and national consumer advocates, medical advisors, and researchers. Some of the topics they have investigated include health behaviors (weight management, smoking cessation), access to health care, violence, and abuse.

Minnesota Chemical Dependency Program for Deaf and Hard of Hearing Individuals

http://www.mncddeaf.org

This program was started in 1989 to provide services for the deaf community who are struggling with any form of chemical dependency. They provide direct services as well as train providers to deliver specialized care to this population.

Yale–CASA National Center on Addiction and Substance Abuse

http://www.casacolumbia.org/

CASA–Columbia is teaming up with Yale University's Medical School and Public Health to form a new research, policy, and education center on addiction.

National Institute on Drug Abuse (NIDA)

http://www.drugabuse.gov/about-nida

This is the federal government's preeminent organization to fund research on addiction. Their role is to also disseminate results of research to improve prevention and intervention services as well as to inform policy makers.

National Institute on Alcohol Abuse (NIAA)

http://www.niaaa.nih.gov/

The mission of this federal government institute, which is part of NIH, is to lead the nation's efforts on clinical and basic science intramural and extramural research on alcohol addiction through grants, contracts, and cooperative agreements. NIAA coordinates research with national and international bodies. In addition, its research mission is to discover the basic science of alcohol addiction in order to establish evidence-based programs of prevention, treatment, and health services.

Substance Abuse Mental Health Services Administration (SAMHSA)

http://www.samhsa.gov/

This is the agency within the federal Department of Health and Human Services charged with the public health agenda of prioritizing the behavioral health of the US population. Its purpose is to fund and organize a national effort to reduce the impact of substance abuse and mental illness on individuals and communities by making research, information, and services more easily accessible. Its primary purpose is to facilitate recovery for these populations. Its online site is home to easily accessible and valuable evidence-based resources for consumers, families, and professionals.

REFERENCES

Adams, W. L., Barry, K. L., & Fleming, M. F. (1996). Screening for problem drinking in older primary care patients. *Journal of the American Medical Association, 276,* 1964–1967.

American Occupational Therapy Association. (2014). Occupational therapy practice framework: Domain and process (3rd ed.). *American Journal of Occupational Therapy, 68*(1), S1–S48. Retrieved from http://dx.doi.org/10.5014/ajot.2014.682006

American Psychiatric Association (APA). (2000). *Diagnostic and statistical manual of mental disorders* (4th ed., text rev.). Washington, DC: Author.

American Psychiatric Association (APA). (2013). Substance-related and addictive disorders. In *Diagnostic and statistical manual of mental disorders* (5th ed.). Author. doi: 10.1176/appi.books.9780890425596.249120

Atchinson, B. J., & Dirette, D. K. (2012). *Conditions in occupational therapy: Effect on occupational performance* (4th ed.). Philadelphia, PA: Lippincott Williams & Wilkins.

Bonder, B. R. (2015). *Substance-related and addictive disorders. Psychopathology and function* (5th ed., pp. 315–350.).Thorofare, NJ: Slack.

Boisvert, R. A., Martin, L. M., Grosek, M., Clarie, A. J. (2008). Effectiveness of a peer-support community in addiction recovery: Participation as intervention. *Occupational Therapy International, 15*(4), 205–220.

Carifio, C. M. (2014). Substance use disorders. In B.A. Boyt Schell, G. Gillen, & M. E. Scaffa (Eds.), *Willard & Spackman's occupational therapy* (12th ed., pp 1182–1184). Philadelphia, PA: Lippincott, Williams and Wilkins.

Center for Substance Abuse Treatment. (2007). *The epidemiology of co-occurring substance use and mental disorders. COCE Overview Paper 8.* (DHHS Publication No. (SMA) 07–4308). Rockville, MD: Substance Abuse and Mental Health Services Administration and Center for Mental Health Services.

Center for Substance Abuse Treatment. (2009). *Emerging issues in the use of methadone: Substance Abuse Treatment Advisory.* (HHS Publication No. (SMA) 09–4368). *8*(1).

Clay, S. W., Allen, J., & Parran, T. (2008). A review of addiction. *Postgraduate Medicine, 120*(2), E01–E07.

Cousijn, J., Wiers, R. W., Ridderinkhof, K. R., van den Brink,W., Veltman, D. J., & Goudriaan, A. E. (2012). Grey matter alterations associated with cannabis use: Results of a VBM study in heavy cannabis users and healthy controls. *Neuroimage, 59*(4), 3845–3851.

D'Souza, D. C., Sewell, R. A., & Ranganathan, M. (2009). Cannabis and psychosis/schizophrenia: Human studies. *European archives of psychiatry and clinical neuroscience, 259*(7), 413–431.

Elliott, D. Y., Geyer, C., Lionetti, T., & Doty, L. (2012). Managing alcohol withdrawal in hospitalized patients. *Nursing, 42*(4), 22–30. doi: 10.1097/01.NURSE.0000412922.97512.07

Gutman, S. A. (2006). Why addiction has a chronic, relapsing course. The neurobiology of addiction: Implications for occupational therapy practice. *Occupational Therapy in Mental Health, 22*(2), 1–29.

Hart, K. (2013). *High price: A neuroscientist's journey of self-discovery that challenges everything you know about drugs and society.* New York, NY: Harper Collins.

Higdon, J. V., & Frei, B. (2006). Coffee and health: A review of recent human research. *Critical Reviews in Food Science and Nutrition, 46,*101–123. doi: 10.1080/10408390500400009.

Heuchemer, B., & Staffan, J. (2006). Leaving homelessness and addiction: Narratives of an occupational transition. *Scandinavian Journal of Occupational Therapy, 13*(3), 160–169.

Hoppes, S., Bryce, H. R., & Peloquin, S. M. (2013). Substance abuse and occupational therapy. In E. Cara & A. MacRae (Eds.), *Psychosocial occupational therapy: An evolving practice* (3rd ed., Chapter 24). Albany, NY: Delmar.

Jones, K. L., & Streissguth, A. P. (2010). Fetal alcohol syndrome and fetal alcohol spectrum disorders: A brief history. *Journal of Psychiatry & Law, Special Issue: Fetal Alcohol Syndrome and Fetal Alcohol Spectrum Disorders: A Brief History, 38*(4), 373–382.

Juliano, L. M., & Roland R. G. (2004). A critical review of caffeine withdrawal: Empirical validation of symptoms and signs, incidence, severity, and associated features. *Psychopharmacology, 176*(1), 1–29.

Knis-Matthews, L. (2003). A parenting program for women who are substance dependent. *Mental Health Special Interest Section Quarterly, 26,* 1–4.

Maniglio, R. (2011). The role of child sexual abuse in the etiology of substance-related disorders. *Journal of Addictive Diseases, 30*(3), 216–228.

Martin, L. M., Bliven, M., & Boisvert, R. (2008). Occupational performance, self-esteem, and quality of life in substance addictions recovery. *OTJR: Occupation, Participation and Health, 28,* 81–88.

Monti, P. M., Miranda, R., Nixon, K., Sher, K. J., Swartzwelder, H. S., Tapert, S. F., … Crews,

F. T. (2005). Adolescence: Booze, brains, and behavior. *Alcoholism: Clinical and Experimental Research, 29*(2), 207–220. doi 10.1097/01. ALC.0000153551.11000.F3

Moyers, P. A. (2011). Co-occurring disorders. In C. Brown & V. C. Stoffel. (Eds.). *Occupational therapy in mental health: A vision for participation* (pp. 211–224). Philadelphia, PA: F.A. Davis.

National Center on Addiction and Substance Abuse at Columbia University. (2007). *Wasting the best and brightest: Substance abuse at America's colleges and universities.* New York, NY: Author.

National Center on Addiction and Substance Abuse at Columbia University. (2011). *Adolescent substance use: America's No. #1 public health problem.* New York, NY: Author.

National Institute on Alcohol Abuse and Alcoholism (NIAAA). (2005a). *Social work curriculum on alcohol use disorders.* Bethesda, MD: Author. Retrieved from http://pubs. Niaa.nih.gov/publications/Social/main.html on June 27, 2015.

National Institute on Alcohol Abuse and Alcoholism (NIAAA). (2005b). *Helping patients who drink too much: A clinician's guide.* Washington, DC: Author.

National Institute on Alcohol Abuse and Alcoholism (NIAAA). (2010). *Rethinking drinking: Alcohol and your health.* Bethesda, MD: Author. Retrieved from http://rethinkingdrinking.niaaa.nih.gov/ NIH Publication No. 13–3770 on June 27, 2015.

National Institute on Drug Abuse (NIDA). (2011). *Comorbidity: Addiction and other mental disorders.* Author. Retrieved from http://www. drugabuse.gov/publications/drugfacts/comorbidity-addiction-other-mental-disorders on July 23, 2015.

National Institute on Drug Abuse (NIDA). (2012a). *Drug facts: Spice ("synthetic marijuana").* Author. Retrieved from http://www.drugabuse.gov/publications/drugfacts/k2spice-synthetic-marijuana on June 27, 2015.

National Institute on Drug Abuse (NIDA). (2012b). *Principles of drug addiction treatment: A research-based guide.* (NIH Publication No. 12–4180). Author.

National Institute on Drug Abuse (NIDA). (2013). *Drug facts: Cocaine.* Author. Retrieved from www. drugabuse.gov/publications/drugfacts/cocaine on June 27, 2015.

National Institute on Drug Abuse (NIDA). (2014a). *Prescription drug abuse: How do opioids affect the brain and body?* Retrieved from http://www. drugabuse.gov/publications/research-reports/prescriptiondrugs/opioids/how-do-opioids-affect-brain-body on July 26, 2015.

National Institute on Drug Abuse (NIDA). (2014b). *Drug facts: Hallucinogens.* Author. Retrieved from http://www.drugabuse.gov/publications/drugfacts/hallucinogens-lsd-peyote-psilocybin-pcp on June 29, 2015.

National Institute on Drug Abuse (NIDA). (2014c). *Drug facts: Cigarettes and other tobacco products.* Author. Retrieved from http://www.drugabuse.gov/publications/drugfacts/cigarettes-other-tobacco-products on July 8, 2015.

National Institute on Drug Abuse (NIDA). (2014d). *Drug facts: Heroin.* Author. Retrieved from http:// www.drugabuse.gov/publications/drugfacts/heroin on June 29, 2015.

National Institute on Drug Abuse (NIDA). (2014e). *Prescription drug abuse: CNS depressants.* Author. Retrieved from http://www.drugabuse. gov/publications/research-reports/prescription-drugs/cns-depressants/what-are-cns-depressants on July 8, 2015.

National Institute on Drug Abuse (NIDA). (2015a): *Drug facts: Marijuana.* Author. Retrieved from http://www.drugabuse.gov/publications/drugfacts/marijuana on June 27, 2015.

National Institute on Drug Abuse (NIDA). (2015b). *Research report series: Marijuana.* (NIH Publication Number 15–3859). Author. Retrieved from http://www.drugabuse.gov/publications/research-reports/marijuana/letter-director on June 27, 2015.

Paxos, C. & Dugan, S. E. (2015). Psychopharmacology. In B. Bonder (Ed.), *Psychopathology and function,* (5th ed., pp. 413–455). Thorofare, NJ: Slack.

Quadling, A., Maree, K., Mountjoy, L., Bosch, G., & Kotkin, Z. (1999). An investigation into a relationship between sensory modulation disorder and substance abuse. *South African Journal of Occupational Therapy, 29*(1), 10–13.

Rabin, R. C. (2014). Healthy consumer: New painkiller rekindles addiction concerns. *The New York Times,* April 21.

Radhakrishnan, R., Wilkinson, S. T., & D'Souza, D. C. (2014). Gone to pot: A review of the association between cannabis and psychosis. *Front Psychiatry, 5,* 54.

Sells, C. H., Stoffel, V. C., & Plach, H. (2011). Substance-related disorders. In C. Brown & V. C. Stoffel (Eds.). *Occupational therapy in mental health: A vision for participation* (pp. 192–210). Philadelphia, PA: F.A. Davis

Silver, M. (2015). Alcohol use in older adults: How occupational therapy can help. *OT Practice,* May 25.

Stoffel, V. C., & Moyers, P. A. (2001). *Occupational therapy practice guidelines for substance use disorder* (3rd ed.). Bethesda, MD: American Occupational Therapy Association.

Stoffel, V. C., & Moyers, P. A. (2004). An evidence-based and occupational perspective of interventions for persons with substance-use disorders. *American Journal of Occupational Therapy, 58*(5), 570–586.

Substance Abuse and Mental Health Services Administration (SAMHSA). (2003). *Inhalants: Substance abuse treatment advisory, 3*(1). (DHHS Publication No. (SMA) 03–3788 NCADI Publication No. MS922). Rockville, MD: Author.

Substance Abuse and Mental Health Services Administration (SAMHSA). (2007). *Fetal alcohol spectrum disorder: Curriculum for addiction professionals, Level 2*. (DHHS Publication No. (SMA) 07–4297). Rockville, MD: Author.

Substance Abuse and Mental Health Services Administration (SAMHSA). (2010). *Quick guide for counselors: Based on TIP 49 incorporating alcohol pharmacotherapies into medical practice*. (HHS Publication No. (SMA) 10–4542). Rockville, MD: Author.

Substance Abuse and Mental Health Services Administration (SAMHSA). (2011). *Substance use disorders in people with physical and sensory disabilities, In Brief* (Volume 6, Issue 1). HHS Publication No. (SMA) 11-4648. Rockville, MD: Author.

Substance Abuse and Mental Health Services Administration (SAMHSA). (2014). *Results from the 2013 National survey on drug use and health: Summary of national findings*. (HHS Publication No. (SMA) 14–4887. NSDUH Series H-49). Rockville, MD: Author.

Thompson, K. (2007). Occupational therapy and substance use disorders: Are practitioners addressing these disorders in practice? *Occupational Therapy in Health Care, 21*(3), 61–77.

Volkow, N. D., Baler, R. D., Compton, W. M., & Weiss, S. R. (2014). Adverse health effects of marijuana use. *New England Journal of Medicine, 370*(23), 2219–2227.

Wall, T. L., Luczak, S. E., & Hiller-Sturmhöfel, S. (2016). Biology, genetics, and environment: Underlying factors influencing alcohol metabolism. *Alcohol Research: Current Reviews, 38*(1), 1–10.

World Health Organization (WHO). (2008). *MH GAP: Mental Health Gap Action Programme—scaling up care for mental, neurological, and substance use disorders*. Geneva, Switzerland: Author.

Physical Conditions

The Physical Conditions Unit includes the most common physical conditions that clients have who are treated by occupational therapists as determined by the National Board of Certification in Occupational Therapy. These chapters focus on conditions that are typically diagnosed in adults, but may also be seen in pediatrics. People with these conditions are typically referred to occupational therapy for the specified physical condition as a primary diagnosis, but they may also have the physical condition as a secondary diagnosis. Each chapter provides information about the etiology, incidence and prevalence, signs and symptoms, course and prognosis, diagnosis, medical/surgical management and impact on occupational performance of these conditions. Case illustrations are used to provide examples of lives affected by the condition. The conditions included in this unit are the following:

17 Cerebrovascular Accident

Mylene Schriner and Joan Ziegler Delahunt

KEY TERMS

Agnosia
Aneurysm
Apraxia (motor
  planning)
Associated reactions
Ataxia
Atherosclerosis
Deep vein thrombosis
Dysarthria
Dysphagia
Embolism
Flaccidity
Hematoma
Homonymous
  hemianopsia
  (hemianopia)
Hemiparesis
Hemiplegia
Hemorrhagic stroke
Hypotonus
Ischemia
Neural plasticity
Spasticity
Thrombus
Transient ischemic
  attacks (TIAs)
Unilateral inattention
  (neglect)

M.V. is a 68-year-old native New Yorker. She was born to Irish and Italian parents on the lower eastside of Manhattan. She attended private preparatory schools and readily was accepted at Columbia University, where she studied fashion marketing and design. She received a second undergraduate degree in business from Barnard College and immediately entered the hectic, high-energy world of finance, within the world of women's fashion and apparel. M.V. never married, finding her life fulfillment more in the glitter and glass world than in diapers and the seeming melancholia of suburbia. She worked ungodly hours, often never stopping for lunch, and sometimes missing dinner altogether. Timelines, deadlines, corporate demands, and the constant need to exceed quotas in order to appease shareholders made her job monetarily rewarding but extremely stressful in overt as well as insidious ways. M.V.'s weight was a constant stressor for her. She seemed to gain 2 to 3 lb each time she walked past a Baskin-Robbins ice cream store. She was always dieting, or going to diet, or thinking that she should be on a diet, but the Coke Zero did not make a discernible dent in her ever-increasing midriff. In addition to her weight, she also had an ongoing relationship with cigarettes. She continued to be a pack-a-day smoker despite all of the Relays for Life, pink ribbons, and St. Jude's commercials that seemed to trumpet their anticancer messages directly at her whenever she gave them a second glance. M.V. was 30 lb overweight and has had high blood pressure since she was a sophomore in college. M.V. was on her usual path from the subway station at 54th St. and Lexington Avenue to her office, when she began to sense that something was happening to her that she had never before experienced. The first sensation was one of a warm drape being pulled over her head; the air she was breathing became thick and difficult for her to draw into her chest. Then there was a bit of a tingle in her right hand, as though the pinky and ring fingers suddenly decided to fall asleep together, the bag of bagels she was carrying to share with her co-workers slipped to the pavement unnoticed by M.V. As she attempted to make sense of what was happening to her, breathing became more challenging, like drawing thick soup through a too-thin straw. She leaned on a nearby storefront and vomited. As she leaned there for a moment, a man came to her side and spoke in a language she seemingly had never heard before, she thought "was he speaking Russian, Latvian, certainly someone here speaks English?" Within a minute or two, M.V. was being guided to the pavement by two people who appeared to be wearing uniforms; possibly they worked for a Russian circus? She was now lying on the pavement feeling frightened, embarrassed, and very, very confused. There was no way she could move her right hand or arm, and her right lower body seemed to have floated away from her and onto another part of the universe. M.V. was taken to a hospital by ambulance, with much of that event lost to her memory. What is happening to M.V.? Is there enough evidence to suspect that a stroke may be evolving? This chapter will provide insight into M.V.'s condition and help provide answers to these questions.

DESCRIPTION AND DEFINITIONS

A stroke, or brain attack, results from an interruption in the blood flow to the brain from either a blocked or ruptured blood vessel. The consequence is an inadequate supply of oxygen and nutrients to this vital organ. Even a brief disruption of this blood flow can lead to brain damage. Medical practitioners use the term "cerebrovascular accident," often abbreviated as CVA, for stroke. A CVA can occur in any part of the brain, the cerebral hemispheres, the cerebellum, or the brainstem. The site and extent of the affected area, or infarct, determines loss of function.

CVAs are divided into two main types: **ischemic** and **hemorrhagic**. Ischemic strokes are characterized by blockages (the term **ischemia** refers to the lack of blood supply) and include atherothrombotic, lacunar, and embolic infarctions, in that order of frequency. Hemorrhagic strokes include intracerebral and subarachnoid hemorrhages (Broderick et al., 2007). Both types of stroke lead to the death, or infarction, of brain tissue. CVA terminology involves a complex composition of pathophysiological entities that include thrombosis, **embolism**, and hemorrhage (Saenger & Christenson, 2011). In most cases, a loss of blood supply is the result of long-standing degeneration of the body's blood vessels. Less commonly, a CVA occurs because of an inborn abnormality or weakness of the brain's vascular supply (Ferguson, 2010). A brief review of cerebral circulation will help understand the impact of each type of stroke.

■ Cerebral Circulatory System

The blood supply of the brain is extremely important because the brain is one of the most metabolically active organs of the body. Although it constitutes only 2% of the body's weight, the brain receives approximately 17% of the cardiac output and consumes about 20% of the oxygen used by the entire body (Lundy-Ekman, 2007).

In the brain, the arteries of the anterior circulation supply the front, top, and side portions of the cerebral hemispheres. The brainstem and cerebellum, as well as the back and undersurface of the cerebral hemispheres, are supplied by the posterior circulation. These two areas of circulation are further categorized into the extracranial portions (arising from outside the skull and traveling toward the brain) and the intracranial portions (arising from within the skull) (Lundy-Ekman, 2007).

■ Extracranial Vessels

Extracranial anterior circulation consists of the two carotid arteries, which travel in the front of the neck on each side of the trachea and esophagus (Lundy-Ekman, 2007). The word "carotid" is derived from the Greek word "karos" meaning "to stupefy," or render unconscious, indicating the significance of this main artery in maintaining consciousness and brain function (Qureshi et al., 2007). The right common carotid artery arises from the innominate artery. The left common carotid artery originates directly from the aortic arch. Around the fifth or sixth vertebrae, these common carotid arteries divide into external carotid arteries, whose branches supply the face and its structures, and the internal carotid arteries, which supply the eyes and the cerebral hemispheres (Lundy-Ekman, 2007; Qureshi, 2007).

The vertebral arteries arise from the subclavian arteries and make up the extracranial posterior circulation. They remain within the vertebral column for part of their course from about C6 to C2. The vertebral arteries enter the cranium through the foramen magnum (Lundy-Ekman, 2007; Qureshi, 2007).

■ Intracranial Vessels

The internal carotid arteries enter the skull through the carotid canal and form an S-shaped curve called the carotid siphon (Qureshi et al., 2007). The artery then enters the subarachnoid space by piercing the dura mater. It gives rise to the ophthalmic arteries, which supply the eyes; the posterior communicating arteries, which join with the posterior circulation; and the anterior cerebral arteries, which supply the orbital and medial surfaces of the frontal lobes and part of the basal frontal lobe white matter and caudate nucleus. The internal carotid artery also branches off to create the middle cerebral arteries, which supply almost the entire lateral surface of the frontal, parietal, and temporal lobes, as well as the underlying white matter and basal ganglia (Lundy-Ekman, 2007). The middle cerebral artery is the largest of the terminal branches of the internal carotid artery and is the direct continuation of this vessel.

The vertebral arteries enter the cranium within the posterior fossa and travel along the side of the medulla, where they produce their longest branch, the posterior inferior cerebellar artery. This artery supplies the lateral medulla and the back of the undersurface of the cerebellum (Alastruey, Parker, Peiró, Byrd, & Sherwin, 2007). The two vertebral arteries then join at the junction between the medulla and pons to form the single midline basilar artery (Alastruey et al., 2007). The basilar artery gives off penetrating arteries to the base of the pons and two vessels (the anterior inferior and superior cerebellar arteries), which supply the upper and anterior undersurfaces of the cerebellum (Alastruey et al., 2007). At the level of the midbrain, the basilar artery bifurcates into the two posterior cerebral arteries (Alastruey et al., 2007). As they circle the brainstem, these two arteries give off penetrating branches to the midbrain and thalamus and then divide into branches that supply the occipital lobes as well as the medial and undersurfaces of the temporal lobes (Alastruey et al., 2007). One of the branches of the posterior cerebral artery, the calcarine artery, is of special significance because it is the main supplier of blood for the visual area of the cortex (Lundy-Ekman, 2007).

■ Communicating Arteries

The right and left carotid vessels connect with each other when they enter the brain, each sending out a small lateral branch that meets in the space between them. These are the anterior communicating arteries. They also branch backward to join with the right and left posterior cerebral arteries, called the posterior communicating arteries. This communicating vascular interchange is known as the circle of Willis, which is pictured in Figure 17.1. It protects the brain

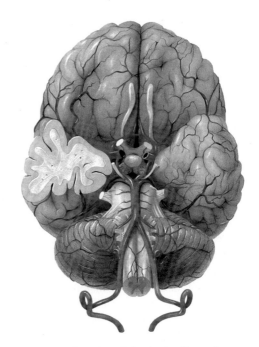

Figure 17.1 Arteries of the brain. (From the American Chart Co.)

should one of the four major supplying arteries coming up through the neck be blocked (Alastruey et al., 2007). This important anatomical feature is named for Dr. Thomas Willis and was first described in the mid-17th century (Zazulia, 2009). Starting from the midline anteriorly, the circle consists of the anterior communicating, anterior cerebral, internal carotid, posterior communicating, and posterior cerebral arteries, from which it continues to the starting point in reverse order (Zazulia, 2009).

When one major vessel supplying the brain is slowly occluded, either within the circle of Willis or proximal to it, the normally small communicating arteries may slowly enlarge to compensate for the occlusion (Lundy-Ekman, 2007). This system is imperfect, however, and it often fails to prevent strokes. In many individuals, the same atherosclerotic processes that caused a stroke also may damage communicating arteries. In addition, only about one-fourth of strokes are caused by a blockage of the major neck vessels (Qureshi et al., 2007). For approximately one-third of the population, the communicating artery may be insufficient or even absent (Alastruey et al., 2007). Such anomalies are more common in those who have strokes than in the general population and may be linked to increased risk of stroke in persons who also have **atherosclerosis** (Van Kooij, Hendrikse, Benders, De Vries, & Groenendaal, 2010).

TYPES OF CEREBROVASCULAR ACCIDENT

■ Ischemic Stroke

Ischemic stroke is the most common type of CVA accounting for 88% of cases (Go et al., 2013). Cerebral infarction, or brain tissue death, results when circulation to an area of the brain is obstructed, with the result being ischemia. Ischemic strokes are classified as thrombotic, embolic, or lacunar strokes. The damaged area has two components: the tissues that have died as a result of blood supply loss and the peripheral area in which there may be temporary dysfunction as a result of edema. Edematous brain tissue sometimes recovers slowly and gradually, resulting in a reappearance of function after a period of 4 to 5 months (Go et al., 2013). In the past, prognoses for functional recovery have been limited to this time frame. However, recent research offers

promising evidence that recovery is possible months and even years post CVA (Hankey et al., 2007). Explanations focus on the brain's ability to reroute neural pathways, a phenomenon known as **neural plasticity** (Huttenlocher, 2009; Takatsuru et al., 2009). Current research supports that recent advances in functional imaging of human brain activity of clients with a CVA demonstrate that the cortical hemisphere contralateral to the infarction lesion serves a vital role in the recovery process and that the most optimal recoveries are linked with the greatest return toward the normal state of brain functional organization (Hara et al., 2015). Further, neural plasticity is evident with positively impacting functional outcomes for clients with past CVA (Rodríguez-Mutuberría et al., 2011).

The actual physiologic events that follow an ischemic stroke occur in characteristic steps. First, the membrane surrounding each affected neuron leaks potassium (a mineral necessary for producing electrical impulses) and adenosine triphosphate (ATP, an energy-producing biochemical found in the body). Fluid quickly accumulates between the blood vessel and neuron, making it difficult for oxygen and nutrients to pass from the bloodstream into the damaged neuron. The initial injury produces a vicious cycle in which more cellular injury results. Irreversible cell death will occur in 5 to 10 minutes if oxygen and nutrients are unable to reach them from the bloodstream or in a slightly longer period if blood flow is only partially interrupted. These dead cells form a zone of infarction that will not regenerate (Minger et al., 2007). Downstream from the infarct zone is a zone of injury (penumbra) (Bose et al., 2008; Gonzalez, 2006). This area may be served by collateral blood vessels and is capable of returning to normal functioning. A third area that reacts differently to the stroke process may also exist. In this area of hyperemia, the blood vessels are congested and swollen and also may have the potential for recovery.

Thrombosis

Cerebral thrombosis occurs when a blood clot forms in one of the arteries supplying the brain, causing vascular obstruction at the point of its formation. The size and location of the infarct depends on which vessel is occluded and the amount of collateral circulation. Thrombosis occurs most frequently in blood vessels that have already been damaged by atherosclerosis (Ho, Huang, Khor, & Tay, 2008).

Atherosclerosis is a gradual degenerative disease of the blood vessel walls. It is a pathologic process rather than a normal effect of human aging (Ho et al., 2008). Rough, irregular fatty deposits form within the intima and inner media of the arteries and often lead to the generation of a **thrombus**, or blood clot. This is the most common cause of CVA, with stenosis, or narrowing of the blood vessels, resulting in much fewer cases (Ho et al., 2008). Large-vessel atherosclerosis accounts for 60% of ischemic stroke (Bang et al., 2010). Because the body's blood vessels have a significant reserve capacity, ischemic strokes do not usually occur until the vessel is two-thirds blocked (Bang et al., 2010). The impact of atherosclerosis on the vascular system is considerable; it is also a major risk factor for heart disease.

To understand the process that produces a mass of degenerated, thickened material (plaque) called atheromas, imagine a glue bottle that has been allowed to collect the residuals of dried glue. The more clogged the cap of the bottle becomes, the more difficult it is for the glue to flow through. Squeezing the glue through the opening can push already dried glue more firmly against the opening. The opening will become smaller and smaller until it closes completely or bursts from the increased pressure.

In the cerebral circulation, atherosclerosis and thrombus formation are most likely to occur in areas where blood vessels turn or divide, such as the origins of the internal carotid artery and the middle cerebral artery and the junction of the vertebral and basilar arteries (van Kooij et al., 2010).

Cerebral thrombosis often causes stuttering or progressive symptoms that occur over several hours or days. Onset during sleep is common. Often, a patient notices mild arm numbness at night and then awakens the next morning with paralysis. **Transient ischemic attacks** (TIAs) precede actual infarction about half the time (van Kooij et al., 2010).

Lacunar Strokes/Penetrating Artery Disease

Lacunar strokes are small infarcts, usually lying in the deep brain structures, such as the basal ganglia, thalamus, pons, internal capsule, and deep white matter (Porter & Kaplan, 2010). Approximately 25% of ischemic strokes are the

result of damage to these deep structures (Porter & Kaplan, 2010). Within a few months of onset of a lacunar stroke, a small cavity ("lacune" in French) is left (Porter & Kaplan, 2010).

Lacunar infarcts or lacunes result from occlusion of a single penetrating artery and account for approximately a quarter of cerebral infarctions (Arboix, 2011). Lacunar infarcts range in size from 2 to 15 mm (Porter, 2010). Because of their small size, minimal neurological symptoms are often present, and many such strokes go undetected. Recent findings indicate, however, that long-term prognosis is not good for lacunar strokes, and the recovery rate is similar to that for other types of CVA (Basile et al., 2006). Typically, lacunar strokes produce purely motor deficits (weakness or **ataxia**), purely sensory deficits, or a combination of sensory and motor deficits (Arboix, Blanco-Rojas, & Martí-Vilalta, 2014; Sacio, 2006). Symptoms do not usually include aphasia, changes in cognition or personality, loss of consciousness, **homonymous hemianopsia**, or seizures (Basile et al., 2006). The most consistently identified risk factor for lacunar infarction is hypertension, and treatment is aimed at controlling it (Basile et al., 2006).

Embolism

Embolism occurs when a clot that has formed elsewhere (thrombus) breaks off (embolus), travels up the bloodstream until it reaches an artery too small to pass through, and blocks the artery (Montaner et al., 2008). At this point, the effects of the embolus are similar to those produced by thrombosis. Embolic materials that travel to the arteries of the brain can originate from many sources, including the aortic arch and arteries arising from it, the extracranial carotid and vertebral arteries, and thrombi in the heart. Cardiac-source emboli occur in approximately 20% of ischemic strokes and are referred to as cardiogenic (Cho et al., 2009). Many cardiac abnormalities can give rise to a cerebral embolism, including atrial fibrillation (AF), coronary artery disease, valvular heart disease, and arrhythmias. Cardiac surgery is also a cause (Cho et al., 2009). The middle cerebral artery is by far the most common destination of cardiac emboli, followed by the posterior cerebral artery (Cho et al., 2009).

In contrast to thrombotic strokes, embolic strokes typically occur during daytime activity (Cho, 2007; Montaner et al., 2008). The embolism

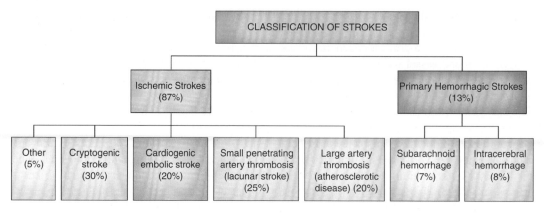

Figure 17.2 Types of stroke. (From Hickey, J. (2013). *Clinical practice of neurological and neurosurgical nursing* (7th ed.). Philadelphia, PA: Lippincott Williams & Wilkins.)

can be precipitated by a sudden movement, or even a sneeze, which raises blood pressure and dislodges the clot. Clinical symptoms are usually maximal at onset, but in some cases, the neurological symptoms improve or stabilize somewhat and then worsen as the embolus moves and blocks a more distal artery. A history of TIAs is rare. Seizures may be associated with embolic strokes (Cho et al., 2007) (Fig. 17.2).

■ Hemorrhagic Stroke

Approximately 20% of CVAs are hemorrhagic (Amarenco, Bogousslavsky, Caplan, Donnan, & Hennerici, 2009). **Hemorrhagic strokes** are caused by a rupture in a blood vessel or an **aneurysm**, with resultant bleeding into or around cerebral tissue. An aneurysm is a bulging or outpouching of a wall of an artery as a result of weakness in the vessel wall; it is prone to rupture at any time. While fatality rates for hemorrhagic strokes are higher than are those for ischemic strokes, recent findings indicate that patients often make a better recovery after a hemorrhagic stroke (Amarenco et al., 2009). Hemorrhagic strokes are more common in young people than are ischemic strokes as the vessel wall anomaly is often congenital. There are two types of hemorrhagic strokes. An intracerebral hemorrhage refers to bleeding directly into brain substance, whereas a subarachnoid hemorrhage is bleeding occurring within the brain's surrounding membranes and cerebrospinal fluid (CSF) (Feigin, Lawes, Bennett, Barker-Collo, & Parag, 2009). These two types of hemorrhage differ in incidence, etiology, clinical signs, and treatment. Age, ethnicity, and hypertension are strongly linked to

intracerebral hemorrhagic stroke (Grysiewicz, Thomas, & Pandey, 2008).

Intracerebral Hemorrhages

Intracerebral hemorrhage results in bleeding directly into the brain and accounts for a high percentage of deaths because of CVA (Feigin et al., 2009). It may occur in any part of the brain and is most commonly linked to hypertension. Other causes include blood vessel abnormalities, such as arteriovenous malformations or aneurysms, or trauma (Locksley, 2010). Release of blood into brain tissue and surrounding edema will then disrupt the function of that particular brain region (Locksley, 2010). Blood irritates the brain tissue and causes swelling, or it may form a mass called a **hematoma**. In either case, the increased pressure on brain tissue can rapidly destroy them. Factors that increase the risk of intracerebral hemorrhage include blood and bleeding disorders such as hemophilia, sickle cell anemia, and leukemia; use of anticoagulants; and liver disease (Porter & Kaplan, 2010).

Clinical signs of intracerebral hemorrhage are usually focal, that is, unlike cerebral infarcts, hemorrhagic bleeds do not follow the anatomic distribution of blood vessels but move spherically through the tissue planes (Locksley, 2010). Typically, they develop suddenly, often during activity (Amarenco et al., 2009). While extremely small hemorrhages may go undetected, a large hematoma causes headache, vomiting, convulsions, and decreased levels of alertness (Ohwaki et al., 2004). Stupor and coma are common signs of very large hemorrhages and indicate a poor prognosis, especially among individuals over 85

(Grysiewicz et al., 2008). Nevertheless, recovery is possible.

Cerebral injury caused by intracerebral bleeding is a result of the damaging effect that the abnormal presence of blood has on the neurons. In addition to the irritant of the blood, abnormal pressure on neurons distorts their normal architecture. It also prevents oxygen and nutrients from passing to the cells from the bloodstream. Eventually, bleeding will stop and a hard clot will form. During a period of months, the clot slowly recedes, breaks down, and is absorbed by the body's white blood cells (Zhao, Grotta, Gonzales, & Aronowski, 2009). If not damaged by increased pressure, the tissues irritated by the blood may heal, leading to a positive outcome, perhaps even full recovery (Zhao et al., 2009).

Subarachnoid Hemorrhages

Subarachnoid hemorrhages account for about 3% of all CVAs and are slightly more common in women (De Rooij et al., 2007). About 95% are caused by the leakage of blood from aneurysms (Grysiewicz et al., 2008). A combination of congenital and degenerative factors, usually at the points of origin or bifurcations of arteries, can precipitate formation of an aneurysm (Ohwaki et al., 2004). Blood may break through the weak point of the aneurysm at any time and, because of the force of arterial pressure, spread quickly

into the CSF surrounding the brain. A subarachnoid hemorrhage also may be caused by bleeding from an arteriovenous malformation, which is an abnormal collection of vessels near the surface of the brain. Other less common causes of subarachnoid hemorrhages are hemophilia, excessive anticoagulation therapy, and trauma to the skull and brain (Amarenco et al., 2009). The extravasated, or escaped, blood irritates the meninges, and intracranial pressure is increased owing to extra fluid in the closed cranial cavity. This can lead to headache, vomiting, and an altered state of consciousness. Sleepiness, stupor, agitation, restlessness, and actual coma are various manifestations of reduced consciousness. Headaches are usually severe and are described as the worst in the patient's life (Perry et al., 2013). Subarachnoid hemorrhages are diagnosed through one of these three methods subarachnoid blood on computed tomography (CT) scan, xanthochromia in CSF, or red blood cells in the final tube of CSF, with positive angiography findings (Perry et al., 2013) (Fig. 17.3).

ETIOLOGY

Research suggests that ten risk factors are associated with 90% of the risk of CVA including history of hypertension, smoking, waist-to-hip

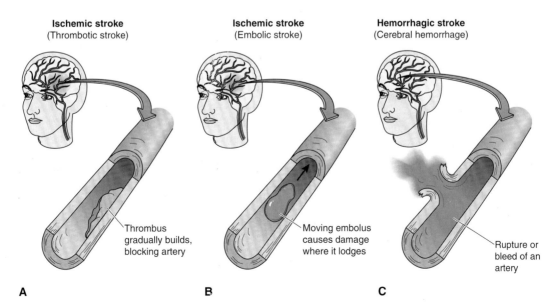

Figure 17.3 Ischemic versus hemorrhagic stroke. (From Walton, T. (2010). *Medical conditions and massage therapy.* Philadelphia, PA: Lippincott Williams & Wilkins.)

ratio, diet risk score, regular physical activity, diabetes mellitus, alcohol intake, psychological stress, and cardiac problems. These risk factors were all significant for ischemic stroke, whereas hypertension, smoking, waist-to-hip ratio, diet, and alcohol intake were significant risk factors for intracerebral hemorrhagic stroke (O'Donnell et al., 2010). A number of risk factors are associated with the likelihood of CVA and resemble those for heart disease, which stands to reason as atherosclerosis is an underlying cause for both conditions. While some of these risk factors are inborn or otherwise unavoidable, many are related to lifestyle and behavioral choices. Specific interventions that lower blood pressure, eliminate smoking, and promote physical activity and a healthy diet could substantially reduce the burden of CVA (O'Donnell et al., 2010).

- Ethnicity—Although all minority groups are at risk, CVA death rates for African Americans is more than twice the risk of stroke compared with other ethnicity groups, and women are at a greater risk for CVA than men (Saenger & Christenson, 2009). Recent data also indicate that blacks living in the South have a greater risk of dying from CVA than do those who live in the northern states (Voeks et al., 2008).
- Age—Risk for CVA increases with age, especially after age 65. People with high blood pressure and who exhibit the other risk factors listed in this chapter are increasingly vulnerable as they age. Younger people are not immune, either: approximately 28% of CVAs occur in individuals younger than age 65 (Bhat et al., 2008; Goldstein et al., 2011).
- Heredity—A family history of CVA, particularly on the father's side, increases one's risk (Bhat et al., 2008). Genetic factors account for 7% to 20% of cases of subarachnoid hemorrhage, and some researchers recommend that people with more than one close relative who suffered a hemorrhagic stroke be screened for aneurysms (Locksley, 2010).
- Obesity—Being overweight is a known risk factor for hypertension and diabetes mellitus and also is associated with CVA. Weight that is centered in the abdomen (so-called apple shape) has a particularly high association with CVA as well as heart disease, while

individuals whose weight is distributed around the hips are less at risk (Lavie, Milani, & Ventura, 2009). A sedentary lifestyle is associated with rising levels of obesity and has been implicated in occurrence of CVAs, as well as hypertension (Bhat et al., 2008).
- Hypertension—Called the "silent disease," hypertension has long been acknowledged as the most significant controllable risk factor for both CVA and heart attack (Bhat et al., 2008). Hypertension occurs in 25% to 40% of the US population (Bhat et al., 2008). Symptoms of hypertension are not clearly identifiable: an occasional headache, dizziness, or light-headedness, which may indicate hypertension, can easily be attributed to other factors. Chronically elevated blood pressure exerts pressure on cerebral vessels, often resulting in lacunar infarctions or intracerebral hemorrhage (Amarenco et al., 2009; Ohira et al., 2006). Hypertension also has been implicated in the atherosclerotic process because it drives fatty substances into the arterial walls, making them brittle, narrowed, and hardened (Zazulia, 2009). The impact of hypertension increases with age (Bhat et al., 2008).
- Smoking—Smoking doubles the risk of CVA (Goldstein et al., 2011). Quitting smoking reduces the likelihood of CVA, and there is some evidence to suggest that 5 years after quitting smoking, individuals lower their risk of having a CVA to nearly that of people of whom have never smoked (Basu, Glantz, Bitton, & Millett, 2013).
- TIAs—A TIA is considered an important risk factor for an impending CVA. Survivors of a TIA represent a population at increased risk of subsequent stroke (Furie et al., 2011). Approximately 30% of all patients who have had a TIA are at risk of having a CVA within 2 years.
- Geographic location—The highest death rates from CVAs in the United States are in North and South Carolina, Georgia, Northern Florida, Alabama, Mississippi, and Tennessee. Specific pockets of high death rates in Texas, Oklahoma, and all of the Hawaiian Islands have been noted (Voeks et al., 2008). This geographical strip, often termed the "stroke belt," is the source of numerous studies on environmental, cultural, or other geographically determined risk factors.

A person who grows up in a high-risk area and then moves to a lower-risk area as an adult continues to carry the greater likelihood of having a CVA. This has led to speculation that the causes may be diet related, cultural, or possibly even related to water supply or altitude (Glymour, Avendaño, & Berkman, 2007).

- Diabetes mellitus—This disease is more common in CVA patients than in a normal population of similar age (Sarwar et al., 2010). Duration of diabetes is independently associated with ischemic stroke risk adjusting for risk factors. The risk increases 3% each year and triples with diabetes ≥10 years (Banerjee et al., 2012).
- Oral contraceptives—Women who have taken birth control pills, especially those with a high estrogen content, have an increased risk for CVA as they become older. Current use of combined oral contraceptive pills is associated with increased odds of venous thromboembolism and ischemic stroke, but not hemorrhagic stroke or myocardial infarction (Urrutia et al., 2013).
- Hyperlipidemia—Hyperlipidemia, including elevated triglycerides and LDL cholesterol, has long been suspected to be a risk factor for CVA (Furie et al., 2011).
- AF is increasing in incidence in the United States and its presence increases the risk of developing CVA (Nichols, 2014).
- Asymptomatic carotid bruits—Bruit is an abnormal sound or murmur heard when a stethoscope is placed over the carotid artery. This slushing noise indicates turbulent blood, often caused by a significant degree of stenosis. Carotid bruit clearly indicates increased CVA risk. Complete occlusion of the carotid artery sometimes follows, resulting in a CVA (Bhat et al., 2008).
- Prior CVA—Approximately one-quarter of the 795,000 CVAs that occur each year are secondary incidents (Furie et al., 2011).
- Heart disease—Diseased heart (whether it be chronic disease, acute heart attacks, or prosthetic heart valves) increases the risk of CVA. Independent of hypertension, people with heart disease have more than twice the risk of CVA than do people with normally functioning hearts (Ohira et al., 2006).
- AF, a condition in which the heart produces an irregular rhythm, is also a known risk factor for CVA. Both persistent and paroxysmal AFs are strong predictors of first as well as recurrent CVA. In the United States, 75,000 cases of CVA per year are attributed to AF (Furie et al., 2011).
- Infections and inflammation—Inflammation occurring with various infections, often mild, has been associated with CVA. Studies examining the relationship between periodontal disease and CVA are inconclusive (Lockhart et al., 2012). Research is under way to determine whether other infections that produce arterial inflammation can lead to CVA or heart disease. For example, chronic infection with *Chlamydia pneumoniae*, which causes mild pneumonia in adults, has been linked with higher risk for CVA (Elkind et al., 2006a).
- Alcohol and drug abuse—Numerous studies indicate that moderate consumption of alcohol decreases the risk of CVA and heart disease; however, excessive consumption and total abstinence are associated with higher risk (Elkind et al., 2006b). Studies have demonstrated an association between alcohol and ischemic stroke, ranging from a definite independent effect to no effect (Furie et al., 2011). Cocaine and methamphetamine abuse are major factors in the incidence of CVA in young adults (Westover, McBride, & Haley, 2007). Use of anabolic steroids for bodybuilding is also associated with increased risk of CVA (Santamarina, Besocke, Romano, Loli, & Gonorazky, 2008).
- Sleep apnea—Sleep apnea is a common disorder in which the throat becomes obstructed during sleep, interfering with normal breathing and sleep. Sleep apnea is worsened by obesity and may contribute to the narrowing of the carotid artery. Obstructive sleep apnea impacts 15 million American adults and is most commonly associated with CVA and cardiovascular disorders including hypertension and arrhythmia (Somers et al., 2008) (Fig. 17.4).

INCIDENCE AND PREVALENCE

CVA is the fourth leading cause of death in the United States, killing nearly 130,000 Americans each year or 1 of every 20 deaths (CDC, 2015;

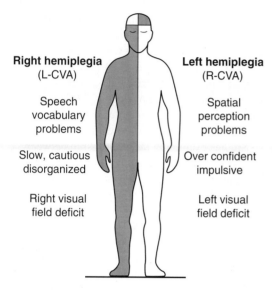

Right hemiplegia
(L-CVA)

Speech
vocabulary
problems

Slow, cautious
disorganized

Right visual
field deficit

Left hemiplegia
(R-CVA)

Spatial
perception
problems

Over confident
impulsive

Left visual
field deficit

Figure 17.4 Left and right hemiplegia. (From Wilkins, E. M. (2011). *Clinical practice of the dental hygienist.* Philadelphia, PA: Lippincott Williams & Wilkins.)

Towfighi & Saver, 2011), surpassed only by heart diseases, cancer, chronic lower respiratory disease, and accidents (Kochanek, Murphy, Xu, & Arias, 2014). The most common cause of disability, CVA is the most widespread diagnosis among clients seen by occupational therapists for the treatment of physically disabled adults (Legg et al., 2007). An estimated 600,000 to 730,000 people in the United States suffer an episode each year, and about 4.5 million stroke survivors are alive today (Xie et al., 2006). Approximately 50% to 70% of people regain functional independence after a CVA; however, 15% to 30% of those who survive an ischemic or hemorrhagic stroke suffer some permanent disability (Xie et al., 2006). Of the two main types, hemorrhagic strokes occur much less frequently (20% of all strokes) than do ischemic strokes, which account for about 80% of all strokes (Xie et al., 2006). Depression affects approximately one-third of stroke survivors (Hackett, Yapa, Parag, & Anderson, 2005; Townend, Tinson, Kwan, & Sharpe, 2010). Impact on family and caregivers is also enormous. If adequate social services and support are not available, caregivers assume the burden for functional tasks that the patient is unable to perform. Numerous studies identified caregiver mental health and the amount of time and effort necessary of the caregiver as significant

determinants of caregiver burden (Rigby, Gubitz, & Phillips, 2009).

Despite these grim statistics, there is some good news. With the exception of subarachnoid hemorrhage, between 1950 and 1990, all types of CVA have shown a significantly decreased incidence (Chiuve et al., 2008). This may be partly the result of increased control of risk factors such as hypertension, diabetes mellitus, and heart disease (Chiuve et al., 2008). Individuals who have had a CVA now live almost twice as long; interestingly, one study even reported that long-term survivors appeared to be less depressed than did the comparison group (Patel, McKevitt, Lawrence, Rudd, & Wolfe, 2007). Fewer people now die of CVA, notwithstanding the continuing debate as to whether this decline is the result of the occurrence of fewer CVAs or better medical treatment (Carandang et al., 2006). However, it should be noted that the absolute number of CVAs occurring in the United States is rising, probably a result of the aging of the population (Carandang et al., 2006). Moreover, dramatic increases in obesity, among children as well as adults, offer grave cause for concern, given the close links determined between obesity and vascular disease (Grysiewicz et al., 2008; Lawlor & Leon, 2005).

■ Pediatric Stroke

CVA in young children occurs in about 1.2 to 13 cases per 100,000 children per year as compared to 240 cases per 100,000 in the adult population (Grysiewicz et al., 2008; Tsze & Valente, 2011). It is more frequent in children younger than 2 years of age, as CVA is 17 times more common in the perinatal period than later in childhood and beyond (Nelson, 2007). Childhood CVA incidence is 5 to 8 per 100,000 children annually with approximately 50% ischemic including arterial ischemic stroke (AIS) or cerebral sinovenous thrombosis (CSVT) (Kitchen et al., 2012). The effects of CVA among children are similar to those described in adults. Sickle cell disease, which affects blood-clotting mechanisms, and genetic disorders are the next most common known causes. Additional risk factors for pediatric stroke include infection, vascular, vasculitis, oncologic, trauma, and drugs (Tsze & Valente, 2011). Residual neurological deficits, which extend into adulthood, are reported in 50% to 90% of children and include motor, language, and cognitive deficits (Kitchen et al., 2012) (Fig. 17.5).

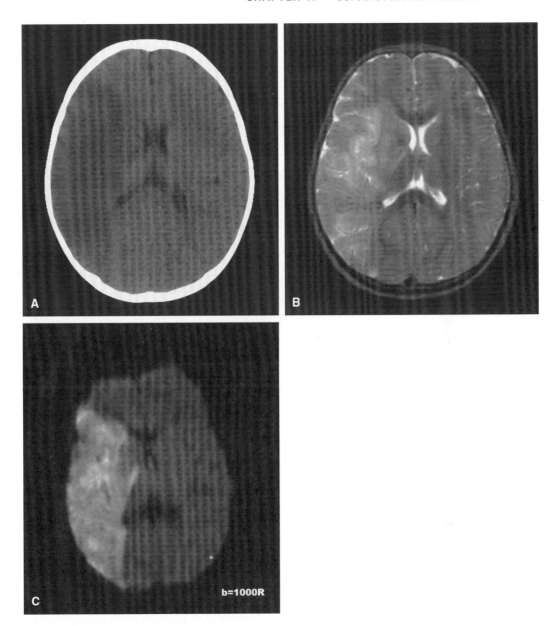

Figure 17.5 Pediatric stroke CT and MRI of a 2-year-old girl who awoke with left hemiparesis and right-gaze preference. **A.** A wedge-shaped area of hypodensity is seen on axial CT. MRI shows **(B)** T2 hyperintensity and **(C)** corresponding diffusion restriction, indicative of an ischemic stroke in the distribution of the right middle cerebral artery. (From Kline, A. M., & Haut, C. (2015). *Lippincott certification review: Pediatric acute care nurse practitioner*. Philadelphia, PA: Lippincott Williams & Wilkins.)

SIGNS AND SYMPTOMS

■ Neurological Effects of CVA

An occlusion that causes a serious CVA can occur anywhere in the extracranial or intracranial system, but the most common site is in the distribution of the middle cerebral artery and its branches in the cerebrum. The majority of cerebral CVAs occur in the left hemisphere compared to right hemispheric (Hedna et al., 2013). It is important to note that even in individuals with the same neurological deficit, the impact of disability is different, depending on the individual's life situation.

Stroke Warning Signs

To educate the public, the American Heart Association and National Stroke Association distribute pamphlets listing the warning signs of an impending serious CVA (American Heart Association [AHA], 2010). Public knowledge of the FAST (Face drooping, Arm weakness, Speech difficulty, Time to call 911) CVA warning signs awareness campaign is effective (Robinson, Reid, Haunton, Wilson, & Naylor, 2012). These include

- Sudden numbness or weakness of the face, arm, or leg; especially on one side of the body
- Sudden confusion, trouble speaking, or understanding
- Sudden trouble seeing in one or both eyes
- Sudden trouble walking, dizziness, and loss of balance or coordination
- Sudden severe headache with no known cause

Some general medical symptoms related to type of CVA were discussed under Etiology. Signs and symptoms also depend on the size and location of the injury, and neurologists can often predict location by the symptoms the individual displays. However, it is important to remember that a CVA is complex, and each individual may experience a unique constellation of symptoms. Relying on stereotypical models of CVA leads to generalized and often inappropriate therapy.

■ Left-Sided Cerebral Injuries: Middle Cerebral Artery

The left cerebral hemisphere controls most functions on the right side of the body because of the decussation of motor fibers (decussation of the pyramids) in the medulla. These fibers that cross, or decussate to the opposite side, form the lateral corticospinal tract. The rest of the fibers descend ipsilaterally, forming the anterior corticospinal tract (Fujimura, Kaneta, Mugikura, Shimizu, & Tominaga, 2007). The proportion of crossing fibers varies from person to person, averaging about 85% (Fujimura et al., 2007).

A CVA in the region of the middle cerebral artery in the left cerebral hemisphere may produce the following symptoms:

1. Loss of voluntary movement and coordination on the right side of the face, trunk, and extremities.
2. Impaired sensation, including temperature discrimination, pain, and proprioception on the right side (hemianesthesia).

3. Language deficits, called aphasia, in which the patient may be unable to speak or understand speech, writing, or gestures. The breakdown of language function is complex; the many types of aphasia will be discussed later in this chapter.
4. Problems with articulation of speech because of disturbances in muscle control of the lips, mouth, tongue, and vocal cords (**dysarthria**).
5. Blind spots in the visual field, usually on the right side.
6. Slow and cautious personality.
7. Memory deficits for recent or past events (Boyd & Winstein, 2003).

■ Right-Sided Cerebral Injuries: Middle Cerebral Artery

The right cerebral hemisphere controls most of the functions on the left side of the body and also is responsible for spatial sensation, perception, and judgment. Injury to the middle cerebral artery of the right cerebral hemisphere may produce a combination of the following deficits:

1. Weakness (**hemiparesis**) or paralysis (**hemiplegia**) on the left side of the body (face, arm, trunk, and leg)
2. Impairment of sensation (touch, pain, temperature, and proprioception) on the left side of the body
3. Spatial and perceptual deficits
4. **Unilateral inattention** (neglect), in which the patient neglects the left side of the body and/or the left side of the environment
5. Dressing apraxia, in which the patient is unable to relate the articles of clothes to the body (Suzuki et al., 2006)
6. Defective vision in the left halves of visual fields or left homonymous hemianopsia in which there is defective vision in each eye (the temporal half of the left eye and the nasal half of the right eye)
7. Impulsive behavior, quick and imprecise movements, and errors of judgment (Suzuki et al., 2006)

■ Anterior Cerebral Artery Stroke

The territory of the anterior cerebral artery is rarely infarcted because of the side-to-side communication provided by the anterior communicating artery in the circle of Willis (Young, 2009). Symptoms of an anterior cerebral artery CVA include

1. Paralysis of the lower extremity, usually more severe than that of the upper extremity, contralateral to the occluded vessel
2. Loss of sensation in the contralateral toes, foot, and leg
3. Loss of conscious control of bowel or bladder
4. Balance problems in sitting, standing, and walking
5. Lack of spontaneity of emotion, whispered speech, or loss of all communication
6. Memory impairment (Thompson & Morgan, 2013)

■ Vertebrobasilar Stroke

The vertebrobasilar system of arteries supplies blood primarily to the posterior portions of the brain, including the brainstem, cerebellum, thalamus, and parts of the occipital and temporal lobes. This posterior circulation is not divided into right and left halves, as in the anterior circulation (Coward et al., 2007; Schneider & Olshaker, 2012). An occlusion here might produce

1. A variety of visual disturbances, including impaired coordination of the eyes
2. Impaired temperature sensation
3. Impaired ability to read and/or name objects
4. Vertigo, dizziness
5. Disturbances in balance when standing or walking (ataxia)
6. Paralysis of the face, limbs, or tongue
7. Clumsy movements of the hands
8. Difficulty judging distance when trying to coordinate limb movements (dysmetria)
9. Drooling and difficulty swallowing (**dysphagia**)
10. Localized numbness
11. Loss of memory (Boyd & Winstein, 2003)
12. Drop attacks in which there is a sudden loss of motor and postural control resulting in collapse, but the individual remains conscious (Parry et al., 2009).

TIAs in this area are common in the elderly. The vertebral arteries travel up to the brainstem through a bony channel in the cervical vertebrae. In older adults, osteoarthritis may develop in the cervical bones, causing narrowing of the cervical canal, especially when the head is extended or rotated (Parry et al., 2009).

■ Wallenberg's Syndrome

Wallenberg's syndrome is a classic brainstem stroke that also is referred to as lateral medullary syndrome (Chen, Khor, Chen, & Huang, 2011). It occurs as the result of an occlusion of a vertebral or cerebellar artery. CVAs in this area may produce contralateral pain and temperature loss, ipsilateral Horner's syndrome (sinking of the eyeball, ptosis of the upper eyelid, and a dry, cool face on the affected side), ataxia, and facial sensory loss. Ischemia to the ipsilateral cranial nerve fibers VIII, IX, and X results in palatal paralysis, hoarseness, dysphagia, and vertigo with no significant weakness (Raymond & Louis, 2015). Brainstem strokes often result in coma because of damage to the centers involved with alertness and wakefulness (reticular system) (Young, Aminoff, Hockberger, & Wilterdink, 2012). A hemorrhage into the brainstem area is rare, quickly accompanied by loss of consciousness, and usually fatal. Among patients who survive brainstem stroke, however, recovery is often good (Young et al., 2012).

■ Other Complications of CVA

Secondary conditions may occur in addition to these deficits. These are important manifestations of the patient's recovery and rehabilitation and may actually be more disabling than the CVA itself (Creutzfeldt, Holloway, & Walker, 2012). Awareness is key to reducing the risk of the following complications.

Seizures

Seizures are among the most common neurological sequelae of CVA. About 10% of all individuals who experience a CVA experience seizures, from CVA onset until several years later (Silverman, Restrepo, & Mathews, 2002). Brain scars that result from CVA may irritate the cortex and cause a spontaneous discharge of nerve impulses that may generalize to a full grand mal convulsion (Leone et al., 2009). Seizures develop in up to 10% of patients with CVA and are more common with embolic than thrombotic infarcts (Leone et al., 2009). Anticonvulsant drugs are sometimes used in patients with early seizures, but their use is controversial (De Reuck, Hemelsoet, & Van Maele, 2007).

Infection

Alteration of swallowing function, aspiration, hypoventilation, and immobility in the patient with CVA often lead to pneumonia (Prass, Braun, Dirnagl, Meisel, & Meisel, 2006). Changes in bladder function may lead to bladder distention and urinary tract infection (Westendorp, Nederkoorn, Vermeij, Dijkgraaf, & van de Beek, 2011). Impaired sensation and inadequate position changes may result in pressure sores (decubitus) and consequent infection of these areas (Turhan, Atalay, & Atabek, 2006).

Thromboembolism

Immobility of the legs and prolonged bed rest often lead to thrombosis of dependent leg veins (MacDougall, Feliu, Boccuzzi, & Lin, 2006). In **deep vein thrombosis** (DVT), local pain and tenderness may develop in the calf, with some swelling and a slight increase in temperature. If the thrombosis is confined to the calf, it may not be serious. However, if the thrombosis spreads up toward the groin to involve the veins in the pelvis, there is a very real possibility of a clot breaking off into the bloodstream. The clot will then travel through the right side of the heart and enter the lungs through the pulmonary arteries, resulting in sudden collapse and death owing to obstruction of the pulmonary arteries (MacDougall et al., 2006). Early mobilization of the patient is of utmost importance in preventing DVT and subsequent pulmonary embolism.

In addition to the above list, it is important to be aware that symptoms resulting from a partial reduction or temporary change in the blood flow to the brain are extremely important warning signs for CVA (Fogle et al., 2008). Several of these conditions are discussed below.

■ Transient Ischemic Attacks

TIAs result from a temporary blockage of the blood supply to the brain. The symptoms occur rapidly and last for <24 hours. Seventy-five percent of TIAs last <5 minutes. The specific signs and symptoms depend on the portion of the brain affected but may include fleeting blindness in one eye, hemiparesis, hemiplegia, aphasia, dizziness, double vision, and staggering. Carotid artery disease and vertebral basilar artery disease may lead to TIAs (Dharmasaroja & Intharakham, 2010). The main distinction between TIAs and CVA is the short duration of the symptoms and the lack of permanent neurological damage. Ten to fifteen percent of clients who experience a TIA will have a CVA within 3 months, with half occurring within 48 hours (Easton et al., 2009; Giles & Rothwell, 2007; Wu et al., 2007). Without preventive treatment, a third of those who suffer TIAs will go on to have a CVA within 5 years (Mattace-Raso et al., 2006). Thus, it is crucial to detect the cause of a TIA and begin appropriate intervention promptly (Sehatzadeh, 2015). The long-term impact of TIAs have been found to be more debilitating (Croot et al., 2014; Moran et al., 2013). Residual problems include anxiety, depression, and fatigue, which need to be addressed before they become disabling. Rehabilitation can play a significant role in decreasing the impact of this type of neurological event (Heron, Kee, Donnelly, & Cupples, 2015).

■ Small Strokes

In some cases, the symptoms of a TIA may last longer than 24 hours. If they last a day or more and then completely resolve, or if they leave only minor neurological deficits, they are called small strokes, or lengthy TIAs (Easton et al., 2009). Often, the remaining neurological deficits are barely noticeable. Like TIAs, however, these small strokes are important warning signs that a more serious CVA may occur (Fogle et al., 2008). A small stroke that completely resolves is called a reversible ischemic neurological deficit (RIND). An episode that lasts more than 72 hours and leaves some minor neurological impairments is called a partially reversible ischemic neurologic deficit (PRIND). The mechanism of injury in RIND and PRIND is the same as that for a CVA or TIA. Like ischemic strokes, RINDs typically occur in the morning; since blood pressure is low during sleep, sudden increases in blood pressure upon arising may cause problems (Metoki et al., 2006).

Many small strokes are not reported to a medical practitioner, which makes the exact frequency of occurrence of these strokes difficult to determine. It is important to recognize the symptoms of a small stroke so that it can be treated early, reducing the risk of more permanent injury.

■ Subclavian Steal Syndrome

This is a rare condition caused by a narrowing of the subclavian artery that runs under the clavicle. Symptoms occur when the arm on the side of the narrowed vessel is exercised. Usually, movement of the arm produces light-headedness, numbness, and weakness. Other neurological symptoms also may be present. In this syndrome, blood is "stolen" from the brain and instead is delivered to the exercised arm. It is a warning sign that advanced atherosclerosis may be present in the arteries throughout the body, including the cerebral arteries (McIntyre, 2009).

COURSE AND PROGNOSIS

CVAs result in anoxic damage to nervous tissue that causes various neurological deficits, depending on where the blood supply was lost. If neuronal cell death occurs, it is considered irreparable and permanent, as no way has yet been found to regenerate nerve cells (Yuan, Lipinski, & Degterev, 2003). However, the nervous system has a high level of plasticity, especially during early development, and individual differences in neural connections and learned behaviors play a major role in functional recovery. No two brains can be expected to be structurally or functionally identical (Carmichael, 2006). Spontaneous recovery may occur as edema subsides or viable neurons reactivate. Recovery also may occur with physiologic reorganization of neural connections or developmental strategies. Reorganization of surviving central nervous system structures facilitates behavioral recovery, such as changes in interhemispheric lateralization, activity of association cortices linked to injured zones, and the organization of cortical representational maps (Hara et al., 2015). Any injury brings different factors into play, affecting axonal and dendritic sprouting or collateral rearrangement, synaptic formation, the excitability of neurons, "substitution of parallel channels," and "mobilization of redundant capacity" (Huang, Shen, & Duong, 2010). Recovery from neurological deficits thus depends on the etiology and size of the infarct (Carmichael, 2006). Approximately 90% of neurological recovery occurs within 3 months, with the rest occurring over a more extended time (Fonarow et al., 2014). It should be noted that recovery from hemorrhagic strokes proceeds more slowly, however (Steiner et al., 2011).

Accuracy in the prediction of function or rate of return is difficult because of individual variability of anatomy and extent of brain damage, as well as differences in types of CVA, learning ability, premorbid personality and intelligence, and motivation (Fonarow et al., 2014). Generally, the prognosis for recovery of function is greater in young clients, possibly because the young brain has more plasticity or because the young are generally in better physical condition.

Secondary complications are important to recovery and rehabilitation as the occurrence of these complications may impact CVA outcomes (Al-Khaled & Eggers, 2013). These complications are discussed in this chapter and include depression, seizures, infection, bowel/bladder incontinence, thromboembolism, shoulder subluxation, painful shoulder, shoulder-hand syndrome, abnormal muscle tone, and **associated reactions** and movements.

Individuals with good sensation, minimal **spasticity**, some selective motor control, and no fixed contractures seem to make the greatest improvements in functional abilities. If an individual has no concept of the affected side and cannot localize stimuli to the affected side, or if he or she has fecal or urinary incontinence, the outlook for independence is generally poor. A small percentage of clients may experience additional CVAs, which affect their recovery outcomes (Bhalla & Birns, 2015).

Long-term complications are associated with CVA (Kuptniratsaikul, Kovindha, Suethanapornkul, Manimmanakorn, & Archongka, 2013). It has been estimated that three-quarters of all clients affected by CVA will have at least one physical or cognitive issue within 1 year of the diagnosis. Different diagnostic conditions, which have been documented, involve musculoskeletal issues including pain, spasticity, shoulder subluxation, and contractures as well as psychological disorders (Kuptniratsaikul et al., 2013).

DIAGNOSIS

The diagnosis of CVA requires knowledge of the incidence of the different types of stroke and awareness of the presence of the complicating factors mentioned above. Symptoms must be carefully noted from the patient or, if the patient is too ill, frightened, or confused, from the family (Hand, Kwan, Lindley, Dennis, & Wardlaw, 2006). Neurologists, neurosurgeons, and some internists are the specialists usually involved in this acute diagnostic phase of treatment (Hand et al., 2006). A number of diagnostic techniques are used to distinguish CVA from other potential causes of observed symptoms and to assist in determining the location of lesions (Sacco et al., 2013).

The physical examination of the client with a suspected CVA or TIA includes a search for possible cardiac sources of emboli by listening to the heart and arteries of the neck. Also useful in the determination of cardiac-source emboli are electrocardiography (ECG), echocardiography, and monitoring for arrhythmias. In addition to cardiac testing, various neuroimaging techniques (see below) and analysis of blood and CSF may be performed (Feldmann et al., 2007). A neurological examination assists in determining the neurological disability and usually includes evaluation of higher cortical function (memory and language), level of alertness, reflexes, visual and oculomotor system, behavior, and gait (Feldmann et al., 2007). Other diagnostic methods include noninvasive studies of blood vessels and invasive techniques requiring injection of dye into the arterial system, for example.

■ Neuroimaging Techniques

CT and magnetic resonance imaging (MRI) are invaluable noninvasive tools that depict pathological changes in the brain in clients with CVA (Tarpley, Frank, Tansy, & Liebeskind, 2013). One or the other of these is almost always used at some point for every client with a suspected CVA. CT and MRI are also capable of showing zones of edema and the shifting of intracranial material (Kidwell & Wintermark, 2010). Negative results of these tests may indicate that the ischemia is reversible (Feldmann et al., 2007). CT scans and MRI are the most reliable tools for determining intracranial hemorrhages and infarctions (Tarpley et al., 2013).

Computed Tomography

CT is a type of radiographic examination that is widely used for analysis of cerebral injury (Kidwell & Wintermark, 2010). CT scans are employed to differentiate between a hemorrhagic stroke and an ischemic stroke (Kidwell & Wintermark, 2010). While they are useful in clarifying the location and the mechanism and severity of CVA, they are not particularly sensitive to subtle ischemic changes such as lacunar strokes and microbleeds (Kidwell & Wintermark, 2010). It is the most common tool used in the diagnosis of CVA caused by hemorrhage, but research is finding that MRI is more effective (Kidwell & Wintermark, 2010). It can be diagnostic in clients with TIAs, but MRI is the preferred method of

evaluation if available (Sidorov, Feng, & Selim, 2014).

Magnetic Resonance Imaging

MRI is more sensitive than a CT scan and does not expose the client to radiation. It provides detailed pictures of the brain by using a magnetic field. MRI provides better detection for ischemic areas than does a CT scan as well as distinguishes whether a hemorrhage is new or chronic (Arsava, 2012). MRI can provide information about all aspects that are being affected when the CVA is detected from tissue health to the circulatory system of the brain, which in turn can help determine the best CVA treatment for the client (Arsava, 2012). Research also shows that MRI may assist in determining the candidacy of the patient for CVA treatment when the length of time the CVA has been occurring is unknown (Tarpley et al., 2013).

Positron Emission Tomography (PET scan)

Positron emission tomography, or PET scan, is being used experimentally. This scan shows how the brain uses oxygen and glucose, which are the main energy elements of the brain, and can indicate the effects of CVA on the brain (Bunevicius, Yuan, & Lin, 2013). Currently, PET scans are seldom used in the management of acute CVA, but research exists supporting the use of PET as another tool in assessing CVA progression to determine management (Bunevicius et al., 2013). The use of PET/MRI together has been found to be particularly sensitive and more precise in guiding treatment decisions (Werner et al., 2015).

Noninvasive Study of Blood Vessels

Noninvasive procedures used to evaluate both extracranial and intracranial blood flow include duplex ultrasonography as well as color-flow and transcranial Doppler ultrasound. These techniques can localize and determine the approximate size of the lesions within the arteries (Aaslid, Huber, & Nornes, 2010).

Duplex ultrasonography is useful in detecting the presence and severity of disease in the common and internal carotid arteries and in the subclavian and vertebral arteries in the neck. This scan can reliably differentiate between minor plaque disease, stenosis, and occlusive lesions. It is an excellent method of monitoring the progression or regression of atherosclerotic disease in the neck (Vassileva, Daskalov, & Stamenova, 2015).

Color-flow Doppler ultrasound is used because it is effective in showing lesions of the carotid and vertebral arteries (Nasr, Ssi-Yan-Kai, Guidolin, Bonneville, & Larrue, 2013). Transcranial Doppler ultrasound gives information about pressure and flow in the intracranial arteries (Dwedar et al., 2014). A recent study found that use of this type of ultrasound may play a therapeutic role in restoring blood flow velocity even before the use of thrombolytic therapy (tPA) and, due to the noninvasive nature provided, it may be another viable method to utilize (Dwedar et al., 2014).

■ Invasive Techniques

Cerebral angiography involves radiography of the vascular system of the brain after injecting a dye or other contrast medium into the arterial blood system. Computer-generated images are then produced that can show the entire visible length of cerebral arteries, as well as, the nature, location, and extent of pathological changes. This technique is now safer than before (<1% incidence of mortality and serious morbidity); however, it is recommended when noninvasive techniques have failed to yield a conclusive diagnosis or when surgery is being planned or considered (Kaufmann et al., 2007). The use of angiography has been found to be effective when decisions about the best therapeutic method are required in terms of delivering thrombolytic agents intravenously or intra-arterially (Porelli et al., 2013).

Analysis of CSF can be helpful in determining the severity and functional outcome of an acute ischemic stroke within the first few hours by examining the levels of cytokines and nitrates present (Beridze, Sanikidze, Shakarishvili, Intskirveli, & Bornstein, 2011). These elements are associated with inflammatory damage, which can occur from the ischemia.

■ Other Diagnostic Techniques

ECG is another diagnostic technique, which can be used due to the high incidence of heart disease in clients with CVA (Salmani, Prarthana, Bandelkar, & Varghese, 2014). With acute stroke patients, changes are noted with ECG recordings, and different wave patterns may be indicative of mortality rates (Salmani et al., 2014); however, more research needs to be performed. Other diagnostic techniques used for CVA include

electroencephalography (EEG), single photon emission tomography (SPET), and other special cardiac and coagulation tests that are useful in detecting unusual heart and blood disorders that can bring on a CVA (Petrella, Coleman, & Doraiswamy, 2003). After the type of CVA has been determined based on the diagnostic tools used, further management may be indicated in the form of medical or surgery. If not, a neurologist will evaluate the brain-damaged person's ability to function. Rehabilitation often will begin at that point to return the client to the highest possible level of independent functioning (Rodríguez-Mutuberría et al., 2011).

MEDICAL/SURGICAL MANAGEMENT

At present, the treatment of acute CVA is limited to management of the results of the primary event and preventive measures against further injury or occurrence (Zhao et al., 2009). The most effective management of CVAs is constantly evolving as new drugs, imaging techniques, and surgical interventions are being developed (Sacks et al., 2013). Before the CVA can be treated, it must be accurately identified as either cerebral infarction or cerebral hemorrhage, since interventions that are beneficial with one type of CVA may be potentially dangerous to the other (Tansy et al., 2015). Therefore, careful and exact diagnosis must be made first. Drug management of CVA is constantly evolving. Common categories of drugs used to minimize the damage of cerebral infarction are described in the following sections.

■ Antiplatelet Therapy

Aspirin is often prescribed to patients when the vascular lesion is not severely stenotic and the individual has not had a CVA (Bégot et al., 2013). Use of two antiplatelets including aspirin reduces the possibility of a CVA in those who have had a previous CVA or TIA, as well as those who are at high risk for CVA more significantly than does just aspirin use in the short term (Tan et al., 2015). But long-term efficacy of dual use of antiplatelets has been found to be detrimental (Xie, Zheng, Zhong, & Song, 2015). There is an additional concern with increased risk of hemorrhage so the benefits must be examined to ensure they outweigh the risk (Tan et al., 2015). It also benefits clients who have had a mild CVA but is not as effective in those with moderate or severe CVAs (Sacco et al., 2006a, 2006b). Aspirin is clearly not suitable for clients with cerebral hemorrhage or those at risk of bleeding. Aspirin is relatively safe and inexpensive. Studies have looked at the efficacy of aspirin use in low doses as a preemptive therapy and found a benefit in the prevention of cardiovascular diseases (Stegeman, Bossuyt, Yu, Boyd, & Puhan, 2015).

■ Anticoagulants

Anticoagulants inhibit clotting by interfering with the activity of chemicals in the liquid portion of blood that are essential for the coagulation process (Mant et al., 2007). Short-term (2 to 3 weeks) heparin therapy is prescribed for clients with complete blockages of large arteries, as heparin is effective in preventing the formation of emboli (Diener et al., 2006). For longer-term treatment (1 to 3 months), the drug warfarin may be used to prevent blockages in areas that cannot be treated by surgery (Mant et al., 2007).

■ Thrombolytics (tPA)

Thrombolytic therapy (tPA), used for dissolution of an occluding thrombus, is frequently applied in the acute treatment of myocardial infarction as well as in the treatment of CVA. It is effective before extensive brain infarction has occurred, so it is only appropriate in CVA patients whose arterial damage has been identified early (Demchuk & Bal, 2012). The potential benefit must be weighed against reperfusion damage, a bleeding tendency, and the possibility of reocclusion. The Food and Drug Administration (FDA) has approved the use of tPA for treatment of acute CVA within 3 hours of onset (Demchuk & Bal, 2012). However, studies are researching whether administration of thrombolytics beyond the 3-hour limit will still produce favorable outcomes in CVA recovery (Emberson et al., 2014). At this time, there is an indication that clients will still improve in their functional outcomes after receiving thrombolytics up to 5 hours after initial CVA symptoms appeared (Emberson et al., 2014). Much more research needs to occur in regard to the time of administration as well as methods of administration. Another area of recent interest is determining the location of the infarct to administer thrombolytics either intravenously or intra-arterially, which can affect how well a client recovers (Berkhemer et al., 2015). Also, newer research is examining the efficacy of moving from using time limits to analyzing the health of brain tissue in determining the administration of thrombolytics (Demchuk & Bal, 2012; Leiva-Salinas et al., 2013).

■ Surgical Interventions

In some cases, surgical treatment may be the best choice for the client. The neurosurgeon must carefully consider many factors before surgery is performed, including the client's overall health and life expectancy. Carotid endarterectomy (CEA) was among the most commonly performed vascular surgeries in the United States, but now, carotid artery stenting (CAS) is used more often due to the lower invasive properties of the procedure (Al-Damluji, Nagpal, Stilp, Remetz, & Mena, 2013). During the CEA procedure, the diseased vessel is opened, the clot is removed, and an artificial graft is put in place (Mendonça et al., 2014). During CAS, a stent, which is a narrow tube, is inserted in the carotid to expand the artery and, in turn, increase the blood flow. CEA has become a less common treatment option for patients with moderate to severe stenosis of the carotid artery due to the common use of statins in the United States (Al-Damluji et al., 2013). Statins are a preemptive medication used to lower blood cholesterol, which decreases the risk of a CVA occurring.

Subarachnoid hemorrhages are often caused by ruptured aneurysms or AVMs. Surgical clipping or coiling is the most effective treatment of these anomalies. If the patient survives the initial bleeding, the goal of surgery is to correct the problem before bleeding recurs. If surgery is performed, there is an increased probability of a successful outcome for the client (Garbossa et al., 2012). In intracerebral hemorrhage, small hematomas usually resolve spontaneously, but the chance of a recurrence is greatly increased (Chou et al., 2012). Surgery of these smaller hematomas has been investigated, but there are increased risks and more research needs to be performed (Kim & Ko, 2014). Clipping versus coiling can affect the patient cognitive outcomes (Latimer, Wilson, McCuskey, Caldwell, & Rennie, 2013). Endovascular coiling appears to affect the patient less cognitively than those patients who underwent neurosurgical clipping and demonstrated more global deficits.

Large hematomas, however, often produce death. Some lesions may expand, causing gradually increasing neurological signs. These expanding lesions can be drained surgically if they are near the surface of the brain, especially in the cerebral or cerebellar white matter. Generally, hemorrhages are evacuated only if they are large and life threatening or when surgery is necessary to treat an aneurysm, tumor, or AVM, but of those who experience this type of bleed, 66% do not undergo surgery (Hobson et al., 2014).

Superficial temporal artery bypass is a new, more delicate surgical therapy for preventing future CVAs (Chou et al., 2012). The procedure begins with craniotomy to expose the brain; then a scalp artery is connected to an intracranial artery microsurgically. This operation is extremely challenging to perform and is thus performed less frequently than CEA. Surgeons who do the procedure, however, are enthusiastic about the results and claim that it revascularizes the brain better than does endarterectomy, and studies have determined that there is a 0% chance of a recurrent CVA (Chou et al., 2012).

■ Treatment of Secondary Effects

Specific pathophysiologic sequelae, or outcomes, follow the occurrence of any type of CVA. Treating these secondary effects is crucial to medical and functional recovery. Two of these are cerebral edema and ischemia. Oxygen therapy to reduce hypoxia, vasodilation to improve blood flow through ischemic areas, therapeutic hypertension, and hemodilution therapy are some of the treatments used for ischemia. Hemodilution results in a significant rise in cerebral blood flow and increased oxygen transfer (Vilela & Newell, 2008).

Edema often complicates ischemic strokes and must be controlled, because most deaths during the first week after a massive CVA are caused by extensive cerebral edema and increased intracranial pressure (Treggiari, Walder, Suter, & Romand, 2003). This pressure can displace the cerebrum downward and interfere with the functioning of the midbrain and lower brainstem, which control such basic vital functions as respiration and heart action (Treggiari et al., 2003).

Corticosteroid therapy can cause a significant reduction in interstitial cerebral edema, reducing swelling and improving outcomes after CVA (Thomas et al., 2007). However, a review of the literature indicates that there is no clear basis for evaluating the effect of corticosteroid treatment for people with acute ischemic strokes (Veltkamp et al., 2005).

IMPACT ON OCCUPATIONAL PERFORMANCE

The Occupational Therapy Practice Framework (OTPF) 3rd edition includes client factors, which are particular capacities, characteristics, or beliefs that define a person and influence performance in occupations (American Occupational Therapy Association [AOTA], 2014). The impact of CVA on an individual is unique and may affect client factors. Deficits in sensory, motor, mental, communication, and emotional client factors may be compounded by secondary complications, such as infection or depression. Together, these significantly impact an individual's performance in all areas of occupation: activities of daily living (both basic and instrumental), work, play, leisure, and social participation.

■ Sensory Functions

Sensory functions can be affected at the very basic level of awareness and at the point of processing and modulation of sensory input. Loss of protective tactile functions, such as diminished awareness of temperature and pain, is a common concern for an individual with a CVA. Loss of these functions poses a safety risk. Individuals with proprioceptive dysfunction may show asymmetrical posture, have difficulty maintaining balance, appear to forget affected body parts, be unable to describe position or movement of limbs, and be susceptible to joint damage (Lima et al., 2015). Individuals with a loss of tactile sensation may demonstrate a lack of awareness of body parts simply because they forget what they cannot feel. They are also vulnerable to damage of affected body parts, particularly skin breakdown. Moreover, diminished tactile function hinders resumption of motor activities. Depending on the location of the infarct, individuals may experience diminished vestibular function, which will limit mobility efficiency and safety. Impaired balance may cause difficulties in assuming and maintaining a vertical posture and in automatic adjustments to changes of position and antigravity movement. As a result, individuals demonstrate an asymmetrical posture at rest, leaning or falling to the hemiplegic side during mobility, or fail to use normal protective reactions when falling (Kim, Kim, & Kang, 2015; Mitsutake et al., 2014).

Defects in visual field functions may impair reading, even in the absence of language dysfunction. For example, clients with right cerebral lesions may find reading difficult or impossible, because visuospatial deficits hinder tracking or following the line of print across the page. Clients with homonymous hemianopsia on either side are unable to respond to people, objects, or the environment on the affected side. They may bump into objects or be startled by their sudden appearance. Individuals experiencing visual inattention have difficulty scanning and shifting their gaze, particularly toward the affected side (Goodwin, 2014) (Fig. 17.6).

Perceptual deficits may be difficult to understand for patient and family alike, but their impact on the client's ability to resume independent function may be profound. Depending on the location of the lesion, or infarct, such deficits include visual **agnosia** and visuospatial agnosia—difficulty in understanding the relationship between objects and between self and objects (Zhang, Kedar, Lynn, Newman, & Biousse, 2006). Individuals affected in this manner are unable to find their way in a familiar environment; they cannot trace a route on a map, cannot pick out objects from a cluttered environment, cannot copy drawings or simple construction, and may have difficulty in functional (spatial) tasks, such as dressing and reading a newspaper. A condition where the client "pushes" away from the nonhemiparetic side is thought to be due to an impairment in the client's perception of their vertical orientation (Mansfield et al., 2015). This behavior could affect participation in occupations by impairing client factors such as mobility.

Agnosia for sounds may also occur, so that the individual cannot understand or confuses nonverbal sounds (Jang, Kim, Park, & Lee, 2014; Tabuchi, 2014; Urbanski, Coubard, & Bourlon, 2014). Another important loss is astereognosis, which affects functional use of the affected hand whenever vision is occluded: tasks such as finding keys or coins in a pocket or a glass on a bedside table when it is dark may be difficult (Murray, Camen, Gonzalez, Bovet, & Clarke, 2006).

The location of the infarct determines which functions are lost and which remain intact. For example, somatagnosia, in which an individual has no awareness of his or her own body and its condition, is commonly seen in right parietal lobe lesions. Deficits that result from right cerebral injuries often cause unilateral perceptual problems of the left body side and space, such as unilateral body inattention. Unilateral body inattention (or neglect) is different from unilateral spatial (or visual) inattention as the first represents a lack of awareness of one side of the body, usually the left side, and the latter is a visual unawareness of part of the visual field. Lesions in the left cerebral hemisphere, however, cause bilateral problems, such as right/left discrimination (Connell, 2008). Impairment of the left parietal lobe results in reduced motor planning (**apraxia**), whereby individuals are unable to adjust movement of their own body parts for intentional movements. Yet impairment of the right parietal lobe causes an inability to adjust the position of external objects. Frontal lobe lesions may also result in impaired motor planning, in which sequencing

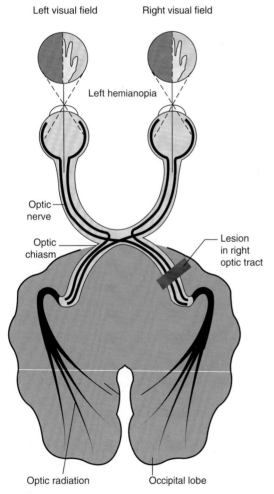

Figure 17.6 Homonymous hemianopsia. (From Timby, B. K., Smith, N. E. (2013). *Introductory medical-surgical nursing* (11th ed.). Philadelphia, PA: Lippincott Williams & Wilkins.)

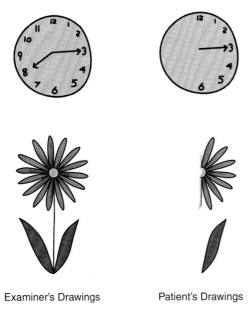

Examiner's Drawings   Patient's Drawings

Figure 17.7 Examples of impaired performance on a test for copying given to a patient with unilateral neglect. (From Hickey, J. (2013). *Clinical practice of neurological and neurosurgical nursing* (7th ed.). Philadelphia, PA: Lippincott Williams & Wilkins.)

of movement becomes difficult. Individuals with impaired motor planning may be unable to carry out a verbal request (for even a simple task such as combing the hair), although often they can perform such tasks automatically (Jax, Rosa-Leyra, & Buxbaum, 2014). They may perseverate, that is, persist in purposeless movement, or they may be unable to complete a required sequence of acts, copy gestures and drawings, or carry out simple spatial constructional tasks (Beis et al., 2004) (Fig. 17.7).

■ Motor Functions

Sensory loss seldom occurs in isolation but typically accompanies the loss of motor functions. The combination of sensory and motor loss impairs limb recovery and overall participation in occupations (Meyer, Karttunen, Thijs, Feys, & Verheyden, 2014). Motor dysfunction because of CVA usually results in changes in muscle tone that render normal movement impossible. It has been commonly said that hypotonicity (flaccid hemiplegia) gives way to hypertonicity (spastic hemiplegia); occasionally, there is progress into a final stage, in which normal movement patterns re-emerge (Mikołajewska, 2012).

The muscle tone of individuals with an intact central nervous system operates within a range that permits effective voluntary movement. Normal muscle tone is high enough to stabilize and maintain a person through an activity, while at the same time low enough to allow ease of movement. This variability of tone allows mobility to be superimposed on stability (Gogola, Saulicz, Kuszewski, Matyja, & Myśliwiec, 2014).

Abnormal tone may be termed either low or high. **Hypotonus**, or **flaccidity**, is felt as too little resistance, or floppiness. When released, the extremity will drop. At the other extreme, when there is too much resistance, hypertonus, or spasticity, is felt. Spasticity is the result of hyperactive reflexes and loss of moderating or inhibiting influences from higher brain centers (Florman, Duffau, & Rughani, 2013; Trompetto et al., 2014). Spasticity may be aggravated by pain, emotional upset, or efforts to hurry. Spasticity is never isolated to one muscle group but is always a part of what is known as either an extensor or flexor synergy, that is, a grouping of stereotypical movements. These movement patterns usually consist of a flexion pattern in the arm (scapular retraction and depression, shoulder adduction and internal rotation, elbow flexion, forearm pronation, wrist flexion, finger and thumb flexion and adduction) and an extension pattern in the leg (pelvis rotated back and internal rotation, knee extension, foot plantar flexion and inversion, toe flexion and adduction).

Abnormal tone is not limited to the extremities, however, and is manifested in the head and trunk. The head is usually flexed toward the hemiplegic side and rotated so that the face is toward the unaffected side. The trunk is rotated back on the hemiplegic side with side flexion of the hemiplegic side (Karthikbabu et al., 2012; Liao, Liaw, Wang, Su, & Hsu, 2015). These typical patterns of spasticity interfere with the normal, smooth, efficient, and coordinated movement necessary for locomotion in and manipulation of the environment including daily occupations (Fujita et al., 2015) (Figs. 17.8 and 17.9).

If untreated, spasticity may lead to contractures (Chang et al., 2013). Spasticity can be debilitating for clients if it interferes with participation in occupations or causes pain. Different types of pharmacological approaches can be used including botulinum toxin and diazepam to decrease the effects of the spasticity, and research continues to

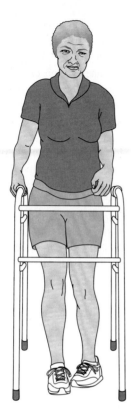

Figure 17.8 Posture of client with right-sided stroke. (From Walton, T. (2010). *Medical conditions and massage therapy.* Philadelphia, PA: Lippincott Williams & Wilkins.)

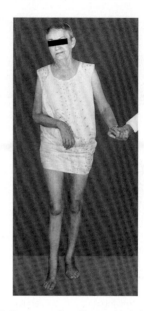

Figure 17.9 Posture of a client with left-sided stroke. (From Salter, R. B. (1998). *Textbook of disorders and injuries of the musculoskeletal system.* Philadelphia, PA: Lippincott Williams & Wilkins.)

investigate different forms of tone management (Dashtipour, Chen, Walker, & Lee, 2015; Francisco & McGuire, 2015). Addressing the return of motor function is an important part of rehabilitation, and a number of theories and treatment methods have been developed. In recent years, one approach that is being studied for its effectiveness is known as constraint-induced therapy (CIMT). CIMT has been found to be highly effective; however, there are questions about its practical use as CIMT is a highly restrictive and time-intensive program and is not a technique that can be used by clients who are severely impaired (Marque, Gasq, Castel-Lacanal, De Boissezon, & Loubinoux, 2014). Modified CIMT (m-CIMT) programs have been studied where the client does not have the unaffected arm restrained for as long as dictated in CIMT programs and success has been documented (Park, Lee, Cho, & Yang, 2015) but this research is ongoing.

The hemiplegic shoulder is also a common concern. Typical problems include shoulder subluxation, pain, and immobility. Because of the unstable nature of the glenohumeral joint, the anatomy of the shoulder is particularly vulnerable to problems. Normally, this lack of stability is partly compensated for by a strong surrounding musculature. However, subluxation is inevitable once the surrounding musculature of the shoulder, especially the so-called rotator cuff muscles, has been damaged (Huang et al., 2012; Kim et al., 2014).

After a CVA, changes in muscle tone and movement, the position of the scapula, and joint capsule stability allow the pull of gravity to draw the head of the humerus out of the glenoid fossa of the scapula, resulting in shoulder subluxation (Huang et al., 2012). Clients with hemiplegia have lost voluntary movement in muscles such as the supraspinatus, infraspinatus, and posterior fibers of the deltoid. In addition, the muscles that support the scapula in its normal alignment are affected, which leads to a change in angulation of the glenoid fossa (Fig. 17.10).

Another typical complication is "the painful shoulder." This condition may either develop quickly after a CVA or at a much later stage. It presents with flaccid or spastic muscle tone and with or without subluxation. In hemiplegia, the normal, coordinated, and timed movement of the scapula and humerus (scapulohumeral rhythm) has been disturbed by abnormal and unbalanced muscle tone (Cho, Kim, & Joo, 2012). The typical

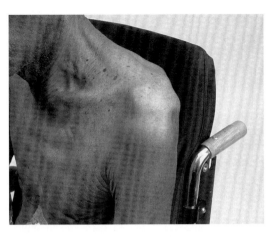

Figure 17.10 Shoulder subluxation. (From Oatis, C. (2008). *Kinesiology: The mechanics and pathomechanics of human movement* (2nd ed.). Philadelphia, PA: Lippincott Williams & Wilkins.)

hemiplegic postural components of depression and retraction of the scapula and internal rotation of the humerus are especially important to the mechanism of pain. Fear of pain during passive movement of the arm will further increase abnormal flexor tone, which can become a vicious cycle (Kim, Jung, Yang, & Paik, 2014). A chronically painful shoulder can lead to shoulder-hand syndrome, also known as reflex sympathetic dystrophy (RSD). This complex condition produces severe pain, edema of the hand, and limitations in range of motion on the involved side (Li et al., 2012). These complications not only interfere with movement, but they may have profound emotional consequences.

Another motor dysfunction caused by CVA is the presence of associated reactions. Associated reactions in hemiplegia are abnormal reflex movements of the affected side that duplicate the synergy patterns of the arm and leg (McMorland, Runnalls, & Byblow, 2015). These movements may be observed when the client moves with effort, is trying to maintain balance, or is afraid of falling. A flexor pattern of involuntary movement in the arm is often observed when the individual yawns, coughs, or sneezes. Associated reactions also are seen when new activities, such as running or putting on socks, are attempted after a CVA. They are stereotyped reactions and may occur even if no active movement is present in the limb. The limb returns to its normal position only after cessation of the stimulus and usually does so gradually (Bhakta, O'Connor, & Cozens, 2008).

Unlike associated reactions, associated movements accompany voluntary movements and are normal, automatic postural adjustments. They reinforce precise movements of other parts of the body or occur when a great amount of strength is required. They are not pathological and can be stopped at will. Associated movements often can be observed in the unaffected extremities of individuals with CVA who are trying new activities (Bhakta et al., 2008).

Other motor dysfunctions include orofacial weakness, which may cause difficulties in expression, speech (dysarthria), mastication, and swallowing (dysphagia) (Yanagida, Fujimoto, Inoue, & Suzuki, 2015; Yang, Choi, & Son, 2015). Additionally, bladder or bowel incontinence may result from a communication disorder or from disruption of normal routine and diet, lack of awareness of body function, or emotional disorder (Daniels et al., 2009; Kovindha, Wyndaele, & Madersbacher, 2010).

■ Mental Functions

Within mental function, the Practice Framework (OTPF) incorporates the areas of affective, cognitive, and perceptual. Cognition encompasses information processing, including attention, comprehension, and formation of speech (Gillen et al., 2015) with cognition being a foundational determinant of occupational performance, social participation, and well-being (AOTA, 2013). Severe CVAs often result in cognitive deficits that affect global and specific mental functions (Hallevi et al., 2009). Statistically, overall prevalence of cerebral infarct resulting in cognitive impairment ranges from 31% to 77% (Jaillard, Naegele, Trabucco-Miguel, LeBas, & Hommel, 2009). Milder CVAs may have a more subtle impact on mental function, however. Commonly used psychometrics are not always sensitive to the wide range of mental functions and process skills that may permit effective occupational performance: initiation, recognition, attention, orientation, sequencing, categorization, concept formation, spatial operations, problem solving, and learning abilities (Nys et al., 2007). Moreover, basic visual deficits also have an impact on cognitive performance. For example, visual attending and scanning deficits lead to a decrease in the efficiency required for cognitive performance (Hoffmann, Bennett, Koh, & McKenna, 2010; Pendlebury, Cuthbertson, Welch, Mehta, & Rothwell, 2010).

In summary, CVAs have the potential to cause deficits in perception and cognition that impact functional independence (Gillen et al., 2015).

■ Emotional Functions

As many as 50% of all clients who experience a CVA may encounter a stroke-related psychological or emotional disorder (Hildebrand, 2015). Carota and Bogousslavsky (2009) organized these disorders into the four categories: (1) affective and mood disorders, such as depression, poststroke emotionalism, and generalized anxiety disorders; (2) behavioral and personality changes such as anger, irritability, apathy, sexual changes, and obsessive-compulsive disorder; (3) cognitive and behavioral disintegration such as acute confusional state and delirium; and (4) perception-identify disorders of the self or of other people and places. Significant depression has been recorded in 30% to 50% of stroke survivors (Berg, Lönnqvist, Palomäki, & Kaste, 2009). These changes often are a major cause of concern to relatives and the individual. While depression is often viewed as a natural and understandable consequence of reduced function caused by CVA, proper treatment can result in observable improvement. Depression is more frequent and severe with lesions in the left hemisphere, as compared with right hemisphere or brainstem strokes (Williams et al., 2007). Both organic and psychological factors are probably involved in poststroke depression (Williams et al., 2007).

Emotional lability, sudden and extreme shifts of mood, may be the result of a release of inhibition. The individual may switch from laughing to crying for no apparent reason. Excessive crying is the most common problem and is frequently the result of organic emotional lability rather than depression or sadness over perceived losses. Organic emotional lability is characterized by little or no obvious relation between the start of emotional expression and what is happening around the person (Provinciali et al., 2008).

Catastrophic reactions are outbursts in which frustration, anger, and depression are combined. When individuals cannot perform tasks that used to be very easy, they may be unable to inhibit emotional expression and may begin sobbing, expressing a sense of hopelessness (Carota, 2008; Thompson & Ryan, 2009). Outbursts and emotional difficulties are to be expected after CVA. Relatives and families should be told that a tendency to cry easily or get upset will improve with time. Families and therapists need to develop a positive, understanding attitude if the individual is to overcome psychological sequelae. The psychosocial impact of CVA on patients and families can be lessened with increased social support and access to services once the individual has been discharged to home and community (Ferro, Caeiro, & Santos, 2009).

CASE STUDY

Initial Presentation

Janet is a 67-year-old female who retired 5 months ago from her occupation of president of a trucking company. She and her husband had built the company from the ground up starting with two trucks 30 years ago. When Janet retired, the company had 500 trucks. She handed the reins to her twin sons who have been "in training" for the past 5 years. Janet's job meant she was at her desk for long hours each day, as well as on call on weekends. The job could be stressful when trailer deliveries did not occur at the time promised or trucks would break down. There was also a high turnover with drivers, and she was always trying to fill positions. Her husband, the CEO, also retired from the same company on the same day. Janet has never been one to exercise. She would just go home and watch TV being so mentally exhausted from her days of dealing with people and problems. Janet has been gaining weight over the past 10 years, but she was not concerned. She eats fast food for dinner at least 4 out of the 5 work days and never has time for breakfast. Her lunch consist of coffee and whatever people have brought in for snacks and desserts. She cooks meals at home on the weekends, but she feels now that she is home more she will be able to start cooking more healthy meals. At this time, she has not been able to start with home cooking since she and her husband have been eating out a lot as their retirement treat. But, she plans to start meal planning soon. Her doctor kept telling her she needed to lose weight and was concerned especially since her BP has been consistently in stage 1 hypertension averaging 150/90 for her past 4 yearly physical exams. Her doctor wants her to take medications to address this issue, but Janet does not want to take any drugs. She just does not believe in pharmaceuticals. Now that she has all this extra time, she believes she will be able to start walking and participate in a consistent exercise program. She feels her BP will be fine and she will be able to lose all the weight. If only she could get motivated to start... "Tomorrow" she tells herself every day.

Sunday afternoon, Janet began to get a headache located in the back of her head. She also began to feel a little nauseated, and as she walked to her bed to take a nap, she ran into the doorway to her bedroom. "That was clumsy of me" she thought as she lay down on her bed and closed her eyes. Two hours later, Janet woke up with a worse headache. She also noticed as she looked up at her ceiling that she could not see her light, which is located to the left of the bed. She turned her head to the left and then saw the light. She thought to herself that maybe she had never been able to see the light and started to get out of bed to go get some aspirin for her headache. As she started to stand up from her bed, she lost her balance and fell to her left side on her bed. "I just can't believe how clumsy I am today" she thought to herself as she tried to stand again. This time she fell to the floor with a crash that brought her husband running into the bedroom. Her husband lifted her up to the bed and asked her what happened. Janet could not figure out why and how she had ended up on the floor. She started to stand again and realized how heavy her left arm felt. Looking at her husband as he stood in front of her, she realized she could only see part of him. So strange she thought to herself, what is going on and why is he standing there? Janet's head was hurting so she tried to lay back down but ended up flopping onto her left side on the bed. Her husband could see something was wrong with her and wondered if she had hit her head when she fell. She was not making sense to him, and she wanted to go back to sleep. He

wondered if she had a concussion. He reached for the phone and dialed 911 asking for an ambulance while trying to keep her talking since he knew that she needed to stay awake if she had hit her head. Janet was not making much sense to him. She was talking about packing for a vacation and going to Mexico. The ambulance arrived in 5 minutes and proceeded to take her and her husband to the emergency room of the local hospital.

Hospital Course

Once in the emergency room, the ER doctor started a preliminary evaluation by asking Janet and her husband questions. Janet was clearly confused by the questions, and her verbalizations were full of made-up words and slurred speech. Her husband expressed his concern that she had hit her head when she fell. The doctor did not see any external signs of trauma and her visual exam showed a left visual homonymous hemianopia. Due to this finding, the doctor activated the stroke response team. Nursing took a finger stick to assess blood sugar and started an IV. The stroke response team arrived and ordered a noncontrast CT scan, cardiac workup, and blood work including CBC, Chem-7, and PT/INR. Results from the CT scan determined an infarct had occurred on the right posterior cerebral artery located in the occipital lobe as well as extending into the right internal capsule and thalamus. Since her husband reported she had complained of a headache about 3 hours ago, tPA was started at the time. Janet was transferred to the ICU where she was monitored by nurses.

Forty-eight hours later, orders were sent to occupational, physical, and speech therapies to evaluate Janet. Occupational therapy noted that she had left homonymous hemianopsia, her left UE strength was weak including her grip and she is left-hand dominant, she had decreased sensation on her left UE, and she was oriented to self only. Janet was able to independently wash her face and brush her teeth after setup using her right hand as she sat in a chair. Since she was in the ICU, the OT did not evaluate her dressing skills. When she spoke, some of her words did not make sense, but she followed all one-step commands consistently. Physical therapy's assessment documented her left LE strength was decreased, but she was able to bear weight on both her legs when she stood up. Her standing and sitting balance were also decreased, and the therapist always had to have her hand on Janet's transfer belt. Ambulation was not attempted. The speech therapist assessed Janet's swallow and found it to be functional. Her speech was slurred, and she appeared to have problems using the correct words. Janet stayed on the ICU unit one more day and was then transferred to the neuro step down unit. The therapists continued to see her for ADLs, mobility, and speech articulation.

Within 3 days, Janet was ready to be transferred to the rehabilitation unit where she would receive at least 3 hours of therapy a day. Janet's husband and sons were very happy with this transition as they all agreed Janet would be going home after an inhospital rehabilitation stay. The goals were to get Janet as independent as possible in her mobility and daily living skills.

CASE STUDY 2

Initial Presentation

During a basketball game, Danny Wiley, a 9-year-old boy developed a sudden onset of weakness and clumsiness on his left side of his body. He quickly noticed that he was unable to dribble the ball using his left hand. At the same time, he felt like his head was going to pop off of his body due to the immense pain and pressure that he felt. Danny's coach noticed that Danny was weaving down the court and that his ball skills were significantly worse than normal. Danny, who was his star forward, was unable to control the ball or his body at all. Danny's coach quickly signaled a time-out to the referee. As soon as Danny's coach ran over to him, Danny had collapsed onto the gym floor. Emergency medical services were called immediately and arrived minutes later.

Hospital Course

Within 30 minutes, Danny and his family were in the emergency room at the local hospital. In the ER, Danny's blood pressure was elevated and he was disoriented. Initial physical examination revealed left-sided weakness and sensory loss more apparent in Danny's arm compared to his leg. The admitting doctor evaluated Danny and advised that he be seen by a pediatric neurologist. The neurological examination revealed decreased grip strength in Danny's left hand, poor finger dexterity, and slowing of rapid alternating movements such as being able to turn his left hand palm up and palm down quickly.

The ER doctor ordered a CT scan of Danny's head, which came back showing internal bleeding. The neurology team advised that Danny be admitted for inpatient hospitalization to allow more testing as they suspected a CVA. Danny and his parents were very worried but trusted the neurology team. MRI with MR angiography (MRA) validated right AIS. A shunt was inserted to relieve the pressure on his brain, and an angiogram revealed an arteriovenous malformation (AVM), an abnormal collection of blood vessels, in the medulla area of the brainstem. Following shunt surgery, Danny recovered in the pediatric intensive care unit or PICU and was kept in a chemically induced coma. He was on a ventilator because doctors were not sure he could breathe on his own. Danny's family was full of worry and questioned how this CVA would affect their son's life. A couple of days later, Danny's eyes opened and he asked his mom, "Where am I?" At that time, Danny's doctor ordered occupational therapy (OT), physical therapy (PT), and speech therapy (SLP) to evaluate Danny's current functioning.

The therapists assessed Danny in the PICU the day the order was received. PT watched how Danny moved his right leg in bed, but noted how he was unable to move his left leg by himself. When PT assisted Danny in sitting at the edge of his bed, Danny required moderate assistance to stay upright and kept leaning his body toward the left. OT observed Danny brushing his teeth and washing his face with his right hand with help to set up the toothbrush with paste and wring out the washcloth. The SLP observed Danny talking and remembering the names of his friends who came by for a visit. Danny's family and doctors were pleased to see that Danny demonstrated no memory impairments. However, Danny was unable to move his left arm and leg without great effort. He was sent to a rehabilitation center for therapy to regain motor functions with the goal of returning to school and basketball.

RECOMMENDED LEARNING RESOURCES

National Stroke Association
www.stroke.org

American Stroke Association
www.strokeassociation.org

National Institute of Neurological Disorders and Stroke
www.ninds.nih.gov

Children's Hemiplegia and Stroke Association
www.chasa.org

Pediatric Stroke Network
www.pediatricstrokenetwork.com

American Heart Association
www.americanheart.org

Family Caregiver Alliance
www.caregiver.org

Stroke Rehabilitation Provider Resource
http://www.stroke-rehab.com/

SURVIVOR AND FAMILY REFERENCES

Gardner, R. (2008). *Take brave steps for stroke survivors and families.* Infinity Publishing Co. ISBN 0-7414-4678-2

Marler, J. R. (2005). *Stroke for dummies.* Wiley Publishing. ISBN-13:978-0-7645-7201-2

PERSONAL STORIES

Berger, P. E., & Mensh, S. (2002). *How to conquer the world with one hand and an attitude* (2nd ed.). Merrifield, VA: Positive Power Publishing.

Bolte-Taylor, J. (2008). *My stroke of insight: A brain scientist's personal journey.* New York: Penguin Group. ISBN 978-0-670-02074-4

Brady, D. (2002). *When I learn. .. Surviving a stroke with pride.* Bloomington, IN: 1st Books Library.

Hutton, C., & Caplan, L. R. (2003). *Striking back at stroke: A doctor-patient journal.* New York: Dana Press.

Robinson, R. (2005). *Peeling the onion: Reversing the ravages of stroke.* Key West, FL: SORA Publishing.

Simon, S. (2001). *A stroke of genius: Messages of hope and healing.* Cedars Group.

REFERENCES

Aaslid, R., Huber, P., & Nornes, H. (2010). Evaluation of cerebrovascular spasm with transcranial Doppler ultrasound. *Journal of Neurosurgery, 55*(2), 112–123. doi: 10.3171/jns.1984.60.1.0037@sup.2010.112.issue-2

Alastruey, J., Parker, K. H., Peiró, J., Byrd, S. M., & Sherwin, S. J. (2007). Modelling the circle of Willis to assess the effects of anatomical variations and occlusions on cerebral flows. *Journal of Biomechanics, 40*(8), 1794–1805.

Al-Damluji, M. S., Nagpal, S., Stilp, E., Remetz, M., & Mena, C. (2013). Carotid revascularization: A systematic review of the evidence. *Journal of Interventional Cardiology, 26*(4), 399–410. doi: 10.1111/joic.12037

Al-Khaled, M., & Eggers, J. (2013). MRI findings and stroke risk in TIA patients with different symptom durations. *Neurology, 80*(21), 1920–1926. doi: 10.1212/WNL.0b013e318293e15f. Epub 2013 Apr 24.

Amarenco, P., Bogousslavsky, J., Caplan, L., Donnan, G., & Hennerici, M. (2009). Classification of stroke subtypes. *Cerebrovascular Diseases, 27,* 493–501. doi: 0.1159/000210432. Epub 2009 Apr 3.

Occupational therapy practice framework: Domain and process (3rd edition) (2014). *American Journal of Occupational Therapy, 68*(Suppl. 1), S1–S48. doi: 10.5014/ajot.2014.682006

Arboix, A. (2011). Lacunar infarct and cognitive decline. *Expert Review of Neurotherapeutics, 11*(9), 1251. doi: 10.1586/ern.11.118

Arboix, A., Blanco-Rojas, L., & Martí-Vilalta, J. L. (2014). Advancements in understanding the mechanisms of symptomatic lacunar ischemic stroke: Translation of knowledge to prevention strategies. *Expert Review of Neurotherapeutics*, *14*(3), 261–276. doi: 10.1586/14737175.2014.884926. Epub 2014 Feb 4.

Arsava, E. M. (2012). The role of MRI as a prognostic tool in ischemic stroke. *Journal of Neurochemistry*, *123*(Suppl. 2), 22–28. doi: 10.1111/j.1471-4159.2012.07940.x.

Bailey, E. L., Smith, C., Sudlow, C. L., & Wardlaw, J. M. (2012). Pathology of lacunar ischemic stroke in humans—A systematic review. *Brain Pathology*, *22*(5), 583–591. doi: 10.1111/j.1750-3639.2012.00575.x. Epub 2012 Mar 16.

Banerjee, C., Moon, Y. P., Paik, M. C., Rundek, T., Mora-McLaughlin, C., Vieira, J. R., ... Elkind, M. S. (2012). Duration of diabetes and risk of ischemic stroke. The Northern Manhattan Study. *Stroke*, *43*(5), 1212–1217. doi: 10.1161/STROKEAHA.111.641381. Epub 2012 Mar 1.

Bang, O. Y. (2014). Intracranial atherosclerosis: Current understanding and perspectives. *Journal of Stroke*, *16*(1), 27–35. Retrieved from http://doi.org/10.5853/jos.2014.16.1.27e

Basile, A. M., Pantoni, L., Pracucci, G., Asplund, K., Chabriat, H., Erkinjuntti, T., ... Inzitari, D. (2006). Age, hypertension, and lacunar stroke are the major determinants of the severity of age-related white matter changes. *Cerebrovascular Diseases*, *21*(5–6), 315–322.

Basu, S., Glantz, S., Bitton, A., & Millett, C. (2013). The effect of tobacco control measures during a period of rising cardiovascular disease risk in India: A mathematical model of myocardial infarction and stroke. *PLoS Medicine*, *10*(7), e1001480. doi: 10.1371/journal.pmed.1001480

Bégot, Y., Aboa-Eboulé, C., de Maistre, E., Jacquin, A., Troisgros, O., Hervieu, M., ... Giroud, M. (2013). Prestroke antiplatelet therapy and early prognosis in stroke patients: The Dijon Stroke Registry. *European Journal of Neurology*, *20*, 879–890. doi: 10.1111/ene.12060. Epub 2012 Dec 24.

Beis, J. M., Keller, C., Morin, N., Bartolomeo, P., Bernati, T., Chokron, S., ... Azouvi, P. (2004). Right spatial neglect after left hemisphere stroke: Qualitative and quantitative study. *Neurology*, *9*(63), 1600–1605.

Berg, A., Lönnqvist, J., Palomäki, H., & Kaste, M. (2009). Assessment of depression after stroke. *Stroke*, *40*, 523–529. doi: 10.1111/ene.12060. Epub 2012 Dec 24.

Beridze, M., Sanikidze, T., Shakarishvili, R., Intskirveli, N., & Bornstein, N. M. (2011). Selected acute phase CSF factors in ischemic stroke: Findings and prognostic value. *BMC Neurology*, *11*, 41. doi: 10.1186/1471-2377-11-41

Berkhemer, O. A., Fransen, P. S., Beumer, D., van den Berg, L. A., Lingsma, H. F., Yoo, A. J., ... Dippel, D. J. (2015). A randomized trial of intraarterial treatment for acute ischemic stroke. *The New England Journal of Medicine*, *372*(1), 11–20. doi: 10.1056/NEJMoa1411587

Bethoux, F. (2015). Spasticity management after stroke. *Physical Medicine and Rehabilitation Clinics of North America*, *26*(4), 625–639. doi: 10.1016/j.pmr.2015.07.003

Bhakta, B., O'Connor, R., & Cozens, J. (2008). Associated reactions after stroke: A randomized controlled trial of the effect of botulinum toxin type a. *Journal of Rehabilitation Medicine*, *40*(1), 36–41.

Bhalla, A., & Birns, J. (2015). *Management of post-stroke complications*. Springer.

Bhat, M., Cole, J., Sorkin, J., Wozniak, M., Malarcher, A., & Wozniak, A. (2008). Dose–response relationship between cigarette smoking and risk of ischemic stroke in young women. *Stroke*, *39*, 2439.

Bose, A. L., Henkes, H., Alfke, K., Reith, W., Mayer, T. E., Berlis, A., ... Sit, S. P. (2008). The Penumbra System: A mechanical device for the treatment of acute stroke due to thromboembolism. *American Journal of Neuroradiology*, *29*(7), 1409–1413. doi: 10.3174/ajnr.A1110. Epub 2008 May 22.

Boyd, L., & Winstein, C. (2003). Impact of explicit information on implicit motor-sequence learning following middle cerebral artery stroke. *Physical Therapy*, *83*(11), 976–989.

Broderick, J., Connolly, S., Feldmann, E., Hanley, D., Kase, C., Krieger, D., ... Zuccarello, M. (2007). Guidelines for the management of spontaneous intracerebral hemorrhage in adults: 2007 update: A guideline from the American Heart Association/American Stroke Association Stroke Council, High Blood Pressure Research Council, and the Quality of Care and Outcomes in Research Interdisciplinary Working Group. *Circulation*, *2007*(116), 391–413.

Bunevicius, A., Yuan, H., & Lin, W. (2013). The potential roles of 18F-FDG-PET in management of acute stroke patients. *BioMed Research International*, *2013*(4), 1–14. doi: 10.1155/2013/634598. Epub 2013 May 15.

Carandang, R., Seshadri, S., Beiser, A., Kelly-Hayes, M., Kase, C., Kannel, W., & Carmichael, S. (2006). Cellular and molecular mechanisms of neural repair after stroke: Making waves. *Annals of Neurology*, *59*(5), 735–742.

Carmichael, S. T. (2006). Cellular and molecular mechanisms of neural repair after stroke: Making waves. *Annals of Neurology*, *59*(5), 735–742.

Carota, A., & Bogousslavsky, J. (2009). *Stroke related psychiatric disorders. Handbook of clinical neurology. Stroke Part II: Clinical manifestations and pathogenesis* (pp. 623–651). Retrieved from http://www.sciencedirect.com

CDC, NCHS. *Underlying Cause of Death 1999–2013 on CDC WONDER Online Database, released 2015. Data are from the Multiple Cause of Death Files, 1999–2013, as compiled from data provided by the 57 vital statistics jurisdictions through the Vital Statistics Cooperative Program. Accessed September 13, 2015.*

Chang, E., Ghosh, N., Yanni, D., Lee, S., Alexandru, D., & Mozaffar, T. (2013). A review of spasticity treatments: Pharmacological and interventional approaches. *Critical Reviews in Physical and Rehabilitation Medicine, 25*(1–2), 11–22. doi: 10.1615/CritRevPhysRehabilMed.2013007945

Chen, C. N., Khor, G. T., Chen, C. H., & Huang, P. (2011). Wallenberg's syndrome with proximal quadriparesis. *The Neurologist, 17*(1), 44–46. doi: 10.1097/NRL.0b013e3181ebe5b2

Chiuve, S., Rexrode, K., Spiegelman, D., Logroscino, G., Manson, J., & Rimm, E. (2008). Primary prevention of stroke by healthy lifestyle. *Circulation, 118*, 947–954.

Cho, H. J., Choi, H. Y., Kim, Y. D., Nam, H. S., Han, S. W., Ha, J. W., … Heo, J. H. (2009). Transesophageal echocardiography in acute stroke patients with sinus rhythm and no cardiac disease history. *Journal of Neurology, Neurosurgery & Psychiatry, 81*, 412–415. doi: 10.1136/jnnp.2009.190322. Epub 2009 Dec 3.

Cho, H. K., Kim, H. S., & Joo, S. H. (2012). Sonography of affected and unaffected shoulders in hemiplegic patients: Analysis of the relationship between sonographic imaging data and clinical variables. *Annals of Rehabilitation Medicine, 36*(6), 828–835. doi: 10.5535/arm.2012.36.6.828

Chou, C., Chang, J., Lin, S., Cho, D., Cheng, Y., & Chen, C. (2012). Extracranial–intracranial (EC–IC) bypass of symptomatic middle cerebral artery (MCA) total occlusion for haemodynamic impairment patients. *British Journal of Neurosurgery, 26*(6), 823–826. doi: 10.3109/02688697.2012.690910

Coward, L., McCabe, D., Ederle, J., Featherstone, R., Clifton, A., & Brown, M. (2007). Long-term outcome after angioplasty and stenting for symptomatic vertebral artery stenosis compared with medical treatment in the carotid and vertebral artery transluminal angioplasty study (CAVATAS): A randomized trial. *Stroke, 38*(5), 1526–1530.

Creutzfeldt, C. J., Holloway, R. G., & Walker, M. (2012). Symptomatic and palliative care for stroke survivors. *Journal of General Internal Medicine,*
27(7), 853–860. doi: 10.1007/s11606-011-1966-4. Epub 2012 Jan 19.

Croot, E. J., Ryan, T. W., Read, J., Campbell, F., O'Cathain, A., & Venables, G. (2014). Transient ischemic attack: A qualitative study of the long term consequences for patients. *BMC Family Practice, 15*, 174. doi: 10.1186/s12875-014-0174-9

Daniels, S., Schroeder, M., DeGeorge, P., Corey, D., Foundas, A., & Rosenbek, J. (2009). Defining and measuring dysphagia following stroke. *American Journal of Speech-Language Pathology, 18*, 74–81. doi: 10.1044/1058-0360(2008/07-0040). Epub 2008 Oct 16.

Dashtipour, K., Chen, J. J., Walker, H. W., & Lee, M. Y. (2015). Systematic literature review of abobotulinumtoxin A in clinical trials for adult upper limb spasticity. *American Journal of Physical Medicine & Rehabilitation/Association of Academic Physiatrists, 94*(3), 229–238. doi: 10.1097/PHM.0000000000000208

De Reuck, J., Hemelsoet, D., & Van Maele, G. (2007). Seizures and epilepsy in patients with a spontaneous intracerebral haematoma. *Clinical Neurology and Neurosurgery, 109*(6), 501–504.

De Rooij, N. K., Linn, F. H., van der Plas, J. A., Algra, A., & Rinkel, G. J. (2007). Incidence of subarachnoid haemorrhage: A systematic review with emphasis on region, age, gender and time trends. *Journal of Neurology, Neurosurgery & Psychiatry, 78*(12), 1365–1372.

Demchuk, A. M., & Bal, S. (2012). Thrombolytic therapy for acute ischemic stroke: What can we do to improve outcomes? *Drugs, 72*(14), 1833–1845. doi: 10.2165/11635740-000000000-00000.

Dharmasaroja, P. A., & Intharakham, K. (2010). Risk factors for carotid stenosis in Thai patients with ischemic stroke/TIA. *Angiology, 6*(8), 789–792. doi: 10.1177/0003319710369793. Epub 2010 May 12.

Diener, H., Ringelstein, E., von Kummer, R., Landgraf, H., Koppenhagen, K., Harenberg, J., … Weidinger, G. (2006). Prophylaxis of thrombotic and embolic events in acute ischemic stroke with the low-molecular-weight heparin certoparin. *Stroke, 37*, 139–144.

Dwedar, A. Z., Ashour, S., Haroun, M., El Nasser, A. A., Moustafa, R. R., Ibrahim, M. H. & Elsadek, A. (2014). Sonothrombolysis in acute middle cerebral artery stroke. *Neurology India, 62*(1), 62–65. doi: 10.4103/0028-3886.128308

Easton, J. D., Saver, J. L., Albers, G. W., Alberts, M. J., Chaturvedi, S., Feldmann, E., & Sacco, R. L. (2009). Definition and Evaluation of Transient Ischemic Attack a Scientific Statement for Healthcare Professionals from the American Heart

Association/American Stroke Association Stroke Council; Council on Cardiovascular Surgery and Anesthesia; Council on Cardiovascular Radiology and Intervention; Council on Cardiovascular Nursing; and the Interdisciplinary Council on Peripheral Vascular Disease: The American Academy of Neurology affirms the value of this statement as an educational tool for neurologists. *Stroke, 40*(6), 2276–2293. doi: 10.1161/STROKEAHA.108.192218

Elkind, M., Sciacca, R., Boden-Albala, B., Rundek, T., Paik, M., & Sacco, R. (2006a). Moderate alcohol consumption reduces risk of ischemic stroke: The northern Manhattan study. *Stroke, 37*, 13–19.

Elkind, M., Tondella, M., Feikin, D., Fields, B., Homma, S., & Di Tullio, M. (2006b). Seropositivity to chlamydia pneumoniae is associated with risk of first ischemic stroke. *Stroke, 37*, 790–795.

Emberson, J., Lees, K. R., Lyden, P., Blackwell, L., Albers, G., Bluhmki, E., ... Hacke, W. (2014). Effect of treatment delay, age, and stroke severity on the effects of intravenous thrombolysis with alteplase for acute ischemic stroke: A meta-analysis of individual patient data from randomised trials. *Lancet, 384*(9958), 1929–1935. doi: 10.1016/S0140-6736(14)60584-5

Feigin, V., Lawes, C., Bennett, D., Barker-Collo, S., & Parag, V. (2009). Worldwide stroke incidence and early case fatality reported in 56 population-based studies: A systematic review. *The Lancet Neurology, 8*(4), 355–369. doi: 10.1016/S1474-4422(09)70025-0. Epub 2009 Feb 21.

Feldmann, E., Wilterdink, J., Kosinski, A., Lynn, M., Chimowitz, M., Sarafin, J., ... Sloan, M. (2007). The stroke outcomes and neuroimaging of intracranial atherosclerosis (SONIA) trial. *Neurology, 68*, 2099–2106.

Ferro, J., Caeiro, L., & Santos, C. (2009). Post stroke emotional and behavior impairment: A narrative review. *Cerebrovascular Diseases, 27*(Suppl. 1), 197–203. doi: 10.1159/000200460. Epub 2009 Apr 3.

Florman, J. E., Duffau, H., & Rughani, A. I. (2013). Lower motor neuron findings after upper motor neuron injury: Insights from postoperative supplementary motor area syndrome. *Frontiers in Human Neuroscience, 7*, 85. doi: 10.3389/fnhum.2013.00085

Fogle, C. C., Oser, C. S., Troutman, T. P., McNamara, M., Williamson, A. P., Keller, M., ... Harwell, T. S. (2008). Public education strategies to increase awareness of stroke warning signs and the need to call 911. *Journal of Public Health Management and Practice, 14*(3), e17–e22.

Fonarow, G. C., Alberts, M. J., Broderick, J. P., Jauch, E. C., Kleindorfer, D. O., Saver, J. L., ...

Schwamm, L. H. (2014). Stroke outcomes measures must be appropriately risk adjusted to ensure quality care of patients a presidential advisory from the American Heart Association/American Stroke Association. *Stroke, 45*(5), 1589–1601. doi: 10.1093/eurheartj/ehv527

Fujimura, M., Kaneta, T., Mugikura, S., Shimizu, H., & Tominaga, T. (2007). Temporary neurologic deterioration due to cerebral hyperperfusion after superficial temporal artery-middle cerebral artery anastomosis in patients with adult-onset moyamoya disease. *Surgical Neurology, 67*(3), 273–282.

Fujita, T., Sato, A., Togashi, Y., Kasahara, R., Ohashi, T., Tsuchiya, K., ... Otsuki, K. (2015). Identification of the affected lower limb and unaffected side motor functions as determinants of activities of daily living performance in stroke patients using partial correlation analysis. *Journal of Physical Therapy Science, 27*(7), 2217–2220. Retrieved from http://doi.org/10.1589/jpts.27.2217

Furie, K. L., Kasner, S. E., Adams, R. J., Albers, G. W., Bush, R. L., Fagan, S. C., ... Wentworth, D. (2011). Guidelines for the prevention of stroke in patients with stroke or transient ischemic attack a guideline for healthcare professionals from the American Heart Association/American Stroke Association. *Stroke, 42*(1), 227–276. doi: 10.1161/STR.0b013e3181f7d043. Epub 2010 Oct 21.

Garbossa, D., Panciani, P. P., Fornaro, R., Crobeddu, E., Marengo, N., Fronda, C., ... Fontanella, M. (2012). Subarachnoid hemorrhage in elderly: Advantages of the endovascular treatment. *Geriatrics & Gerontology International, 12*(1), 46–49. doi: 10.1111/j.1447-0594.2011.00725.x

Giles, M. F., & Rothwell, P. M. (2007). Risk of stroke early after transient ischaemic attack: A systematic review and meta-analysis. *Lancet Neurology, 6*, 1063–1072.

Giles, M. F., & Rothwell, P. M. (2009). Transient ischaemic attack: Clinical relevance, risk prediction and urgency of secondary prevention. *Current Opinion in Neurology, 22*, 46–53. doi: 10.1097/WCO.0b013e32831f1977

Gillen, G., Nilsen, D. M., Attridge, J., Banakos, E., Morgan, M., Winterbottom, L., & York, W. (2015). Effectiveness of interventions to improve occupational performance of people with cognitive impairments after stroke: An evidence-based review. *The American Journal of Occupational Therapy, 69*(1), 1–4A. doi: 10.5014/ajot.2015.012138

Glymour, M., Avendaño, M., & Berkman, L. (2007). Is the 'stroke belt' worn from childhood? Risk of first stroke and state of residence in childhood and adulthood. *Stroke, 38*, 2415–2421.

Go, A. S., Mozaffarian, D., Roger, V. L., Benjamin, E. J., Berry, J. D., Borden, W. B., ... Stroke, S. S.

(2013). Heart disease and stroke statistics—2013 update: A report from the American Heart Association. *Circulation*, *127*(1), e6. doi: 10.1161/CIR.0b013e31828124ad. Epub 2012 Dec 12.

Gogola, A., Saulicz, E., Kuszewski, M., Matyja, M., & Myśliwiec, A. (2014). Development of low postural tone compensatory patterns—Predicted dysfunction patterns in upper part of the body. *Developmental Period Medicine*, *18*(3), 380–385.

Goldstein, L. B., Bushnell, C. D., Adams, R. J., Appel, L. J., Braun, L. T., Chaturvedi, S, & Pearson, T. A. (2011). Guidelines for the primary prevention of stroke a guideline for healthcare professionals from the American Heart Association/American Stroke Association. *Stroke*, *42*(2), 517–584. doi: 10.1161/STR.0b013e31829734f2

Gonzalez, R. (2006). Imaging-guided acute ischemic stroke therapy: From "time is brain" to "physiology is brain". *American Journal of Neuroradiology*, *27*(4), 728–735.

Goodwin, D. (2014). Homonymous hemianopia: challenges and solutions. *Clinical Ophthalmology*, *8*, 1919–1927. doi: 10.2147/OPTH.S59452. eCollection 2014.

Grysiewicz, R. A., Thomas, K., & Pandey, D. K. (2008). Epidemiology of ischemic and hemorrhagic stroke: Incidence, prevalence, mortality, and risk factors. *Neurologic Clinics*, *26*(4), 871–895. doi: 10.1016/j.ncl.2008.07.003

Hackett, M., Yapa, C., Parag, V., & Anderson, C. (2005).Frequency of depression after stroke: A systematic review of observational studies. *Stroke*, *36*(10), 2296–2301.

Hallevi, H., Albright, K., Martin-Schild, S., Barreto, A., Morales, M., Bornstein, N., … Savitz, S. (2009). Recovery after ischemic stroke: Criteria for good outcome by level of disability at day 7. *Cerebrovascular Diseases*, *28*, 341–348. doi: 10.1159/000229552. Epub 2009 Jul 24.

Hand, P., Kwan, J., Lindley, R., Dennis, M., & Wardlaw, J. (2006). Distinguishing between stroke and mimic at the bedside: The brain attack study. *Stroke*, *37*, 769–775.

Hankey, G. J., Spiesser, J., Hakimi, Z., Bego, G., Carita, P., & Gabriel, S. (2007). Rate, degree, and predictors of recovery from disability following ischemic stroke. *Neurology*, *68*, 1583–1587.

Hara, T., Abo, M., Kobayashi, K., Watanabe, M., Kakuda, W., & Senoo, A. (2015). Effects of low-frequency repetitive transcranial magnetic stimulation combined with intensive speech therapy on cerebral blood flow in post-stroke aphasia. *Translational Stroke Research*, *6*(5), 365–374. doi: 10.1007/s12975-015-0417-7. Epub 2015 Aug 7.

Hedna, V. S., Bodhit, A. N., Ansari, S., Falchook, A. D., Stead, L., Heilman, K. M., & Waters, M. F. (2013). Hemispheric differences in ischemic stroke: Is left-hemisphere stroke more common? *Journal of Clinical Neurology*, *9*(2), 97–102. doi: 10.3988/jcn.2013.9.2.97. Epub 2013 Apr 4.

Heron, N., Kee, F., Donnelly, M., & Cupples, M. E. (2015). Systematic review of rehabilitation programmes initiated within 90 days of a transient ischaemic attack or "minor" stroke: A protocol. *BMJ Open*, *5*, e007849. doi: 10.1136/bmjopen-2015-007849

Hildebrand, M. W. (2015). Effectiveness of interventions for adults with psychological or emotional impairment after stroke: An evidence-based review. *American Journal of Occupational Therapy*, *69*(1). doi: 10.5014/ajot.2015.012054.

Ho, B. L., Huang, P., Khor, G. T. & Tay, R. (2008). Lin simultaneous thrombosis of cerebral artery and venous sinus. *Acta Neurologica Taiwanica*, *17*(2), 112–116.

Hobson, C., Dortch, J., Ozrazgat Baslanti, T., Layon, D. R., Roche, A., Rioux, A., … Bihorac, A. (2014). Insurance status is associated with treatment allocation and outcomes after subarachnoid hemorrhage. *PLoS One*, *9*(8), e105124. doi: 10.1371/journal.pone.0105124

Hoffmann, T., Bennett, S., Koh, C., & McKenna, K. (2010). A systematic review of cognitive interventions to improve functional ability in people who have cognitive impairment following stroke. *Topics in Stroke Rehabilitation*, *17*(2), 398–412. doi: 10.1310/tsr1702-99

Huang, S., Liu, S., Tang, H., Wei, T., Wang, W., & Yang, C. (2012). Relationship between severity of shoulder subluxation and soft-tissue injury in hemiplegic stroke patients. *Journal of Rehabilitation Medicine*, *44*(9), 733–739. doi: 10.2340/16501977-1026.

Huang, S., Shen, Q., & Duong, T. Q. (2010). Artificial neural network prediction of ischemic tissue fate in acute stroke imaging. *Journal of Cerebral Blood Flow & Metabolism*, *30*(9), 1661–1670. doi: 10.1038/jcbfm.2010.56. Epub 2010 Apr 28.

Huttenlocher, P. R. (2009). *Neural plasticity*. Cambridge, MA: Harvard University Press.

Jaillard, A., Naegele, B., Trabucco-Miguel, S., LeBas, J. F., & Hommel, M. (2009). Hidden dysfunctioning in subacute stroke. *Stroke*, *40*(7), 2473–2479. doi: 10.1161/STROKEAHA.108.541144. Epub 2009 May 21.

Jang, D., Kim, M., Park, K., & Lee, J. (2014). Language-specific dysgraphia in Korean patients with right brain stroke: Influence of unilateral spatial neglect. *Journal of Korean Medical Science*, *30*, 323–327. doi: 10.3346/jkms.2015.30.3.323. Epub 2015 Feb 16.

Jax, S. A., Rosa-Leyra, D. L., & Buxbaum, L. J. (2014). Conceptual- and production-related predictors of pantomimed tool use deficits in apraxia.

Neuropsychologia, 62, 194–201. doi: 10.1016/j. neuropsychologia.2014.07.014

Karthikbabu, S., Chakrapani, M., Ganeshan, S., Rakshith, K. C., Nafeez, S., & Prem, V. (2012). A review on assessment and treatment of the trunk in stroke: A need or luxury. *Neural Regeneration Research, 7*(25), 1974–1977. Retrieved from http:// doi.org/10.3969/j.issn.1673-5374.2012.25.008

Kaufmann, T., Huston, J., Mandrekar, J., Schleck, C., Thielen, K., & Kallmes, D. (2007). Complications of diagnostic cerebral angiography: Evaluation of 19826 consecutive patients. *Radiology, 243*, 812–819. Retrieved from http://radiology.rsna.org/ content/243/3/812.abstract.

Kidwell, C. S., & Wintermark, M. (2010). The role of CT and MRI in the emergency evaluation of persons with suspected stroke. *Current Neurology and Neuroscience Reports, 10*, 21–28. doi: 10.1007/ s11910-009-0075-9

Kim, Y., & Ko, J. (2014). Sole stenting with large cell stents for very small ruptured intracranial aneurysms. *Interventional Neuroradiology, 20*, 45–53. doi: 10.15274/INR-2014-10007

Kim, Y. H., Jung, S. J., Yang, E. J., & Paik, N. J. (2014). Clinical and sonographic risk factors for hemiplegic shoulder pain: A longitudinal observational study. *Journal of Rehabilitation Medicine, 46*(1), 81–87. doi: 10.2340/16501977-1238

Kim, K., Kim, Y. M., & Kang, D. Y. (2015). Repetitive sit-to-stand training with the step-foot position on the non-paretic side, and its effects on the balance and foot pressure of chronic stroke subjects. *Journal of Physical Therapy Science, 27*(8), 2621–2624. doi: 10.1589/jpts.27.2621. Epub 2015 Aug 21.

Kitchen, L., Westmacott, R., Friefeld, S., MacGregor, D., Curtis, R., Allen, A., ... Domi, T. (2012). The pediatric stroke outcome measure a validation and reliability study. *Stroke, 43*(6), 1602–1608. doi: 10.1161/STROKEAHA.111.639583. Epub 2012 Apr 3.

Kochanek, K. D., Murphy, S. L., Xu, J., & Arias, E. (2014). Mortality in the United States, 2013. *NCHS Data Brief, 178*, 1–8.

Kovindha, A., Wyndaele, J. J., & Madersbacher, H. (2010). Prevalence of incontinence during rehabilitation in patients following a stroke. *Current Bladder Dysfunction Reports.*

Kuptniratsaikul, V., Kovindha, A., Suethanapornkul, S., Manimmanakorn, N., & Archongka, Y. (2013). Long-term morbidities in stroke survivors: a prospective multicenter study of Thai stroke rehabilitation registry. *BMC Geriatrics, 13*, 33. doi: 10.1186/1471-2318-13-33

Latimer, S. F., Wilson, F. C., McCuskey, C. G., Caldwell, S. B., & Rennie, I. (2013). Subarachnoid haemorrhage (SAH): Long-term cognitive outcome in patients treated with surgical clipping or endovascular coiling. *Disability and Rehabilitation, 35*(10), 845–850. doi: 10.3109/09638288.2012.709909

Lavie, C. J., Milani, R. V., & Ventura, H. O. (2009). Obesity and cardiovascular disease: Risk factor, paradox, and impact of weight loss. *Journal of the American College of Cardiology, 53*(21), 1925–1932. doi: 10.1016/j.jacc.2008.12.068

Lawlor, D. A., & Leon, D. A. (2005). Association of body mass index and obesity measured in early childhood with risk of coronary heart disease and stroke in middle age findings from the aberdeen children of the 1950s prospective cohort study. *Circulation, 111*(15), 1891–1896.

Legg, L., Drummond, A., Leonardi-Bee, J., Gladman, J. R. F., Corr, S., Donkervoort, M., ... Langhorne, P. (2007). Occupational therapy for patients with problems in personal activities of daily living after stroke: Systematic review of randomised trials. *British Medical Journal, 335*(7626), 922.

Leiva-Salinas, C., Aghaebrahim, A., Zhu, G., Patrie, J. T., Xin, W., Lau, B. C., ... Wintermark, M. (2013). Tissue at risk in acute stroke patients treated beyond 8 h after symptom onset. *Neuroradiology, 55*(7), 807–812. doi: 10.1007/s00234-013-1164-7

Leone, M. A., Tonini, M. C., Bogliun, G., Gionco, M., Tassinari, T., Bottacchi, E., Beghi, E., ARES (Alcohol Related Seizures) Study Group. (2009). Risk factors for a first epileptic seizure after stroke: A case control study. *Journal of the Neurological Sciences, 277*(1), 138–142.

Li, N., Tian, F., Yu, P., Zhou, X., Wen, Q., Qiao, X., & Huang, L. (2012). Therapeutic effect of acupuncture and massage for shoulder-hand syndrome in hemiplegia patients: A clinical two-center randomized controlled trial. *Journal of Traditional Chinese Medicine, 32*(3), 343–349. PMID: 23297553

Liao, C., Liaw, L., Wang, R., Su, F., & Hsu, A. (2015). Relationship between trunk stability during voluntary limb and trunk movements and clinical measurements of patients with chronic stroke. *Journal of Physical Therapy Science, 27*(7), 2201–2206. doi: 10.1589/jpts.27.2201

Lima, N. M., Menegatti, K. C., Yu, É., Sacomoto, N. Y., Oberg, T. D., & Honorato, D. C. (2015). Motor and sensory effects of ipsilesional upper extremity hypothermia and contralesional sensory training for chronic stroke patients. *Topics in Stroke Rehabilitation, 22*(1), 44–55. doi: 10.1590/004-282X20150128

Lockhart, P. B., Bolger, A. F., Papapanou, P. N., Osinbowale, O., Trevisan, M., Levison, M. E., ... Baddour, L. M. (2012). Periodontal disease and atherosclerotic vascular disease: Does the evidence support an independent association? A scientific statement from the American Heart Association. *Circulation, 125*(20), 2520–2544. doi: 10.1161/CIR.0b013e31825719f3

Locksley, H. (2010). Natural history of subarachnoid hemorrhage, intracranial aneurysms and arteriovenous malformations: Based on 6368 cases in the cooperative study. *Journal of Neurosurgery, 112*(2). doi: 10.3171/jns.1966.25.3.0321

Lundy-Ekman, L. (2007). *Neuroscience: Fundamentals for rehabilitation* (3rd ed.). Philadelphia, PA: WB Saunders.

MacDougall, D., Feliu, A. Boccuzzi, S., & Lin, J. (2006). Economic burden of deep-vein thrombosis, pulmonary embolism, and post-thrombotic syndrome. *American Journal of Health-System Pharmacy, 63*(20), 5–15.

Mansfield, A., Fraser, L., Rajachandrakumar, R., Danells, C. J., Knorr, S., & Campos, J. (2015). Is perception of vertical impaired in individuals with chronic stroke with a history of 'pushing'? *Neuroscience Letters, 590*, 172–177. doi: 10.1016/j.neulet.2015.02.007

Mant, J., Hobbs, F. R., Fletcher, K., Roalfe, A., Fitzmaurice, D., Lip, G. Y., Murray, E.; BAFTA Investigators, Midland Research Practices Network (MidReC). (2007). Warfarin versus aspirin for stroke prevention in an elderly community population with atrial fibrillation (the Birmingham Atrial Fibrillation Treatment of the Aged Study, BAFTA): A randomised controlled trial. *The Lancet, 370*(9586), 493–503.

Marque, P., Gasq, D., Castel-Lacanal, E., De Boissezon, X., & Loubinoux, I. (2014). Post-stroke hemiplegia rehabilitation: Evolution of the concepts. *Annals of Physical and Rehabilitation Medicine, 57*(8), 520–529. doi: 10.1016/j.rehab.2014.08.004

Martinaud, O., Pouliquen, D., Gérardin, E., Loubeyre, M., Hirsbein, D., Hannequin, D., & Cohen, L. (2012). Visual agnosia and posterior cerebral artery infarcts: An anatomical-clinical study. *PLoS One, 7*(1), e30433v. doi: 10.1371/journal.pone.0030433

Mattace-Raso, F., Van der Cammen, T., Hofman, A., van Popele, N., Bos, M., Schalekamp, M., … Witteman, J. (2006). Arterial stiffness and risk of coronary heart disease and stroke: The Rotterdam Study. *Circulation, 113*, 657–663.

Mayo Clinic Staff. (2009). *Brain aneurysm overview*. Retrieved August 16, 2010, from http://www.mayoclinic.com/health/brain-aneurysm/DS00582

McIntyre, K. E. (2009). Subclavian steal syndrome. *eMedicine Vascular Surgery: Medscape.*

McMorland, A. C., Runnalls, K. D., & Byblow, W. D. (2015). A neuroanatomical framework for upper limb synergies after stroke. *Frontiers in Human Neuroscience, 9*, 82. doi: 10.3389/fnhum.2015.00082

Mendonça, C. T., Fortunato, J. J., Carvalho, C. D., Weingartner, J., Filho, O. M., Rezende, F. F., & Bertinato, L. P. (2014). Carotid endarterectomy in awake patients: Safety, tolerability and results. *Revista Brasileira De Cirurgia Cardiovascular: Órgão Oficial Da Sociedade Brasileira De Cirurgia Cardiovascular, 29*(4), 574–580. doi: 10.5935/1678-9741.20140053

Metoki, H., Ohkubo, T., Kikuya, M., Asayama, K., Obara, T., Hashimoto, J., … Imai, Y. (2006). Prognostic significance for stroke of a morning pressor surge and a nocturnal blood pressure decline: The Ohasama study. *Hypertension, 47*(2), 149–154.

Meyer, S., Karttunen, A. H., Thijs, V., Feys, H., & Verheyden, G. (2014). How do somatosensory deficits in the arm and hand relate to upper limb impairment, activity, and participation problems after stroke? A systematic review. *Physical Therapy, 94*(9), 1220–1231. doi: 10.2522/ptj.20130271

Mikołajewska, E. (2012). NDT-Bobath method in normalization of muscle tone in post-stroke patients. *Advances in Clinical and Experimental Medicine: Official Organ Wroclaw Medical University, 21*(4), 513–517.

Minger, S. L., Ekonomou, A., Carta, E. M., Chinoy, A., Perry, R. H., & Ballard, C. G. (2007). Endogenous neurogenesis in the human brain following cerebral infarction. *Regenerative Medicine, 2*(1), 69–74.

Mitsutake, T., Chuda, Y., Oka, S., Hirata, H., Matsuo, T., & Horikawa, E. (2014). The control of postural stability during standing is decreased in stroke patients during active head rotation. *Journal of Physical Therapy Science, 26*(11), 1799–1801. doi: 10.1589/jpts.26.1799. Epub 2014 Nov 13.

Montaner, J., Perea-Gainza, M., Delgado, P., Ribó, M., Chacón, P. Rosell, A., … Sabín, J. (2008). Etiologic diagnosis of ischemic stroke subtypes with plasma biomarkers. *Stroke, 39*, 2280–2287.

Moran, G. M., Fletcher, B., Calvert, M., Feltham, M. G., Sackley, C., & Marshall, T. (2013). A systematic review investigating fatigue, psychological and cognitive impairment following TIA and minor stroke: Protocol paper. *Systematic Reviews, 2*, 72. doi: 10.1186/2046-4053-2-72

Murray, M., Camen, C., Gonzalez, A., Bovet, P., & Clarke, S. (2006). Rapid brain discrimination of sounds of objects. *The Journal of Neuroscience, 26*(4), 1293–1302.

Nasr, N., Ssi-Yan-Kai, G., Guidolin, B., Bonneville, F., & Larrue, V. (2013). Transcranial color-coded sonography to predict recurrent transient ischaemic attack/stroke. *European Journal of Neurology*, *20*, 1212–1217. National Stroke Association. doi: 10.1111/ene.12178. Epub 2013 May 6. Retrieved from http://www.stroke.org/site/PageServer?pagename=STROKE

Nelson, K. B. (2007). Perinatal ischemic stroke. *Stroke*, *38*(2), 742–745.

Nichols, E. H. (2014). Atrial fibrillation and stroke. In *MD Conference Express* (Vol. *14*(6), pp. 15–17). SAGE Publications.

Nys, G., van Zandvoort, M., de Kort, P., Jansen, B., de Haan, E., & Kappelle, L. (2007). Cognitive disorders in acute stroke: Prevalence and clinical determinants. *Cerebrovascular Diseases*, *23*, 408–416. doi: 10.1159/000101464

O'Donnell, M. J., Xavier, D., Liu, L., Zhang, H., Chin, S. L., Rao-Melacini, P., ... Yusuf, S. (2010). Risk factors for ischaemic and intracerebral haemorrhagic stroke in 22 countries (the INTERSTROKE study): A case–control study. *The Lancet*, *376*(9735), 112–123. doi: 10.1016/S0140-6736(10)60834-3

Ohira, T., Shahar, E., Chambless, L., Rosamond, W., Mosley, T., & Folsom, A. (2006). Risk factors for ischemic stroke subtypes: The atherosclerosis risk in communities study. *Stroke*, *37*, 2493–2498.

Ohwaki, K., Yano, E., Nagashima, H., Hirata, M., Nakagomi, T., & Tamura, A. (2004). Blood pressure management in acute intracerebral hemorrhage relationship between elevated blood pressure and hematoma enlargement. *Stroke*, *35*, 1364–1367.

Paci, M., Nannetti, L., Taiti, P., Baccini, M., Pasquini, J., & Rinaldi, L. (2007). Shoulder subluxation after stroke: Relationships with pain and motor recovery. *Physiotherapy Research International*, *12*, 95–104.

Park, J., Lee, N., Cho, Y., & Yang, Y. (2015). Modified constraint-induced movement therapy for clients with chronic stroke: Interrupted time series (ITS) design. *Journal of Physical Therapy Science*, *27*(3), 963. doi: 10.1589/jpts.27.963. Epub 2015 Mar 31.

Parry, W., Reeve, L., Shaw, F., Davison, J., Norton, M., Frearson, R., ... Newton, J. (2009). The Newcastle protocols 2008: An update on head-up tilt table testing and the management of vasovagal syncope and related disorders. *Heart*, *95*, 416–420. doi: 10.1136/hrt.2007.136457. Epub 2008 Aug 13.

Patel, M., McKevitt, C., Lawrence, E., Rudd, A., & Wolfe, C. (2007). Clinical determinants of long-term quality of life after stroke. *Age and Aging*, *36*(3), 316–322.

Pendlebury, S., Cuthbertson, F., Welch, S., Mehta, Z., & Rothwell, P. (2010). Underestimation of cognitive impairment by Mini-Mental State examination versus the Montreal Cognitive Assessment in patients with transient ischemic attack and stroke: Population-based study. *Stroke*, *41*, 1290–1293. doi: 10.1161/STROKEAHA.110.579888

Perry, J. J., Stiell, I. G., Sivilotti, M. L., Bullard, M. J., Hohl, C. M., Sutherland, J., ... Wells, G. A. (2013). Clinical decision rules to rule out subarachnoid hemorrhage for acute headache. *JAMA*, *310*(12), 1248–1255. doi: 10.1001/jama.2013.278018

Petrella, J., Coleman, R., & Doraiswamy, P. (2009). Neuroimaging and early diagnosis of Alzheimer disease: A look to the future. *Radiology*, *226*, 315–336. Retrieved from http://radiology.rsna.org/content/226/2/315.abstract

Porelli, S., Leonardi, M., Stafa, A., Barbara, C., Procaccianti, G., & Simonetti, L. (2013). CT angiography in an acute stroke protocol: Correlation between occlusion site and outcome of intravenous thrombolysis. *Interventional Neuroradiology*, *19*, 87–96.

Prass, K., Braun, J., Dirnagl, U., Meisel, C., & Meisel, A. (2006). Stroke propagates bacterial aspiration to pneumonia in a model of cerebral ischemia. *Stroke*, *37*, 2607–2612.

Provinciali, L., Paolucci, S., Torta, R., Toso, V., Gobbi, B., & Gandolfo, C. (2008). Depression after first-ever ischemic stroke: The prognostic role of neuroanatomic subtypes in clinical practice. *Cerebrovascular Diseases*, *26*, 592–599.

Purushothaman, S., Salmani, D., Prarthana, K. G., Bandelkar, S. M. G., & Varghese, S. (2014). Study of ECG changes and its relation to mortality in cases of cerebrovascular accidents. *Journal of Natural Science, Biology, and Medicine*, *5*(2), 434–436. doi: 10.4103/0976-9668.136225

Qureshi, A. I., Alexandrov, A. V., Tegeler, C. H., Hobson II, R. W., Baker, J. D., & Hopkins, L. N. (2007). MD guidelines for screening of extracranial carotid artery disease: A statement for Healthcare Professionals from the Multidisciplinary Practice Guidelines Committee of the American Society of Neuroimaging; Cosponsored by the Society of Vascular and Interventional Neurology. *Journal of Neuroimaging*, *17*(1), 19–47.

Raymond, M., & Louis, D. (2015). Neurological and neuropsychiatric disorders: Cerebrovascular diseasea-03 left vertebral artery dissection with left medullary infarct and associated wallenberg syndrome: A clinical case study. *Archives of Clinical Neuropsychology*, *30*(6), 487–487.

Rigby, H., Gubitz, G., & Phillips, S. (2009). A systematic review of caregiver burden following stroke. *International Journal of Stroke*, *4*(4), 285–292.

Riggs, R., Andrews, K., Roberts, P., & Gilewski, M. (2007). Visual deficit interventions in adult stroke and brain injury: A systematic review. *American Journal of Physical Medicine & Rehabilitation*, *86*(10), 853–860.

Robinson, T. G., Reid, A., Haunton, V. J., Wilson, A., & Naylor, A. R. (2012). The face arm speech test: Does it encourage rapid recognition of important stroke warning symptoms? *Emergency Medicine Journal*, *30*(6), 467–471.

Rodríguez-Mutuberría, L., Álvarez-González, L., López, M., Bender-del Busto, J. E., Fernández-Martínez, E., Martínez-Segón, S., & Bergado, J. A. (2011). Efficacy and tolerance of a neurological restoration program in stroke patients. *Neurorehabilitation*, *29*, 381–391. doi: 10.3233/NRE-2011-0716

Sacco, R. L., Kasner, S. E., Broderick, J. P., Caplan, L. R., Connors, J. J., Culebras, A., … Vinters, H. V. (2013). on behalf of the American Heart Association Stroke Council, Council on Cardiovascular Surgery and Anesthesia, Council on Cardiovascular Radiology and Intervention, Council on Cardiovascular and Stroke Nursing, Council on Epidemiology and Prevention, Council on Peripheral Vascular Disease, and Council on Nutrition, Physical Activity and Metabolism. An updated definition of stroke for the 21st century: A statement for healthcare professionals from the American Heart Association/American Stroke Association. *Stroke*, *44*(7), 2064–2089. doi: 10.1161/STR.0b013e318296aeca

Sacco, S., Marini, C., Totaro, R., Russo, T., Cerone, D., & Carolei, A. (2006a). A population-based study of the incidence and prognosis of lacunar stroke. *Neurology*, *66*(9), 1335–1338.

Sacco, R., Prabhakaran, S., Thompson, J., Murphy, A., Sciacca, R., Levin, B., & Mohr, J. (2006b). Comparison of warfarin versus aspirin for the prevention of recurrent stroke or death: Subgroup analyses from the Warfarin-Aspirin Recurrent Stroke Study. *Cerebrovascular Diseases*, *22*, 4–12.

Sacks, D., Black, C. M., Cognard, C., Connors, J. J. III, Frei, D., Gupta, R., … Vorwerk, D. (2013). Multisociety consensus quality improvement guidelines for intra-arterial catheter-directed treatment of acute ischemic stroke. *American Journal of Neuroradiology*, *34*, E0.

Saenger, A. K., & Christenson, R. H. (2010). Stroke biomarkers: Progress and challenges for diagnosis, prognosis, differentiation, and treatment. *Clinical Chemistry*, *56*(1), 21–33.

Santamarina, R., Besocke, A., Romano, L., Loli, P., & Gonorazky, S. (2008). Ischemic stroke related to anabolic abuse. *Clinical Neuropharmacology*, *31*, 2.

Sarwar, N., Gao, P., Seshasai, S. R., Gobin, R., Kaptoge, S., Di Angelantonio, E., … Danesh, J.; Emerging Risk Factors Collaboration. (2010). Diabetes mellitus, fasting blood glucose concentration, and risk of vascular disease: A collaborative meta-analysis of 102 prospective studies. *Lancet*, *375*, 2215–2222.

Schneider, J. I., & Olshaker, J. S. (2012). Vertigo, vertebrobasilar disease, and posterior circulation ischemic stroke. *Emergency Medicine Clinics of North America*, *30*(3), 681–693.

Sehatzadeh, S. (2015). Is transient ischemic attack a medical emergency? An evidence based analysis. *Ontario Health Technology Assessment Series*, *15*(3), 1–45.

Sidorov, E. V., Feng, W., & Selim, M. (2014). Cost-minimization analysis of computed tomography versus magnetic resonance imaging in the evaluation of patients with transient ischemic attacks at a large academic center. *Cerebrovascular Diseases Extra*, *4*(1), 69–76. doi: 10.1159/000360521. eCollection 2014.

Silverman, I. E., Restrepo, L., & Mathews, G. C. (2002). Poststroke seizures. *Archives of Neurology*, *59*(2), 195–201.

Somers, V. K., White, D. P., Amin, R., Abraham, W. T., Costa, F., Culebras, A., … Young, T. (2008). Sleep apnea and cardiovascular disease: An American heart association/American College of Cardiology Foundation scientific statement from the American Heart Association Council for high blood pressure research professional education committee, council on clinical cardiology, stroke council, and council on cardiovascular nursing in collaboration with the national heart, lung, and blood institute national center on sleep disorders research (national institutes of health). *Journal of the American College of Cardiology*, *52*(8), 686–717.

Stegeman, I., Bossuyt, P. M., Yu, T., Boyd, C., & Puhan, M. A. (2015). Aspirin for primary prevention of cardiovascular disease and cancer. A benefit and harm analysis. *PLoS One*, *10*(7), e0127194. doi: 10.1371/journal.pone.0127194

Steiner, T., Vincent, C., Morris, S., Davis, S., Vallejo-Torres, L., & Christensen, M. C. (2011). Neurosurgical outcomes after intracerebral hemorrhage: results of the Factor Seven for Acute Hemorrhagic Stroke Trial (FAST). *Journal of Stroke and Cerebrovascular Diseases*, *20*(4), 287–294. doi: 10.1016/j.jstrokecerebrovasdis.2009.12.008. Epub 2010 May 8.

Suzuki, M., Omori, M., Hatakeyama, M., Yamada, S., Matsushita, K., & Iijima, S. (2006). Predicting recovery of upper-body dressing ability after stroke. *Archives of Physical Medicine and Rehabilitation*, *87*(11), 1496–1502.

Tabuchi, S. (2014). Auditory dysfunction in patients with cerebrovascular disease. *The Scientific World*

Journal, 261824. doi: 10.1155/2014/261824. Epub 2014 Oct 23.

Takatsuru, D., Fukumoto, M., Yoshitomo, T., Nemoto, H., Tsukada, R., & Nabekurak, L. (2009). Neuronal circuit remodeling in the contralateral cortical hemisphere during functional recovery from cerebral infarction. *Journal of Neuroscience, 29*(32), 10081–10086. doi: 10.1523/JNEUROSCI.1638-09.2009

Tan, S., Xiao, X., Ma, H., Zhang, Z., Chen, J., Ding, L., ... Hong, H. (2015). Clopidogrel and aspirin versus aspirin alone for stroke prevention: A meta-analysis. *PLoS One, 10*(8), e0135372. doi: 10.1371/journal.pone.0135372

Tansy, A. P., Hinman, J. D., Ng, K. L., Calderon-Arnulphi, M., Modir, R., Chatfield, F., Liebeskind, D. S. (2015). Image more to save more. *Frontiers in Neurology, 6*, 156. doi: 10.3389/fneur.2015.00156. eCollection 2015.

Tarpley, J., Frank, D., Tansy, A. P., & Liebeskind. (2013). Use of perfusion imaging and other imaging techniques to assess risks/benefits of acute stroke interventions. *Current Atherosclerosis Reports, 15*(7), 336.

Thomas, K., Gerlach, S., Jorn, H., Larson, J., Brott, T., & Files, J. (2007). Advances in the care of patients with intracerebral hemorrhage. *Mayo Clinic Proceedings, 82*(8), 987–990.

Thompson, S. B., & Morgan, M. (2013). *Occupational therapy for stroke rehabilitation*. Springer.

Thompson, H., & Ryan, A. (2009). The impact of stroke consequences on spousal relationships from the perspective of the person with stroke. *Journal of Clinical Nursing, 18*(12), 1803–1811. doi: 10.1111/j.1365-2702.2008.02694.x

Towfighi, A., & Saver, J. L. (2011). Stroke declines from third to fourth leading cause of death in the United States historical perspective and challenges ahead. *Stroke, 42*(8), 2351–2355. doi: 10.1161/STROKEAHA.111.621904. Epub 2011 Jul 21.

Townend, E., Tinson, D., Kwan, J., & Sharpe, M. (2010) Feeling sad and useless: An investigation into personal acceptance of disability and its association with depression following stroke. *Clinical Rehabilitation, 24*(6), 555–564. doi: 10.1155/2014/354906

Treggiari, M., Walder, B., Suter, P., & Romand, J. (2003). A systematic review of the prevention of delayed ischemic neurological deficits with hypertension, hypervolemia, and hemodilution therapy following subarachnoid hemorrhage. *Journal of Neurosurgery, 98*(5), 978–984.

Trivedi, M. M., Ryan, K. A., & Cole, J. W. (2015). Ethnic differences in ischemic stroke subtypes in young-onset stroke: The Stroke Prevention in Young Adults Study. *BMC Neurology, 15*(1), 221. doi: 10.1186/s12883-015-0461-7

Trompetto, C., Marinelli, L., Mori, L., Pelosin, E., Currà, A., Molfetta, L., & Abbruzzese, G. (2014). Pathophysiology of spasticity: Implications for neurorehabilitation. *BioMed Research International, 2014*(3), 1. doi: 10.1155/2014/354906

Tsze, D. S., & Valente, J. H. (2011). Pediatric stroke: A review. *Emergency Medicine International, 2011*, 734506. doi: 10.1155/2011/734506. Epub 2011 Dec 27.

Turhan, N., Atalay, A., & Atabek, H. (2006). Impact of stroke etiology, lesion location and aging on post-stroke urinary incontinence as a predictor of functional recovery. *International Journal of Rehabilitation Research, 29*(4), 353–358.

Urbanski, M., Coubard, O. A., & Bourlon, C. (2014). Visualizing the blind brain: Brain imaging of visual field defects from early recovery to rehabilitation techniques. *Frontiers in Integrative Neuroscience, 8*, 74. doi: 10.3389/fnint.2014.00074

Urrutia, R. P., Coeytaux, R. R., McBroom, A. J., Gierisch, J. M., Havrilesky, L. J., Moorman, P. G., ... Myers, E. R. (2013). Risk of acute thromboembolic events with oral contraceptive use: A systematic review and meta-analysis. *Obstetrics & Gynecology, 122*(2, PART 1), 380–389. doi: 10.1097/AOG.0b013e3182994c43

Van Kooij, B. J. M., Hendrikse, J., Benders, M. J. N. L., De Vries, L. S., & Groenendaal, F. (2010). Anatomy of the circle of Willis and blood flow in the brain-feeding vasculature in prematurely born infants. *Neonatology, 97*(3), 235–241. doi: 10.1159/000253754. Epub 2009 Oct 30.

Vassileva, E., Daskalov, M. & Stamenova, P. (2015). Free-floating thrombus in stroke patients with nonstenotic internal carotid artery—An ultra-sonographic study. *Journal of Clinical Ultrasound, 43*(1), 34–38.

Veltkamp, R., Siebing, D., Sun, L., Heiland, S., Bieber, K., Marti, H., Nagel, S., & Schwaninger, M. (2005). Hyperbaric oxygen reduces blood–brain barrier damage and edema after transient focal cerebral ischemia. *Stroke, 36*, 1679–1683.

Vilela, M., & Newell, D. (2008). Superficial temporal artery to middle cerebral artery bypass: Past, present, and future. *Neurosurgery, 24*(6), 566–579.

Voeks, J., McClure, L., Go, R., Prineas, R., Cushman, M., Kissela, B., & Roseman, J. (2008). Regional differences in diabetes as a possible contributor to the geographic disparity in stroke mortality: The reasons for geographic and racial differences in stroke study. *Stroke, 39*, 1675–1680.

Warning signs of a heart attack. (n.d.). Retrieved from American Heart Association website, http://www.heart.org/HEARTORG/General/911—Warnings-Signs-of-a-Heart-Attack_UCM_305346_SubHomePage.jsp on September 10, 2015.

Werner, P., Saur, D., Zeisig, V., Ettrich, B., Patt, M., Sattler, B., … Barthel, H. (2015). Simultaneous PET/MRI in stroke: A case series. *Journal of Cerebral Blood Flow & Metabolism*, *35*, 1421–1425. doi: 10.1038/jcbfm.2015.158. Epub 2015 Jul 15.

Westendorp, W. F., Nederkoorn, P. J., Vermeij, J. D., Dijkgraaf, M. G., & van de Beek, D. (2011). Post-stroke infection: A systematic review and meta-analysis. *BMC Neurology*, *11*(1), 110. doi: 10.1186/1471-2377-11-110

Westover, A., McBride, S., & Haley, R. (2007). Stroke in young adults who abuse amphetamines or cocaine: A population-based study of hospitalized patients. *Archives of General Psychiatry*, *64*(4), 495–502.

Williams, L., Kroenke, K., Bakas, T., Plue, L., Brizendine, E., Tu, W., & Hendrie, H. (2007). Care management of post stroke depression. *Stroke*, *38*, 998–1003.

Wolf, P. (2006). Trends in incidence, lifetime risk, severity, and 30-day mortality of stroke over the past 50 years. *Journal of the American Medical Association*, *296*, 2939–2946.

Wu, C. M., McLaughlin, K., Lorenzetti, D. L., Hill, M. D., Manns, B. J., & Ghali, W. A. (2007). Early risk of stroke after transient ischemic attack: A systematic review and meta-analysis. *Archives of Internal Medicine*, *167*(22), 2417–2422.

Xie, J., Wu, E., Zheng, Z., Croft, J., Greenlund, K., Mensah, G., & Labarthe, D. (2006). Impact of stroke on health-related quality of Life in the noninstitutionalized population in the United States. *Stroke*, *37*, 2567–2572.

Xie, W., Zheng, F., Zhong, B., & Song, X. (2015). Long-term antiplatelet mono- and dual therapies after ischemic stroke or transient ischemic attack: Network meta-analysis. *Journal of the American Heart Association*, *4*(8), e002259. doi: 10.1161/JAHA.115.002259

Yanagida, T., Fujimoto, S., Inoue, T., & Suzuki, S. (2015). Prehospital delay and stroke-related symptoms. *Internal Medicine (Tokyo, Japan)*, *54*(2), 171–177. doi: 10.2169/internalmedicine.54.2684.

Yang, S., Choi, K. H., & Son, Y. R. (2015). The effect of stroke on pharyngeal laterality during swallowing. *Annals of Rehabilitation Medicine*, *39*(4), 509–516. doi: 10.5535/arm.2015.39.4.509

Yuan, J., Lipinski, M., & Degterev, A. (2003). Diversity in the mechanisms of neuronal cell death. *Neuron*, *40*(2), 401–413.

Zazulia, A. R. (2009). Critical care management of acute ischemic stroke. *Continuum: Lifelong Learning in Neurology*, *15*(3), 68–82.

Zhang, X., Kedar, S., Lynn, M., Newman, N., & Biousse, V. (2006). Natural history of homonymous hemianopia. *Neurology*, *66*, 90–905.

Zhao, X., Grotta, J., Gonzales, N., & Aronowski, J. (2009). Hematoma resolution as a therapeutic target the role of microglia/macrophages. *Stroke*, *40*(3 Suppl. 1), S92–S94.

18 Cardiopulmonary Disorders

Reese Martin

Nadine looked down at her feet and saw that they were really swollen today. She also felt more short of breath than she did a couple of days ago but assumed it was because she had been working hard to move some of her belongings into her daughter's home as she was going to help take care of her grandchildren for a few weeks. A couple of months ago, her doctor had told her that she had signs of congestive heart failure (CHF), and although she thought the name of the condition sounded serious, she was told she could control it. She had no time to think about it at the moment though, as she was focused on helping her daughter. Over the next few days, her shortness of breath and fatigue worsened—and so did her swollen ankles. One night, Nadine felt like she couldn't breathe if she lay flat in her bed, so she decided to sleep in her recliner. The next morning, she decided to go see her doctor. While being weighed prior to her session, Nadine noticed that she had gained 4 lb even though she had been eating less. During their meeting, her doctor explained that her heart was not pumping hard enough to circulate her blood normally and that fluid was building up in her lungs and other parts of her body.

Occupational therapists often work with clients who have either a primary or secondary diagnosis that involves the cardiopulmonary system. This chapter reviews introductory anatomy and physiology information about the lungs and heart and defines common conditions that negatively impact these important structures. Common conditions to be further discussed in this chapter include coronary artery disease (CAD), CHF, chronic obstructive pulmonary disorder, myocardial infarctions (MIs), and hypertension.

DEFINITIONS AND DESCRIPTION

■ The Cardiopulmonary System: An Overview

The cardiopulmonary system consists of the lungs, the heart, and their interconnections. Cardiopulmonary function enables the heart and lung to maintain flow and regulation of blood between these vital organs—a process that relies on their connection via the pulmonary artery. In this section of the chapter, a brief overview of these systems and their connections, as well as the interaction of these organs as a functional unit that is the cardiopulmonary system, are discussed. In addition, cardiopulmonary vital signs will be discussed, which are essential in understanding how the heart and lungs function.

Lungs

The respiratory system includes the nose, throat, trachea, and lungs. Inhalation of air contains oxygen and other gases. Oxygen is a basic gas that every cell in the body requires to maintain life. To begin the inhalation process, the diaphragm muscle pulls down into the chest cavity creating a vacuum for air to enter. Air moves through the lungs, where small sacs called alveoli perform the gas exchange. The lungs consist of two spongy, balloon-like parts. The right lung contains three lobes and is slightly larger than the left lung, which contains two lobes. In the lungs, the oxygen from each breath is transferred to the bloodstream and sent to all the body's cells as life-sustaining fuel. Each cell in the body exchanges oxygen cells for waste, gas, and carbon dioxide. The carbon dioxide travels back to the lungs where the waste gas is removed from the bloodstream and exhaled from the body. This vital process, called gas exchange, occurs automatically within the body (Fig. 18.1). The respiratory system has several protective mechanisms. The epiglottis, a thin flap of tissue that covers the trachea during each episode of swallowing, prevents foreign materials from entering the air passages that lead to the lungs. Inhaled air is warmed and moistened for optimal humidity within the nose and mouth and then cleaned by mucus, which lines the airway structures. Cilia, hairlike structures, remove the mucus up and out of the system (American Lung Association, n.d.).

Heart

The heart is the main pumping station of the circulatory system, working to provide needed nutrients and oxygen to all organs of the body. The heart attempts to provide the right amount of blood at the proper rate to make sure an adequate amount of oxygen is delivered to all of the organs. The amount of oxygen needed throughout the body varies depends on the tasks being completed. For example, increased oxygen is needed in the gastrointestinal system when digesting after a meal. Also, voluntary muscle groups require more oxygen while exercising. Heart rate changes in order to meet these needs.

The heart contains four chambers: the two upper chambers (atria) that collect blood and the two lower chambers (ventricles) that pump blood out of the heart. Beginning with the right atrium, oxygen-depleted blood enters the upper chamber after circulating through the body, continuing to the right ventricle and then entering the lung to receive oxygen. Oxygen-rich blood returns from the lungs to the left atrium, continues to the left ventricle, and is then expelled to the body via the bloodstream. Muscular walls surround the four chambers and valves of the heart to keep the blood moving in the right direction and prevent backflow. Refer to Figure 18.2 for a visualization of the process of the blood flow through the heart.

Combination of Lungs and Heart

It is vital that the heart and lungs work in tandem in order to efficiently transport oxygen and nutrients to all systems of the body. The lungs receive deoxygenated blood from the heart, where the blood circulates through the alveoli within the lungs in order to gather oxygen from air inhaled into the lungs and remove the carbon dioxide waste. The lungs then return the oxygenated blood to the heart in order to be pumped back out to the rest of the body. Due to the direct connection between these two organs, conditions impacting one can cause impairments of the other.

■ Cardiopulmonary Vital Signs

Cardiopulmonary vital signs measure cardiac pulse rate, respiratory rate, blood pressure, oxygen saturation, and temperature. These measurements help detect potential medical issues as well as monitor how the body tolerates activities. When working with various cardiopulmonary disorders, vital signs are often monitored closely

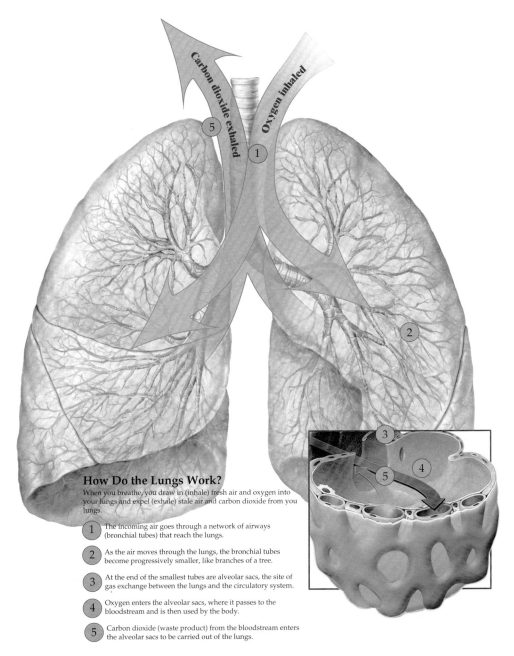

How Do the Lungs Work?

When you breathe, you draw in (inhale) fresh air and oxygen into your lungs and expel (exhale) stale air and carbon dioxide from you lungs.

(1) The incoming air goes through a network of airways (bronchial tubes) that reach the lungs.

(2) As the air moves through the lungs, the bronchial tubes become progressively smaller, like branches of a tree.

(3) At the end of the smallest tubes are alveolar sacs, the site of gas exchange between the lungs and the circulatory system.

(4) Oxygen enters the alveolar sacs, where it passes to the bloodstream and is then used by the body.

(5) Carbon dioxide (waste product) from the bloodstream enters the alveolar sacs to be carried out of the lungs.

Figure 18.1 How lungs function. (From Anatomical Chart Company.)

to determine a patient's tolerance to activities (John Hopkins Medicine, n.d.).

Pulse Rate

The pulse rate, often referred to as a heart rate, is the number of times the heart beats per minute (BPM). As the heart pushes blood through the arteries, the arteries expand and contract with the flow of the blood. This can be measured by palpation, or the manual pressing of the examiner's fingers on arteries located close to the surface of the skin. The outcome of this is the heart sounds that occur as the heart forces blood through the arteries. The pulse can be found on the wrist, inside of the elbow, or neck. To check a pulse rate, count the beats felt in 60 seconds by firmly pressing the fingertips of your first and second digits. A normal resting heart rate

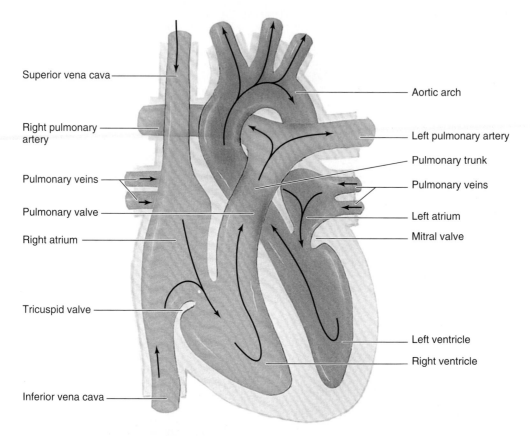

Figure 18.2 Blood flow through the heart. The *arrows* show the direction of blood flow. Red vessels carry oxygen-rich blood and blue vessels carry oxygen-poor blood. (From Anatomical Chart Company.)

The image labels read, from top left: Superior vena cava, Right pulmonary artery, Pulmonary veins, Pulmonary valve, Right atrium, Tricuspid valve, Inferior vena cava. From top right: Aortic arch, Left pulmonary artery, Pulmonary trunk, Pulmonary veins, Left atrium, Mitral valve, Left ventricle, Right ventricle.

for healthy adults ranges from 60 to 100 BPM. Adult females tend to have a higher resting heart rate than do adult males. **Arrhythmias** are any changes from the normal sequence of electrical impulses in the heart, causing the heart to beat too slow, too quickly, or irregularly. If the heart doesn't beat appropriately, blood is not adequately pumped throughout the body, which may lead to organs inefficiently working or becoming damaged ("Tachycardia, Fast Heart Rate," 2015). Although 60 to 100 BPM is considered normal, athletes may have a heart rate as low as 40 BPM without experiencing problems. A heart rate <60 BPM in adults is called **bradycardia**. A heart rate higher than 100 BPM in adults is called **tachycardia**. **Atrial fibrillation** (AFib) is an irregular, rapid heart rate that can lead to poor blood flow to the body. This occurs when the upper chambers of the heart quiver and beat irregularly, leading to ineffectively moving the blood to the ventricles. This can cause the blood to slow down and pool, which increases the risk for blood clots, stroke,

and heart-related complications, including heart failure (Mayo Clinic Staff, 2015).

Respiratory Rate

The number of breaths a person takes per minute is the respiratory rate. The rate is measured by counting the number of breaths for 1 minute by counting how many times the chest rises typically when a person is at rest. The average adult takes 15 to 20 breaths per minute (American Lung Association, n.d.).

Blood Pressure

Blood pressure is the force of blood pushing against the artery walls. Blood pressure consists of two numbers written as a fraction and is recorded as millimeters of mercury (mm Hg). The recording represents how high the mercury column on a mercury manometer, an older manual blood pressure device, is raised by the pressure of the blood. Blood pressures are now commonly taken with a blood pressure cuff with a simple dial and a stethoscope. The top number, also known as the **systolic**, measures the pressure in the arteries when the heart muscle contracts or beats. The systolic factor is usually the higher of the two numbers. **Diastolic**, the bottom number, measures the pressure in the arteries when the heart muscle is resting between beats and refilling with blood. One's blood pressure rises with each heartbeat and falls when the heart relaxes between beats. For an adult over 20, a normal blood pressure should be <120/80 mm Hg. **Hypertension**, or high blood pressure, is a prevalent chronic disease that is often asymptomatic. Early-stage hypertension may present with dull headaches, dizzy spells, or increased nosebleeds. These signs and symptoms usually do not occur until high blood pressure has become severe or life threatening. Hypertension will be discussed in further detail later in this chapter. Hypotension, low blood pressure, can cause symptoms of dizziness and light-headedness, and severe cases can be life threatening. Blood pressure is considered low if the systolic (top number) is 90 mm Hg or below or if the diastolic (bottom number) is 60 mm Hg or less. Hypotension can occur for various reasons, such as dehydration or pregnancy, but is generally treatable once the cause of the low blood pressure is identified (American Heart Association, 2014).

Oxygen Saturation

In order to function properly, your body needs a certain level of oxygen circulating in the blood to cells and tissues. Oxygen saturation is a percentage measure of the amount of oxygen in which the blood is carrying. Oxygen saturation can be measured by testing a sample of blood from an artery by way of a pulse oximeter, which is a small device that usually clips to a finger. Normal pulse oximeter readings range from 95% to 100%. Values under 90% are considered low, or hypoxemic. **Hypoxemia**, or low blood oxygen, describes a lower than normal level of oxygen in your blood (Mayo Clinic, n.d.).

PREVALENT CARDIOPULMONARY DISORDERS

■ Coronary Artery Disease

Description and Definition

CAD develops when your coronary arteries, the blood vessels that supply the heart with blood, oxygen, and nutrients, become damaged. CAD occurs when plaque, which is the by-product of cholesterol, fat, and calcium deposits and other substances, builds up in the arteries that supply blood to the heart. Over time, the plaque hardens and leads to narrowing of arteries, or stenosis, reducing the rate of blood flow to the heart. This process is also known as **atherosclerosis** (Fig. 18.3).

Etiology

Causes of the CAD are thought to be a combination of lifestyle choice and genetics. CAD is thought to begin with damage or injury to the inner layer of a coronary artery. The damage may be caused by smoking, high cholesterol, high blood pressure, diabetes, and obesity or sedentary lifestyle, or radiation therapy to the chest. Age and family history are additional risk factors.

Incidence and Prevalence

According to the Center for Disease Control (2015), heart disease is the leading cause of death for both men and women. Coronary heart disease is the most common type of heart disease in the United States, resulting in death in over three hundred and seventy thousand people annually (Center for Disease Control, 2015).

Signs and Symptoms

At first, the decreased blood flow to the heart may not cause any symptoms. As plaque builds up in the coronary arteries, a patient may develop angina (chest pain), shortness of breath, and/or fatigue with exertion. A complete blockage of a coronary artery may lead to a heart attack.

Course and Prognosis

CAD progresses and slowly worsens with time; the disease can go unnoticed until an artery is blocked to the point of a heart attack. Over time, the disease can weaken the heart muscle, which may lead to heart failure, a serious condition where the heart cannot adequately pump blood. Arrhythmias can also develop as the disease progresses.

Medical/Surgical Management

Medical management for CAD is commonly a combination of lifestyle changes, medication, and, if severe enough, surgical interventions. Lifestyle changes include smoking cessation, healthy diet, and active lifestyle, losing weight, and stress reduction. Medications utilized for

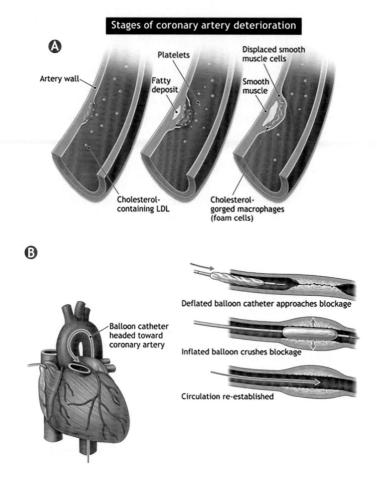

Figure 18.3 A. Deterioration of a coronary artery from deposits of fatty substances that roughen the vessel's center. When a thrombus (blood clot) forms above the plaque, complete blockage of the artery produces a myocardial infarction or heart attack. A coronary artery bypass graft (CABG) creates a new "transportation route" around the blocked region to allow the required blood flow to deliver oxygen and nutrients to the previously "starved" surrounding heart muscle. The saphenous vein from the leg is the most commonly used bypass vessel. CABG involves sewing the graft vessels to the coronary arteries beyond the narrowing or blockage, with the other end of the vein attached to the aorta. Medications (statins) lower total and LDL cholesterol, and daily low-dose aspirin (81 mg) reduces post-CABG artery narrowing beyond the insertion site of the graft. Repeat CABG surgical mortality averages 5% to 10%. **B.** Angioplasty procedure to fix a blocked coronary artery. (From McArdle, W. D., Katch, I., & Katch, V. L. (2013). *Exercise physiology* (8th ed.). Philadelphia, PA: Lippincott Williams & Wilkins.)

CAD include cholesterol-modifying medications; aspirin or a blood thinner; beta-blockers, which can slow the heart rate and decrease blood pressure; and nitroglycerin tablets to open coronary arteries and decrease chest pain. When the artery blockage is severe enough, certain procedures to restore and improve blood flow are needed. An **angioplasty** is a procedure in which a catheter with a deflated balloon is inserted into the blocked artery (Fig. 18.3). Once in place, the balloon is inflated, compressing the plaque to the sides of the artery, opening up the artery, and improving blood flow to the heart. A stent, a small metal mesh tube, is then inserted into the narrowed artery. Some stents release medicine to help keep the artery open. When CAD is causing significant blockage, one may have a **coronary artery bypass graft** (CABG) (Fig. 18.4).

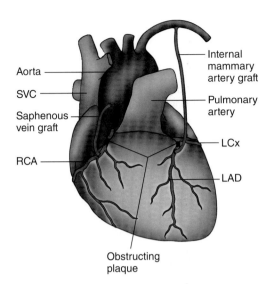

Aorta

SVC

Saphenous vein graft

RCA

Internal mammary artery graft

Pulmonary artery

LCx

LAD

Obstructing plaque

Figure 18.4 Coronary artery bypass surgery. Two types of bypasses are illustrated: (1) the left internal mammary artery originates from the left subclavian artery, and in this schematic, it is anastomosed to the left anterior descending (LAD) coronary artery distal to obstructing plaque; (2) one end of a saphenous vein graft is sutured to the proximal aorta and the other end to the right coronary artery (RCA) distal to a stenotic segment. (From Lilly, L. S. (2015). *Pathophysiology of heart disease* (6th ed.). Philadelphia, PA: Wolters Kluwer.)

A CABG is a procedure in which arteries or veins from other parts of the body, oftentimes from the leg, are removed and surgically attached to bypass the blocked arteries in the heart. In order to perform surgery on a patient's heart, the sternum is often cracked open and wired back together after surgery. After the surgery, patients generally have sternal precautions: no pushing, pulling, or lifting anything more than 5 to 10 lb (surgeon dependent) in order for the sternum to adequately heal. Patients with CAD often attend cardiac rehabilitation, a medically supervised program consisting of exercise training as well as educating the patient about the disease. Occupational therapists are often involved in these programs (National Heart, Lung, and Blood Institute, 2014).

■ Congestive heart failure

Description and Definition

Congestive heart failure, or heart failure (CHF), is a chronic, noncurable condition where the heart does not beat strongly enough to maintain adequate blood flow throughout the body causing organs to become oxygen deprived and leading to fluid retention throughout the body.

Etiology

Certain conditions such as narrowed arteries (CAD) or chronic high blood flow can gradually lead to the heart muscles becoming too weak or stiff to fill and pump blood efficiently. According to the American Heart Association (2014), CAD is the most common cause of CHF. Other common risk factors that may lead to CHF include heart attacks causing damage to the heart muscles, congenital birth defects, arrhythmias, high blood pressure, infection of the heart, diabetes, thyroid problems, obesity, alcohol or drug abuse, or certain types of chemotherapy.

Incidence and Prevalence

According to CDC, about 5.1 million Americans are diagnosed with heart failure. Heart failure is one of the most common reasons people aged 65 and older go into the hospital. In 2009, heart failure was a contributing cause of death for one in nine deaths in the United States (Center for Disease Control, 2015).

Signs and Symptoms

Signs and symptoms of CHF include **dyspnea**, a sensation of having impaired breathing such as shortness of breath, due to exertion or when lying down, fatigue and weakness, and reduced activity/exercise tolerance. A patient may also experience chest pain, arrhythmias, coughing, or wheezing. Patients diagnosed with CHF often suffer from fluid retention causing sudden weight gain, edema in lower extremities, ascites (swelling of the abdomen), and increased need to urinate at night. Additional symptoms include lack of appetite, nausea, as well as difficulty concentrating or decreased alertness (Mayo Clinic, n.d.).

Course and Prognosis

CHF is a chronic diagnosis that requires lifelong management. Shortness of breath, an initial symptom of the condition, is often mistaken for a normal process of aging. As the condition progresses, shortness of breath worsens and overall endurance declines. Although treatment may improve various symptoms, the disease slowly progresses depriving the body of much needed oxygen and may eventually lead to death. The Center for Disease Control (2015) estimates that about half of people who develop heart failure in the United States die within 5 years of diagnosis. Early diagnosis and treatment can improve quality and length of life.

Medical/Surgical Management

Treatment can help improve the various symptoms associated with the disease leading to an increased quality of life, increase lifespan, and reduce the chances of sudden death. Specific treatment is determined via identifying and treating the underlying cause of the heart failure. Similar to all cardiopulmonary conditions, lifestyle changes can decrease the rate of progression of the disease. Lifestyle changes include diet modifications such as limiting sodium intake and monitoring portions, exercising regularly, and smoking cessation. According to a systematic review of various research articles, authors report that although length of life was not significantly impacted, men with mild to moderate CHF who participated in regular exercise had a better quality of life and better overall fitness than did those who did not (Davies et al., 2010). Medications are often utilized to help minimize the symptoms associated with CHF. Medications may include angiotensin-converting enzyme (ACE) inhibitors, which expand the blood vessels to decrease the heart's workload, diuretics to reduce fluid overload, and dioxin to help the heart contract properly. When CHF becomes severe, surgical interventions may be indicated. If the CHF is caused by inadequate blood flow to the muscles in the heart, a CABG surgery or angioplasty (stent placement) or heart valve replacement or repair may be considered in order to improve blood circulation. A pacemaker insertion may also be indicated to help maintain a consistent heartbeat.

■ Chronic Obstructive Pulmonary Disease

Definition and Description

Chronic obstructive pulmonary disease (COPD) is an overarching term, which refers to a group of lung diseases characterized by airflow obstruction that interferes with normal breathing. Emphysema and chronic bronchitis are the most prevalent conditions that compose COPD, and they often coexist. A normal functioning lung resembles an inflated balloon with tension and pressure to allow for proper air exchange. COPD may cause the lungs to lose their elasticity, resembling a somewhat deflated balloon. Walls of the airways may also become inflamed or damaged, or mucus within the airways can build up and lead to a blockage. The damage of COPD leads to decreased airflow. With **emphysema**, the walls between air sacs are damaged causing the air sacs to lose their shape. Damage can also destroy the walls of the air sacs, leading to fewer and larger air sacs instead of many tiny ones in a normal lung. When this occurs, the quantity of gas exchange in the lungs is reduced. **Bronchitis** causes the lining of the airways to become irritated and inflamed causing the lining to thicken. Buildup of mucus leads to difficulty breathing.

Etiology

The National Heart, Lung, and Blood Institute (n.d.) consistently indicates that cigarette smoking is the leading cause of COPD. Long-term exposure to other lung irritants—such as air pollution, chemical fumes, or dust—may also contribute to COPD.

Incidence and Prevalence

The Center for Disease Control reports that chronic lower respiratory disease, primarily COPD, was the third leading cause of death in the United States in 2011. Fifteen million Americans report that they have been diagnosed with COPD. Chronic bronchitis affects people of all ages, although people aged 65 years or more have the highest rate at 64.2 per 1,000 persons. In 2011, more women reported a diagnosis of emphysema than did men and were twice as likely to be diagnosed with chronic bronchitis. In 2011, 3.3 million men (29.6 per 1,000 population) had a diagnosis of chronic bronchitis compared to 6.8 million women (56.7 per 1,000 population). Prevalence seems to be highest in the Midwest and Southeast states (Center for Disease Control, 2014).

Signs and Symptoms

Typical symptoms of COPD include persistent chronic cough with increased mucus production, dyspnea (especially with exertion), wheezing, chest tightness, frequent respiratory infections, and fatigue. COPD often goes undetected until the condition is moderately to severely advanced. Severe COPD may cause edema in the lower extremities, weight loss, or decreased muscle endurance. **Cyanosis**, a bluish color to the skin (usually evident in lips and fingernails), is usually due to decreased oxygen levels. The severity of symptoms is dependent on the severity of lung damage. An American Lung Association (n.d.) survey revealed that half of all COPD patients (51%) indicate that their condition limits their ability to work. It also limits them in normal physical exertion (70%), household chores (56%), social activities (53%), sleeping (50%), and family activities (46%).

Course and Prognosis

COPD is a progressive and irreversible disease. As the disease worsens, increased difficulty breathing leads to decreased oxygen levels throughout the body. The heart may become enlarged due to the strain with decreased oxygen levels, and changes in blood pressures may also be present. Increased shortness of breath and difficulty with daily tasks are often thought as symptoms of normal aging leading to a delay in accurate diagnosis and medical management. With the delay in diagnosis, decreased lung function has already occurred or began. The progression of the disease can be slowed and quality of life maintained via lifestyle changes such as smoking cessation or avoiding irritants, managing symptoms, medication management, and simplifying daily tasks by way of energy conservation techniques.

Medical/Surgical Management

COPD is diagnosed through a history of exposure to toxins and lifestyle choices as well as a series of functional pulmonary tests to determine lung function. A spirometry test, the most common pulmonary measure, is used to assess how well the lungs work by measuring how much air is inhaled and exhaled and the pace of exhalation. A chest radiograph and computerized tomography (CT) scan can visualize emphysema and lead to a diagnosis of COPD.

Although COPD is a progressive disease, medical management can help manage symptoms, reduce the risk for exacerbations or complications, and improve quality of life. The most critical treatment of managing COPD is smoking cessation to prevent the disease from continuing to worsen. Various medications may be utilized to help manage symptoms. Bronchodilators, often prescribed as inhalers, relax the muscles around the airways to alleviate coughing and decrease dyspnea. Inhaled and oral steroids reduce airway inflammation and help prevent exacerbations. Antibiotics are often prescribed to prevent exacerbations as respiratory infections such as pneumonia can aggravate symptoms of COPD. Oxygen therapy may be indicated with moderate to severe COPD to help maintain adequate oxygen levels. Patients with COPD may be referred to a Pulmonary Rehabilitation Program, which combines education, exercise training, nutrition advice, and personal counseling to improve quality of life and decrease hospitalizations.

Despite consistent management, acute exacerbations (worsening of symptoms for days to weeks) may occur and lead to lung failure if not adequately and promptly treated. Respiratory infections or exposure to irritants are often the cause of COPD exacerbations. Some forms of severe emphysema that are not adequately managed with medications and lifestyle changes may undergo surgical interventions such as lung volume reduction surgery or a lung transplant.

■ Myocardial Infarction
Definition and Description

A **myocardial infarction** (MI), commonly referred to as a heart attack, occurs when the blood flow that brings oxygen to the heart muscle is severely reduced or completely occluded causing the heart muscle tissue to be without oxygen. This results in varying degrees of physical destruction to that tissue (Fig. 18.5). Atherosclerosis, which is the formation of plaque within the arterial wall, is the leading cause of MI. Atherosclerosis may rupture and leak cholesterol and other substances into the bloodstream. A blood clot, or thrombus, forms at the site of the rupture, which can occlude all blood flow through that coronary artery. A spasm of a coronary artery is an additional cause of MI, which shuts down blood flow to the heart muscle. These spasms are often a result of tobacco or illicit drug use. Spontaneous coronary artery dissection, or a tear in the arterial wall, may also lead to an MI (Mayo Clinic, 2015).

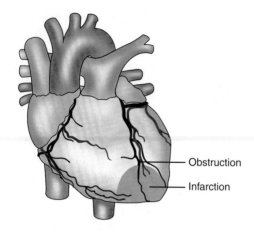

Obstruction

Infarction

Figure 18.5 A heart attack occurs when one or more of the coronary arteries become blocked, preventing blood from reaching the myocardium. The lack of oxygen and nutrients causes the tissue that is supplied by the affected artery to die. (From Carter, P. J. (2011). *Lippincott textbook for nursing assistants* (3rd ed.). Philadelphia, PA: Lippincott Williams & Wilkins.)

Etiology

Key risk factors for heart attacks include smoking, high blood pressure, elevated levels of cholesterol, diabetes, obesity and poor diet, sedentary lifestyles, and excessive alcohol intake (Mayo Clinic, 2014).

Incidence and Prevalence

About every 34 seconds, a single incident of MI occurs in the United States (American Heart Association, 2014). The Center for Disease Control (2015) reports that every year, about seven hundred and thirty five thousand Americans are diagnosed.

Signs and Symptoms

The most common sign of a heart attack is chest discomfort or pain, which may spread to the arm, neck, or jaw. Shortness of breath, nausea/vomiting, cold sweats, and fatigue are additional warning signs of a heart attack (Fig. 18.6). The American Heart Association reports that women, more often than men, experience shortness of breath, neck/jaw or back pain, and nausea or vomiting. Knowing the warning signs of a heart attack is essential to prevent death. A study in 2005 revealed that 92% of respondents recognized chest pain as a major sign of a heart attack, and only 27% of those in the

study were aware of the additional signs of a heart attack (Center for Disease Control, 2008).

Course and Prognosis

Cardiac damage caused by an MI can be limited if adequate medical management is acquired in an appropriate amount of time. With adequate medical management and lifestyle modifications, many people survive heart attacks and recover to return to full, active lives. Given a cardiac event, one is at higher risk for additional MIs (Mozzafarian & Benjamin, 2015).

Medical/Surgical Management

Early medical management can prevent or limit heart muscle damage. Medical personnel can initiate treatment of an MI prior to admission to the hospital. Aspirin is a first-line treatment to thin blood and prevent further clotting. Nitroglycerin, typically a sublingual medication, is used for chest pain and reduction of cardiac output and acts to improve blood flow through the coronary arteries. An MI is often diagnosed via electrocardiogram (ECG) and blood tests following admission. An ECG records the electric activity of the heart and confirms, in part, that a cardiac event has occurred or is in process, as injured heart muscles do not create normal electrical impulses. When the heart has been damaged, certain enzymes slowly leak into the bloodstream, which can be identified in a blood test. Once the diagnosis is confirmed, treatment is initiated to restore blood flow to the heart. Thrombolytic medicine, commonly referred to as "clot busting" medicine, is used to dissolve blood clots that are blocking the coronary arteries. For best results, the medicines should be administered within hours of the start of the symptoms of a heart attack. Once the location of the blockage is identified, a patient may undergo a coronary angioplasty, a procedure used to open blocked arteries. Smoking cessation, like all cardiac diseases, is encouraged. Lifestyle changes may also be recommended, such as increasing exercise/activity.

■ Hypertension
Definition and Description

Hypertension, or high blood pressure, is an increase in the amount of force that is pushing against the artery walls as the heart pumps blood. A blood pressure consists of two readings,

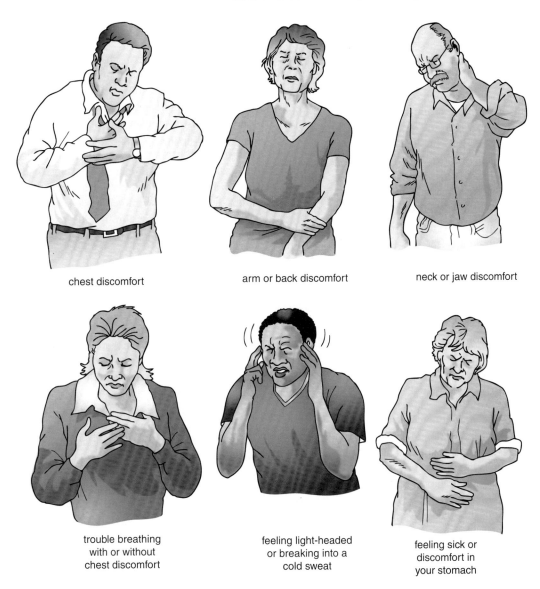

chest discomfort

arm or back discomfort

neck or jaw discomfort

trouble breathing
with or without
chest discomfort

feeling light-headed
or breaking into a
cold sweat

feeling sick or
discomfort in
your stomach

Figure 18.6 Heart attack symptoms include chest pain, possible arm pain, sweating, shortness of breath, nausea, and light-headedness. (From Delaet, R. (2011). *Introduction to health care & careers*. Philadelphia, PA: Lippincott Williams & Wilkins.)

a diastolic and systolic number. Normal blood pressure is considered to be 120/80 mm Hg. Hypertension is likely to be diagnosed when one or both of the numbers are persistently above 140/90. Blood pressures above 120/80 mm Hg but below 140/90 mm Hg will result in a diagnosis of prehypertension.

Etiology

There are two types of hypertension—primary and secondary. Primary hypertension is diagnosed when there is no identifiable cause and tends to develop gradually over years. Secondary hypertension is caused by an underlying condition, tends to have a sudden onset, and causes higher blood pressures than does primary hypertension. Various conditions that may lead to secondary hypertension include kidney problems, adrenal gland problems, thyroid problems, congenital blood vessel defects, certain medications, illegal drugs, chronic alcohol use, and sleep apnea (Mayo Clinic, n.d.).

Incidence and Prevalence

It is estimated that 29% or one of three American adults has high blood pressure. Hypertension is most prevalent in African American women and older populations as blood vessels become increasingly compromised with age. High blood pressure increases the risk for various life-threatening conditions such as heart attack, stroke, heart failure, and kidney disease (Mozzafarian & Benjamin, 2015).

Signs and Symptoms

Hypertension is often asymptomatic and can be undiagnosed and, therefore, untreated for several years. Although asymptomatic, high blood pressure can cause damage to the heart, kidneys, and other body structures. Those with early-stage hypertension may present with dull headaches, dizzy spells, or increased nosebleeds. These signs and symptoms usually do not occur until high blood pressure has become severe or life threatening (Mayo Clinic, n.d.). Someone experiencing a hypertensive crisis, which is defined as a systolic measure of 180 or higher or diastolic of 110 or higher, may present with severe headache and anxiety, shortness of breath, and nosebleeds. Because hypertension often has no signs or symptoms, high blood pressure is often identified when readings are taken by a health care provider. Several blood pressure readings will be taken at various times before a diagnosis is made as blood pressures can fluctuate throughout the day (American Heart Association, 2014).

Course and Prognosis

Hypertension can often be adequately controlled with medication and lifestyle changes. Uncontrolled hypertension increases risk for various life-threatening conditions such as heart attack, stroke, heart failure, and kidney disease.

Medical/Surgical Management

The goal of treating hypertension is to lower blood pressure to decrease risk of various complications described above. Lifestyle change is the first defense line when treating hypertension. These changes include dietary changes (decreasing salt intake, drinking water), increasing physical activity, smoking cessation, and limiting alcohol intake. Medications can also help maintain a lower blood pressure. Medications prescribed depend on the type of hypertension as well as other medical conditions. Diuretics are commonly utilized to help the kidneys eliminate water and sodium, which reduces blood volume. Various other medications help relax the blood vessels making it easier for blood to flow through, decreasing the workload on the heart (Mayo Clinic, n.d.).

IMPACT ON OCCUPATIONAL PERFORMANCE

Each of the cardiopulmonary disorders impacts occupational performance across all domains. Common symptoms throughout the cardiac disorders described here include shortness of breath, fatigue, and decreased activity tolerance. These symptoms may cause increased difficulty managing all occupations and lead to a decreased quality of life. Additionally, patients commonly have precautions after cardiac procedures, which may impact occupational performance. Common precautions after a coronary artery bypass grafting surgery and angioplasties include no pushing, pulling, or lifting anything more than 5 to 10 lb. Functional transfers and bed mobility are modified to maintain these precautions. Household chores, work tasks, and play/leisure activities are often limited after these procedures due to lifting restrictions. Occupational therapists play a lead role when working with patients with cardiac disorders including assessing one's ability to safely complete activities of daily living, educating patients regarding energy conservation and work simplification techniques, and assisting with progressing back to normal activity by a program of strengthening and endurance training.

CASE STUDY

Kenny, a 58-year-old male, worked as a tow truck driver who spent 50 to 60 hours a week on the road towing cars after accidents. In the middle of a high-stress 12-hour workday, Kenny began to feel severe chest heaviness while on his way to his next job. Kenny did not think much of the pain, figured it was heartburn from lunch, and continued on with his workday. The chest heaviness, however, did not go away and began traveling to his arms and neck. Kenny began having cold sweats and feeling nauseous. He decided to go to the emergency room.

Once Kenny arrived at the emergency room, Kenny was given medicine to alleviate chest pain and decrease workflow for the heart. Blood draws and an EKG were completed and both came back abnormal; Kenny was diagnosed with an acute MI. Kenny was given medicine to help break up the blood clot that was preventing blood flow. Once his condition was stabilized, Kenny was taken to the cardiac catheter lab and underwent a coronary angioplasty in order to open the blocked arteries.

Kenny had to stay in the hospital for 2 days in order to be monitored by cardiologists. Kenny was seen by cardiac rehabilitation therapists to provide education and guidelines for home as well as dieticians to discuss diet recommendations such as limiting salt intake. Kenny was able to go home and continue living independently after a couple of short days in the hospital. Once he completed outpatient cardiac rehabilitation and had a follow-up appointment with his cardiologist, Kenny was able to return to work.

CASE STUDY

Ruth, a 71-year-old female, is a retired secretary who lives with her spouse. Over the past several weeks, she has been experiencing increased shortness of breath with activities and increased overall fatigue. The shortness of breath and decreased activity level lead to significant overall weakness, and Ruth made an appointment with her doctor to discuss her concerns. The doctor ordered a cardiac stress test, which came back abnormal, so a cardiac catheter procedure was completed. The procedure revealed severe multivessel coronary artery disease. Due to the severity of the blockages to the arteries, the doctor recommended a coronary artery bypass graft.

After discussion with her doctors and family, Ruth decided to have the surgery and was admitted to the hospital. After the surgery, Ruth remained in the hospital for approximately 1 week where she was monitored by the cardiologists. After the surgery, Ruth worked with therapists. Because of her surgery, Ruth was unable to use her arms to help herself get in and out of bed or on and off the toilet. Because Ruth required more help with her basic care and was having difficulty with transfers and mobility, she went to a rehabilitation facility (skilled nursing facility) when she was medically stable to leave the hospital.

Ruth stayed at the skilled nursing facility for 2 weeks until she was able to safely care for herself and return home. Once she was home, her spouse continued to assist her as needed, such as providing transportation to and from appointments and helping with household chores and meal preparation.

RESOURCE LIST

American Heart Association
http://www.heart.org/HEARTORG/

American Lung Association
http://www.lung.org/lung-disease/

National Heart, Lung, and Blood Institute
http://www.nhlbi.nih.gov/

The Mayo Clinic
http://www.mayoclinic.org/

Center for Disease Control
http://www.cdc.gov/heartdisease/index.htm

REFERENCES

American Heart Association. (2014). *Why blood pressure matters*. Retrieved from http://www.heart.org/HEARTORG/Conditions/HighBloodPressure/WhyBloodPressureMatters/Why-Blood-Pressure-Matters_UCM_002051_Article.jsp, on August 4, 2014.

American Heart Association. (n.d.). *About heart attacks*. Retrieved from http://www.heart.org/HEARTORG/Conditions/HeartAttack/AboutHeartAttacks/About-Heart-Attacks_UCM_002038_Article.jsp

American Lung Association. (n.d.). *Chronic obstructive pulmonary disease (COPD) fact sheet*. American Lung Association. Retrieved from http://www.lung.org/lung-disease/copd/resources/facts-figures/COPD-Fact-Sheet.html

CDC. (2008). Disparities in adult awareness of heart attack warning signs and symptoms—14 states, 2005. *MMWR, 57*(7), 175–179.

Center for Disease Control. (2015). *Heart disease fact sheet*. Retrieved from http://www.cdc.gov/dhdsp/data_statistics/fact_sheets/docs/fs_heart_disease.pdf, on February 19, 2015.

Centers for Disease Control and Prevention. *National Center for Health Statistics: National Health Interview Survey Raw Data, 2011*. Analysis performed by the American Lung Association Research and Health Education Division using SPSS and SUDAAN software.

Davies, E. J., Moxham, T., Rees, K., Singh, S., Coats, A. J. S., Ebrahim, S., et al. (2010). Exercise training for systolic heart failure: Cochrane systematic review and meta-analysis. *European Journal of Heart Failure, 12*, 706–715. doi: 10.1093/eurjhf/hfq056

John Hopkins Medicine. (n.d.). Retrieved from www.Hopkinsmedicine.orghealthlibrary/conditions/cardiovascular_diseases/vital_signs_body_temperature_pulse_rate_respiration_rate_blood_pressure_85,P00866/

Mayo Clinic. (2014). *Heart attack causes*. Mayo Clinic Retrieved from http://www.mayoclinic.org/diseases-conditions/heart-attack/basics/causes/con-20019520, on November 2014.

Mayo Clinic. (2015). *Heart failure symptoms*. Mayo Clinic. Retrieved from http://www.mayoclinic.org/diseases-conditions/heart-failure/basics/symptoms/con-20029801, on January 17, 2015.

Mayo Clinic. (n.d.-a). *Low blood pressure (hypotension)*. Mayo Clinic. Retrieved from http://www.mayoclinic.org/diseases-conditions/low-blood-pressure/basics/definition/con-20032298

Mayo Clinic. (n.d.-b). *High blood pressure (hypertension) treatments and drugs*. Mayo Clinic. Retrieved from http://www.mayoclinic.org/diseases-conditions/high-blood-pressure/basics/treatment/con-20019580

Mayo Clinic Staff. (2015) *Atrial fibrillation*. Mayo Clinic. Retrieved March 18, 2015 from http://www.mayoclinic.org/diseases-conditions/atrial-fibrillation/basics/definition/con-20027014

Mozzafarian, D., & Benjamin E. (2015). Heart Disease and Stroke Statistics—2015 Update: A report from the American Heart Association. *Circulation, 131*, e29–322. doi: 10.1161/CIR.0000000000000152

National Heart, Lung, and Blood Institute. (2014). *How is coronary heart disease treated?*. NHLBI, NIH. Retrieved from http://www.nhlbi.nih.gov/health/health-topics/topics/cad/treatment, on September 29, 2014.

National Heart, Lung, and Blood Institute. (n.d.-a). *Life after a heart attack*. NHLBI, NIH. Retrieved from http://www.nhlbi.nih.gov/health/health-topics/topics/heartattack/lifeafter

National Heart, Lung, and Blood Institute. (n.d.-b). *What is COPD?*. NHLBI, NIH. Retrieved from http://www.nhlbi.nih.gov/health/health-topics/topics/copd

Tachycardia | Fast Heart Rate. (2015). Retrieved from http://www.heart.org/HEARTORG/Conditions/Arrhythmia/AboutArrhythmia/Tachycardia-Fast-Heart-Rate_UCM_302018_Article.jsp#, on April 21, 2015.

19 Diabetes

Joanne Phillips Estes

Autonomic neuropathy
Diabetic foot
Diabetic ketoacidosis
End-stage renal disease
Fasting plasma glucose
Hemoglobin **A**1c
Hygiene hypothesis
Hyperglycemia
Hypertension
Hypotension
Insulin
Nephropathy
Nocturia
Peripheral artery
    disease
Peripheral neuropathy
Polydipsia
Polyphagia
Polyuria
Prediabetes
Retinopathy
Type 1 diabetes
Type 2 diabetes

Stella is a 61-year-old white female who retired from her job as a grocery clerk about a year ago. Since retiring, Stella spends most of her time watching TV and reading. She also replaced cooking balanced meals with eating processed convenience foods, which contributed to an 80-lb. weight gain. Her children have been encouraging Stella to see her physician for a long-overdue checkup, but Stella has resisted doing so. She maintained that she does not need to see a doctor because other than being thirsty and needing to urinate often, she feels fine and perceives herself to be healthy. Ultimately, Stella agreed to have a physical exam in order for her and her husband to be able to purchase life insurance policies.

Stella saw her physician for a complete physical exam, including fasting blood tests. The results of her checkup stunned Stella. Her weight of 258 lb and body mass index of 29 kg/m^2 classifies Stella as obese. Stella's blood pressure reading of 155/99 mm Hg resulted in a diagnosis of hypertension. Additionally, results of her blood tests produced diagnoses of hyperlipidemia (total serum cholesterol level = 250 mg/dL) and type 2 diabetes mellitus (HbA$_{1c}$ = 7.1%). Stella's doctor prescribed antihypertensive, cholesterol-lowering, and glucose-reducing medications. He also strongly advised her to add a moderate exercise routine such as walking 30 minutes per day in order to increase her activity level.

DESCRIPTION AND DEFINITIONS

Diabetes mellitus, more commonly known as diabetes, refers to a group of metabolic conditions characterized by a malfunction in the body's ability to make insulin, to use insulin, or a combination of both (Canivell & Gomis, 2014). **Insulin** is a hormone produced by the pancreas and functions to regulate glucose metabolism. Insulin transports glucose into the body's cells where it is used for growth and energy. Without insulin, glucose builds up in the bloodstream producing a condition known as **hyperglycemia**. The excess glucose is ultimately excreted in the urine (Fig. 19.1). Without insulin to transport it, organs and tissues do not receive glucose causing the body to break down its own fat or lipids to produce an energy source. The by-products of this process are known as ketones that are released in the bloodstream. Total lack of insulin

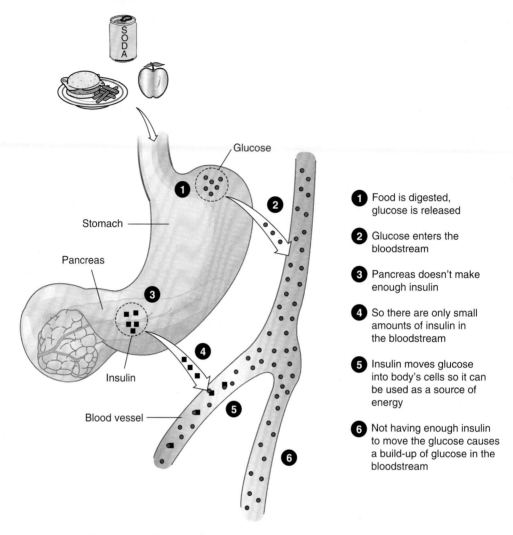

Figure 19.1 Type 1 diabetes mechanism of hyperglycemia.

is potentially lethal, and a chronic high blood glucose level has devastating effects on multiple tissues and organ systems. The American Diabetes Association (ADA) classifies diabetes into four disease entities (i.e., type 1, type 2, gestational diabetes, and other specific types) plus a prediabetes entity (ADA, 2015a). Historically, the two most prevalent entities (type 1 and type 2 diabetes) were distinguished by etiology and age of onset (Tuomi et al., 2014). Advances in understanding of the underlying pathophysiology along with sociocultural trends have led to the creation of subclassifications (Thomas & Philipson, 2015) and deem age to continue to be an important but no longer a discriminating factor (ADA, 2015a; Ducloux, Safraou, & Altman, 2015).

■ Type 1 Diabetes

Type 1 diabetes, formerly known as insulin-dependent or juvenile-onset diabetes mellitus, most frequently occurs in children and accounts for 5% to 10% of people with diabetes (ADA, 2015b). Type 1 diabetes is a condition of complete insulin deficiency and requires insulin replacement for survival (Craig et al., 2014). Onset of the disease is abrupt with the individual initially presenting in an acutely ill state and oftentimes with a life-threatening condition known as **diabetic ketoacidosis** (Fritsch et al., 2011) resulting from a buildup of ketones in the bloodstream. Type 1 diabetes is further classified according to pathogenesis with type 1A associated with an autoimmune destruction of pancreatic beta cells and type 1B lacking the same (Canivell & Gomis, 2014). A third subtype, latent autoimmune diabetes of adults (LADA), refers to an autoimmune-based form of diabetes that occurs in adults aged 35 years or older (Thomas & Philipson, 2015).

Type 2 Diabetes

In **type 2** (formerly known as non–insulin-dependent or adult-onset) **diabetes** mellitus, the pancreas secretes insulin but insulin resistance is present and the amount of insulin may be insufficient, producing a chronic state of hyperglycemia (ADA, 2015a). Type 2 accounts for 90% to 95% of all cases of diabetes (ADA, 2015b) and typically occurs with increasing age and in people who are obese (Ducloux et al., 2015). Onset of type 2 diabetes is gradual, and in asymptomatic cases, the disease may go undetected for years (ADA, 2015a). Historically, type 2 diabetes diagnoses were limited to adults. A marked increase in prevalence of obesity in children and adolescents both in the United States and globally has resulted in dramatic increases in type 2 diabetes for these age groups (Pulgaron & Delamater, 2014).

Gestational Diabetes

Gestational diabetes is a transient form of diabetes mellitus that first appears during pregnancy and typically requires no further treatment after delivery (ADA, 2015a). Women with gestational diabetes are seven times more likely to develop type 2 diabetes at some future point as compared to non–gestational diabetes counterparts (Bellamy, Cases, Hingorani, & Williams, 2009). Postpartum weight loss is associated with mitigating deterioration in glucose metabolism and perhaps delaying a future diagnosis of type 2 diabetes (Ehrlich et al., 2014).

Other Specific Types

The ADA (2015a) classifies other types of diabetes according to etiology. Genetic defects of the beta cell include two subtypes: maturity-onset diabetes of the young (MODY) and neonatal diabetes. MODY presents in people before age 25 as hyperglycemia due to impaired insulin secretion (ADA, 2015a). Neonatal diabetes appears in the first 6 months of life and may be transient (ADA, 2015a). Other etiologic-based conditions include those resulting from pancreatic trauma or diseases (e.g., pancreatitis, cystic fibrosis, carcinoma),

drugs (e.g., glucocorticoids, thyroid hormone), infections (e.g., congenital rubella), or genetic syndromes (e.g., Down's syndrome, Klinefelter's syndrome) (Craig et al., 2014).

Prediabetes

People with **prediabetes** are in an intermediate zone between normal blood glucose levels and meeting diagnostic criteria for diabetes (Egan & Dinneen, 2014). These individuals present with impaired fasting glucose levels (100 to 125 mg/dL) and impaired glucose tolerance levels (140 to 199 mg/dL) and are at risk for developing diabetes in the future (ADA, 2015a). Prediabetes is also associated with obesity and increased risk for cardiovascular disease (ADA, 2015a). Lifestyle modifications such as increasing one's physical activity level and losing weight (Tabák, Herder, Rathmann, Brunner, & Kivimäki, 2012) and eating a healthy diet (Ley, Hamdy, Mohan, & Hu, 2014) can delay or prevent progression to type 2 diabetes.

ETIOLOGY

Type 1

The type 1 diabetes disease process is precipitated by an autoimmune response whereby antibodies are produced that destroy pancreatic insulin-producing cells known as beta cells (Canivell & Gomis, 2014). Etiological factors are multifaceted and overlapping; however, specific roles of some remain unknown, unclear, or controversial (Atkinson, Eisenbarth, & Michels, 2014; Canivell & Gomis, 2014; Craig et al., 2014; Nielson, Krych, Buschard, Hansen, & Hansen, 2014). Current theories include etiological factors focusing on a strong genetic susceptibility coupled with a variety of environmental factors thought to trigger or drive the disease process. Three categories of environmental factors include viral infections, infant diet, and exposure to microbial toxins. Some research points to a clinically significant association between viral infections such as the Enterovirus and the autoimmune response in type 1 diabetes (Yeung, Rawlinson, & Craig, 2011). However, other studies have found no association (Canivell & Gomis, 2014). Infant diet, specifically ingestion of cow's milk; a short duration of breast-feeding; and early introduction of gluten-based cereals are thought to be inciting factors (Nielson et al., 2014). Exposure to microbial toxins in the form of ingested nitrites and nitrates in food (e.g., processed meat products) and water may also be triggering factors (Akerblom et al., 2002). Theories relating the **hygiene hypothesis** (Liu, 2015) to the autoimmune response in diabetes are emerging in the literature (Canivell & Gomis, 2014). The hygiene hypothesis purports that improved hygiene practices are decreasing childhood exposure to infectious agents and subsequent opportunities for immune system development leading to a rise in autoimmune diseases (Liu, 2015). At the same time, exposure to environmental pollutants (Janghorbani, Momeni, & Mansourian, 2014) and vitamin D deficiency are also thought to play a role; however, evidence for the same is weak (Canivell & Gomis, 2014).

■ Type 2

Beta cell malfunction in type 2 diabetes has a clear genetic element (Kahn, Cooper, & Del Prato, 2014). Nevertheless, etiological factors related to age, obesity, sedentary lifestyle (ADA, 2015a), and other lifestyle factors are prevalent in the literature. Obesity affects metabolism by releasing certain substances including nonesterified fatty acids (NEFAs) that are associated with insulin resistance (Al-Goblan et al., 2014). From 1994 to 2010, the percentage of adults with diagnosed diabetes who were obese increased from 34.9% to 56.9% (Centers for Disease Control [CDC], 2015). Body fat distribution is also associated with insulin resistance such that those with more abdominal fat are at higher risk (Al-Goblan et al., 2014). Lifestyle choices such as prolonged television watching (Grøntved & Hu, 2011) and habitual consumption of sugar beverages (Imamura et al., 2015) are associated with new-onset diabetes. Finally, the pathophysiology of obstructive sleep apnea may also play a part in abnormal insulin metabolism (Morgenstern et al., 2014).

INCIDENCE AND PREVALENCE

■ Children and Adolescence Incidence

The 2014 National Diabetes Statistics Report provides data based on 2009 to 2012 data (CDC, 2014a). Approximately 18,346 (ADA, 2015b) youth (rate of 22 per 1,000) (CDC, 2014a) are newly diagnosed with type 1 diabetes and 5,089 (ADA, 2015b) youth (rate of 10 per 1,000) (CDC, 2014a) with type 2 diabetes annually.

Non-Hispanic White youth had the highest rate of newly diagnosed cases of type 1 diabetes (28 per 100,000), with type 2 being extremely rare in this group of youth under age 10 (CDC, 2014a). The highest rates of newly diagnosed type 2 cases occurred in American Indians/Alaskan natives (28 per 100,000), non-Hispanic African Americans (23 per 100,000), and Hispanics (17 per 100,000) (CDC, 2014a). For these groups, the incidence of type 2 diabetes was greater than that of type 1.

■ Adult Incidence

In 2012, 1.7 million new cases of diabetes were diagnosed in people aged 20 or older in the United States, with the majority of cases in the 45- to 64-year-old age range (CDC, 2014a). The age-adjusted incidence of diabetes was slightly higher for men (11.2 per 100,000) than for women (7.5 per 100,000) aged 20 to 74 years from 2007 to 2010 (Menke et al., 2014). Incidence for African American, Hispanic, and Asian Americans is 2 to 3 times that of Caucasian Americans (Kanaya et al., 2014).

Prevalence of Diabetes

Approximately 29.1 million Americans or approximately 9.3% of the population now have diabetes (ADA, 2015b). Trends in prevalence of diabetes have steadily risen such that there was a fourfold increase in the number of adults diagnosed between 1980 and 2012 (CDC, 2014b), and if present trends continue, 1 in 3 adult Americans could have diabetes by 2050 (CDC, 2014b). Prevalence is associated with race and ethnicity. For type 1 diabetes, non-Hispanic White people have the highest while African Americans and people of Asian descent have the lowest prevalence (CDC, 2014b). Prevalence of type 2 diabetes is highest among American Indians/Alaskan natives (15.9%), followed by non-Hispanic African Americans (13.2%), Hispanics (12.8%), Asian Americans (9.0%), and non-Hispanic Caucasians (7.6%) (CDC, 2014a). Type 1 diabetes occurs equally among males and females (Dabelea et al., 2014), with type 2 prevalence slightly higher for men (10.6%) than women (7.6%) (Menke et al., 2014).

SIGNS AND SYMPTOMS

Classic symptoms of type 1 diabetes are those caused by hyperglycemia: **polydipsia** (increased thirst), **polyuria** (frequent urination), **polyphagia** (increased hunger), weight loss, and blurred vision (ADA, 2015a). Additional symptoms of type 1 may include muscle cramps, irritability, emotional lability, headaches, anxiety attacks, abdominal pain or discomfort, diarrhea or constipation, and altered school and work behaviors. The individual may also present with ketonuria. Ketones are waste products from the body's breakdown of fat for energy, high concentrations of which leads to DKA (ADA, 2015a). DKA is an acute and potentially life-threatening condition that may appear as the first symptom of previously undiagnosed diabetes (Demirci, Cosar, Ciftci, & Sari, 2015). Clinical signs of DKA include dehydration; tachycardia (rapid heart rate); tachypnea (rapid breathing); deep, sighing respirations with fruity breath odor; nausea and vomiting; abdominal pain; and confusion or drowsiness (Wolfsdorf et al., 2014). The number of deaths due to DKA decreased by 19.8% from 1980 to 2009 (CDC, 2015).

Because onset of type 2 diabetes is gradual, levels of hyperglycemia may not be severe enough to produce noticeable symptoms (ADA, 2015b). DKA is rare in type 2 diabetes but can present concurrently with other conditions such as infections, stroke, or pancreatitis (Demirci et al., 2015). However, symptoms related to chronic hyperglycemia and subsequent systemic complications can occur, for example, nephropathy, neuropathy, and retinopathy. These symptoms may be present upon diagnosis if preceded by long periods of hyperglycemia (Powers, 2008).

COURSE AND PROGNOSIS

For people diagnosed with diabetes, longevity and quality of life are currently better than in the past owing to improvements in insulin delivery regimens, medication treatment for **hyperlipidemia** (i.e., excessive concentration of fats or lipids in the bloodstream), and lifestyle modifications (Miller et al., 2012). However, life expectancy remains lower overall for persons with diabetes as compared to those who do not have the disease (Jørgensen, Almdal, & Carstensen, 2013). Duration of diabetes and advancing age are predictive of morbidity and mortality rates (Huang et al., 2013). From 2002 to 2011, mortality rates declined for males with type 1 diabetes by 6.6% and for

females by 4.8% (Jørgensen et al., 2013). One study approximated an 11-year lower life expectancy for men with type 1 diabetes and a 13-year lower life expectancy for women (Livingstone et al., 2015). Children and young adults diagnosed with type 2 diabetes lose approximately 15 years of remaining life expectancy (Rhodes et al., 2012). For people with type 2 diabetes, mortality is associated with onset and duration of complications, especially macrovascular-related complications (ADA, 2015a).

■ Hypoglycemia

During the course of the disease, people with diabetes may experience periods of hypoglycemia. **Hypoglycemia** or insulin shock is a condition of too much insulin or oral hypoglycemic medication and not enough glucose in the bloodstream (Powers, 2008). Risk factors for severe hypoglycemia include hypoglycemia unawareness, longer durations of insulin replacement therapy, cognitive deficits, age (e.g., early childhood or adolescence), and low socioeconomic status or health literacy (Canadian Diabetes Association [CDA], 2013). Symptoms include, but are not limited to, trembling, sweating, hunger, anxiety, confusion, drowsiness, dizziness, and difficulty concentrating (CDA, 2013). Mild hypoglycemia can be frightening to patients (ADA, 2015a) and lead to less-than-optimal blood glucose control. Severe hypoglycemic states are dangerous as they can result in falls or automobile accidents (ADA, 2015a). To treat hypoglycemia, the individual needs to ingest some form of carbohydrate that contains sugar, for example, orange juice, cola, and candy (CDA, 2013). Some strategies that can prevent hypoglycemia are education, careful self-monitoring of blood glucose levels, diet and exercise adjustments, and medication modifications (Seaquist et al., 2013).

■ Hyperglycemia

Hyperglycemia is a condition of too little insulin causing abnormally high blood glucose levels. If untreated, the patient is at risk for entering into a diabetic coma. Mortality from hyperglycemia increases with age typically due to the presence of a comorbid condition (myocardial infarction, cerebral vascular accident, sepsis). Treatment depends on insulin to reverse metabolic abnormalities and successful treatment of the comorbid conditions.

Hyperglycemia has a direct toxic effect on body tissues (Powers, 2008). Few diseases have the same potential for damaging as many organ systems and producing impairments as does diabetes (Fig. 19.2). In 1993, the National Institutes of Health completed a 9-year study called the "Diabetes Control and Complications Trial (DCCT)." Results of this study showed that intensive insulin therapy slows the development of long-term complications (Nathan, 2014). Prior to this landmark study, it was unclear whether tight glucose control was beneficial. Damage occurs in microvascular and macrovascular structures as well as autonomic and peripheral nerves. These complications are acute and chronic and affect the quality and duration of life for people with diabetes. However, rates of major complications have substantially declined since 1990 (Gregg et al., 2014).

■ Macrovascular Complications
Hypertension

Stage 1 **hypertension** (HTN) is defined as blood pressure > 140/90 mm Hg (Powers, 2008). Although it varies according to age, type of diabetes, racial and ethnic groups, and obesity, HTN affects over two-thirds of people with type 2 (Ferrannini & Cushman, 2012) as well as young adults with type 1 diabetes who have an underlying disorder such

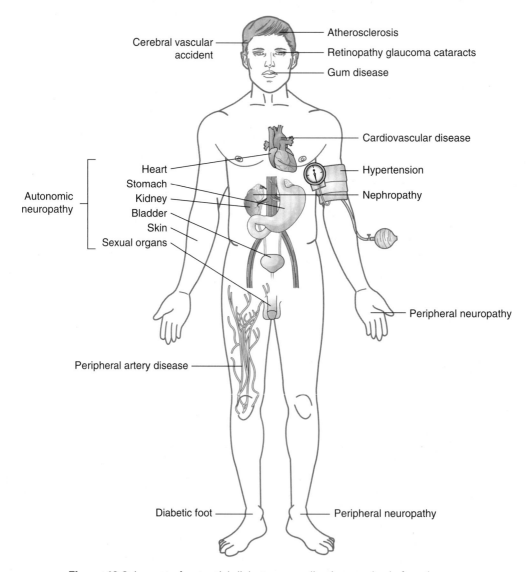

Figure 19.2 Impact of potential diabetes complications on body functions.

as nephropathy (ADA, 2015a). Those with type 2 diabetes commonly develop HTN associated with central obesity (Lago, Singhy, & Nesto, 2007). HTN combined with diabetes produces significant risk for cerebrovascular disease, retinopathy, and end-stage renal disease (ADA, 2015a). The ADA recommends that people with diabetes should generally target blood pressure goals at <140/90 mm Hg; however, lower targets (i.e., <130/80 mm Hg) may be appropriate for younger people (ADA, 2015a).

Cardiovascular Disease

People with diabetes have a higher risk for cardiovascular disease (CVD) and CVD is a major cause of morbidity and mortality (ADA, 2015a; Wannamethee, Shaper, Wincup, Lennon, & Sattar, 2011). Along with accelerated atherosclerosis, typical cardiac risk factors (e.g., HTN, smoking, abnormal cholesterol level, obesity, and inactivity) are common in people with type 2 diabetes (ADA, 2015a). Having diabetes for longer duration (Wannamethee et al., 2011) and older age (Halter et al., 2014) further the risk of CVD for people with diabetes. Thus, CVD is becoming more common in people with type 1 diabetes as these individuals are living longer (Melendez-Ramirez, Richards, & Cefalu, 2010). Women with diabetes have a 40% greater chance of developing CVD as compared to men (Peters, Huxley, & Woodward, 2014). Despite these trends, the number of people with diabetes diagnosed with acute myocardial infarction (MI) decreased by 67.8% from 1990 to 2010 (Gregg et al., 2014).

Cerebrovascular Disease

Similarly, accelerated atherosclerosis is an important risk factor for cerebrovascular accident (CVA) as having diabetes doubles the risk of CVA and 1 in 8 to 9 cases of CVA is attributable to diabetes (Luitse, Biessels, Rutten, & Kappelle, 2012). The rates of CVA in people with diabetes dramatically decreased (58.9 fewer cases per 10,000 people) from 1990 to 2010 (Gregg et al., 2014); however, women have a 27% greater relative risk as compared to men (Peters et al., 2014). Despite a general decline in incidence, people with diabetes and comorbid CVA have poorer long-term outcomes especially if they present in a hyperglycemic state (Luitse et al., 2012). Dyslipidemia (i.e., elevated cholesterol) and HTN (Powers, 2008) combined with lifestyle

choices such as smoking, inactivity, heavy alcohol consumption, and unhealthy diets increase the risk of CVA (Luitse et al., 2012).

Peripheral Artery Disease

Peripheral artery disease (PAD) is a condition of decreased arterial blood flow to the extremities, stomach, and kidneys (Deshpande, Harris-Hayes, & Schootman, 2008; Neschis & Golden, 2015). PAD occurs at an earlier age and at a faster rate in people with diabetes (Deshpande et al., 2008; McDermott, 2015) with those in the age 40- to 49-year-old age range who have at least one other risk factor for atherosclerosis at higher risk (Neschis & Golden, 2015). Severity of PAD increases with duration of diabetes and presence of neuropathy (Deshpande et al., 2008). Two categories of symptoms include intermittent claudication (pain or discomfort during walking or exercise that resolves with rest) and resting pain (Neschis & Golden, 2015). PAD predisposes people with diabetes to impaired wound healing (Kolluru, Bir, & Kevil, 2012), tissue hypoxia, and decreased mobilization of white blood cells to infected tissues (Goodman, 2009), all of which contribute to diabetes being the leading cause of nontraumatic lower extremity amputation (Powers, 2008).

■ Microvascular Complications

Diabetic Retinopathy

Retinopathy, or damage to the eye producing visual impairment, is a key indicator of microvascular complications and as such of the impact of diabetes. Diabetic retinopathy (DR) is the leading cause of blindness in adults aged 20 to 65 years (Ding & Wong, 2012). In 2011, approximately 19% of adults aged 18 years or older with diabetes had DR, which represented a 6% drop since 1997 (CDC, 2015). Of this same group, 15.6% of Hispanics, 17% of Caucasians, and 20.7% of African Americans with diabetes reported visual impairment (CDC, 2015). Similarly, females (19%) were more likely than males (16%) with diabetes to report visual impairment (CDC, 2015). Mechanisms leading to visual loss include macular edema, new vessel hemorrhage, retinal detachment, or neovascular glaucoma (Fraser & D'Amico, 2015). Risk factors include longer duration of diabetes, HTN, hyperglycemia, obesity, and puberty (Olafsdottir, Anderson, Dedorsson, & Stefánsson, 2014). Most people with DR are asymptomatic until late stages, and rate of progression can be rapid. Regular screening and early diagnosis and treatment, including intensive insulin control (McCulloch, 2015), can slow the disease process (Fraser & D'Amico, 2015).

Diabetic Nephropathy

Diabetic **nephropathy** results from structural and functional changes in the kidney that lead to chronic kidney disease, the progression of which can be slowed by optimal interventions (Bakris, 2015) of strict blood pressure and glycemic control (Mailoux, 2015). Diabetes is the leading cause of **end-stage renal disease** (ESRD), a condition of nonfunctioning kidneys. Twenty to forty percent of people with diabetes were diagnosed with kidney disease (ADA, 2015a) with equal risk for type 1 and type 2 diabetes (Bakris, 2015). However, the number of people with diabetes and comorbid ESRD dropped 28% from 1990 to 2010 (Gregg et al., 2014) likely due to advances in treatment. Family history of diabetes, Black race, Mexican American or Pima Indian heritage, poor blood glucose control, HTN, and cigarette smoking increase the risk for diabetic nephropathy (Bakris, 2015). The presence of diabetic retinopathy can be used to screen for and diagnose diabetic nephropathy (He et al., 2013). For people with ESRD, renal replacement therapy in the form of dialysis or kidney transplant is required for survival with transplantation offering the most optimal outcomes (Mailoux, 2015).

■ Neurologic Complications

Peripheral Neuropathy

Up to 50% of people with long-standing type 1 or type 2 diabetes have damage to peripheral nerves, a condition known as diabetic **peripheral neuropathy** (DPN) (Powers, 2008; Tesfaye & Selvarajah, 2012) with painful DPN affecting up to 25% of people with diabetes (Tesfaye et al., 2011). Risk factors include duration of diabetes, poor glycemic control, and cardiovascular risk factors such as abdominal obesity, hypertension, and hyperlipidemia (Singh, Kishore, & Kaur, 2014; Jaiswal et al., 2013; Tesfaye & Selvarajah, 2012). Cigarette smoking is also positively associated with DPN (Clair, Cohen, Eichler, Selby, & Rigotti, 2015). The most common symptoms include burning pain; stabbing, prickly, or tingling sensation; or numbness and lack of pro-

tective sensation (ADA, 2015a; Martin et al., 2014). Pain is worse at night, and symptoms are more common in lower extremities than in upper (Tesfaye et al., 2011). Severe pain can interfere with sleep, and subsequent daytime sleep debt and daytime pain negatively impact daily functioning (Tessfaye et al., 2011). Intensive insulin therapy and tight glycemic control reduce the risk of DPN (Martin, Albers, & Pop-Busui, 2014).

Autonomic Neuropathy

Damage to autonomic nerves that innervate organs leads to diabetic **autonomic neuropathy** (DAN) that affects multiple systems in the body including the cardiovascular, gastrointestinal, and genitourinary systems (ADA, 2015a). DAN produces a wide spectrum of symptoms and onset is gradual and progressive (Freeman, 2013; Vinik & Erbas, 2013). Cardiac autonomic neuropathy (CAN) is a serious complication that affects up to one-third of people with type 2 diabetes and increases risk of cardiovascular complications and sudden death (Vinik, Erbas, & Casellini, 2013). Clinical manifestations of CAN include resting tachycardia (rapid heart rate), orthostatic **hypotension** (i.e., drop in blood pressure upon standing), exercise intolerance, greater risk for intraoperative or perioperative cardiovascular incidents, increased incidence of myocardial infarction (MI), and lower rate of post-MI survival (ADA, 2015a; Vinik et al., 2013).

Autonomic neuropathy of the gastrointestinal system produces mild to severe symptoms that occur more in people with long-standing diabetes and poorly controlled hyperglycemia (Vinik & Erbas, 2013). Diabetes can cause an increase or decrease in gastric motility. The latter leads to gastroparesis, a condition of delayed gastric emptying (Freeman, 2013). Gastroparesis interferes with the relationship between glucose absorption and insulin administration and influences absorption of orally ingested medications (Freeman, 2013). Patients may experience cramping, bloating, heartburn, loss of appetite, nausea, vomiting, constipation, and diarrhea (Vinik & Erbas, 2013). Genitourinary involvement produces bladder dysfunction in the form of decreased sensation that results in decreased voiding frequency, urinary retention, and subsequent increased risk of urinary tract infections (Vinik & Erbas, 2013). Sexual dysfunction is common in men with diabetes over the age of 50 with erectile dysfunction the most frequent issue (Isidro, 2012). Erectile dysfunction is typically the first sign of DAN for this age group (Isidro, 2012).

Neurodegeneration

Recent literature provides evidentiary support for a link between type 2 diabetes and neurodegenerative diseases such as Alzheimer's disease (Verdile, Fuller, & Martins, 2015) in that people with **type** 2 diabetes are at higher risk for developing Alzheimer's disease (Hao et al., 2015). Current thought postulates that type 2 diabetes can exacerbate the neurodegenerative process but the exact mechanism is not well understood (Verdile et al., 2015). Metabolic abnormalities linked with diabetes (e.g., hyperglycemia, hypercholesterolemia) are also associated with AD (Verdile et al., 2015). Although more research is needed, one hypothesis points to shared genetic risk factors that cross both conditions (Hao et al., 2015).

■ Other Complications

Diabetic Foot

Multiple sequelae of diabetes merge to make foot ulcers and infections common leading to a condition known as **diabetic foot**. Etiological factors leading to foot ulcers include repetitive stress on the skin with body weight and activity level increasing the pressure (Noor, Zubair, & Ahmad, 2015). Autonomic neuropathy results in dry, cracked skin making it more prone to ulceration and allowing easier access for infection entry (Powers, 2008). Sensory polyneuropathy diminishes pain and temperature perceptions causing lesions to go unnoticed (Noor et al., 2015). PAD impairs blood supply needed for healing, and hyperglycemia reduces host defenses (Powers, 2008). Trauma to the foot combined with these risk factors results in lesions that can be slow to heal and subject to a secondary infection (Noor et al., 2015). Infections may extend to deeper soft tissues, bones, joints, and systemic circulation (Noor et al., 2015) (Fig. 19.3). Management of mild infections involves antimicrobial therapy with surgical intervention in the form of debridement or revascularization (Powers, 2008). Severe infections leading to gangrene tissues require limb amputation. Risk factors for foot ulcers or amputation include being male; having diabetes > 10 years; smoking; and presence of PAD, peripheral neuropathy, nephropathy, or foot structure abnormalities (ADA, 2015a; Powers, 2008).

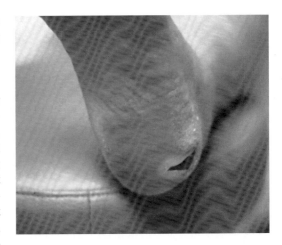

Figure 19.3 Diabetic ulcer of the heel. (From Goodheart, H. P. (2003). *Goodheart's photoguide of common skin disorders* (2nd ed.). Philadelphia, PA: Lippincott Williams & Wilkins.)

The CDC reports a 3.3/1,000 incidence rate of lower extremity amputation–related hospital discharges for people with diabetes, which represents a 5.6/1,000 drop since 1988 (CDC, 2015). Despite this decline in incidence rates, the number of lower extremity amputation–related hospital discharges for people with diabetes increased by 24% from 1988 to 2009 (CDC, 2015). This increase is likely due to the increasing numbers of people diagnosed with diabetes.

Periodontal Disease

Diabetes and periodontal disease have a bidirectional relationship (Chapple & Genco, 2013) in that diabetes increases the risk of periodontitis especially for people with type 2 diabetes (Bascones-Martinez et al., 2011) and periodontitis negatively affects diabetes outcomes (Borgnakke, Ylostalo, Taylor, & Genco, 2013). It has been suggested that increased incidence of periodontal disease in this population is due to inhibition of cellular mechanisms that destroy bacteria in the mouth or to impaired functioning of reparative (i.e., wound-healing) cells (Álamo, Soriano, & Pérez, 2011).

DIAGNOSIS

Abnormal plasma glucose levels serve to screen for and diagnose both type 1 and type 2 diabetes (ADA, 2015a). The ADA (2015a) published threshold levels for four types of blood glucose

TABLE 19.1 American Diabetes Association Plasma Glucose Level Diagnostic Thresholds				
	HBA$_{1c}$	FPG	2-h PG	RPG
Diabetes	≥6.5%	≥126 mg/dL	≥200 mg/dL	≥200 mg/dL
Prediabetes	5.7%–6.4%	100–125 mg/dL	140–199 mg/dL	

Note: American Diabetes Association (ADA). (2015a). Standards of medical care in diabetes—2015. *Diabetes Care, 38*(Suppl. 1), S1–S90. Retrieved from http://professional.diabetes.org/admin/UserFiles/0%20-%20Sean/Documents/January%20Supplement%20Combined_Final.pdf.

tests, any of which may affirm a diagnosis of diabetes or prediabetes (Fig. 19.4). In 2009, the ADA added glycated **hemoglobin A**$_{1c}$ (HbA$_{1c}$) as a diagnostic indicator for diabetes (Atkinson et al., 2014). An HbA$_{1c}$ level shows the average blood glucose concentration level over a 3-month period (Atkinson et al., 2014) and is commonly used to screen for and diagnose diabetes in adults. Some research has raised questions as to the validity of HbA$_{1c}$ levels for diagnosing type 2 diabetes in children and adolescents (Buse et al., 2013). The ADA acknowledges this limitation but still recommends using HbA$_{1c}$ as a diagnostic indicator for children and adolescents (ADA, 2015a). **Fasting plasma glucose** (FPG) levels are measured following a minimum of an 8-hour period of no caloric intake (ADA, 2015a). For the 2-hour plasma glucose (2-h PG), blood glucose levels are checked following a 75-g oral glucose tolerance test (OGGT). Finally, random plasma glucose (RPG) levels that exceed the diagnostic threshold concurrent with presentation of hyperglycemic crisis or classic symptoms indicate a clinical diagnosis of diabetes (ADA, 2015a). One additional blood test result indicative of type 1 diabetes is the presence of pancreatic autoantibodies; however, most laboratories are not equipped to measure all autoantibodies and may produce false-negative results (Chiang, Kirkman, Laffel, & Peters, 2014) (Table 19.1).

MEDICAL MANAGEMENT

■ Type 1

Management Regimens

There is no known cure for diabetes; therefore, medical management focuses on developing individually tailored, culturally sensitive, and age and developmentally appropriate care plans (Chiang

et al., 2014). Management regimens center on insulin replacement, glycemic control, assessment of and prevention of complications, and attention to lifestyle and psychosocial issues. The ADA recommends intense and ongoing diabetes self-management education (DSME) to promote knowledge and skills necessary for effective glycemic control and self-care (ADA, 2015b). DSME topics include medications, self-monitoring of blood glucose levels (SMBG), physical activity, complications, nutrition, risk reduction (e.g., foot care, smoking), and psychosocial issues (Powers et al., 2015).

Insulin Replacement and Glycemic Control

Until insulin was characterized and manufactured in 1921, diabetes was a death sentence. Insulin replacement uses combinations of rapid-acting (e.g., Humalog), short-acting (Humulin S), intermediate-acting (Humulin I), and long-acting (Lantus) insulin that can be delivered by syringe, pen, continuous subcutaneous insulin infusion (CSII) or insulin pump, or inhalation (Leong, Velusamy, & Choudhary, 2014). For children, the goal of insulin replacement is to achieve as near-normal glycemic control as possible as indicated by HbA$_{1c}$ levels targeted at <7.5% for all pediatric age groups (Chiang et al., 2014). Insulin injection schedules depend on the individual's age, compliance level, and severity of disease, with the ADA recommending three or more injections of prandial (rapid-acting or mealtime) insulin and one to two injections of basal (long-acting) insulin daily (Chiang et al., 2014). Approximately 40% of people with type 1 diabetes use CSII (Pickup, 2011), advantages of which include the ability to alter insulin infusion to meet physiological requirements, provide more precise insulin delivery, and be connected to continuous glucose monitoring sensors (Leong et al., 2014). Inhaled insulin advantages include simple delivery and rapid action; however, concerns related to precision of dose and secondary effects on lungs remain (Leong et al., 2014).

Surgical options include pancreatic transplants or pancreatic islet cell transplants. Pancreatic transplants occur in one of three categories: simultaneous kidney/pancreas transplant (SKP), pancreas after kidney transplant (PAK), or pancreas alone transplant (PAT) (Gruessner, Sutherland, & Gruessner, 2012). Long-term follow-up studies show positive trends in pancreatic function (i.e., insulin secretion) that have steadily improved over time (Gruessner et al., 2012) and improvements in glycemic control following all three categories of transplants (Gruessner et al., 2012; Lehman et al., 2015). The benefits of being free of insulin dependency and avoiding secondary complications of diabetes outweigh transplant surgical risks (Gruessner et al., 2012). Although currently considered experimental (Atkinson et al., 2014), islet cell transplantation may be a less-risky option for those who are poor candidates for organ transplantation (Chiang et al., 2014). Short-term outcomes are more favorable than long-term as patients are insulin free for 3 years on average (Barton et al., 2012).

Management of Lifestyle and Psychosocial Issues

Attention to lifestyle factors such as diet and physical activity levels/exercise along with psychosocial issues is important to the management of type 1 diabetes. People with type 1 diabetes should participate in nutrition therapy comprised of education related to how food impacts blood glucose, how to avoid hypoglycemia or hyperglycemia resulting from food-exercise-insulin interactions, and how to adapt food-related plans to a various situations (Chiang et al., 2014). The ADA has published nutrition guidelines (ADA, 2015a) that recommend a healthy, balanced diet and monitoring intake of carbohydrates for people with type 1 diabetes (Chiang et al., 2014). Long delays between meals should be avoided, as not eating in a predictable pattern consistent with one's insulin regimen may cause hypoglycemia. Frequent, small snacks at the time of peak insulin action should also be taken to avoid hypoglycemia. The many health benefits associated with increased physical activity and exercise along with recommendations that all children engage in 60 minutes of physical activity per day apply to people with type 1 diabetes (Chiang et al., 2014). However, for those with type 1 diabetes, exercise may induce states of hyperglycemia or hypoglycemia and thus requires diligence in frequently monitoring blood glucose levels and adjusting insulin dosages and/or food intake accordingly (Chiang et al., 2014). Finally, assessment and management of psychosocial issues (e.g., depression, anxiety related to hypoglycemia or hyperglycemia, eating disorders, family tensions) are important to ensure that individuals with type 1 diabetes can responsibly and effectively manage their diabetes care (Chiang et al., 2014).

■ Type 2

Management of type 2 diabetes focuses on supporting lifestyle changes related to nutritional strategies, exercise programs, and prevention and/or treatment of complications, along with glycemic control (Chatterjee & Davies, 2015). As with type 1 diabetes management, patient education plays a crucial role in effectively managing type 2 diabetes (Coppola, Sasso, Bagnasco, Giustina, & Gazzaruso, 2015). Medical nutritional therapy in the form of controlling the amount and types of fats, carbohydrates, and proteins is recommended for weight reduction and prevention or reduction of atherosclerotic vascular disease (ADA, 2015a). A Mediterranean-style diet (i.e., consumption of monosaturated and omega-3 fatty acids, fresh fruits and vegetables, high fiber, and vegetable protein) can reduce insulin resistance in people with type 2 diabetes (Esposito & Guigliano, 2014).

The health-promoting benefits of increased physical activity and regular exercise are well documented. The ADA recommends a minim of 150 minutes of moderately intense exercise physical activity or exercise per week (ADA, 2015a). For patients with type 2 diabetes, regular exercise reduces insulin resistance, promotes cardiovascular health, and prevents/improves obesity, anxiety, and depression (Inzucchi et al., 2012).

The targets for glycemic control are HbA_{1c} levels of ≤7.5% for children and adolescents with type 2 diabetes and ≤7.0% for most adults (ADA, 2015a). A more stringent goal (i.e., <6.5%) may be recommended for certain individuals (e.g., those with recent diagnosis, long life expectancy, or those without cardiovascular disease) if the goal can be met without risk of hypoglycemia (ADA, 2015a). Less stringent targets (≤8.5%) may be indicated for older adults who have advanced complications, are in otherwise poor health, or have shorter life expectancy (Chiang et al., 2014). When diet and exercise are ineffective in controlling blood glucose levels, individuals take oral glucose-lowering agents. Several classes of these medications are prescribed and dosages individualized for patients. Metformin (Glucophage) is typically the first line of intervention (Chatterjee & Davies, 2015) and is used to decrease liver output of glucose (ADA, 2015a). Glimepiride (Amaryl) and repaglinide (Prandin) stimulate insulin secretion and pioglitazone (Acta) increases sensitivity of skeletal muscle tissues to insulin (ADA, 2015a). Individuals with type 2 diabetes may initially respond to oral hypoglycemics but then not respond well after years of therapy. This could be the result of decreased compliance with diet and exercise programs, progression of pancreatic failure to produce insulin, complications from comorbid medical conditions or medications, or development of tolerance to medications. Insulin therapy is indicated at that point.

■ Self-Monitoring of Blood Glucose Levels

SMBG is crucial for both type 1 and type 2 diabetes. Self-monitoring requires that individuals with diabetes take active control of their own health and well-being, increases understanding of the impact of diet and physical activity, and allows for more immediate adjustments to insulin therapy in order to prevent hypoglycemia (Chiang et al., 2014). People with type 1 diabetes should monitor their blood glucose levels up to 6 to 10 times per day including but not limited to before and after meals and exercise, before bedtime, when they suspect low blood glucose levels, and oftentimes prior to driving (Chiang et al., 2014). People with type 2 diabetes who are insulin dependent should monitor before breakfast, dinner, and bedtime, with the goal of monitoring being to avoid hyperglycemia.

Technology plays an important role in SMBG. Portable glucose meters are available that take blood for sampling, give a digital readout of glucose levels, and have a computerized memory for record keeping. Newer intermittent glucose monitoring devices can be preprogrammed to calculate rapid-acting insulin doses (Cavan et al., 2014) and connect to insulin pumps and mobile phones (Leong et al., 2014). The use of mobile phone apps to assist with diabetes management is becoming more prevalent, and research shows promising trends in some patient outcomes, for example, self-efficacy and self-management behaviors (Holtz & Lauckner, 2012). However, further research is needed to establish evidence as to the impact of their usage on glycemic outcomes especially for people with type 1 diabetes (Peterson, 2014).

IMPACT ON CLIENT FACTORS AND OCCUPATIONAL PERFORMANCE

■ Body Functions

Diabetes and its subsequent complications potentially affect most body functions. Specifically, diabetes affects mental functioning in several ways due to both acute and chronic complications. Acutely, insulin and blood glucose levels influence the level of arousal. Symptoms of hypoglycemia include drowsiness and fatigue. Variations in blood glucose levels can also cause mood swings and irritability.

Chronic complications affect those with both type 1 and type 2 diabetes. Adults with type 1 diabetes are prone to diminished intelligence, attention, psychomotor speed, cognitive flexibility, and visual perception (McCrimmon, Ryan, & Frier, 2012). Adults with type 2 diabetes are more prone to learning and memory deficits (McCrimmon et al., 2012) and at higher risk for developing Alzheimer's disease (Verdile et al., 2015). Emotional regulation is also impacted. Depression and diabetes are common comorbid conditions (Holt, de Groot, & Hill Gordon, 2014), especially for females with type 1 diabetes over the age of 40 (Navmenova, Mokhort, & Makhlina, 2014), and youth (Walders-Abramson, 2013) and adults with type 2 diabetes (Saddiqui, 2014). Some research points to stresses related to living with diabetes as partially responsible for this comorbidity (Holt et al., 2014) in that the presence of complications increased the risk for depression (Saddiqui, 2014). At the same time, while other research showed an increase prevalence of mild to moderate depression in people with diabetes, there was no correlation between a diagnosis of depression and disease duration and presence of complications (Trento et al., 2012).

Sensory functions are affected by retinopathies and neuropathies. Retinopathy visual impairment can ultimately lead to blindness (Fraser & D'Amico 2015). Neuropathy affects sensory functioning such that people with diabetes often experience pain that may be severe (Tesfaye et al., 2011) along with diminished touch and pressure sensations in the upper and lower extremities (Noor et al., 2015; Shah, Clark, McGill, & Mueller, 2015). In one study, people with diabetes had greater prevalence of decreased shoulder range of motion and muscle strength and decreased grip and pinch strength than those without diabetes (Shah et al., 2015). Autonomic neuropathy leads to compromised functioning of cardiovascular (Freeman, 2013), gastrointestinal (Vinik & Erbas, 2013), genitourinary (Isidro, 2012), and integumentary systems (Powers, 2008).

■ Occupational Performance

Effective functioning in multiple occupational performance areas impacts the disease process and subsequent quality of life and is also impacted by living with diabetes. Functioning in specific activities of daily living (ADLs) that affect disease outcomes includes personal hygiene and grooming (i.e., personal hygiene, dental care) and personal device care (i.e., blood glucose meters, insulin syringes). Risk of diabetic foot complications can be reduced by daily inspection and care of feet. The link between periodontal disease and diabetes (Álamo et al., 2011) makes proper dental hygiene imperative. The disease process also impacts ADL functioning as approximately 10% of adults age 60 years or older reported needing assistance with ADLs in 2011 (CDC, 2015). Lower extremity neuropathies affect functional mobility. Percentages of adults over age 18 living with diabetes reported difficulty with the following functional mobility tasks in 2011: 37% walking a quarter mile, 28% climbing 10 steps, 38% standing for 2 hours, and 44% stooping, bending, or kneeling (CDC, 2015). Sexual activity dysfunction is reported for women and men. Women with diabetes are more likely to experience problems with sexual functioning and satisfaction (Copeland et al., 2012) and men problems with low desire and erectile dysfunction (Isidro, 2012).

Successful management of multiple instrumental activities of daily living (IADLs) tasks affects the diabetes disease process and is affected by the same. Almost 16% of adults over age 60 with diabetes report needing assistance with IADLs (CDC, 2015). Meal preparation must meet dietary guidelines. Tasks that require cognitive functioning (e.g., managing medication routines, financial management) may be difficult due to fluctuations in blood glucose levels. Neuropathies can impact the ability to use communication devices (e.g., writing or typing) or perform home management tasks (e.g., meal preparation). Retinopathy, neuropathy, and fluctuating blood glucose levels may make driving and community mobility difficult or prohibitive. Health management and maintenance are perhaps the most important IADL tasks for people with diabetes (Powers et al., 2015). People with diabetes must develop and adhere to effective routines to manage the multifaceted care demands (Fritz, 2014; Pyatak, 2011), including dietary and nutritional issues (Ley et al., 2014), physical fitness (Balducci et al., 2014), medication management (Strom Williams et al., 2014), and reduction of health risk behaviors such as smoking cessation (Clair et al., 2015).

People with diabetes are at higher risk for sleep problems than those without diabetes (Plantinga, Rao, & Schillinger, 2012) that can interfere with glycemic control and limit quality of life (Surani, Brito, Surani, & Ghamande, 2015). Problems include **nocturia** (nighttime urination), restless leg syndrome, apnea, and inadequate amount of sleep (Plantinga et al., 2012). Education, work, play, and leisure participation routines must incorporate diabetes self-management including SMBG and adhering to insulin regimens. This may be challenging for children and young adults with type 1 diabetes whose activity levels directly influence blood glucose levels and insulin needs (Pyatak, 2011) and for whom peer acceptance and pressures are issues (Chiang et al., 2014). Finally, social participation may be limited by fatigue and decreased mobility (Schmader, 2001); however, one study in China showed a positive association between cognitive social capital (i.e., support, reciprocity, cohesion) and quality of life for people with type 2 diabetes (Hu et al., 2015).

CASE STUDY 1

Jalen is a 15-year-old African American male diagnosed with obesity (weight of 270 lb) and HTN during a mandatory presports physical exam. The physician referred him to an internal medicine doctor for a more thorough exam. The results of this checkup confirmed the previous diagnosis of HTN (BP reading of 160/100 mm Hg). Blood test results produced additional diagnoses of hyperlipidemia (total cholesterol level of 260 mg/dL) and type 2 diabetes (FPG = 138 mg/dL). His physician prescribed Lipitor (atorvastatin; cholesterol lowering), 20 mg per day; Maxzide (hydrochlorothiazide; anti-HTN), 50 mg twice per day; and Glucophage (metformin; glucose lowering), 500 mg twice per day medications. He further recommended that Jalen routinely check his blood glucose levels and lose weight. Jalen met with a nurse and a dietician for a series of intensive training sessions for diabetes self-management education (DSME). Training topics centered on medications, SMBG, physical activity, complications, nutrition, risk reduction (e.g., foot care, smoking), and psychosocial issues (Powers et al., 2015). Jalen attended some but not all of the scheduled sessions. During several of the training sessions, he appeared to be drowsy and occasionally drifted off to sleep. When asked about his apparent lack of interest in the education, Jalen stated that having diabetes is no big deal for his mother and grandmother, so it will be no big deal for him.

Jalen's mother is single and works two part-time jobs to support him and his older sister and younger brother. Together with his maternal grandparents, they live in a subsidized, three-bedroom apartment in a large, inner-city urban neighborhood. Family history is significant as both Jalen's mother and maternal grandmother are obese and have a long-standing history of HTN and type 2 diabetes. Jalen's grandmother is living with several complications of diabetes, including retinopathy and lower extremity PAD that causes pain and diminished sensation. She has ESRD and receives hemodialysis treatment 3 d/wk. Due to his own poor health issues, Jalen's grandfather can provide only minimal assistance with his wife's care. Jalen's mother is overwhelmed with work and parental care-taking responsibilities. She is exhausted by the end of the day, so meals consist of fast or processed foods.

Recently, Jalen's school attendance has been erratic as he often skips to hang out with his friends. When not with his friends, Jalen isolates himself in his bedroom playing computer games and listening to music through earbuds. Lacking parental guidance, Jalen typically eats convenience foods and drinks sugary soft drinks. His medication compliance is poor as he often forgets to take his pills or does not take the prescribed dosages. Jalen continues to smoke cigarettes (1 pack/d) and drink alcohol with his friends (3 to 4 d/wk). His mother is worried about him because he seems sad all the time.

Jalen presently shows no signs of systemic complications from hyperglycemia. However, his weight, HTN, smoking, alcohol abuse, and poor compliance with medication regimen place him at high risk for rapid development of the same (e.g., cardiovascular disease, peripheral artery disease, peripheral neuropathies, and end-stage renal disease). His lack of parental support and adult supervision contributes to a high risk of morbidity and mortality from diabetic complications.

CASE STUDY 2

Tammy is a 39-year-old Caucasian female diagnosed with type 1 diabetes at age 11. Her medical history includes long-standing history of HTN and hyperlipidemia, and she was diagnosed with ESRD at age 36. Since then, she has been on a three times per week regimen of outpatient hemodialysis. Tammy has decreased vision due to retinopathy, and she complains of leg pain due to lower extremity peripheral neuropathy. Six months ago, Tammy had an acute myocardial infarction. Since then, she complains of fatigue and lack of interest in participating in activities that she used to enjoy.

Tammy's medication regimen is extensive. She injects 10 units of Lantus (long-acting insulin)

BID and Humulin (short-acting insulin) three to four times per day as indicated by SMBG results. Tammy takes 20 mg of Lipitor (cholesterol lowering), 5 mg of amlodipine (anti-HTN), 1 Nephrocap (prescription multivitamin), 17 g MiraLax (laxative) dissolved in water, 325 g ferrous sulfate (anemia) twice a day, and 3,667 PhosLo (phosphate binder) three times per day with meals. Calcium binds phosphorus with ingested foods to prevent phosphorus from going into the body; normal kidney function eliminates extra phosphorus in the body.

Tammy must also adhere to fluid and diet restrictions. Fluids are restricted to 1,800 mL/d. Dietary restrictions consist of limiting phosphorus (i.e., dairy foods, cola), potassium, salt, and carbohydrates. Tammy has a history of poor adherence to these restrictions, especially the fluid restrictions as she typically starts hemodialysis in a state of fluid overload. This raises her blood pressure, and the dialysis staff has difficulty removing the excess fluid without risks of cramping and hypotension. She communicates little information to the staff or her physician during dialysis, spending most of the time trying to sleep.

Tammy lives with her parents who transport her to dialysis. She has never been married and is currently unemployed, although her employment history consisted of several part-time jobs, primarily as a retail clerk. She has two older sisters and one younger brother, all of whom are married and have children of their own. Tammy's social interactions are centered on her family as she enjoys spending time with her nieces and nephews and often attends their sporting events with her parents. She has few friends of her own age as her past friends are busy with family responsibilities of their own and Tammy finds that she has little in common with them now. Tammy's hobbies consist of watching TV and occasionally knitting.

Tammy is right-hand dominant and receives dialysis through her LUE. She has moderate pain and numbness in her LUE because of an ischemic neuropathy that is the result of decreased blood flow because blood is diverted to her dialysis access site. She has full bilateral upper extremity active range of motion but decreased peripheral sensation (tactile, pain, and temperature). Tammy has a moderate decrease in bilateral grip and pinch strength, with her left side weaker than her right. Tammy recently stepped on a tack, did not feel it, and subsequently developed an infection that is not responding to antimicrobial medication. Her physician told her that she will likely have to undergo a below-knee amputation.

Tammy's parents transport her to and from dialysis as declining vision and lower extremity neuropathy deem her unsafe to drive. She ambulates and transfers independently but with increasing difficulty. Tammy is independent in all activities of daily living (ADLs) and prefers to prepare her own meals rather than eat food her mother prepares. She lives in a double-story house with a half bathroom on the main level and her bedroom and full bathroom on the upper level. Climbing the steps is becoming difficult such that Tammy only does so to go to bed at night.

Tammy is moderately but increasingly disabled by the physical and emotional ramifications of diabetes, retinopathy, neuropathies, renal failure, and cardiac status. This affects her roles as daughter, sister, and aunt. Her parents are concerned about Tammy's declining health and her future ability to care for herself as they are aging and dealing with their own health issues. While she can currently access her home environment, she may not be able to do so in the near future. Socially, Tammy is becoming withdrawn and disinterested in participating in the few previous activities she used to enjoy. The context of her occupational performance further reflects the impact that diabetes has on decreasing her quality of life.

RECOMMENDED LEARNING RESOURCES

American Diabetes Association (ADA)
www.diabetes.org)

Centers for Disease Control (CDC)
www.cdc.gov)

The Mayo Clinic
http://www.mayoclinic.org/diseases-conditions/diabetes/basics/definition/con-20033091

National Institute of Diabetes and Digestive and Kidney Disease (NIDDK)
www.niddk.nih.gov)

National Kidney Foundation (NKF)
www.kidney.org)

REFERENCES

Akerblom, H. K., Vaarala, O., Hyoty, H., Ilonen, J., & Knip, M. (2002). Environmental factors in the etiology of type 1 diabetes. *American Journal of Medical Genetics, 115*, 18–29. doi: 10.2337/dc07-S042

Álamo, S. M., Soriano, Y. J., & Pérez, M. G. S. (2011). Dental considerations for the patient with diabetes. *Journal of Clinical and Experimental Dentistry, 3*(1), e25–e30. doi: 10.4317/jced.3.e25

Al-Goblan, A. S., Al-Alfi, M. A., & Khan, M. Z. (2014). Mechanism linking diabetes mellitus and obesity. *Diabetes, Metabolic Syndrome, and Obesity: Targets and Therapy, 7*, 587–591.

American Diabetes Association (ADA). (2015a). Standards of medical care in diabetes—2015. *Diabetes Care, 38*(Suppl. 1), S1–S90. Retrieved from http://professional.diabetes.org/admin/UserFiles/0%20-%20Sean/Documents/January%20Supplement%20Combined_Final.pdf

American Diabetes Association (ADA). (2015b). Fast facts: Data and statistics about diabetes. Retrieved from http://professional.diabetes.org/ResourcesForProfessionals.aspx?cid=91777

Atkinson, M. A., Eisenbarth, G. S., & Michels, A. W. (2014). Type 1 diabetes. *The Lancet, 383*(9911), 69–82. doi: 10.1016/s0140-6736(13)60591-7

Bakris, G. L. (2015). Overview of diabetic nephropathy. *Up to Date.* Retrieved from http://www.uptodate.com/contents/overview-of-diabetic-nephropathy?source=search_result&search=diabetic+nephropathy&selectedTitle=1~150

Balducci, S., Sacchetti, M., Haxhi, J., Orlando, G., D'Errico, V., Fallucca, S., ... Pugliese, G. (2014). Physical exercise as therapy for type 2 diabetes management. *Diabetes/Metabolism Research and Reviews, 30*(S1), 13–23. doi: 10.1002/dmrr.2514

Barton, F. B., Rickels, M. R., Alejandro, R., Hering, B. J., Wease, S., Naziruddin, J., ... Shapiro, A. M. J. (2012). Improvement in outcomes of clinical islet transplantation: 1999–2010. *Diabetes Care, 35*(7), 1436–1445. doi: 10.2337/dc12-006

Bascones-Martinez, A., Matesanz-Perez, Escribano-Bermego, Gonalez-Moles, M., Bascones-Ilundain, J., & Meurman, J. (2011). Periodontal disease and diabetes: Review of the literature. *Medicina Oral Patología Oral y Cirugia Bucal, 16*(6), e722–e729. doi: 10.4317/medoral.17032

Bellamy, L., Cases, J., Hingorani, A. D., & Williams, D. (2009). Type 2 diabetes mellitus after gestational diabetes: A systematic review and meta-analysis. *The Lancet, 373*(9677), 1773–1779. doi: 10.1016/s0140-6736(09)60731-5

Borgnakke, W. S., Ylostalo, P. V., Taylor, G. W., & Genco, R. J. (2013). Effect of periodontal disease on diabetes: Systematic review of epidemiologic observational evidence. *Journal of Clinical Periodontology, 40*(Suppl. 14), S135–S152. doi: 10.1111/jcpe.12080

Buse, J., Bergenstal, R., Glass, L., Cory Heilmann, C., Lewis, M., & Rosenstock, J. (2011). Use of twice-daily exenatide in basal insulin–treated patients with type 2 diabetes: A randomized, controlled trial. *Annals of Internal Medicine, 154*, 103–112.

Canadian Diabetes Association. (2013). Hypoglycemia. *Canadian Journal of Diabetes, 37*, S69–S71. doi: 10.1016/j.jcjd.2013.01.022

Canivell, S., & Gomis, R. (2014). Diagnosis and classification of autoimmune diabetes mellitus. *Autoimmunity Reviews, 13*(3–4), 403–407. doi: 10.1016/j.autrev.2014.01.020

Cavan, D. A., Ziegler, R., Cranston, I., Barnard, K., Ryder, J., Vogel, C., ... Wagner, R. S. (2014). Use of an insulin bolus advisor facilitates earlier and more frequent changes in insulin therapy parameters in sub optimally controlled patients with diabetes treated with multiple daily insulin injection therapy: Results of the ABACUS trial. *Diabetes Technology Therapy, 16*, 310–316. doi: 10.1089/dia.2013.0280

Centers for Disease Control and Prevention. (2015). Diabetes home: National data. Retrieved from http://www.cdc.gov/diabetes/data/national.html

Centers for Disease Control and Prevention. (2014). *National Diabetes Statistics Report: Estimates of Diabetes and Its Burden in the United States, 2014.* Atlanta, GA: US Department of Health and Human Services.

Centers for Disease Control and Prevention. (2014). *Diabetes Report Card 2014.* Atlanta, GA: US Department of Health and Human Services.

Chapple, I. L., Genco, R.; Working group 2 of joint EFP/AAP workshop. (2013). Diabetes and periodontal diseases: Consensus report of the joint EFP/AAP workshop on periodontitis and systemic diseases. *Journal of Clinical Periodontology, 40*(Suppl. 14), S106–S112. doi: 10.1111/jcpe.12077

Chatterjee, S., & Davies, M. (2015). Type 2 diabetes: Recent advances in diagnosis and management. *Prescriber, 26*(10), 15–21. doi: 10.1002/psb.1355

Chiang, J. L., Kirkman, M. S., Laffell, L. M. B., & Peters, A. L. (2014). Type 1 diabetes through the life span: A position statement of the American Diabetes Association. *Diabetes Care, 37*(7), 2034–2054. doi: 10.2337/dc14-1140

Clair, C., Cohen, M. J., Eichler, F., Selby, K. J., & Rigotti, N. A. (2015). The effect of cigarette smoking on diabetic peripheral neuropathy: A systematic review and meta-analysis. *Journal of General Internal Medicine, 30*(8), 1193–1203. doi: 10.1007/x11606-015-3345-y

Copeland, K. L., Brown, J. S., Creasman, J. M., Van Den Eeden, S. K., Subak, L. L., Thom, D. H., … Huang, A. J. (2012). Diabetes mellitus and sexual function in middle-aged older women. *Obstetrics & Gynecology, 120*(2), 331–340. doi: 10.1097/AOG.Ob013e31825ec5fa

Coppola, A., Sasso, L., Bagnasco, A., Giustina, A., & Gazzaruso, C. (2015). The role of patient education in the prevention and management of type 2 diabetes: A review. *Endocrine.* Advance online publication. doi: 10.1007/s12020-015-0775-7

Craig, M. E., Jefferies, C., Dabelea, D., Balde, N., Seth, A., & Donaghue, K. C. (2014). Definition, epidemiology, and classification of diabetes in children and adolescents. *Pediatric Diabetes, 15*(Suppl. 20), 4–17. doi: 10.1111/pedi.12186

Dabelea, D., Mayer-Davis, E. J., Saydah, S., Imperatore, G., Linder, B., Divers, J., … Hamman, R. F. (2014). Prevalence of type 1 and type 2 diabetes among children and adolescents from 2001 to 2009. *Journal of the American Medical Association, 311*(17), 1778–1786. doi: 10.1001/jama.2014.3201

Demirci, H., Cosar, R., Ciftci, O., & Sari, I. K. (2015). Atypical diabetic ketoacidosis: Case report. *Balkan Medical Journal, 32*(1), 124–126. doi: 10.5152/balkanmedj.2015.15123

Deshpande, A. D., Harris-Hayes, M., & Schootman, M. (2008). Epidemiology of diabetes and diabetes-related complications. *Physical Therapy, 88*(11), 1254–1264. doi: 10.2522/ptj.20080020

Ding, J., & Wong, T. Y. (2012). Current epidemiology of diabetic retinopathy and diabetic macular edema. *Current Diabetes Reports, 12*(4), 346–354. doi: 10.1007/s11892-012-0283-6

Ducloux, R., Safraou, M., & Altman, J. (2015). Etiologic diagnosis of diabetes mellitus in adults: Questions to ask, tests to request. *International Journal of Diabetes in Developing Countries, 35*(4), 604–611. doi: 10.1007/s13410-015-0336-x

Egan, A. M., & Dinneen, S. F. (2014). What is diabetes? *Medicine, 42*(12), 679–681. doi: 10.1016/j.mpmed.2014.09.005

Ehrlich, S. F., Hedderson, M. M., Quesenberry, C. P., Feng, J., Brown, S. D., Crites, Y., & Ferrara, A. (2014). Post-partum weight loss and glucose metabolism in women with gestational diabetes: The DEBI study. *Diabetic Medicine, 31*, 862–867. doi: 10.1111/dme.12425

Esposito, K., & Guigliano, D. (2014). Mediterranean diet and type 2 diabetes. *Diabetes/Metabolism Research and Reviews, 30*(Suppl. 1), 34–40. doi: 10.1002/dmrr.2516

Ferrannini, E., & Cushman, W. C. (2012). Diabetes and hypertension: The bad companions. *The Lancet, 380*(9841), 601–610. doi: 10.1016/s0140-6736(12)60987-8

Fraser, C. E., & D'Amico, D. J. (2015). Diabetic retinopathy: Classification and clinical features. *Up to Date.* Retrieved from http://www.uptodate.com/contents/diabetic-retinopathy-classification-and-clinical-features?source=search_result&search=diabetic+retinopathy&selectedTitle=1~95

Freeman, R. (2013). Diabetic autonomic neuropathy. In D. W. Zochodne & R. A. Malik (Eds.), *Handbook of clinical neurology, Vol. 126,* (pp. 63–79). Atlanta, GA: Elsevier B. V.

Fritsch, M., Rosenbauer, A., Schober, E., Neu, J., Placzek, K., & Holl, R. W. (2011). Predictors of diabetic ketoacidosis in children and adolescents with type 1 diabetes: Experience from a large multicentre database. *Pediatric Diabetes, 12*(4), 307–312. doi: 10.1111/j.1399-5448.2010.00728.x

Fritz, H. (2014). The influence of daily routines on engaging in diabetes self-management. *Scandinavian Journal of Occupational Therapy, 21*, 232–240. doi: 10.3109/11038128.2013.868033

Goodman, C. C. (2009). The endocrine and metabolic systems. In C. C. Goodman & K. S. Fuller (Eds.), *Pathology: Implications for physical therapists* (3rd ed., pp. 453–518). Philadelphia, PA: Saunders.

Gregg, E. W., Li, Y., Wang, J., Burrows, N. R., Ali, M. K., Rolka, D., … Geiss, L. (2014). Changes in diabetes-related complications in the United States, 1990–2010. *New England Journal of Medicine, 370*(16), 1514–1523. doi: 10.1056/nejmoa1310799

Grøntved, A., & Hu, F. B. (2011). Television watching and risk of Type 2 diabetes, cardiovascular disease, and all-cause mortality. *Journal of the American Medical Association, 305*(23), 2448–2455. doi: 10.1001/jama.2011.812

Gruessner, A. C., Sutherland, D. E. R., & Gruessner, R. W. G. (2012). Long-term outcome after pancreas transplant. *Current Opinion in Organ Transplantation, 17*(1), 100–105. doi: 10.1097/mot.0b013e32834ee700

Halter, J. B., Musi, N., McFarland Horne, F., Crandall, J. P., Goldberg, A., Harkless, L., … High, K. P. (2014). Diabetes and cardiovascular disease in older adults: Current status and future directions. *Diabetes, 63*, 2578–2589. doi: 10.2337/db14-0020

Hao, K., DiNarzo, A. F., Ho, L., Luo, W., Li, S., Chen, R., … Pasinetti, G. M. (2015). Shared genetic etiology underlying Alzheimer's disease and type 2 diabetes. *Molecular aspects of medicine, 43–44*, 66–76. doi: 10.1016/j.mam.2015.06.006

He, F., Xia, X., Wu, X. F., Yu, X. Q., & Huang, F. X. (2013). Diabetic retinopathy in predicting diabetic nephropathy in patients with type 2 diabetes and renal disease: A meta-analysis. *Diabetologia, 56*(3), 457–456. doi: 10.1007/s00125-012-2796-6

Holt, R. I. G., de Groot, M., Hill Gordon, S. (2014). Diabetes and depression. *Current Diabetes Reports, 14*(6), 491–500. doi: 10.1007/s11892-014-0491-3

Holtz, B., & Lauckner, C. (2012). Diabetes management via mobile phones: A systematic review. *Telemedicine and e-Health, 18*(3), 175–184. doi: 10.1089/tmj.2011.0119.

Hu, F., Niu, L., Chen, R., Ma, Y., Qin, X., & Hu,. Z. (2015). The association between social capital and quality of life among type 2 diabetes patients in Anhui province, China: A cross-sectional study. *BMC Public Health, 15*, 786–781. doi: 10.1186/s12889-015-2138-y

Huang, E. S., Laiteerapong, N., Liu, J. Y., John, P. M., Moffet, H. J. (2013). Rates of complications and mortality in older patients with diabetes mellitus. *Journal of the American Medical Association, 174*(2), 251–258. doi: 10.1001/jamainternmed.2013.12956

Imamura, F., O'Connor, L., Ye, Z., Mursu, J., Hayashina, Y., Bhupathiraju, S. N., & Forouhi, N. G. (2015). Consumption of sugar sweetened beverages, artificially sweetened beverages, and fruit juice and incidence of type 2 diabetes: Systematic review, meta-analysis, and estimation of population attribution fraction. *British Medical Journal, 351*, 1–12. doi: 10.1136/bmj.h3576

Inzucchi, S. E., Bergenstal, R. M., Buse, J. B., Diamant, M., Ferrannini, E., Nauck, M., ... Matthews, D. R. (2012). Management of hyperglycemia in type 2 diabetes: A patient-centered approach. *Diabetes Care, 35*(6), 1364–1379. doi: 10.2337/dc13-er02

Isidro, M. L. (2012). Sexual dysfunction in men with type 2 diabetes. *Postgraduate Medicine, 88*, 152–159. doi: 10.1136/postgradmedj-2011-1300069

Jaiswal, M., Lauer, A., Martin, C. L., Bell, R. A., Divers, J., Dabelea, D., ... Feldman, E. L. (2013). Peripheral neuropathy in adolescents and young adults with type 1 and type 2 diabetes from the SEARCH for diabetes in youth follow-up cohort. *Diabetes Care, 36*(12), 3903–3908. doi: 10.2337/dc13-1213

Janghorbani, M., Momeni, F., & Mansourian, M. (2014). Systematic review and metaanalysis of air pollution exposure and risk of diabetes. *European Journal of Epidemiology, 29*(4), 231–242. doi: 10.1007/s10654-014-9907-2

Jørgensen, M. E., Almdal, T. P., & Carstensen, B. (2013). Time trends in mortality rates in type 1 diabetes from 2002 to 2011. *Diabetologia, 56*(11), 2401–2404. doi: 10.1007/s00124-013-3025-7

Kahn, S. E., Cooper, M. E., & Del Prato, S. (2014). Pathophysiology and treatment of type 2 diabetes: Perspectives on the past, present, and future. *The Lancet, 383*(9922), 1068–1083. doi: 10.1016/s0140-6736(13)62154-6

Kanaya, A. M., Herrington, D., Vittinghoff, E., Ewing, S. K., Liu, K., Blaha, M. J., ... Kandula, N. R. (2014). Understanding the high prevalence of diabetes in U. S. South Asians compared with four racial/ethnic groups: The MASALA and MESA studies. *Diabetes Care, 37*, 1621–1628. doi: 10.2337/dc13-2656

Kolluru, G. K., Bir, S. C., & Kevil, C. G. (2012). Endothelial dysfunction and diabetes: Effects on vascular remodeling and wound healing. *International Journal of Vascular Medicine, 2012*, 1–30. doi: 10.1155/2012/918267

Lago, R. M., Singhy, P. P., & Nesto, R. W. (2007). Diabetes and hypertension. *Nature Clinical Practice, 3*(10), 667. doi: 10.1038/ncpendme0638

Lehmann, R., Graziano, J., Brockmann, J., Pfammatter, T., Kron, P., de Rougemont, O., ... Gerber, P. A. (2015). Glycemic control in simultaneous islet-kidney versus pancreas-kidney transplantation in type 1 diabetes: A prospective 13-year follow-up. *Diabetes Care, 38*, 752–759. doi: 10.2337/dc14-1686

Leong, C. H. M., Velusamy, A., & Choudhary, P. (2014). Modern technologies for glucose monitoring and insulin replacement. *Medicine, 42*(12), 703–706. doi: 10.1016/j.mpmed.2014.09.004

Ley, S. H., Hamdy, O., Mohan, V., & Hu, F. B. (2014). Prevention and management of type 2 diabetes: Dietary components and nutritional strategies. *The Lancet, 383*(9933), 1999–2007. doi: 10.1016/s0140-6736(14)60613-9

Liu, A. H. (2015). Revisiting the hygiene hypothesis for allergy and asthma. *Journal of Allergy and Clinical Immunology, 136*(4), 860–865. doi: 10.1016/j.jaci.2015.08.012

Livingstone, S. J., Levin, D., Looker, H. C., Lindsay, R. S., Wild, S. H., Joss, N., ... Colhoun, H. M. (2015). Estimated life expectancy in a Scottish cohort with type 1 diabetes, 2008–2010. *Journal of the American Medical Association, 313*(1), 37–44. doi: 10.1001/jama.2014.16425

Luitse, M. J. A., Biessels, G. A., Rutten, G. E. H. M., & Kappelle, L. J. (2012). Diabetes, hyperglycemia, and acute ischemic stroke. *Lancet Neurology, 11*(3), 261–271. doi: 10.1016/s1474-4422(12)70005-4

Mailoux, L. U. (2015). Dialysis in diabetic nephropathy. *Up to Date*. Retrieved from http://www.uptodate.com/contents/dialysis-in-diabetic-nephropathy?source=search_result&search=diabetic+kidney+dialysis&selectedTitle=1~150

Martin, C. L., Albers, J. W., & Pop-Busui, R. (2014). Neuropathy and related findings in the Diabetes Control and Complications Trial/Epidemiology of

Diabetes Interventions and Complications study. *Diabetes Care, 37*(1), 31–38. doi: 10.2337/dc13-2114

McCrimmon, R. J., Ryan, M., & Frier, B. M. (2012). Diabetes and cognitive function. *The Lancet, 379*(9833), 2291–2299. doi: 10.1016/s0140-6736(12)60360-2

McCulloch, D. K. (2015). Glycemic control and vascular complications in type 2 diabetes. *Up to Date.* Retrieved from http://www.uptodate.com/contents/glycemic-control-and-vascular-complications-in-type-2-diabetes-mellitus?source=search_result&search=diabetic+vascular&selectedTitle=1~150

McDermott, M. M. (2015). Lower extremity manifestations of peripheral artery disease. *Circulation Research, 116*(9), 1540–1550. doi: 10.1161/circresaha.114.303517

Melendez-Ramirez, L. Y., Richards, R. J., & Cefalu, W. T. (2010). Complications of type 1 diabetes. *Endocrinology Metabolism Clinics North America, 39*(3), 625–640. doi: 10.1016/j.ecl.2010.05.009

Menke, A., Rust, K. F., Fradkin, J., Cheng, Y. J., Cowie, C. C. (2014). Associations between trends in race/ethnicity, aging, and body mass index with diabetes prevalence in the United States. *Annals of Internal Medicine, 161*(5), 328–336. doi: 10.7326/M14-0286

Miller, R. G., Secrest, A. M., Sharma, R. K., Songer, T. J., & Orchard, T. J. (2012). Improvements in the life expectancy of type 1 diabetes. *Diabetes, 61*(11), 2987–2992. doi: 10.2337/db11-1625

Morgenstern, M., Wang, J., Beatty, N., Batemarco, T., Sica, A. L., & Greenberg, H. (2014). Obstructive sleep apnea: An unexpected cause of insulin resistance and diabetes. *Endocrinology Metabolism Clinics North America, 43*(1), 187–204. doi: 10.1016/j.ecl.2013.09.002

Navmenova, Y., Mokhort, T., & Makhlina, E. (2014). Depression risk factors in type 1 diabetes mellitus. *Endocrine Abstracts, 35*, 410. doi: 10.1530/endoabs.35.P410

Neschis, D. G., & Golden, M. A. (2015). Clinical features and diagnosis of lower extremity peripheral artery disease. *Up to Date.* Retrieved from http://www.uptodate.com/contents/clinical-features-and-diagnosis-of-lower-extremity-peripheral-artery-disease?source=search_result&search=diabetic+peripheral+artery+disease&selectedTitle=1~150

Nielson, D. S., Krych, L., Buschard, K., Hansen, C. H. F., & Hansen, A. K. (2014). Beyond genetics: Influence of dietary factors and gut microbiota on type 1 diabetes. *FEBS Letters, 588*(22), 4234–4243. doi: 10.1016/j.febslet.2014.04.010

Noor, S., Zubair, M., & Ahmad, J. (2015). Diabetic foot ulcer: A review on pathophysiology, classification and microbial etiology. *Diabetes & Metabolic Syndrome: Clinical Research & Reviews, 9*(3), 192–199. doi: 10.1016/j.dsx.2015.04.007

Olafsdottir, E., Andersson, D. K. G., Dedorsson, I., Stefánsson, E. (2014). The prevalence of retinopathy in subjects with and without type 2 diabetes mellitus. *Acta Ophthalmologica, 92*(2), 133–137. doi: 10.1111/aos.12095

Peters, S. A. E., Huxley, R. R., & Woodward, M. (2014). Diabetes as a risk factor for stroke in women compared with men: A systematic review and meta-analysis of 64 cohorts, including 775,385 individuals and 12, 539 strokes. *Lancet, 383*(9933), 1973–1980. doi: 10.1016/s0140-6736(14)60040-4

Peterson, A. (2014). Improving Type 1 diabetes management with mobile tools: A systematic review. *Journal of Diabetes Science and Technology, 8*(4), 859–864. doi: 10.1177/1932296814529885

Pickup, J. (2011). Insulin pumps. *International Journal of Clinical Practice, 65*, 16–19. doi: 10.1111/j.1742-1241.2010.02574.x

Plantinga, L., Rao, M. N., & Schillinger, D. (2012). Prevalence of self-reported sleep problems among people with diabetes in the United States, 2005–2008. *Preventing Chronic Disease, 9*(110244), 1–12. doi: 10.5888/pcd9.110244

Powers, A. (2008). Diabetes mellitus. In A. Fauci, E. Braunwalk, D. Kasper, S. Hauser, D. Longo, J. Jameson, & J. Loscalzo (Eds.), *Harrison's principles of internal medicine*, (17th ed., pp. 2275–2304). New York, NY: McGraw-Hill.

Powers, M. A., Bardsley, J., Cypress, M., Duker, P., Funnell, M. M., Fischl, A. H., … Vivan, E. (2015). Diabetes self-management education and support in type 2 diabetes. *Journal of the Academy of Nutrition and Dietetics, 115*(8), 1323–1334. doi: 10.1016/j.jand.2015.05.012

Pulgaron, E. R., & Delamater, A. M. (2014). Obesity and Type 2 diabetes in children: Epidemiology and treatment. *Current Diabetes Reports, 14*(8), 508–520. doi: 10.1007/s11892-014-0508-y

Pyatak, E. (2011). Participation in occupation and diabetes self-management in emerging adulthood. *American Journal of Occupational Therapy, 65*, 462–469. doi: 10.5014/ajot2011.001453

Rhodes, E. T., Prosser, L. A., Hoerger, T. J., Lieu, T., Ludwig, D. S., & Laffel, L. M. (2012). Estimated morbidity and mortality in adolescents and young adults diagnosed with type 2 diabetes. *Diabetic Medicine, 29*(4), 453–463. doi: 10.1111/j.1464-5491.2011.03542.x

Saddiqui, S. (2014). Depression in type 2 diabetes: A brief review. *Diabetes and Metabolic Syndrome, 8*(1), 62–65. doi: 10.1016/j.dsx.2013.06.010

Schmader, K. E. (2001). Epidemiology and impact on quality of life of postherpetic neuralgia and painful diabetic neuropathy. *The Clinical Journal of Pain, 18*(6), 350–353. doi: 10.1097/00002508-200211000-00002

Seaquist, E. R., Anderson, J., Childs, B., Cryer, P., Dagogo-Jack, S., Fish, L., ... Vigersky, R. (2013). Hypoglycemia and diabetes: A report of a workgroup of the American Diabetes Association and The Endocrine Society. *Diabetes Care*, *36*(5), 1384–1395. doi: 10.2337/dc12-2480

Shah, K. M., Clark, B. R., McGill, J. B., & Mueller, M. J. (2015). Upper extremity impairments, pain, and disability in patients with diabetes mellitus. *Physiotherapy*, *101*, 147–154. doi: 10.1016/j.physio.2014.007.003

Singh, R., Kishore, L., & Kaur, N. (2014). Diabetic peripheral neuropathy: Current perspective and future directions. *Pharmacological Research*, *80*, 21–35. doi: 10.1016/j.phrs.2013.12.005

Strom Williams, J. L., Walker, R. J., Smalls, B. L., Campbell, J. A., & Egede, L. E. (2014). Effective interventions to improve medication adherence in type 2 diabetes: A systematic review. *Diabetes Management*, *4*(1), 29048. doi: 10.2217/dmt.13.62

Surani, S., Brito, V., Surani, A., & Ghamande, S. (2015). Effect of diabetes mellitus on sleep quality. *World Journal of Diabetes*, *6*(6), 868–873. doi: 10.4239/wjd.v6.i6.868

Tabák, A. G., Herder, C., Rathmann, W., Brunner, E. J., & Kivimäki, M. (2012). Prediabetes: A high-risk state for diabetes development. *The Lancet*, *673*(12), 2279–2290. doi: 10.1016/s0140-6736(12)60283-9

Tesfaye, S., & Selvarajah, D. (2012). Advances in the epidemiology, pathogenesis and management of diabetic peripheral neuropathy. *Diabetes/Metabolism Research and Reviews*, *28*(Suppl. 1), 8–14. doi: 10.1002/dmrr.2239

Tesfaye, S., Vileikyte, L., Rayman, G., Sindrup, S. H., Perkins, B. A., Baconja, M., ... Boulton, A. J. M. (2011). Painful diabetic peripheral neuropathy: Consensus recommendations on diagnosis, assessment and management. *Diabetes/Metabolism Research and Reviews*, *27*(7), 629–638. doi: 10.1002/dmrr.1225

Thomas, C. C., & Philipson, L. H. (2015). Update on diabetes classification. *Medical Clinics of North America*, *99*, 1–16. doi: 10.1016/j.mcna.2014.08.015

Trento, M., Raballo, M., Trevisan, J., Sicuro, P., Passera, L. Cirio, L., ... Porta, M. (2012). A cross-sectional survey of depression, anxiety, and cognitive function in patients with type 2 diabetes. *Acta Diabetology*, *49*, 199–203. doi: 10.1007/s00592-011-0275-z

Tuomi, T., Santoro, N., Caprio, S., Cai, M., Weng, J., & Groop, L. (2014). The many faces of diabetes: A disease with increasing heterogeneity. *The Lancet*, *383*(9922), 1084–1094. doi: 10.1016/s0140-6736(13)62219-9

Verdile, G., Fuller, S. J., & Martins, R. N. (2015). The role of type 2 diabetes in neurodegeneration. *Neurobiology of disease*, *84*, 22–38. doi: 10.1016/j.nbd.2015.04.008

Vinik, A. I., & Erbas, T. (2013). Diabetic autonomic neuropathy. In R. M. Bujs & F. Swaab (Eds.), *Handbook of clinical neurology, Vol. 117* (pp. 279–294). Atlanta, GA: Elsevier B. V.

Vinik, A. I., Erbas, T., & Casellini, C. M. (2013). Diabetic cardiac autonomic neuropathy, inflammation and cardiovascular disease. *Journal of Diabetes Investigation*, *4*(1), 4–18. doi:10.1111/jdi.12042

Walders-Abramson, N. (2013). Depression and quality of life in youth-onset type 2 diabetes mellitus. *Current Diabetes Reports*, *14*(1), 449–454. doi: 10.1007/s11892-013-0449-x

Wannamethee, S. G., Shaper, A. G., Wincup, P. H., Lennon, L., & Sattar, N. (2011). Impact of diabetes on cardiovascular disease risk and all-cause mortality in older men. *Archives of Internal Medicine*, *171*(5), 404–410. doi: 10.1001/archinternmed.2011.2

Wolfsdorf, J. I., Allgrove, J., Craig, M. E., Edge, J., Glaser, N., Jain, V., ... Hanas, R. (2014). Diabetic ketoacidosis and hyperglycemia and hyperosmolar state. *Pediatric Diabetes*, *15*(Suppl. 20), 154–179. doi: 10.1111/pedi.12165

Yueng, W-C. G., Rawlinson, W. D., & Craig, M. E. (2011). Enterovirus infection and type 1 diabetes mellitus: Systematic review and meta-analysis of observational molecular studies. *British Medical Journal*, *342*, 1–9. doi: 10.1136/bmj.d35

Acquired Brain Injury

Gerry E. Conti

It had been a hot summer day, the work was hard, and J.D.'s construction job required every ounce of his strength and endurance. He'd missed lunch and was roofing in the heat as the final part of his day, the tar radiating heat upward while the sun beat down on this back. At last it was over. J.D. picked up Kathy, his girlfriend of 4 years, and headed for the beach. Five hours and many beers later, they sped home on familiar secondary roads. He negotiated the first part of an S-curve fine, but his reflexes were too slow to manage the second curve when a rabbit ran into the road. Overcompensating, he lost control of the car, slamming it up against a tree. In an instant, his life changed. Kathy was killed. J.D., age 20, survived. At the hospital, he was diagnosed with a traumatic brain injury.

Acquired brain injury (ABI) is defined by the World Health Organization as "damage to the brain, which occurs after birth and is not related to a congenital or a degenerative disease." These impairments may be temporary or permanent and cause partial or functional disability or psychosocial maladjustment (Brain Trauma Foundation, 2007). ABI includes the conditions of traumatic brain injury (TBI), brain tumors, and cerebrovascular accidents (CVA). This chapter will address TBI and brain tumors; CVA is discussed in a separate chapter.

TRAUMATIC BRAIN INJURY

■ Description and Definition

TBI is defined by the Diagnostic and Statistical Manual of Mental Disorders (American Psychiatric Association, 2013) as a mild, moderate, or severe

brain trauma with specific characteristics that include at least one of the following: loss of consciousness, posttraumatic amnesia, disorientation and confusion, or, in more severe cases, neurological signs (e.g., positive neuroimaging,

a new onset of seizures or a marked worsening of a preexisting seizure disorder, visual field cuts, anosmia, hemiparesis). To be attributable to TBI, the neurocognitive disorder must present immediately after the brain injury occurs or immediately after the individual recovers consciousness after the injury and persist past the acute post-injury period.

TBI therefore involves a complex matrix of physical, cognitive, and neurobehavioral changes that may have a lifetime effect on a person's ability to participate in necessary and preferred occupations. Many functions are compromised, including the ability to produce coordinated movement, speak, remember, reason, and alter behavior in response to the environment (Wehman et al., 2003a). The combination of these changes makes TBI a major public health problem (Rutland-Brown, Langlois, Thomas, & Xi, 2006).

The extent of disability is typically identified within 48 hours of medical evaluation and is based on loss of consciousness or **coma**, posttraumatic amnesia, and disorientation and confusion at initial assessment (American Psychiatric Association, 2013). The following definitions will be used for this chapter.

Mild TBI: Loss of consciousness of
<30 minutes, posttraumatic amnesia of
<24 hours and disorientation and confusion, and a Glasgow Coma Scale (GCS) score of
13 to 15.
Moderate TBI: Loss of consciousness
of 30 minutes to 24 hours, posttraumatic
amnesia of 24 hours to 7 days, and a GCS
score of 9 to 12.
Severe TBI: Loss of consciousness of more
than 24 hours, posttraumatic amnesia of
more than 7 days, and a GCS score of 3 to 8
(American Psychiatric Association, 2013).

Mild TBI represents 80% of all brain injury, and about 85% of these people will recover without intervention over a 3-month period (Greenwald & Rigg, 2009). Persons with mild TBI typically report symptoms such as headaches, dizziness, fatigue, visual disturbance, memory, and **executive function** difficulties during the first week following injury. However, for some individuals, these difficulties persist from 3 months to a lifetime, causing significant distress and disruption of daily activities (Ponsford, Willmott, & Rothwell, 2000).

The onset of TBI is sudden, following a single-incident neurologic insult, and results in both primary and secondary brain damage. Primary brain damage may be focal (localized) or diffuse and is created by direct impact, acceleration, deceleration, and rotation of the brain; by intrusion into the brain by a penetrating object, such as a gunshot; or by blast waves from an explosion (Maas, Stochetti, & Bullock, 2008). Focal lesions are limited in scope and are associated with direct impact of short duration such as occurs with gunshot. Diffuse lesions occur throughout multiple brain areas and may result from an explosion, motor vehicle accidents, or sport collisions. Diffuse axonal injuries (DAI) may occur with head collisions at about 15 miles per hour or greater (Meythaler, Peduzzi, & Eleftheriou, 2001). DAI therefore can occur with high-speed running collisions with others, as in football, soccer, or hockey, as well as with higher-speed motor vehicle accidents. Motor vehicle accidents typically result in both coup and **contrecoup** injuries. With these injuries, direct damage is incurred as the cerebrum rotates on the more stable brainstem while accelerating from the force of impact. The cerebrum strikes the skull (coup), and then reaccelerates in the opposite direction to strike the skull at an opposite location (contrecoup). This continues until the force of impact has been absorbed (Drew & Drew, 2004).

The mechanism for DAI is stretching and shearing of brain cell axons, and typically results in profound coma and a poor outcome (Maas et al., 2008). Injury to the tracts leading from the hypothalamus and/or pituitary stalk results in medical complications of hyperventilation, hormonal changes, electrolyte disturbances of salt and water, altered temperature regulation, and dysfunctional awareness of hunger (Adams, Graham, & Murray, 1982; Dawodu, 2005; Meythaler et al., 2001). DAI is characterized by small lesions in and shearing of white matter tracts of the cerebral cortex, such as the sensory and motor cortices and the frontal lobe, and the corpus callosum, brainstem, and cerebellum (Maas et al., 2008). Common cognitive deficits associated with these structures include deficits in working memory and processing speed and memory, as well as limited planning and executive functions (Meythaler et al., 2001; Salmond & Sahakian, 2005). A common motor deficit is difficulty with bilateral integration due to callosal damage, which is frequently disrupted in TBI (Hulkower, Poliak, Rosenbaum, Zimmerman, & Lipton, 2013).

Secondary damage, with differing pathophysiological mechanisms, occurs within hours and days of impact. Factors leading to secondary damage may include inflammatory responses, raised intracranial pressure, and decreased cerebral blood flow or ischemia (Maas et al., 2008). Increased intracranial pressure results in swelling, which cannot be accommodated within the rigid structure of the skull. Ischemia occurs when blood vessels can no longer provide sufficient blood to the brain.

Medical complications are frequent and impair recovery following TBI. Following a high-impact TBI, such as occurs with a motor vehicle accident, persons may have single or multiple seizures (Frey, 2003), and **hydrocephalus** (De Bonis, Pompucci, Mangiola, Rigante, & Anile, 2010). Fifty percent of people with severe TBI have extremity injuries including lacerations and fractures (Probst et al., 2009), resulting in casting of extremities. The incidence of deep vein thrombosis following TBI is up to 54% (Cifu, Kaelin, & Wall, 1996; Probst et al., 2009; Rimel & Jane, 1983). Systemic complications may include the cardiovascular, respiratory, immunological, hematological, and endocrinological systems (Wijayatilake, Sherren, & Jigajinni, 2015). As a result of respiratory dysfunction, nasal intubation or tracheostomy may be required, and the person is at risk for pneumonia. Neurogenic bowel and bladder disorders require catheterization, while limited body mobility requires close monitoring to avoid the development of decubiti (Dijkstra, Kazimier, & Halfens, 2015).

■ Etiology

The three leading causes of TBI are falls, motor vehicle accidents, and violence. Falls are the most common cause of TBI, but motor vehicle accidents are the most common cause of severe TBI. Children below the age of 5 and elderly adults over 85 years are the most commonly seen groups with TBI in hospital emergency departments (Gordon et al., 2006). According to a major statewide study from 2003 to 2006, males accounted for about 61% of all motor vehicle accidents, both with and without the presence of alcohol or substance use (Rochette, Conner, & Smith, 2009). Among children involved in motor vehicle accidents resulting in moderate to severe injury, half were unrestrained at the time of injury (National Highway Traffic Safety Agency, 2006). In the United States, survivors of violence, the second major cause of TBI, are more likely to be men, single, unemployed, and from a minority background (Bogner, Corrigan, & Mysiw, 2001; Bushnik, Hanks, Kreutzer, & Rosenthal, 2003).

Severity of injury is related to cause. Surviving vehicle crash victims tend to be injured more severely than do survivors of either falls or violence and to have additional injuries such as long bone fractures and plexopathies; falls are more often associated with mild injury. Intoxication, which is present in one-third to one-half of individuals at the time of injury, and substance use are significantly negatively correlated with outcome. Persons who were intoxicated when injured also tend to be hospitalized longer and have greater severity of injury, greater incidence of death, and a lower cognitive status at the time of discharge, as well as greater periods of post-acquired amnesia (Bogner et al., 2001; Corrigan, 1995; Cummings, Rivara, Olson, & Smith, 2006; Cunningham, Maio, Hill, & Zink, 2002). People injured by violence tend to have more severe injuries and poorer community reintegration after injury (Gordon et al., 2006).

■ Incidence and Prevalence

The great incidence of TBI around the world has led the World Health Organization to refer to TBI as a "silent epidemic" (Binder, Corrigan, & Langlois, 2005). An estimated 1.7 million Americans sustain a TBI each year. Of these, about 52,000 will die, 275,000 will be hospitalized, and between 80,000 and 90,000 persons will experience lifetime disability (American Psychiatric Association, 2013).

The incidence of disability increases with the severity of brain injury. Permanent disability occurs in about 10% of those with mild TBI, 66% of those with moderate TBI, and 100% of those with severe TBI (Jallo & Narayan, 2000). Additionally, age, gender, and ethnicity affect the incidence rate. At greatest risk for injury are young men between the ages of 15 and 24, who are twice as likely as women of the same age to sustain a TBI (American Psychiatric Association, 2013). It is not known, however, whether gender affects the severity of and outcome from TBI (Ragnarsson, 2006). Age groups that show an increased incidence of TBI include adults older than 75 years and children below the age of 5 (Centers for Disease Control and Prevention, 2001). A review of current evidence suggests that injury in older adults may result in greater impairment and more limited recovery (Ragnarsson, 2006). Inner-city environments have higher incidence rates (Bruns, 2003), with persons of American Indian/ Alaskan and African American ethnicity having the highest rates from TBI of all races (Corrigan, Selassie, & Orman, 2010). It is uncertain whether this incidence is due to issues related to socioeconomic status or to lack of medical and rehabilitation opportunities (Ragnarsson, 2006).

The costs of TBI, both individually and for society, are staggering. The estimated economic cost of TBI in the United Stated in 2010, including both direct and indirect health care costs, was $76.5 billion (Centers for Disease Control and Prevention, 2014). As only 20% to 50% of TBI survivors are employed (Injury, 1999), an additional $1 billion annually may be incurred due to lost wages, lost income taxes, and increased public assistance (Johnstone, Mount, & Schopp, 2003). However, researchers have used different economic analysis methodologies, and historical results have been inconsistent (Humphreys, Wood, Phillips, & Macey, 2013). Nevertheless, it is clear that TBI results in significant costs to society, the individual, and the family during the acute phase of recovery and through lifetime costs.

■ Signs and Symptoms

People with TBI experience a wide range of deficits, depending on the location and severity of their injuries. The following is a description of the medical, motor, cognitive, psychosocial, and cranial nerve signs and symptoms associated with TBI.

Medical Complications

Seizures are a frequent medical complication of moderate or severe TBI (Ragnarsson, 2006) and are typically classified as immediate, early, or late seizures, depending on whether they occur within 24 hours, 1 week or after 1 week, respectively (Najafi, Tabesh, Hosseini, Akbari, & Najafi, 2015). Risk factors for seizures include the severity of the injury, time since injury, decompressive craniectomy, and brain contusion with subdural hematoma, and being older than 65 (Huang, Liao, Chen, & Ou, 2015; Najafi et al., 2015). The risk of seizures varies for different groups, however. For example, seizure rates of up to 53% have been identified after military injuries, while a 4% seizure incidence may occur with a small intracranial injury (Frey, 2003). The overall incidence of not-inflicted TBI seizures in children is 15% to 17%, while the incidence for inflicted TBI seizures is 48% to 65% (Park & Chugani, 2015). The risk of a first seizure for someone of any age continues to be elevated for more than 10 years after brain injury (Annegers, Hauser, & Coan, 1998).

Posttraumatic hydrocephalus is the most common medical complication following TBI, with rates of incidence varying from approximately 2% to 45% (Gordon et al., 2006). Those with more severe injuries and those who have undergone decompressive craniotomies are at more risk to develop posttraumatic hydrocephalus (Fig. 20.1).

Dysautonomia is also frequently seen after severe TBI and is characterized by hypertension, tachycardia, increased body temperature and blood pressure, profuse sweating, and decerebrate or decorticate posturing (Gordon et al., 2006; Hendricks, Heeren, & Vos, 2010). People experiencing dysautonomia have been shown to have longer rehabilitation lengths of stay, longer periods of posttraumatic amnesia, and lower Glasgow Outcome Scale scores (Baguley, Nicholls, & Felmingham, 1999; Gordon et al., 2006). (Table 20.1)

It has been estimated that up to 20% of people with TBI have deep vein thrombosis on admission to the hospital (Carlile et al., 2010). Deep venous thrombosis (DVT) results from prolonged immobilization. DVT can give rise to pulmonary emboli, which is the most common preventable cause of hospital death in TBI (Anderson, Wheeler, & Goldberg, 1991; Gordon et al., 2006). Brain injury involves associated cerebral and brainstem depression or destruction that, in turn, affects the person's level of consciousness. Mild brain injury may result in a relatively short

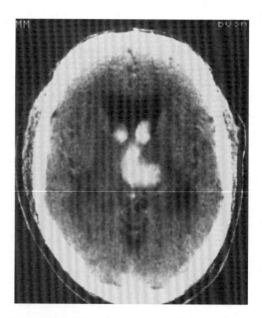

Figure 20.1 Hydrocephalus in a 58-year-old patient. (From Rowland, L. P. (2005). *Merritt's neurology* (11th ed.). Philadelphia, PA: Lippincott Williams & Wilkins.)

TABLE 20.1 Glasgow Coma Scale

Monitored Performance	Reaction	Score
Eye opening	Spontaneous	4
	Open when spoken to	3
	Open at pain stimulus	2
	No reaction	1
Verbal performance	Coherent	5
	Confused, disoriented	4
	Disconnected words	3
	Unintelligible sounds	2
	No verbal reaction	1
Motor responsiveness	Follows instructions	6
	Intentional pain-avoidance	5
	Large motor movement	4
	Flexor synergism	3
	Extensor synergism	2
	No reaction	1

Best possible total score = 15; worst possible total score = 3.

loss of consciousness. Coma, defined as an alteration of consciousness associated with decreased arousal and awareness of all stimuli (Posner, Saper, Schiff, & Plum, 2007), is typically present following moderate to severe TBI.

Either diffuse cerebral hypoxia or extensive cortical damage, with minimal to no impairment of the brainstem, may result in a vegetative state. In this state, the individual's eyes may be open and follow a moving object, and the limbs may move but without apparent purpose. The person will not respond to pain or simple verbal requests, however, and there is no evidence of cortical function related to voluntary movement (Bazarian, McClung, & Shah, 2005). Persons in such a vegetative state may live briefly or for years.

Motor Deficits

Damage to the brainstem between the vestibular nuclei and the red nucleus produces **decerebrate rigidity**, defined as an extensor posture of all extremities and/or the trunk. When the brainstem is intact despite severe cortical damage, **decorticate rigidity** is present, with flexion of the upper extremities and extension of the lower extremities (Fig. 20.2). Abnormal reflexes complicate

movement patterns. During deep coma, brainstem reflexes may result in grimacing to noxious stimuli, which may be accompanied by a change in postural tone in the extremities. These deficits decline as coma lightens, and motor disturbances reflecting neural damage become apparent. These deficits may include quadriparesis, hemiplegia, or monoplegia, with or without fluctuating muscle tone or spasticity, as well as disorders of coordination.

Spasticity is characterized by velocity-dependent increase in muscle tone resulting from hyperexcitability of the stretch reflex (Kandel, Schwartz, Jessell, Siegelbaum, & Hudspeth, 2012). Spasticity is common in adults after moderate and severe TBI, interfering with limb mobility and performance capabilities (Burnett, Watanabe, & Greenwald, 2003; Gordon et al., 2006); 65% of children also have spasticity following TBI (Dumas, Haley, Carey, Ludlow, & Rabin, 2003). With immobility, **heterotopic ossification**, or bone formation at an abnormal soft tissue site, may form at synovial joints surrounded by spastic musculature, particularly the hips, knees, and elbows (Gordon et al., 2006).

Coordination deficits include tremor and ataxia. Tremor types include cerebellar, resting,

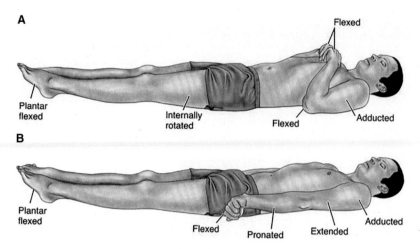

Figure 20.2 Decorticate rigidity **(top)** and decerebrate rigidity **(bottom)**. (From Pellico, L. H. (2012). *Focus on adult health*. Philadelphia, PA: Lippincott Williams & Wilkins.)

essential, and physiologic. Cerebellar or intention tremors are slow tremors that occur at the end of purposeful movement and are associated with ataxia, hypotonia, and balance disorders. They tend to occur in trunk and proximal muscles with intentional movement, at a frequency of approximately 4 to 6 per second. Resting tremors are correlated with striatal damage and involve a pill-rolling movement at rest, occurring at a similar rate. Essential tremors are slow constant tremors that typically affect more distal musculature, occur at a frequency of 8 to 12 per second, and increase with anxiety and maintained positions. Physiologic tremor is present in every person and occurs at the same rate as essential tremor. It can be exacerbated by fatigue, stress, strong emotions, caffeine, and fever. Post acquired ataxia is a result of damage to the sensory, equilibrium, or cerebellar systems and is present in 20% to 30% of persons sustaining DAI (NINDS, 2015).

Cognitive Deficits

Cognitive deficits are among the most common, difficult, and long-lasting consequences of all levels of TBI in both adults and children. Limited memory, especially, is typically present from coma through the person's lifespan. **Retrograde** and **anterograde amnesia** affect learning and cognitive rehabilitation. Retrograde amnesia, or memory loss prior to the accident, may gradually but incompletely improve. Anterograde amnesia, defined as the inability to learn new long-term declarative information, is typically the last to improve.

As coma subsides, cognitive deficits become apparent. These may include difficulties with sustained attention, concentration, memory, comprehension, reasoning, self-monitoring and impulse control, other-awareness, and executive functions. Executive functions involve the ability to formulate context-appropriate goals and to initiate, plan and organize, sequence, and adapt behavior based on the anticipated or actual consequences of actions (Cicerone, Dahlberg, & Kalmar, 2000; Hawley, 2004).

Other effects of cognitive dysfunction are apparent and include difficulty performing routine activities of daily living (ADL), learning new motor routines, and adapting to new or cognitively demanding situations (Cicerone et al., 2000). Motor learning, or the ability to relearn previously well-known or learn new adaptive motor skills, is often functional during the rehabilitation process despite memory loss because it is located in the cerebellum.

Psychosocial Deficits

Neurobehavioral deficits occur as a result of cognitive deficits interacting with brain dysfunction. These deficits are typically seen whether the TBI is mild, moderate, or severe (Cicerone et al., 2000; Hawley, 2004) and include impulsivity, perseveration, irritability, poor control of temper, aggression, disinhibition, and apathy (Noggle & Pierson, 2010; Ylvisaker et al., 2007). Limited self-awareness or a lack of insight may slow rehabilitation progress, as well as the ability to participate successfully in academic, vocational, and/or social roles. Depression and loss of self-esteem are a common problem and may be particularly prevalent in children with TBI as they age. An increasing awareness of their deficits coupled with decreased academic achievement (Fay et al., 1994) may lead to depression in children. In one large sample of 722 outpatients with TBI, major depressive disorder was found in 42% of the sample (Kreutzer, Seel, & Gourley, 2001); another large study of 666 people found the incidence to be 27% (Seel, Kreutzer, & Rosenthal, 2003). Neither time since injury nor severity of injury is correlated with depression (Gordon et al., 2006). With depression comes the potential for suicide. Suicide rates for people with TBI vary between 2.7 and 4.1 times that of the general population when matched for age and gender (Engberg & Teasdale, 2004; Teasdale & Engberg, 2001). A diagnosis of TBI and evidence of aggression and hostility are predictive of suicide attempts (Gordon et al., 2006). Posttraumatic stress disorder is also seen in people with TBI. Studies have found that symptoms of posttraumatic stress disorder were related to the person's level of self-awareness, but not to severity of injury, years of education, intelligence, or memory impairment (Gordon et al., 2006). Additional psychiatric conditions correlated with TBI include substance abuse and aggressive behavior and agitation. Aggressive behavior has been shown to be three times greater in people with TBI compared to people with multiple trauma (Baguley et al., 1999). Other psychiatric diagnoses associated with TBI include borderline, avoidant, paranoid, obsessive-compulsive, and narcissistic personality. The onset of these disorders is independent of severity of injury, age at injury, and time since injury (Gordon et al., 2006).

Visual rather than perceptual deficits are more common in the person with TBI. Such problems may include diplopia, problems with accommodation and convergence, visual field deficits, saccadic dysfunction, and strabismus (Goodrich, Flyg, Kirby, Chang, & Martinsen, 2013).

Cranial Nerve Dysfunction

As the cranial nerves originate from the brainstem, TBI typically results in damage to both the sensory and motor functions of these nerves. Lower levels of coma may permit only assessment of cranial nerves III, VI, and VII (Keane & Baloh, 1992). Pupillary reflexes are important early indicators of brain damage. The absence of a pupillary reflex in response to light by an unconscious patient is an indication of damage to the midbrain, from which the oculomotor nerve (III) originates. A fixed dilated pupil, indicative of pressure on the oculomotor nerve, is frequently seen following moderate to severe TBI (Kandel et al., 2012).

Cranial nerve II is the optic nerve and it transmits visual information from the eye to the brain. The functions of cranial nerve II are acuity and processing of the visual fields. Damage to this nerve may result in homonymous hemianopsia, or difficulty seeing objects on the left or right hemispheres. If the damage occurs at the level of the optic chiasm, bitemporal hemianopsia can occur, which involves loss of the lateral part of vision in both eyes. As coma subsides, significant visual deficits typically become apparent, because of damage to the oculomotor (III), trochlear (IV), and abducens (VI) nerves. These deficits include binocular, oculomotor, accommodative, refractive, and eyelid movement dysfunction, as well as nystagmus, ptosis, and diplopia (Ciuffreda, Ludlam, & Kapoor, 2009). Indeed, the composite signs of diplopia, blurred vision, visual field loss, decreased oculomotor skills, and seeing movement in the stable external environment has been termed posttrauma vision syndrome. Double vision has been called the hallmark of visual deficits for persons with TBI and often results in the individual closing one eye to eliminate double vision.

Loss of the sense of smell (cranial nerve I) occurs in 7% of the people with brain injuries, as a result of damage to the olfactory nerve (Tao & Shenbagamurthi, 2012). Anosmia, or the absence of smell, is especially common following frontal or occipital blows, as nerve endings cross through the thin and easily fractured cribriform plate of the ethmoid bone in the nose (Tao & Shenbagamurthi, 2012). Recovery of smell is not universal and is often incomplete. A study of persons with TBI by Costanzo and Becker found that only 33% of TBI victims improved in smell function. If recovery occurs, it typically occurs between 6 and 12 months postinjury (Burnett et al., 2003; Costanzo & Becker, 1990).

Damage to the ear is recognized as a common deficit associated with TBI; high-frequency hearing loss is correlated with severity of cortical injury (Munjal, Panda, & Pathak, 2010). Eighty to 90% of individuals with TBI who receive a longitudinal fracture of the temporal bone will experience a conductive hearing loss as a result of damage to the vestibulocochlear nerve (VIII). Positional vertigo has been found in 15% to 90% of people with mild brain injury (Ahn et al., 2011).

As oral feeding is attempted, damage to the glossopharyngeal (IX) and vagus (X) nerves in the medulla may become apparent. Dysfunction results in an absent or depressed gag reflex and decreased movement of the palate and uvula. This decreased oral-motor movement makes swallowing hazardous and may necessitate continued use of nasogastric or gastrostomy feeding tubes. In a seminal study of swallowing disorders in brain-injured patients, Lazarus and Logemann found that 81% of patients had a delayed or absent swallowing reflex, 50% demonstrated limited tongue control, and 33% had slowed peristalsis (Lazarus & Logemann, 1987). Morgan, in a more recent study of dysphagia in children with TBI, found that the incidence of dysphagia ranged from 1% in those with mild TBI to 68% to 76% for those with severe TBI (Morgan, 2010). **Aspiration**, or pathologic inhalation of food or mucus into the respiratory tract, was found in one-third of all persons with TBI. The presence of aspiration is highly correlated with the development of pneumonia, which may be life threatening. In later stages of recovery, there may be hypotonia of the oral musculature, resulting in drooling, limited lip closure and tongue control, pocketing of food in the cheek, and a delayed swallow trigger (Morgan, 2010).

Course and Prognosis

Response to and recovery from TBI tend to be highly individual, due to the variety of neuropathological effects that may be present, as well as individual factors of age, gender, and preinjury history. Persons with TBI, in general, may expect a reduced life expectancy by 9 years (Harrison-Felix et al., 2015). Furthermore, TBI "accounts for the greatest number of total years lived with a disability resulting from trauma" (p. 728) (Maas et al., 2008).

Significant functional, emotional, behavioral, and social difficulties remain for many years following injury. Useful factors in determining a person's prognosis are the trauma score, the GCS score, the presence of certain biomarkers, and the presence or absence of hypoxia. In addition,

consideration of neuroimaging studies and electro-diagnostic findings, length of coma and duration of posttraumatic amnesia help determine general psychosocial and functional outcomes (Gordon et al., 2006).

The GCS was the first scale developed to predict both mortality and outcome for the comatose patient and remains the best known and widely accepted scale of coma (Kornbluth & Bhardwaj, 2011). The Disability Rating Scale (DRS) (Fig. 20.3) has expanded on this information to provide a quantitative assessment of the disability of patients with severe brain injury. The DRS includes eight categories, including assessments of the cognitive components of self-care activities, the general level of functioning/dependence on others, and psychosocial skill/employability (Rappaport, Hall, & Hopkins, 1982). The DRS has demonstrated high interrater and test-retest reliability, as well as concurrent and predictive validity (Pretz, Malec, & Hammond, 2013).

The Levels of Cognitive Functioning Scale (LCFS) (Hagan, Malkmus, & Durham, 1972) (Fig. 20.4) is used in many rehabilitation programs. This scale classifies the admitted patient into one of eight levels of cognitive functioning and has been shown to have good interrater and test-retest reliability (Gouvier, Blanton, & LaPorte, 1987). Limitations for the scale are that it does not adequately reflect small changes in recovery, may not accurately place a patient with characteristics of two or more categories, and is less accurate at higher levels (Wright, 2000).

Level I of the LCFS is a period of dense unresponsiveness to all external stimuli. In level II, an inconsistent, nonpurposeful, and often delayed response to external stimuli is seen. Responses may be gross body movements, vocalizations, or physiologic changes such as sweating. Visual tracking of large objects is present, but the eyes appear unfocused. In level III, the level of localized response, there is an inconsistent but specific response to a strong stimulus such as pain or a bright object. An inconsistent response to simple verbal commands may be present. The person may respond to discomfort by pulling at nasogastric or catheter tubing. At level III, observational assessments of deficits of vision and/or visual perception, somatosensation, and movement may become feasible. Level IV is a highly variable stage, which may last for shorter or longer periods of time for the individual person. In level IV, the

TBI NATIONAL DATABASE COLLECTION FORM

Patient Name: _____ **Date of Rating:**_____

Name of Person Completing Form: _____

DISABILITY RATING SCALE:

Disability Rating Scale ratings to be completed within 72 hours after Rehab. Admission. And within 72 hours before Rehab. Discharge.

A. EYE OPENING:

☐ (0) Spontaneous
☐ (1) To Speech
☐ (2) To Pain
☐ (3) None

0-SPONTANEOUS: eyes open with sleep/wake rhythms indicating active arousal mechanisms, does not assume awareness.
1-TO SPEECH AND/OR SENSORY STIMULATION: a response to any verbal approach, whether spoken or shouted, not necessarily the command to open the eyes. Also, response to touch, mild pressure.
2-TO PAIN: tested by a painful stimulus.
3-NONE: no eye opening even to painful stimulation.

B. COMMUNICATION ABILITY:

☐ (0) Oriented
☐ (1) Confused
☐ (2) Inappropriate
☐ (3) Incomprehensible
☐ (4) None

0-ORIENTED: implies awareness of self and the environment. Patient able to tell you a) who he is; b) where he is; c) why he is there; d) year; e) season; f) month; g) day; h) time of day.
1-CONFUSED: attention can be held and patient responds to questions but responses are delayed and/or indicate varying degrees of disorientation and confusion.
2-INAPPROPRIATE: intelligible articulation but speech is used only in an exclamatory or random way (such as shouting and swearing); no sustained communication exchange is possible.
3-INCOMPREHENSIBLE: moaning, groaning or sounds without recognizable words, no consistent communication signs.
4-NONE: no sounds or communications signs from patient.

C. MOTOR RESPONSE:

☐ (0) Obeying
☐ (1) Localizing
☐ (2) Withdrawing
☐ (3) Flexing
☐ (4) Extending
☐ (5) None

0-OBEYING: obeying command to move finger on best side. If no response or not suitable try another command such as "move lips," "blink eyes," etc. Do not include grasp or other reflex responses.
1-LOCALIZING: a painful stimulus at more than one site causes limb to move (even slightly) in an attempt to remove it. It is a deliberate motor act to move away from or remove the source of noxious stimulation. If there is doubt as to whether withdrawal or localization has occurred after 3 or 4 painful stimulations, rate as localization.
2-WITHDRAWING: any generalized movement away from a noxious stimulus that is more than a simple reflex response
3-FLEXING: painful stimulation results in either flexion at the elbow, rapid withdrawal with abduction of the shoulder or a slow withdrawal with adduction of the shoulder. If there is confusion between flexing and withdrawing, then use pinprick on hands.
4-EXTENDING: painful stimulation results in extension of the limb.
5-NONE: no response can be elicited. Usually associated with hypotonia. Exclude spinal transection as an explanation of lack of response; be satisfied that an adequate stimulus has been applied.

D. FEEDING (COGNITIVE ABILITY ONLY)

☐ (0.0) Complete
☐ (1.0) Partial
☐ (2.0) Minimal
☐ (3.0) None

Does the patient show awareness of how and when to perform this activity? Ignore motor disabilities that interfere with carrying out this function. (This is rated under Level of Functioning described below.)
0-COMPLETE: continuously shows awareness that he knows how to feed and can convey unambiguous information that he knows when this activity should occur.
1-PARTIAL: intermittently shows awareness that he knows how to feed and/or can intermittently convey reasonably clearly information that he knows when the activity should occur.
2-MINIMAL: shows questionable or infrequent awareness that he knows in a primitive way how to feed and/or shows infrequently by certain signs, sounds, or activities that he is vaguely aware when the activity should occur.
3-NONE: shows virtually no awareness at anytime that he knows how to feed and cannot convey information by signs, sounds, or activity that he knows when the activity should occur.

E. TOILETING (COGNITIVE ABILITY ONLY)

☐ (0.0) Complete
☐ (1.0) Partial
☐ (2.0) Minimal
☐ (3.0) None

Does the patient show awareness of how and when to perform this activity? Ignore motor disabilities that interfere with carrying out this function. (This is rated under Level of Functioning described below.) Rate best response for toileting based on bowel and bladder behavior
0-COMPLETE: continuously shows awareness that he knows how to toilet and can convey unambiguous information that he knows when this activity should occur.
1-PARTIAL: intermittently shows awareness that he knows how to toilet and/or can intermittently convey reasonably clearly information that he knows when the activity should occur.
2-MINIMAL: shows questionable or infrequent awareness that he knows in a primitive way how to toilet and/or shows infrequently by certain signs, sounds, or activities that he is vaguely aware when the activity should occur.
3-NONE: shows virtually no awareness at anytime that he knows how to toilet and cannot convey information by signs, sounds, or activity that he knows when the activity should occur.

Figure 20.3 Disability rating scale.

F.GROOMING (COGNITIVE ABILITY ONLY)

☐ (0.0) Complete
☐ (1.0) Partial
☐ (2.0) Minimal
☐ (3.0) None

Does the patient show awareness of how and when to perform this activity? Ignore motor disabilities that interfere with carrying out this function. (This is rated under Level of Functioning described below.) Grooming refers to bathing, washing, brushing of teeth, shaving, combing or brushing of hair and dressing.
0-COMPLETE: continuously shows awareness that he knows how to groom self and can convey unambiguous information that he knows when this activity should occur.
1-PARTIAL: intermittently shows awareness that he knows how to groom self and/or can intermittently convey reasonably clearly information that he knows when the activity should occur.
2-MINIMAL: shows questionable or infrequent awareness that he knows in a primitive way how to groom self and/or shows infrequently by certain signs, sounds, or activities that he is vaguely aware when the activity should occur.
3-NONE: shows virtually no awareness at any time that he knows how to groom self and cannot convey information by signs, sounds, or activity that he knows when the activity should occur.

G.LEVEL OF FUNCTIONING (PHYSICAL, MENTAL, EMOTIONAL OR SOCIAL FUNCTION)

☐ (0.0) Completely Independent
☐ (1.0) Independent in special environment
☐ (2.0) Mildly Dependent—limited assistance (non-resid - helper)
☐ (3.0) Moderately Dependent—moderate assist (person in home)
☐ (4.0) markedly Dependent—assist all major activities, all times
☐ (5.0) Totally Dependent—24-hour nursing care

0-COMPLETELY INDEPENDENT: able to live as he wishes, requiring no restriction due to physical, mental, emotional or social problems.
1-INDEPENDENT IN SPECIAL ENVIRONMENT: capable of functioning independently when needed requirements are met (mechanical aids)
2-MILDLY DEPENDENT: able to care for most of own needs but requires limited assistance due to physical, cognitive and/or emotional problems (e.g., needs non-resident helper).
3-MODERATELY DEPENDENT: able to care for self partially but needs another person at all times. (person in home)
4-MARKEDLY DEPENDENT: needs help with all major activities and the assistance of another person at all times.
5-TOTALLY DEPENDENT: not able to assist in own care and requires 24-hour nursing care.

H."EMPLOYABILITY"(AS A FULL TIME WORKER, HOMEMAKER, OR STUDENT)

☐ (0.0) Not restricted
☐ (1.0) Selected jobs, competitive
☐ (2.0) Sheltered workshop, non-competitive
☐ (3.0) Not employable

0-NOT RESTRICTED: can compete in the open market for a relatively wide range of jobs commensurate with existing skills; or can initiate, plan, execute, and assume responsibilities associated with homemaking; or can understand and carry out most age relevant school assignments.
1-SELECTED JOBS, COMPETITIVE: can compete in a limited job market for a relatively narrow range of jobs because of limitations of the type described above and/or because of some physical limitations; or can initiate, plan, execute, and assume many but not all responsibilities associated with homemaking; or can understand and carry out many but not all school assignments.
2-SHELTERED WORKSHOP, NON-COMPETITIVE: cannot compete successfully in a job market because of limitations described above and/or because of moderate or severe physical limitations; or cannot without major assistance initiate, plan, execute, and assume responsibilities for homemaking; or cannot understand and carry out even relatively simple school assignments without assistance.
3-NOT EMPLOYABLE: completely unemployable because of extreme psychosocial limitations of the type described above, or completely unable to initiate, plan, execute, and assume any responsibilities associated with homemaking; or cannot understand or carry out any school assignments.

The psychosocial adaptability or "employability" item takes into account overall cognitive and physical ability to be an employee, homemaker, or student.
This determination should take into account considerations such as the following:
1. Able to understand, remember, and follow instructions.
2. Can plan and carry out tasks at least at the level of an office clerk or in simple routine, repetitive industrial situation or can do school assignments.
3. Ability to remain oriented, relevant, and appropriate in work and other psychosocial situations.
4. Ability to get to and from work or shopping centers using private or public transportation effectively.
5. Ability to deal with number concepts.
6. Ability to make purchases and handle simple money exchange problems
7. Ability to keep track of time and appointments.

Revised 03/2010

Figure 20.3 (Continued)

confused-agitated level, the person is confused and agitated, primarily responsive to internal stimuli, and unable to cooperate with treatment. Behavior may be aggressive, explosive, and nonpurposeful, with incoherent verbalization. As this behavior may be out of character for the person, it can upset family and friends and provide challenges for the treatment team. No short-term memory is present.

Attention is severely limited and is frequently driven by external stimuli. In the absence of motor deficits, sitting, standing, reaching, and ambulating are possible but do not occur purposefully or consistently on request (Hagan et al., 1972).

At level V, the confused-inappropriate-nonagitated level, more consistent motor response to requests becomes possible. Agitated

RANCHO LOS AMIGOS SCALE
AKA level of cognitive functioning scale (LCFS)

___(1)   **Level I** - *No response.*
Patient does not respond to external stimuli and appears asleep.

___(2)   **Level II** - *Generalized response.*
Patient reacts to external stimuli in nonspecific, inconsistent, and nonpurposeful manner with stereotypic and limited responses.

___(3)   **Level III** - *Localized response.*
Patient responds specifically and inconsistently with delays to stimuli, but may follow simple commands for motor action.

___(4)   **Level IV** - *Confused, agitated response.*
Patient exhibits bizarre, nonpurposeful, incoherent or inappropriate behaviors, has no short-term recall, attention is short and nonselective.

___(5)   **Level V** - *Confused, inappropriate, nonagitated response.*
Patient gives random, fragmented, and nonpurposeful responses to complex or unstructured stimuli—simple commands are followed consistently, memory and selective attention are impaired, and new information is not retained.

___(6)   **Level VI** - *Confused, appropriate, response.*
Patient gives context appropriate, goal-directed responses, dependent upon external input for direction. There is carry-over for relearned, but not for new tasks, and recent memory problems persist.

___(7)   **Level VII** - *Automatic, appropriate response.*
Patient behaves appropriately in familiar settings, performs daily routines automatically, and shows carry-over for new learning at lower than normal rates. Patient initiates social interactions, but judgment remains impaired.

___(8)   **Level VIII** - *Purposeful, appropriate response.*
Patient oriented and responds to the environment but abstract reasoning abilities are decreased relative to premorbid levels.

Figure 20.4 Levels of cognitive functioning scale.

and exaggerated behavior may still occur, especially in response to external stimuli. An inability to maintain selective attention is present, and frequent redirection is needed for any task completion. Simple social and automatic communication is possible but only for short periods of time. Memory is severely impaired and initiation is often limited. While the person may be physically able to complete simple self-care and feeding, verbal supervision is needed to accomplish tasks. The use of some selected formal or standardized assessments may become possible at level V.

In stages VI through VIII, the injured person becomes increasingly more aware of his or her person, the external environment, and other persons and is able to intentionally plan movement sequences. Responses to requests become consistently more appropriate, and the supervision level decreases for previously learned tasks. New academic learning is generally impaired until level VIII (Hagan et al., 1972).

Other factors, such as memory loss, age, and intracranial pressure, are also associated with outcome. Postinjury amnesia of <1 day suggests a mild injury, whereas amnesia lasting more than 1 day is indicative of a more severe injury. A younger age at injury improves both the chance of survival and overall outcome in adults. In children, higher death rates are associated with younger ages, and mortality below the age of 1 year is great, with abuse common as the primary cause (Craig, Campbell, Richards, Ventureya, & Hutchison, 2004).

■ Medical/Surgical Management
Acute Phase

Physicians from neurology, neurosurgery, internal medicine, or orthopedics may direct overall medical management in the acute phase. The focus of acute medical management is preservation of life, management of secondary complications and the prevention of secondary damage. Maintaining an effective airway and maintaining circulatory function are critical life-preserving steps immediately after injury. An endotracheal tube is typically placed to support breathing. After arrival at the hospital, diagnostic tests are begun to identify the location and severity of all injuries. The patient typically receives a computerized axial tomography scan (CAT). If this reveals an intracranial hematoma, immediate surgical decompression is performed. Constant monitoring of consciousness occurs, as the duration and depth of coma are significant indicators of both mortality and morbidity (Carlile et al., 2010). Diagnosis and management of secondary diagnoses also occur upon arrival at the hospital. Most persons with severe head injury have additional injuries (Eapen, Allred, O'Rourke, & Cifu, 2015). A common secondary complication from the brain injury is hydrocephalus, which is a serious complication for up to 4five percent of individuals with TBI (Eapen et al., 2015). Fractures are common as well, and 16% to 59% of persons with TBI have a concomitant spinal cord injury (Macciocchi, Seel, Thompson, Byams, & Bowman, 2008). In this case, immediate medical management is needed for both a brain injury and a high-level spinal cord injury .

Intensive care medical management is constant. An indwelling urinary catheter is placed and closely monitored. About one-third of those hospitalized with TBI aspirate food into their lungs, resulting in aspiration pneumonia. These persons usually have a delayed or absent swallowing reflex (Lazarus & Logemann, 1987; Logemann et al., 1994; Mackay et al., 1999). A nasogastric tube is positioned and used for high-caloric feeding for people with swallowing dysfunction. Close attention to skin integrity is essential, and the person's total body position is changed frequently. Vigorous respiratory therapy is typically implemented to prevent additional pulmonary problems (Wijayatilake et al., 2015).

Ongoing management of common medical complications occurs in the acute phase. Prophylactic medication for seizures is provided typically for only the first 7 days following injury and then discontinued unless the person has recurring seizures. As a result of rigid abnormal posturing and other motor disturbances, many persons with TBI develop contractures of the neck, trunk, and/or extremities. The longer the duration of coma, the greater is the potential for the development of contractures, heterotopic ossification, and DVTs. Treatment to prevent these complications commonly includes range of motion and splinting in the acute phase. Medical intervention for spasticity in the acute phase includes physical and pharmacological interventions. Commonly prescribed medications include baclofen, tizanidine, dantrolene, and botulinum toxin (Greenwald & Rigg, 2009).

Rehabilitation interventions in the acute phase may begin as soon as neurological stability is achieved. The focus of acute rehabilitation is to prevent joint deformity and to provide graded and specific sensory stimulation, with the assumption that selective sensory input may speed or improve neurological recovery.

REHABILITATION

Admission to an inpatient rehabilitation unit is needed for people with moderate to severe TBI. Reasonable and necessary requirements for admission to an inpatient rehabilitation facility are (1) medical stability, (2) the need for close medical supervision, and (3) the need for active and ongoing intensive therapy by multiple therapy disciplines (Department of Health and Human Services, 2015). Inpatient rehabilitation requires tolerance for at least 3 hours of two or more therapies 5 to 7 days per week; subacute rehabilitation requires the ability to participate for 0.5 to 2 hours each day. Intensive rehabilitation is usually directed by a physiatrist, a physician specializing in rehabilitation medicine. Goals of the rehabilitation program are to maximize the person's function, minimize additional physical or psychosocial impairments, and prevent complications (Greenwald & Rigg, 2009). Along with the primary physician, core rehabilitation members include specialists in occupational therapy, physical therapy, speech/language pathology, nursing, neuropsychology, and social work. In 2005, a major review of multidisciplinary rehabilitation of adults with TBI found "strong evidence of benefit from formal intervention," with earlier functional gains from more intensive programs (Turner-Stokes, Pick, Disler & Wade, 2015).

The long-term rehabilitation goals in occupational therapy are to re-establish occupational performance skill, sensorimotor integration and control, and the improvement of perceptual, cognitive, and communication skills for daily function. Where remediation is not possible or when maximal neurological recovery is assumed to be complete, the use of compensation strategies may be appropriate. As basic goals are accomplished, discharge from the hospital may occur, with more advanced skills learned on an outpatient basis. Outpatient occupational therapy goals include instrumental ADL, further community reintegration, and work reentry.

■ Impact of TBI on Occupational Performance

All areas identified in the Occupational Therapy Practice Framework are affected with TBI. The deeply comatose person, with cognitive levels I through III, shows depressed function in all areas of meaningful function. With further recovery, improvement in performance skills and patterns, as well as in client factors, may occur and enable the performance of preferred or required occupations. In a study of 1,170 records from the TBI Model Systems database, Bushnik et al. (2003) found that individuals with TBI as a result of a vehicular accident were initially admitted with significantly lower Functional Independence Measure motor scores than those who were admitted because of violence, falls, or other causes. However, at discharge from rehabilitation, no significant differences were found among patients in the four etiology groups for most psychosocial and functional outcome measures. In fact, 85% to 96% of all patients demonstrated sufficient basic ADL skills to live in a supervised private residence upon discharge.

Despite the acquisition of basic ADL skills, independence in community living is difficult for many people after TBI. A study of 147 survivors of severe TBI 4 years after injury found that 12% of participants were still impaired in common ADL after 4 years. These activities included the items of incontinence, grooming, toileting, bathing, dressing, and feeding as well as transfers, walking, and climbing. More than 50% of survivors needed help for activities such as using a bank account, paying household bills, managing appointments, and keeping track of money. Participants reported regular contacts with siblings, other relatives, and closest friends, but less often with other acquaintances. Few people participated in a professional activity (Jourdan et al., 2015).

■ Work

Many people have major difficulties returning to a productive life after TBI whether the injury is mild or severe. Roffolo, Friedland, and Dawson (1999) reported that while 42% of people with mild brain injury returned to work, only 12% returned to their premorbid level of employment. Cognitive and behavioral issues were cited for this decreased function. Bushnik et al. found the unemployment rate for persons with TBI because of violence to be 70%, significantly greater than the rate of approximately 50% for those with TBI from all other causes (Bushnik et al., 2003). An additional factor independently predicting poorer productivity outcomes was preinjury substance abuse (Sherer, Bergloff, & High, 1999).

For those with moderate to severe injuries, the ability to return to work has been inconsistently correlated with self-awareness. Sherer et al. (1998), in a multicenter TBI Model System study, found that limited self-awareness accounted for a substantial proportion (0.31) of the variance in positive vocational outcomes, while Coetzer and du Toit (2002) found no comparable correlation in their study of 40 people with TBI of varying levels of severity. In the absence of definitive findings to date, the difficulty of people with TBI to be aware of their deficits and the effect of their actions on others should be included in planning for return to productivity. Indeed, psychosocial skills that affect social integration show a stronger correlation with successful return to work than do either cognitive or sensorimotor skills, or any combination of the three factors (Conti, 1992).

Neither gender nor race has been consistently linked to productivity outcomes. A review by van Reekum found conflicting evidence that females had poorer outcomes, partly based on varying definitions of productivity (van Reekum, 2001). A major study of race and productivity (Sherer, Nick & Sander, 2003) found that African Americans and other people from minority backgrounds had less productive outcomes than did Whites, but race alone accounted for little of the variance in productivity. Race and productivity had confounding associations with preinjury productivity, educational level, and cause of injury.

The DRS (Rappaport et al., 1982) has been found to predict employment. In a study of 145 persons with TBI, Cope, Cole, and Hall (1999) found that 62% of those with scores of one to three on rehabilitation admission were employed or in school at 1 year after discharge, while 39% of those with scores of 4 to 6 and only 11% of those with a DRS score of 7 to 20 were similarly employed. For those returning to work, supported part-time employment has been shown to be a viable and cost-effective option (Cope et al., 1999). However, limited employment opportunities with typically lower wages and decreased work hours often result in the need for public assistance (Johnstone et al., 2003; Wehman et al., 2003b).

Driving

Physical disabilities; cognitive, visual, or perceptual dysfunction; and self-awareness deficits can significantly impair driving function. A number of studies have attempted to identify factors that predict those persons with TBI who may successfully return to driving, with inconclusive results (Coleman, Rapport, & Ergh, 2002; Pietrapiana et al., 2005; Rapport, Coleman, & Hanks, 2008). Severity of injury and duration of coma have not shown to impact driving consistently. One study found that persons more likely to return to driving included those discharged from rehabilitation with independence or modified independence in scores on the Functional Independence Measure (Fisk, Schneider, & Novak, 1998). Neuropsychological testing may provide insight into driving potential, but these findings may be limited by the person's level of self-awareness (Novack et al., 2010). Nevertheless, about 50% of people with moderate to severe TBI have resumed driving within 5 years, with most driving within the first year of injury (Novack et al., 2010; Rapport, Hanks, & Bryer, 2006). Tamietto and colleagues (2006) note, however, that as many as two-thirds of these may resume driving without any formal examination. In a study comparing nondrivers to drivers with TBI, Rapport et al. (2006) found that nondrivers who wanted to drive rated themselves as physically and cognitively fit to drive, despite cognitive skills that were significantly worse than drivers with TBI. In discussing this finding, Rapport et al. (2006) stated that "even nondrivers rate their current driving abilities as better than average (that) may reflect unawareness of deficit, denial, resistance to role change or accurate self-perception" (p. 42).

TUMORS OF THE CENTRAL NERVOUS SYSTEM

Descriptions and Definitions

Brain tumors, another category of ABI, have increased in the past few decades. Fortunately, this appears to be due to enhanced neuroimaging techniques and improved medical treatment options (Fisher, Schwartzbaum, Wrensch, & Wiemels, 2007) rather than a rise in natural incidence. Tumors are classified as primary or secondary and malignant or benign. The site of origin for the tumor is considered its primary site, even when the tumor has spread to other parts of the body or brain (secondary site). **Malignant tumors** are composed of abnormal cells that multiply rapidly, with the ability to invade, or **metastasize**, into other tissues. Brain tumors, conversely, rarely metastasize beyond the brain. There are four general categories of malignant brain tumors: gliomas, meningiomas, germ cell tumors, and sellar region tumors (Bondy et al., 2008; Fisher, Schwartzbaum, Wrensch, & Berger, 2006). **Benign tumors**, on the other hand, are not cancerous and they do not invade other body tissues or spread to other body parts. Benign tumors may become life threatening as they cause increasing deficits with cell growth, because they press upon nearby structures and tissues (Fisher et al., 2007). This section will discuss malignant primary brain tumors. However, the signs and symptoms of, and diagnosis, and treatment for, a secondary brain tumor are similar.

Etiology

Chemical changes in brain cells lead to the formation of brain tumors. However, why these changes occur is not fully understood. Most brain tumors develop for no apparent reason and are not associated with anything the person did or did not do.

The incidence of brain tumors in the United States has increased over time and differs according to gender, age, race and ethnicity, and geography. In the United States, the median age at diagnosis among all patients diagnosed with a primary brain tumor between 1998 and 2002 was 57 years. Gliomas are approximately twice as common among Caucasians as compared with African-Americans, as are germ cell tumors, while the incidence of glioma among non-Hispanics was greater than that of Hispanics (Fisher et al., 2007). The lowest age-adjusted average annual incidence of all CNS tumors is found in Virginia, while the highest incidence is present in Colorado (Fisher et al., 2007). Gender appears to be associated with risk for varying types of tumors. Men are more susceptible to glioma and germ cell tumors, while women are twice as likely as men to have meningiomas. In addition, relatively consistent research results show that being premenopausal confers a greater meningioma risk than being postmenopausal (Fisher et al., 2007).

High levels of ionizing radiation are strongly associated with tumor development, as was found following the atomic bombing of Hiroshima in World War II (Fisher et al., 2007). Types of tumors associated with radiation include glioma, schwannoma, and pituitary tumors. In the past, infants and children have been treated with radiation in the treatment of tinea capitis and skin hemangioma and have shown increased risk for nerve sheath tumors, meningioma, and pituitary adenoma. Taken as a whole, however, exposure to high levels of radiation is rare.

Many studies suggest that the risk for glioma is reduced as a result of allergies and immune-related conditions. This may arise from the anti-inflammatory effects of cytokines present in allergic and autoimmune diseases (Fisher et al., 2007). Inconsistent results have been found for exposure to other environmental factors. Studies of cell phone use and glioma risk do not generally support the conclusion that cell phone use causes brain tumors (Inskip et al., 2001; Kan, Simonsen, Lyon, & Kestle, 2007). However, long-term studies are needed to determine definitively any risk factor between cell phone use and glioma. Inconsistent, minimal, or no evidence is present to suggest any relationship with increased brain tumor risk and head trauma, certain dietary supplements, alcohol consumption, tobacco smoking, cellular phone use, and exposure to electromagnetic fields (Fisher et al., 2006, 2007). Inconclusive studies suggest that exposure to neurogenic or carcinogenic substances may be a risk factor. Therefore, occupations involving these substances may have a higher risk for brain tumors. Such occupations may include agricultural works, firefighters, petroleum and gas workers, construction workers, and janitors (Wrensch, Minn, Chew, Bondy, & Berger, 2002).

■ Incidence and Prevalence

About 22,070 persons were diagnosed with primary malignant brain tumors in 2009, including 12,060 men and 10,060 women (Central Brain Tumor Registry of the United States, 2014). An estimated 3,420 new cases of primary brain tumors were expected to occur in children in 2015, with the rate higher in boys than girls (Central Brain Tumor Registry of the United States, 2014). Incidence differs according to gender, age, race and ethnicity, and geography. Adult men tend to have higher rates than do women of primary malignant brain tumors, while nonmalignant meningioma is more common in women (Bondy et al., 2008).

Age affects the survival rate for both the youngest and oldest people. Childhood cancer is the second leading cause of death (after accidents) in children between 1 and 14 years (American Cancer Society, 2014). They are also the third leading cause of death in young adults ages 20 to 39 (Jemal, Siegel, Xu, & Ward, 2010). In general, and for most tumors, the 5-year survival rate increases with age (Bondy et al., 2008) through the fifties and early sixties.

Studies of race and ethnicity are confounded by issues related to low socioeconomic status. African Americans are more likely to develop tumors than any other racial or ethnic group, and death rates from cancer are 34% higher for African American men and 17% higher for African American women than their Caucasian counterparts. Hispanic people tend to have lower incidence rates for cancer. These figures must be placed in context with concerns of poverty. About 25% of African Americans and Hispanic Americans lived below the poverty line during the period from 2007 to 2011. By comparison, only 11% of non-Hispanic White people lived below the poverty line (Macartney, Bishaw, & Fontenot, 2013). Furthermore, one in five African Americans and one in three Hispanic persons were uninsured and therefore less able to receive needed treatment. Finally, issues of health disparity may play a role in the provision of health care. Racial and ethnic minorities tend to receive a lower quality of care than do Whites, even when insurance status, income, age, and severity of conditions are comparable (Institute of Medicine, 2002).

Cancer rates tend to be higher in more developed countries, partly due to greater technology resources for evaluation and treatment.

■ Signs and Symptoms

Signs and symptoms of brain tumors include fatigue, sleep disturbance, pain, mood disorders, and cognitive dysfunction. Fatigue may be the single most significant problem with brain tumors, resulting in increased daytime sleep and decreased or interrupted nighttime sleep. Nightly sleep disturbance is reported by up to 50% of people with brain tumors (Liu, Page, Solheim, Fox, & Chang, 2009). One study of people with recurrent malignant gliomas found that as many as 94% reported severe fatigue (Osoba, Brada, Prados & Yung, 2000).

Headache is the most common type of pain experienced, with up to 50% of people with gliomas reporting severe pain. Mood disorders accompanying brain tumors include anxiety and depression. Depression particularly has been linked to survival, and yet, one study found that only 60% of people who reported this to their physician received antidepressants (Litofsky et al., 2004). Problems with memory and executive functions are found in almost half of all people with glioma tumors (Liu et al., 2009).

Course and Prognosis

In general, survival from any tumor is lowest in the oldest age groups. When types of tumors are examined, the relative survival probability of those with glioblastomas is the lowest, with a 37.7% 2-year survival rate and a 30.2% 5-year survival rate. The survival rates for benign meningioma are much less well known but appear to be significantly better. One estimate is that the 5-year survival rate for meningioma may be 81% for people aged 21 to 64 years and 56% for those 65 or older at diagnosis (McCarthy, Davis, & Freels, 1998).

Diagnosis

Diagnosis begins with the onset of unexplained symptoms. As tumor cells multiply in the brain, they create pressure on and irritate normal brain tissue. As a result, two-thirds of those with primary brain tumors report symptoms as just described. Amazingly, about one-third of all people with brain tumors have no symptoms initially.

The presence of symptoms is typically assessed by a neurologist, with the use of such diagnostic procedures as magnetic resonance imaging (MRI), computerized tomography (CT), positron emission tomography (PET), or biopsy. The MRI uses an extremely strong magnet and radio waves to produce brain images. It may or may not be used with angiography, in which a dye is inserted into the bloodstream to differentiate between healthy and tumor tissue. People receiving an MRI may not have pacemakers or metal implants or be allergic to the dye used in angiography. CT scans involve multiple x-rays of the brain from different angles. From this, a computerized three-dimensional model of the brain can be displayed. Iodine is commonly used as a contrast agent to enhance the image. As a result, this may not be the best diagnostic procedure for people with allergies, diabetes, or a heart, kidney, or thyroid condition. PET scans are typically an ancillary diagnostic tool to either the MRI or PET scan. Finally, a biopsy of the suspected brain tissue may be made. Following the biopsy surgery, histologic analysis of brain cell tissue occurs (American Cancer Society, 2015d).

In most cancer, an important next step is to determine the stage of the tumor. However, brain tumors rarely spread to other organs, although they may spread within the brain. Therefore, there is no formal staging system for the prognosis of brain tumor. Instead, the oncologist will use the following information to determine the outlook: the type of tumor, the grade of the tumor (how quickly it can be expected to spread), the person's age, the person's functional status (whether symptoms are present or not), the size and location of the tumor, the feasibility of surgical removal of the tumor, and whether there is evidence of spread to other parts of the brain and/or spinal cord (American Cancer Society, 2015d).

Medical/Surgical Management

Management of brain tumors may involve surgery, radiation therapy, and/or chemotherapy. Surgery is now more sophisticated than in the past. It can now be guided at least partially by the use of MRI, to determine locations of important brain areas and their distance from a tumor. Surgery also may be directly aided by image-guidance, which provides better visualization of the brain area (American Cancer Society, 2015d).

Radiation therapy uses x-rays, gamma rays, electron beams, or protons to destroy cancer cells. Because radiation can be localized, it affects only the body part being treated. It may be used alone or in combination with surgery or chemotherapy, where some drugs may actually make cancer cells more sensitive to radiation. Radiation may be given externally, using a linear accelerator, or internally, where a radioactive source in an implant is surgically placed near the tumor (American Cancer Society, 2015a, 2015d).

Significant improvements have occurred to radiation therapy recently, allowing smaller doses of radiation and more precise placement of the radiation. Stereotactic radiosurgery is not really surgery but the delivery of precise radiation to a brain site guided by MRI or CT scans. Nearby tissue is affected as little as possible. Types of stereotactic radiosurgery include using a moving linear accelerator, the Gamma Knife, or the use of accelerator-delivered proton and helium ions. Stereotactic radiosurgery typically uses just one treatment session to deliver the full radiation dose (American Cancer Society, 2015a).

Common side effects of radiation therapy, requiring medical management, include fatigue, fever/chills, and a sore or dry mouth. Because radiation therapy to the brain may increase the chance of tooth cavities, ongoing dental consultations are advised. Hair loss also is a common side effect (American Cancer Society, 2015b). While this is not a dangerous side effect, it is often distressing to the person.

Newer approaches to chemotherapy are also available. Traditionally, chemotherapy drugs have had difficulty crossing the blood-brain barrier. Research is currently underway to modify these drugs to successfully cross the barrier, so that they can reach more easily the bloodstream in the brain. Some targeted drug treatments have been developed that focus on specific abnormalities within cancer cells. These treatments are very new and are still undergoing rigorous study in clinical trials (American Cancer Society, 2015c).

The schedule for chemotherapy is dependent on a number of factors and may be provided daily, weekly, or even monthly. After each treatment cycle, a break is provided to allow the body time to rebuild healthy new cells and recuperate from the strong chemicals used. Common side effects of chemotherapy include fatigue, nausea, vomiting, sore mouth, diarrhea or constipation, loss of appetite, pain or difficulty swallowing, swelling in hands or feet, itching or rash, shortness of breath, cough, muscle or joint pain, or numbness in hands or feet (American Cancer Society, 2015b).

In addition to chemotherapy, the medications most commonly prescribed for brain tumors are steroids and anti-epileptic drugs. Steroids are used to reduce brain edema and ameliorate the person's symptoms. They may be prescribed at diagnosis or before or after surgery. Common steroids include dexamethasone, Decadron, prednisone, or methylprednisone. Short-term side effects include insomnia, weight gain and increased appetite, mood swings, and irritability. Side effects from long-term use include cataracts, osteoporosis, muscle weakness, and diabetes (University of California San Francisco, 2012).

Antiepileptic medications may be used as a precautionary measure or in response to seizure activity. Common anticonvulsant drugs include Dilantin, Tegretol, Depakote, Keppra, Neurontin, Topamax, phenobarbital and Lamictal. Side effects from these medications include fatigue, weakness, nausea and vomiting, and incoordination.

Complementary and alternative therapies may also be used, not to replace medical treatment but to lessen symptoms. Complementary therapies may include stress management, relaxation and imagery training, meditation, acupuncture, herbal medicine, and massage.

Education and support are critical throughout the course of treatment. Support groups may be helpful to both the person with cancer and his or her caregivers. Additionally, individual or family counseling may provide additional support and individual-specific information.

■ Impact on Occupational Performance

While rates of survival have improved for some types of cancer, most people consider a tumor to be deadly. Values and beliefs may be in conflict. For example, a highly valued commitment to honesty may conflict with the desire not to cause others distress. A basic belief in fairness may be shaken by the timing of the diagnosis. Spiritual beliefs may be overturned, or spirituality may grow.

Mental functions are likely to decline, as well as movement-related skills, vision, and/or communication, depending on the site of the tumor. Pain is likely to increase. Fatigue and side effect from medical treatment may make participation in all daily activities and preferred occupations difficult. While ADL may or may not remain intact for a considerable amount of time, instrumental activities such as work and leisure pursuits are likely to suffer fairly quickly from both physical dysfunction and cognitive deficits. Rest may be disrupted and daytime sleep ineffective in decreasing perceptions of fatigue. In a study comparing people with malignant glioma to age- and gender-matched people with lung cancer, greater problems with vision, motor function, communication, headaches and seizures were identified by the people with glioma (Klein, Taphoorn, & Heimans, 2001).

Both TBI and brain tumors result in physical, cognitive, and social-emotional deficits affecting all areas of occupation. For the occupational therapist, assessment and intervention are challenging, at times frustrating, and ultimately rewarding.

CASE STUDY 1

John, age 20, survived an automobile accident, with a moderate TBI. After 2 weeks each in intensive care and an acute medical unit, he is to begin intensive rehabilitation. His occupational therapist cannot get reliable information from him, so she relies on a medical record review for his medical history and a discussion with his mother to identify his previous occupations.

His mother does not seem to be very aware of his activities. She states that he has had three garage mechanic jobs in the last 2 years. She says he seemed to get tired of a routine and didn't get along well with his bosses. He moved into her two-bedroom apartment about 6 months ago so he could start saving money for a new car. He does not participate in any home care tasks but does help with the rent. Leisure activities included fixing up his old car and "hot-rodding" around. John's mother does not care for many of his friends, but becomes tearful when asked about his relationship with Kathy. She says they were planning to be married in the fall.

The medical record review reveals that John sustained a right tibia-fibula fracture with the TBI. After 3 days of general unresponsiveness, he began to obey simple commands (LCFS III). In a few days, he became agitated and confused. A few words could be understood, including swear words. He persistently pulled out both his urinary catheter and his nasogastric tube.

The agitation has lessened somewhat, but he continues to be intermittently disoriented, as when he calls his occupational therapist "Kathy." There is a 1- to 2-second delay before any requested movement. His gaze appears divergent. When fatigued or perhaps frustrated, he is irritable and the therapist has used protective measures she was taught to protect both herself and John from injury as he jabs his fist out toward her.

Motor deficits include poor sitting balance and right hemiplegia, with moderate to severe spasticity. The left upper extremity is within functional limits in range of motion and strength. Transfers require moderate assistance.

John is independent in eating but requires assistance for all other tasks. He requires moderate assistance and verbal cuing for showering using a shower chair, donning and doffing a T-shirt, and transferring to and from the bed and wheelchair. Wheelchair mobility is slow, but he can wheel himself from one area to another with verbal cuing for the route. John is unable to read, and perseveration is apparent when writing his name. John has come a long way, but there is still a longer way to go to achieve maximal possible independence.

Case Study 2

As a part of routine fourth-grade vision screening, the school nurse noticed that Jesus appeared to have some vision problems that weren't present last year. Jesus said things seemed fuzzy. She sent a note home with Jesus to his mother but never received a response. Six weeks later, his teacher sent Jesus to see the school nurse again, this time because of ongoing complaints of a headache. While with the nurse, Jesus vomited and said that he had been routinely vomiting for the last few weeks. He had no fever. Alarmed, the school nurse drove Jesus home to the trailer in which he and his mother, brother and two sisters lived.

She spoke to the mother and stressed the need for immediate evaluation by a physician. Maria, his mother, stated that she had no physician and no insurance, and that the only medical care she and her family received was at the free clinic, open only on Tuesday afternoons and evenings. The school nurse wrote out information for the doctor there, and Maria promised to take Jesus to the next clinic.

The physician at the clinic examined Jesus and immediately set Jesus up for an evaluation by a pediatric oncologist. Social workers at the clinic assisted in finding transportation, and assured Maria that medical care would be provided despite her inability to pay. The visit to the pediatric oncologist provided a diagnosis of glioma. This message was sent to the social worker at the clinic, where there was a telephone. The social worker drove to Maria's to give Maria this information and to plan how to achieve the medical care

Jesus needed. School was put on the back burner. Jesus entered a regional children's cancer center. Maria arranged for the other children to stay with an aunt and stays near the center.

It was a confusing and fun and sad time for Jesus. He missed his friends and his family, but he enjoyed the activities of the center. He did not like how he felt after radiation therapy, and it was hard to understand that something that made him feel so bad could make him better. He was glad his mother was around and, for the first time in years, spent time sitting on her lap.

Jesus came home, to a great family celebration. Maria ended the celebration after an hour, seeing that Jesus was tired. But Jesus was happy to be home. He didn't care that he had no hair, because he was beginning to feel better, even though he tired easily. He missed his friends at school and hoped to go back soon, but he knew he still couldn't see well. Maria feared for the future of Jesus and her family and worried about bills that would certainly come.

RECOMMENDED LEARNING RESOURCES

Brain Injury Association of America
1608 Spring Hill Road
Suite 110
Vienna, VA 22182
Phone: 703-761-0750
braininjuryinfo@biausa.orghttp://www.biausa.org

National Institute of Neurologic Disorders and Stroke (NINDS).
Traumatic Brain Injury Information Page
http://www.ninds.nih.gov/disorders/tbi/tbi.htm

Family Caregiver Alliance/National Center on Caregiving
785 Market St.
Suite 750
San Francisco, CA 94103
Tel: 415-434-3388, 800-445-8106
info@caregiver.org
http://www.caregiver.org

American Brain Tumor Association
8550 W. Bryn Mawr Ave.
Suite 550
Chicago, IL 60631
773-577-8750, CareLine: 800-866-2282
info@abta.org

REFERENCES

Adams, J. H., Graham, D. I., & Murray, L. S. (1982). Diffuse axonal injury due to non-missile head injury in humans. *Annals of Neurology, 12,* 557–663.

Ahn, S.-K., Jeon, S.-Y., Kim, J.-P., Park, J. J., Hur, D. G., Kim, D.-W., … Kim, J.-Y. (2011). Clinical characteristics and treatment of benign paroxysmal positional vertigo after traumatic brain injury. *Journal of Trauma, 70,* 442–446. doi: 10.1097/TA.0b013e3181d0c3d9

American Cancer Society (Producer). (2014). *Facts and Figures report outlines progress and challenges in childhood cancer.* Retrieved from http://www.cancer.org/cancer/news/news/facts-figures-report-outlines-progress-and-challenges-in-childhood-cancer

American Cancer Society. (2015a). *How are brain and spinal cord tumors in adults treated?* Retrieved from http://www.cancer.org/cancer/braincnstumorsinadults/detailedguide/brain-and-spinal-cord-tumors-in-adults-treating-general-info

American Cancer Society. (2015b). *Treatments and side effects.* Retrieved from http://www.cancer.org/treatment/treatmentsandsideeffects/index

American Cancer Society. (2015c). *What's new in research and treatment for brain and spinal cord tumors in children?* Retrieved from http://www.cancer.org/cancer/braincnstumorsinchildren/detailedguide/brain-and-spinal-cord-tumors-in-children-new-research

American Cancer Society. (2015d). *What do doctors look for in biopsy and cytology specimens?* Retrieved from http://www.cancer.org/treatment/understandingyourdiagnosis/examsandtest-descriptions/testingbiopsyandcytologyspecimensforcancer/testing-biopsy-and-cytology-specimens-for-cancer-what-doctors-look-for

American Psychiatric Association. (2013). *Diagnostic and statistical manual of mental disorders* (5th ed.). Arlington, VA: American Psychiatric Association.

Anderson, F. A. J., Wheeler, H. B., & Goldberg, R. J. (1991). A population-based perspective of the hospital incidence and case-fatality rates of deep vein thrombosis and pulmonary embolism. The Worcester DVT study. *Archives of Internal Medicine, 151,* 933–938.

Annegers, J. F., Hauser, W. A., & Coan, S. P. (1998). A population-based study of seizures after traumatic brain injuries. *New England Journal of Medicine, 338*(1), 20–24.

Baguley, I. J., Nicholls, J. L., & Felmingham, K. L. (1999). Dysautonomia after traumatic brain injury: A forgotten syndrome? *Journal of Neurology, Neurosurgery, and Psychiatry, 67,* 39–43.

Bazarian, J. I., McClung, J., & Shah, M. N. (2005). Mild acquired brain injury in the United States, 1998–2000. *Brain Injury, 19,* 85–91.

Binder, S., Corrigan, J. D., & Langlois, J. A. (2005). The public health approach to traumatic brain injury: An overview of CDC's research and programs. *Journal of Head Trauma Rehabilitation, 20,* 189–195.

Bogner, J. A., Corrigan, J. D., & Mysiw, J. (2001). A comparison of substance abuse and violence in the prediction of long-term rehabilitation outcomes after acquired brain injury. *Archives of Physical Medicine and Rehabilitation, 82,* 571–577.

Bondy, M. L., Scheurer, M. E., Malmer, B., Barnholtz-Sloan, J. S., Davis, F. G., Il'yasova, D., ... Buffler, P. A. (2008). Brain tumor epidemiology: Consensus from the brain tumor epidemiology consortium. *Cancer, 113*(7 Suppl.), 1953–1968.

Bruns, J. J. (2003). The epidemiology of acquired brain injury. *Epilepsia, 44,* 2–10.

Burnett, D. M., Watanabe, T. K., & Greenwald, B. D. (2003). Congenital and acquired brain injury. 2. Brain injury rehabilitation: Medical Management. *Archives of Physical Medicine and Rehabilitation, 84*(Suppl. 1), S8–S11.

Bushnik, T., Hanks, R. A., Kreutzer, J., & Rosenthal, M. (2003). Etiology of brain injury: Characterization of different outcomes up to 1 year postinjury. *Archives of Physical Medicine and Rehabilitation, 84,* 255–262.

Carlile, M., Nicewander, D., Yablon, S. A., Brown, A., Brunner, R., Burke, D., ... Diaz-Arrastia, R. (2010). Prophylaxis for venous thromboembolism during rehabilitation for traumatic brain injury: A multicenter observational study. *Journal of Trauma, 68*(4), 916–923. doi: 10.1097/TA.0b013e3181b16d2d

Costanzo, R. M., & Becker, D. P. (1990). Smell and taste disorders in head injury and neurosurgery patients. In R. L. Meiselman & R. S. Rivlin (Eds.), *Clinical measurement of taste and smell.* New York, NY: Macmillan

Centers for Disease Control and Prevention. (2001). Acquired brain injury in the United States: A report to congress. Retrieved from http://www.cdc.gov/ncipc/TBI/TBI-congress/index.htm

Centers for Disease Control and Prevention. (2014). *Severe Traumatic Brain Injury.* Retrieved from http://www.cdc.gov/TraumaticBrainInjury/severe.html

Central Brain Tumor Registry of the United States. (2014). *2014 CBTRUS Fact Sheet.* Retrieved from http://www.cbtrus.org/2010-NPCR-SEER/CBTRUS-WEBREPORT-Final-3-2-10.pdf

Cicerone, K., Dahlberg, C., & Kalmar, K. (2000). Evidence-based cognitive rehabilitation: Recommendations for clinical practice. *Archives of Physical Medicine and Rehabilitation, 81,* 1596–1615.

Cifu, D. X., Kaelin, D. L., & Wall, B. E. (1996). Deep venous thrombosis: Incidence on admission to a brain-injury rehabilitation program. *Archives of Physical Medicine and Rehabilitation, 77*(11), 1182–1185.

Ciuffreda, K. J., Ludlam, D. P., & Kapoor, N. (2009). Clinical oculomotor training in traumatic brain injury. *Optometry and Vision Development, 40,* 16–23.

Coetzer, B. R., & Du Toit, P. L. (2002). Impaired awareness following brain injury and its relationship to placement and employment outcomes. *Journal of Cognitive Rehabilitation, 20,* 20–24.

Coleman, R. D., Rapport, L. J., & Ergh, T. C. (2002). Predictors of driving outcome after traumatic brain injury. *Archives of Physical Medicine and Rehabilitation, 83,* 1415–1422.

Conti, G. E. (1992). *Factors affecting return to work for persons with traumatic brain injury (Unpublished thesis).* Eastern Michigan University, Michigan.

Cope, D. N., Cole, J. R., & Hall, K. M. (1999). Brain injury: Analysis of outcome in post-acute rehabilitation system. Part I: General analysis. *Brain Injury, 5,* 111–125.

Corrigan, J. D. (1995). Substance abuse as a mediating factor in outcome from acquired brain injury. *Archives of Physical Medicine and Rehabilitation, 76,* 302–309.

Corrigan, J. D., Selassie, A. W., & Orman, J. A. (2010). The epidemiology of traumatic brain injury. *Journal of Head Trauma Rehabilitation, 25*(2), 72–80.

Craig, G. N., Campbell, S. M. K., Richards, P. M. P., Ventureya, E., & Hutchison, J. S. (2004). Medical and cognitive outcome in children with traumatic brain injury. *The Canadian Journal of Neurological Science, 31,* 213–219.

Cummings, P., Rivara, F. P., Olson, E. M., & Smith, K. M. (2006). Chances in traffic crash mortality rates attributed to use of alcohol, or lack of a seat belt, air bag, motorcycle helmet, or bicycle helmet. *Injury Prevention, 12,* 148–154.

Cunningham, R. M., Maio, R. F., Hill, E. M., & Zink, B. J. (2002). The effects of alcohol on head injury in the motor vehicle crash victim. *Alcohol, 37,* 236–240.

Dawodu, S. T. (2005). Acquired brain injury: Definition, epidemiology, pathophysiology. *eMedicine.*

De Bonis, P., Pompucci, A., Mangiola, A., Rigante, I., & Anile, C. (2010). Post-traumatic hydrocephallus after decompressive craniectomy. *Journal of Neurotrauma, 27*(11), 1965–1970.

Department of Health and Human Services. (2015). Inpatient rehabilitation facility prospective payment system. *Payment System Series.* ICN006874.

Dijkstra, A., Kazimier, H., & Halfens, R. J. (2015). Using the care dependency scale for identifying patients at risk for pressure ulcer. *Journal of Advanced Nursing, 71*(11), 2529–2539. doi: 10.1111/jan.12713

Drew, L. B., & Drew, W. E. (2004). The contrecoupcoup phenomenon. A new understanding of the mechanism of closed head injury. *Neurocritical Care, 1,* 385–390.

Dumas, H. M., Haley, S. M., Carey, T. M., Ludlow, L. H., & Rabin, J. P. (2003). Lower extremity spasticity as an early marker of ambulatory recovery following traumatic brain injury. *Childs Nervous System, 19,* 114–118.

Eapen, B. C., Allred, D. B., O'Rourke, J. O., & Cifu, D. X. (2015). Rehabilitation of moderate-to-severe traumatic brain injury. *Seminars in Neurology, 35,* e1–e13. doi: 10.1055/s-0035-1549094

Engberg, A. W., & Teasdale, T. W. (2004). Psychosocial outcome following traumatic brain injury in adults: A long-term population-based follow-up. *Brain Injury, 18,* 533–545.

Fay, G. C., Jaffe, K. M., Polissar, M. L., Liao, S., Rivara, J. B., & Martin, K. M. (1994). Outcome of pediatric traumatic brain injury at 3 years: A cohort study. *Archives of Physical Medicine and Rehabilitation, 75,* 733–741.

Fisher, J. L., Schwartzbaum, J. A., Wrensch, M., & Berger, M. S. (2006). Evaluation of epidemiological evidence for primary adult brain tumor risk factors using evidence-based medicine. *Progressive Neurological Surgery, 19,* 54–79.

Fisher, J. L., Schwartzbaum, J. A., Wrensch, M., & Wiemels, J. L. (2007). Epidemiology of brain tumors. *Neurologic Clinics, 25,* 867–890.

Fisk, G., Schneider, J., & Novak, T. (1998). Driving following traumatic brain injury: Prevalence, exposure, advice, and evaluations. *Brain Injury, 12,* 683–695.

Frey, L. C. (2003). Epidemiology of posttraumatic epilepsy: A critical review. *Epilepsia, 44*(Suppl 10), 11–17.

Goodrich, G. L., Flyg, H. M., Kirby, J. E., Chang, C. Y., & Martinsen, G. L. (2013). Mechanisms of TBI and visual consequences in military and veteran populations. *Optometry and Visual Science, 90*(2), 105–112. doi: 10.1097/OPX.0b013e31827f15a1

Gordon, W. A., Zafonte, R., Cicerone, K., Cantor, J., Brown, M., Lombard, L., … Chandna, T. (2006). Traumatic brain injury rehabilitation: State of the science. *American Journal of Physical Medicine and Rehabilitation, 65*(4), 343–382.

Gouvier, W. D., Blanton, P. D., & LaPorte, K. K. (1987). Reliability and validity of the disability rating scale and the levels of cognitive functioning scale in monitoring recovery from severe head injury. *Archives of Physical Medicine and Rehabilitation, 68,* 94–97.

Guidelines for the management of severe head injury: A joint initiative of the Brain Trauma Foundation, the American Association of Neurological Surgeons, the Joint Section on Neurotrauma and Critical Care: Brain Trauma Foundation. (2007). *Journal of Neurotrauma, 24*(Suppl. 1). doi: 10.1089/neu.2007.9999

Greenwald, B. D., & Rigg, J. L. (2009). Neurorehabilitation in traumatic brain injury: Does it make a difference? *Mount Sinai Journal of Medicine, 76,* 182–189.

Hagan, C., Malkmus, D., & Durham, P. (1972). *Levels of cognitive functioning.* Downey, CA: Rancho Los Amigos Hospital.

Harrison-Felix, C., Pretz, C., Hammond, F., Cuthbert, J. P., Bell, J., Corrigan, J., … Haarbauer-Krupa, J. (2015). Life expectancy after inpatient rehabilitation for traumatic brain injury in the United States. *Journal of Neurotrauma, 32,* 1893–1901. doi: 10.1089/neu.2014.3353

Hawley, C. A. (2004). Behavior and school performance after head injury. *Brain Injury, 18,* 645–659.

Hendricks, H. T., Heeren, A. H., & Vos, P. E. (2010). Dysautonomia after severe traumatic brain injury. *European Journal of Neurology, 17*, 1172–1177.

Huang, Y.-H., Liao, C.-C., Chen, W.-F., & Ou, C.-Y. (2015). Characterization of acute post-craniectomy seizures in traumatically brain-injured patients. *Seizure, 25*, 150–154.

Hulkower, M. B., Poliak, D. B., Rosenbaum, S. B., Zimmerman, M. E., & Lipton, M. L. (2013). A decade of DTI in traumatic brain injury: 10 Years and 100 articles later. *AJNR American Journal of Neuroradiology, 34*, 2064–2074. doi: 10.3174/ajnr. A3395

Humphreys, I., Wood, R. L., Phillips, C. J., & Macey, S. (2013). The costs of traumatic brain injury: A literature. *ClinicoEconomics and Outcomes Research, 5*, 281–287. Retrieved from http://www. ncbi.nlm.nih.gov/pmc/articles/PMC3699059/pdf/ ceor-5-281.pdf

Inskip, P. T., Tarone, R. E., Hatch, E. E., Wilcosky, T. C., Shapiro, W. R., Selker, R. G., … Linet, M. S. (2001). Cellular-telephone use and brain tumors. *The New England Journal of Medicine, 344*(2), 79–86.

Institute of Medicine. (2002). *Unequal treatment: What healthcare providers need to know about racial and ethnic disparities in healthcare.* Retrieved from https://iom.nation- alacademies.org/~/media/Files/Report%20 Files/2003/Unequal-Treatment-Confronting- Racial-and-Ethnic-Disparities-in-Health-Care/ Disparitieshcproviders8pgFINAL.pdf

Jallo, J. I., & Narayan, R. K. (2000). Craniocerebral trauma. In W. G. Bradley, R. B. Daroff, & G. M. Fenichel (Eds.), *Neurology in clinical practice*. Boston, MA: Butterworth-Heinemann.

Jemal, A., Siegel, R., Xu, J., & Ward, E. (2010). Cancer statistics 2010. *CA: A Cancer Journal for Clinicians, 60*, 277–300.

Johnstone, B., Mount, D., & Schopp, L. H. (2003). Financial and vocational outcomes 1 year after acquired brain injury. *Archives of Physical Medicine and Rehabilitation, 84*, 238–241.

Jourdan, C., Bayen, E., Pradat-Diehl, P., Ghout, I., Darnoux, E., Azerad, S., … Azouvi, P. (2015). A comprehensive picture of 4-year outcome of severe brain injuries. Results from the PariS-TBI study. *Annals of Physical and Rehabilitation Medicine.* doi: http://dx.doi.org/10.1016/j.rehab.2015.10.009

Kan, P., Simonsen, S. E., Lyon, J. L., & Kestle, J. R. W. (2007). Cellular phone use and brain tumor: A meta-analysis. *Journal of Neurooncology, 86*, 71–78. doi: 10.1007/s11060-007-9432-1

Kandel, E. R., Schwartz, J. H., Jessell, T. M., Siegelbaum, S. A., & Hudspeth, A. J. (2012). *Principles of neural science* (5th ed.). New York, NY: McGraw-Hill.

Keane, J. R., & Baloh, R. W. (1992). Posttraumatic cranial neuropathies. *The Neurology of Trauma, 10*(4), 849–867.

Klein, M., Taphoorn, M. J., & Heimans, J. J. (2001). Neurobehavioral status and health-related quality of life in newly diagnosed high-grade glioma patients. *Journal of Clinical Oncology, 19*, 4037–4047.

Kornbluth, J., & Bhardwaj, A. (2011). Evaluation of coma: A critical appraisal of popular scoring sys- tems. *Neurocritical Care, 14*(1), 134–143.

Kreutzer, J. S., Seel, R. T., & Gourley, E. (2001). The prevalence and symptom rates of depression after traumatic brain injury: A comprehensive examina- tion. *Brain Injury, 15*(7), 563–576.

Lazarus, C., & Logemann, J. (1987). Swallowing dis- orders in closed head trauma patients. *Archives of Physical Medicine and Rehabilitation, 68*, 79–84.

Litofsky, N. S., Farace, E., Anderson, F. A. J., Meyers, C. A., Huang, W., & Laws, E. R. J. (2004). Depression in patients with high-grade glioma: Results of the glioma outcome project. *Neurosurgery, 54*, 358–367.

Liu, R., Page, M., Solheim, K., Fox, S., & Chang, S. M. (2009). Quality of life in adults with brain tumors: Current knowledge and future directions. *NeuroOncology, 11*, 330–339.

Logemann, J. A., Pepe, J., & Mackey, L. E. (1994). Disorders of nutrition and swallowing: Intervention strategies in the trauma center. *Journal of Head Trauma Rehabilitation, 9*, 43–56.

Maas, A. I. R., Stochetti, N., & Bullock, R. (2008). Moderate and severe traumatic brain injury in adults. *Lancet Neurology, 7*, 738–741.

Macartney, S., Bishaw, A., & Fontenot, K. (2013). *Poverty rates for selected detailed race and hispanic groups by state and place: 2007–2011.* Retrieved from https://www.census.gov/ prod/2013pubs/acsbr11-17.pdf

Macciocchi, S., Seel, R. T., Thompson, N., Byams, R., & Bowman, B. (2008). Spinal cord injury and co-occurring traumatic brain injury: Assessment and incidence. *Archives of Physical Medicine and Rehabilitation, 89*(7), 1350–1357. doi: 10.1016/j. apmr.2007.11.055

Mackay, L. E., Morgan, A. S., & Bernstein, B. A. (1999). Factors affecting oral feeding with severe traumatic brain injury. *Journal of Head Trauma Rehabilitation, 14*(5), 435–437.

McCarthy, B. J., Davis, F. G., & Freels, S. (1998). Factors associated with survival in patients with meningioma. *Journal of Neurosurgery, 88*(5), 831–839.

Meythaler, J. M., Peduzzi, J. D., & Eleftheriou, E. (2001). Current concepts: Diffuse axonal injury—associated acquired brain injury. *Archives of Physical Medicine and Rehabilitation, 82*, 1461–1471.

Morgan, A. T. (2010). Dysphagia in childhood traumatic brain injury: A reflection on the evidence and its implications for practice. *Developmental Neurorehabilitation, 13*(3), 192–203. doi: 10.3109/17518420903289535

Munjal, S. K., Panda, N. K., & Pathak, A. (2010). Relationship between severity of traumatic brain injury (TBI) and extent of auditory dysfunction. *Brain Injury, 24*(3), 525–532. doi: 10.3109/02699050903516872

Najafi, M. R., Tabesh, H., Hosseini, M. H., Akbari, M., & Najafi, A. M. (2015). Early and late post-traumatic seizures following traumatic brain injury: A five-year follow-up national survey. *Advanced Biomedical Research, 4*, 82. doi: 10.4103/2277-9175.156640

National Highway Traffic Safety Agency. (2006). *Traffic safety facts 2006*. Retrieved from http://www.nhtsa.gov/portal/site/

National Institute of Neurological Disorders and Stroke (NINDS). (2015). *Tremor Fact Sheet*. Retrieved from http://www.ninds.nih.gov/disorders/tremor/detail_tremor.htm

Noggle, C. A., & Pierson, E. E. (2010). Psychosocial and behavioral functioning following pediatric TBI: Presentation, assessment, and intervention. *Applied Neuropsychology, 17*(2), 110–115.

Novack, T. A., Labbe, D., Grote, M., Carlson, N., Sherer, M., Arango-Lasprilla, J. C., … Seel, R. T. (2010). Return to driving within 5 years of moderate-severe traumatic brain injury. *Brain Injury, 24*(3), 464–471.

Osoba, D., Brada, M., Prados, M. D., & Yung, W. K. (2000). Effect of disease burden on health-related quality of life in patients with malignant gliomas. *Neuro-Oncology, 2*, 221–228.

Park, J. T., & Chugani, H. T. (2015). Post-traumatic epilepsy in children—experience from a tertiary referral center. *Pediatric Neurology, 52*, 174–181. doi: 10.1016/j.pediatrneurol.2014.09.013

Pietrapiana, P., Tamietto, M., Torrini, G., Mezzanato, T., Rago, R., & Perino, C. (2005). Role of premorbid factors in predicting safe return to driving after severe TBI. *Brain Injury, 19*, 197–211.

Ponsford, J., Willmott, C., & Rothwell, A. (2000). Factors influencing outcome following mild traumatic brain injury in adults. *Journal of the International Neuropsychological Society, 6*, 568–579.

Posner, J. B., Saper, C. B., Schiff, N., & Plum, F. (2007). *Plum and Posner's diagnosis of stupor and coma*. Oxford, England: Oxford University Press, Inc.

Pretz, C. R., Malec, J. F., & Hammond, F. M. (2013). Longitudinal description of the disability rating scale for individuals in the national institute on disability and rehabilitation research traumatic brain injury model systems national database. *Archives of Physical Medicine and Rehabilitation, 94*, 2478–2485. doi: 10.1016/j.apmr.2013.06.019

Probst, C., Pape, H. C., Hildebrand, F., Regel, G., Mahlke, L., Giannoudis, P., … Grotz, M. R. (2009). 30 years of polytrauma care: an analysis of the change in strategies and results of 4849 cases treated at a single institution. *Injury, 40*, 77–83.

Ragnarsson, K. T. (2006). Traumatic brain injury research since the 1998 NIH Consensus Conference. Accomplishments and unmet goals. *Journal of Head Trauma Rehabilitation, 21*(5), 379–387.

Rappaport, M., Hall, K. M., Hopkins, K., Belleza, T., & Cope, D. N. (1982). Disability rating scale for severe head trauma: Coma to community. *Archives of Physical Medicine and Rehabilitation, 63*, 118–123.

Rapport, L. J., Coleman, B. R., & Hanks, R. A. (2008). Driving and community integration after traumatic brain injury. *Archives of Physical Medicine and Rehabilitation, 89*, 922–930.

Rapport, L. J., Hanks, R. A., & Bryer, R. C. (2006). Barriers to driving and community integration after traumatic brain injury. *Journal of Head Trauma Rehabilitation, 21*(1), 34–44.

Rehabilitation of persons with traumatic brain injury (1998). NIH *Consensus Statement Online, 16*(1), 1–41.

Rimel, R. M., & Jane, J. A. (1983). *Characteristics of the head injured patient*. Philadelphia, PA: FA Davis.

Rochette, L. M., Conner, K. A., & Smith, G. A. (2009). The contribution of traumatic brain injury to the medical and economic outcomes motor vehicle-related injuries in Ohio. *Journal of Safety Research, 40*, 353–358.

Roffolo, C. F., Friedland, J. F., & Dawson, D. R. (1999). Mild traumatic brain injury from motor vehicle accidents: Factors associated with return to work. *Archives of Physical Medicine and Rehabilitation, 80*, 392–398.

Rutland-Brown, W., Langlois, J. A., Thomas, K. E., & Xi, Y. L. (2006). Incidence of traumatic brain injury in the United Stated, 2003. *Journal of Head Trauma Rehabilitation, 21*(6), 544–548.

Salmond, C. H., & Sahakian, B. J. (2005). Cognitive outcome in traumatic brain injury survivors. *Current Opinion in Critical Care, 11*, 111–116.

Seel, R. T., Kreutzer, J. S., & Rosenthal, M. (2003). Depression after traumatic brain injury: A National Institute on Disability and Rehabilitation Research Model Systems multicenter investigation. *Archives of Physical Medicine and Rehabilitation, 84*, 177–184.

Sherer, M., Bergloff, P., & High, W. J. (1999). Contribution of functional ratings to prediction of longterm employment outcome after traumatic brain injury. *Brain Injury, 13*, 973–981.

Sherer, M., Bergloff, P., & Levin, E. (1998). Impaired awareness and employment outcome after traumatic brain injury. *Journal of Head Trauma Rehabilitation, 13*, 52–61.

Sherer, M., Nick, T. G., & Sander, A. M. (2003). Race and productivity outcome after traumatic brain injury: Influence of confounding factors. *Journal of Head Trauma Rehabilitation, 18*, 408–424.

Tao, K., & Shenbagamurthi, S. (2012). Coup and contrecoup head injury resulting in anosmia. *The Journal of Emergency Medicine, 42*(2), 180–181.

Tamietto, M., Torrini, G., Adenzato, M., Pietrapiana, P., Rago, R., & Perino, C. (2006). To drive or not to drive (after TBI)? A review of the literature and its implications for rehabilitation and future research. *Neuro Rehabilitation, 21*, 81–92.

Teasdale, T. W., & Engberg, A. W. (2001). Suicide after traumatic brain injury: A population study. *Journal of Neurology, Neurosurgery, and Psychiatry, 71*, 436–440.

Turner-Stokes, L., Pick, A., Disler, P. B., & Wade, D. T. (2015). Multi-disciplinary rehabilitation for acquired brain injury in adults of working age. *Cochrane Database of Systematic Reviews, 12*(CD004170). doi: 10.1002/14651858.CD004170.pub3

University of California San Francisco. (2012). *Orientation to Caregiving. A handbook for family caregivers of patients with brain tumors.* Retrieved from http://www.osher.ucsf.edu/wp-content/uploads/2012/01/caregivers.pdf

van Reekum, R. (2001). Review: Women have worse outcomes than men after traumatic brain injury. *Evidence Based Mental Health, 4*, 58.

Wehman, P., Kregel, J., Keyser-Marcus, L., Sherron-Targett, P., Campbell, L., West, M., & Cifu, D. (2003a). Supported employment for persons with acquired brain injury: A preliminary investigation of long-term follow-up costs and program efficiency. *Archives of Physical Medicine and Rehabilitation, 84*, 192–196.

Wehman, P., Kregel, J., Keyser-Marcus, L., Sherron-Targett, P., Campbell, L., West, M., & Cifu, D. X. (2003b). Supported employment for persons with traumatic brain injury: A preliminary investigation of long-term follow-up costs and program efficiency. *Archives of Physical Medicine and Rehabilitation, 84*(2), 192–196.

Wijayatilake, D. S., Sherren, P., & Jigajinni, S. V. (2015). Systemic complications of traumatic brain injury. *Current Opinion in Anesthesiology, 28*, 525–531. doi: 10.1097/ACO.0000000000000236

Wrensch, M., Minn, Y., Chew, T., Bondy, M., & Berger, M. S. (2002). Epidemiology of primary brain tumors: Current concepts and review of the literature. *Neuro-Oncology, 4*(4), 278–299.

Wright, J. (2000). *Introduction to the disability rating scale. The Center for Outcome Measurement in Brain Injury.* Retrieved from http://www.tbims.org/combi/drs

Ylvisaker, M., Turkstra, L., Coehlo, C., Yorkston, K., Kennedy, M., & Sohlberg, M. M. (2007). Behavioral interventions for children and adults with behavior disorders after TBI: A systematic review of the evidence. *Brain Injury, 21*(8), 769–805.

21 Burns

Rebecca Ozelie

Sam, age 15, is scheduled for a burn dressing change at the outpatient burn clinic. Sam suffered 46% mixed partial- and full-thickness burns to his face, neck, chest, and bilateral arms 4 months ago when he added gasoline to a brush fire. The resulting explosion set Sam's clothes on fire. Sam panicked and started running. A neighbor who heard the explosion from inside his house tackled Sam and smothered the flames with a blanket. Sam spent 2 months as an inpatient on the burn unit where he received extensive grafting to his face, neck, arms, and chest. He was discharged 2 months ago but continues to have scattered small open areas. Sam arrives at the clinic, accompanied by his mother, and immediately requests assistance to remove his coat. When he is asked to try to remove his coat himself, he is able to complete the task but is noted to have extremely limited range of motion (ROM) and severe bilateral axillary contractures. It is noted that both his clothing and temporary compression garment have been cut apart at the arms and shoulder and duct-taped together. When asked why this was done, he replies that it is easier to remove his clothes this way. His mother states, "I told him he shouldn't do that."

DESCRIPTION AND DEFINITIONS

Anatomy and Physiology of the Skin

An understanding of burn injury must begin with a review of the anatomy and physiology of the skin. The skin is the largest organ of the body (Latenser & Kowal-Vern, 2002). The skin has three anatomical layers: **epidermis**, **dermis**, and the **subcutaneous tissue**. The thin nonvascular outer layer, called the epidermis, consists of layers of epithelial cells. This layer serves as a barrier to bacteria and moisture loss. Beneath the epidermis is the thicker dermis, which makes up the bulk of the skin. Housed within the dermis are hair follicles, blood vessels, sweat glands, nerve endings, and sebaceous glands, which play an integral part in the functions of the skin (Fig. 21.1). The functions of the skin include (McGraft & Uitto, 2010)

- Protection against infection
- Prevention loss of body fluid
- Control of body temperature
- Functioning as an excretory organ
- Production of vitamin D
- Helping to determine personal identity

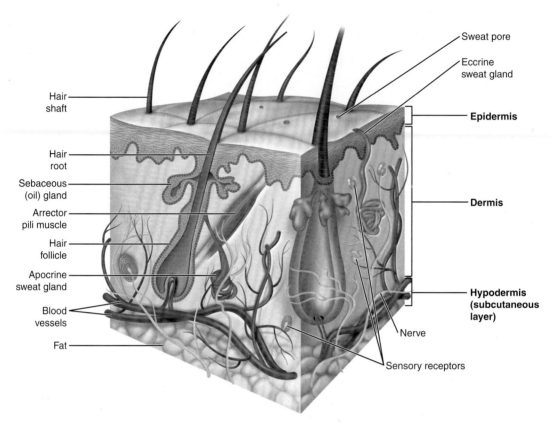

Figure 21.1 Anatomy of the skin. (From Archer, P., & Nelson, L. A. (2012). *Applied anatomy & physiology for manual therapists*. Philadelphia, PA: Lippincott Williams & Wilkins.)

■ Pathophysiology of Burns

In addition to understanding the anatomy and physiology of the skin, it is important to understand the pathophysiology of burns. An understanding of what kind of physiological response a burn will induce is critical to the management of burns. The two primary factors that influence the amount of tissue destruction that occurs following a burn injury are temperature and duration of exposure (McGraft & Uitto, 2010). The tissue damage that occurs following a burn injury can be divided into three zones (Kowalske, 2011). The **zone of coagulation** is the area exposed to the most amount of heat and ensues the most damage. This is the area of irreversible tissue destruction. Surrounding this is the **zone of stasis**, where damage results in decreased tissue perfusion. The tissue in this zone may be salvageable, and the main goal of burn resuscitation is to increase tissue perfusion here and prevent any irreversible damage. The outer zone is referred to as the **zone of hyperemia**.

The tissues in these outer zones are damaged but with proper care should recover and heal. Without proper care of the tissue in the zone of hyperemia, further damage may result and increased tissue loss can occur (Kowalske, 2011; Rowan et al., 2015). The aim of care after a burn injury is to reduce or prevent dermal ischemia, thereby avoiding further tissue death. The residual necrotic layers of skin destroyed by direct heat damage or the injury occurring secondary to heat damage is referred to as eschar.

ETIOLOGY

The most common cause of the burns is fire/flame (43%), scald (34%), contact (9%), electrical (4%), chemical (3%), and other (7%). The majority of burns occur in the home (73%). The other places burns occur include occupational (5%), street/highway (5%), recreational/sport (5%), and other (9%) (American Burn Association, 2015).

INCIDENT AND PREVALENCE

The American Burn Association (2015) reports that 486,000 people seek medical treatment for burns each year. This estimate is derived from hospital admission and emergency department data. It is acknowledged that this number is an estimate range because some burns may have been treated at home, in the community, and at clinics. Sixty percent of the estimated acute hospitalizations for burns were admitted to 128 burn centers and the other 40% to the nation's 4,500 acute care hospitals. Those hospitals average fewer than three burn admissions per year. Of the 60% admitted to the nation's burn centers, there is a 96.7% survival rate with 69% male and 31% female. The mean age is 30 years (Veeravagu et al., 2015). Caucasians represented the largest ethnic group affected (59%) followed by African American (20%), Hispanic (14%), and others (7%).

SIGNS AND SYMPTOMS

■ Depth of Burn

The depth of a burn injury reflects how deep into the skin layers a burn extends and the duration of hot contact (Fig. 21.2). Understanding the depth of burn injury will influence projected survival rates, healing time, treatment, and scar formation.

Superficial Burn Injury

A **superficial** (first-degree) burn injury involves only the epidermal layers of the skin (Kowalske, 2011). This burn is characterized by redness and pain. The wound is dry and does not form blisters. The wound blanches readily and is exquisitely sensitive to air and/or light touch. A superficial burn injury can result from a variety of causes such as a sunburn or flash from an explosion.

Partial-Thickness Burn Injury (Superficial vs. Deep)

A **partial-thickness** (second-degree) injury destroys the epidermal layer and extends down into the dermal layer of the skin. The differentiation between superficial partial thickness and deep partial thickness is dependent on how deep the burn extends into the dermal layer. A superficial partial-thickness burn has damage in the upper layers of the papillary dermis (Lloyd, Rodgers, Michener, & Williams, 2012). A sunburn that peels is the depth of a superficial partial-thickness burn. These burns are characterized by clear blisters and weeping, wet skin. The burn will blanch and is painful when touched.

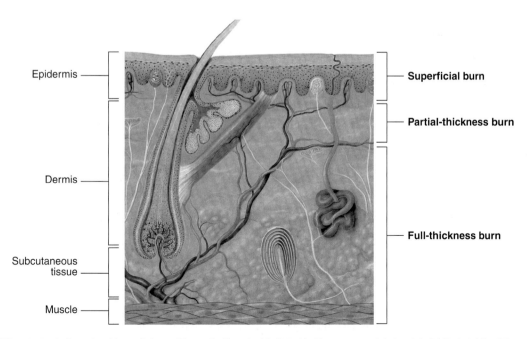

Figure 21.2 Depth of burn injury. (From Pellico, L. H. (2012). *Focus on adult health*. Philadelphia, PA: Lippincott Williams & Wilkins.)

A burn to the deeper layers of the dermis is classified as a deep partial-thickness burn. Deep **partial-thickness burns** affect the entire epidermis and dermis but spare the base of the hair follicle (Kowalske, 2011). This type of burn will appear white and will not blanch when touched. Deep-partial thickness burns are often extremely painful because there can be exposed nerve endings due to the depth of the burn.

Full-Thickness Burn Injury

A **full-thickness** (third-degree) burn injury destroys the entire epidermal and dermal layers of the skin and extends down into subcutaneous fat. A full-thickness injury may be a variety of colors. The wound can be charred black, cherry red, tan, or pearly white in color. This wound may present with small fragile, thin-walled blisters that break easily and do not increase in size. Overall, the wound is dry and leathery hard in texture (Lloyd et al., 2012). Since nerve endings are destroyed, the wound is initially insensate but remains sensitive to deep pressure. Because burn wounds often have a mixture of differing depths, pain is not a good indicator of the depth of wound. This wound will leave a residual scar and is at severe risk for contracture formation (Morgan, Bledsoe, & Barker, 2000).

Deep Full-Thickness Burn Injury

Deep full-thickness (fourth-degree) burns destroy all skin layers and extend into the muscle, tendon, or bone. This type of burn will be characterized by a charred or mummified appearance (Kowalske, 2011). Deep full-thickness wounds are challenging to close and can result in partial or total loss of function (Sahin et al., 2012). When this type of burn involves severe damage to the underlying structures, amputations may be warranted.

■ Inhalation Injury

Inhalation injuries most commonly occur in a setting of thermal injury of an enclosed space. Signs and symptoms of inhalation injuries are typically based on observations of the following: the presence of facial burns, singed nasal hair, darkened oral mucosa, hoarse voice, wheezing, hypoxia, and/or cough (Dries & Endorf, 2013; Mlcak, Suman, & Herndon, 2007). Medical diagnosis of an inhalation injury is typically completed with a fiberoptic bronchoscopy.

A common concurrent form of injury is carbon monoxide toxicity (Mlcak et al., 2007). Almost all products release carbon monoxide during combustion. It is an odorless, colorless gas that has a greater affinity for binding hemoglobin than oxygen, thus displacing oxygen and leading to asphyxia (Dries & Endorf, 2013). During a fire, the concentration of oxygen typically drops to 10% to 15%, at which point death from asphyxia occurs (Barillo, 2009). Hydrogen cyanide is produced during combustion of multiple household materials and can be inhaled during a fire. Hydrogen cyanide also decreases oxygen consumption. Carbon monoxide and cyanide toxicity can interfere with oxygen transport at the cellular level and affect electron transport within cells leading to death (Dries & Endorf, 2013).

■ Burn Shock

A complication that may occur in patients with burns in excess of 20% total body surface area (TBSA) is **burn shock** (Atiyeh, Dibo, Ibrahim, & Zgheib, 2012). Burn shock can occur within 48 to 72 hours after injury (Parihar, Parihar, Milner, & Bhat, 2008). Unlike other causes of shock, the problem is not a loss of blood but rather the fluid or plasma portion of the circulating blood volume. Immediately following a burn injury, an increase in capillary permeability allows fluid in the intravascular space to shift into the interstitial space producing burn wound edema. The effect on the cardiovascular system is a marked increase in peripheral vascular resistance accompanied by a decrease in cardiac output. This shift is greatest in the first 12 hours postinjury but continues for 72 hours postinjury (Atiyeh et al., 2012). After the first 72 hours, capillary wall function returns and gradually burn wound edema will shift back into the intravascular volume and be excreted by the kidneys. In the presence of a burn wound >25%, this fluid shift occurs throughout the body and edema develops in areas that have not been burned (James, 2012). In burns <25%, the fluid shift is usually confined to the burn area.

■ Hypermetabolism

Hypermetabolism is a significant concern for patients with burns. A large burn injury triggers a significant and prolonged stress response in the body and initiates the release of catecholamines, cytokines, and insulin (Abdullahi & Jeschke, 2015). The release of these hormones initiates and mediates a hypermetabolic response and increased energy expenditure and protein turnover in the body. This hypermetabolic state will result in increased energy catabolism, skeletal muscle catabolism, immune deficiencies, peripheral lipolysis, and reduced bone mineralization and growth. Energy expenditure is most significant in the first weeks postburn and then begins to decrease (Lavrentieva, 2016).

■ Infection

The skin provides a barrier to the external environment and offers metabolic and immunological support. Injury to this barrier disrupts the innate immune system and increases susceptibility to infection (Church, Elsayed, Reid, Winston, & Lindsay, 2006). The leading cause of death following a severe burn injury is infection (Chaudhari, Upadhyay, Bambhaniya, & Patel, 2015). The typical systems of an infection (fever, tachycardia, and leukocytosis) are commonly observed in persons with burn injuries, without the presence of an infection. Therefore, the American Burn Association (Greenhalgh et al., 2007) proposed indicators that are more specific for sepsis in burns. These include

- Temperature (>39°C or <36°C), progressive tachypnea (>25 breaths/minute not ventilated or >12 L/minute ventilated)
- Progressive tachycardia (>110 beats/minute)
- Thrombocytopenia (<100,000/μL, applied only after day 3 postresuscitation)
- Hyperglycemia (untreated glucose >200 mg/dL, >7 units/hour insulin infusion, or >25% increase in insulin dosing over 24 hours)
- Enteral feeding intolerance (abdominal distention, residuals over two times the feeding rate, or diarrhea >2,500 mL/24 hours)

In the event three or more of these indicators are present, the infection site should be identified and antibiotics should be initiated. The use of topical antibiotics, early excision and grafting of the wound areas, and strict sterile techniques also aid in the prevention of infections.

■ Scars

Scars are fibrous tissue that replaces normal tissue after injury. Typical scars are initially red in color and fade as the fibrous tissue begins to develop (Heppt et al., 2015). Burn scars begin to form as wounds close. Burn scars are prone to hypertrophic scar formation. **Hypertrophic scars** result from uncontrolled production of fibroblasts and excess in deposition of collagen tissue (Heppt et al., 2015). Collagen is a basic structural fibrous protein found in all tissue. Hypertrophic scars typically present as red, raised, and rigid and generally do not extend past the injury site (Heppt et al., 2015). Hypertrophic scars are differentiated from keloid scar formation by the fact that they remain within the boundary of the original wound and will eventually fade in color, flatten, and become more pliable as they mature.

People who are most susceptible to hypertrophic scars are those who have a genetic predisposition, have African ethnic origin, and have burns in areas of the body involved in stretch or motion such as the shoulders and truck and areas of prolonged healing (Heppt et al., 2015). **Keloids** are excessive fibrosis, nodular proliferations that project beyond the margins of the original injury (Heppt et al., 2015). Keloids are tender and painful and can be difficult to treat. In addition, keloids can cause physical, cosmetic, psychological, and social concerns (Viera, Vivas, & Berman, 2012). Keloids can occur in all skin types, but increased prevalence is noted in the African population, and genetic predisposition may impact keloid formation (Viera et al., 2012).

■ Contractures

Wound healing involves three processes: epithelialization, connective tissue deposition, and contraction. Wound contraction is an active process generated by fibroblasts and myofibroblasts and is one of the most powerful mechanical forces in the body. Burn scar contracture is the shortening and tightening of the burn scar. It is estimated that approximately 40% of those that suffer burn injuries will develop scar contractures (Ehanire et al., 2013). Burn scar contracture deformities are most problematic over large joints. They can severely limit ROM and interfere with the ability to perform activities of daily living (ADLs) (Niedzielski & Chapman, 2015). Additionally, contractures can be disfiguring and painful and cause itching (Ehanire et al., 2013). Mature burn scars do not have the capacity to stretch like normal skin. Children with large full-thickness injuries may develop burn scar contractures years after their initial burn injury as they literally grow out of their skin.

COURSE AND PROGNOSIS

The course and prognosis of a burn injury depends on the depth and surface area of the burn. A superficial burn will generally heal within 3 to 4 days as the epidermis sloughs, and there will not be any residual scarring (Herdon, 2012). A superficial partial-thickness burn will generally heal within 2 weeks, and typically, there is no scarring; however, there are often pigmentation changes (Kowalske, 2011). A deep partial-thickness burn will heal in 3 weeks or longer and commonly result in significant scarring and contractures (Lloyd et al., 2012). Because both layers of the skin are destroyed in the full-thickness burn injury, the wound will not heal spontaneously and the healing time is dependent upon the availability of donor sites. A full-thickness burn injury has the potential to affect all body systems. Organ failure, sepsis, pneumonia, and cellulitis are common complications from burn injuries. Sixty percent of deaths from burn injuries are attributed to multisystem organ failure (Veeravagu et al., 2015).

A common cause of death in persons with burn injuries is inhalation injuries (Mlcak et al., 2007). The presence of an inhalation injury can increase the burn mortality rate by 20%, and there is an increased predisposition to pneumonia (Mlcak et al., 2007). Burn injuries can also lead to a rapid and significant loss of intravascular fluid into the interstitial space. If this is not managed, it can lead to progressive organ dysfunction and ultimately death.

DIAGNOSIS

The depth of the burn wound is not always clear on admission, and burn depth is often not accurately assessed. A clinical examination of burn depth has been found to be only 70% accurate (Bezuhly & Fish, 2012). Laser Doppler scanning, histological assessments, and indocyanine green fluorescence are some of the new technologies being used to increase the accuracy of burn depth determination.

In addition to evaluating the depth of a burn, it is important to accurately estimate the **total body surface area (TBSA)** involved in the burn injury. Burn depth and burn size will guide medical and therapeutic management of the burns. There are three common methods used to estimate extent of burn: the Lund and Browder scale, the rule of nines, and the rule of palms. The Lund and Browder scale (Fig. 21.3) is a diagram that

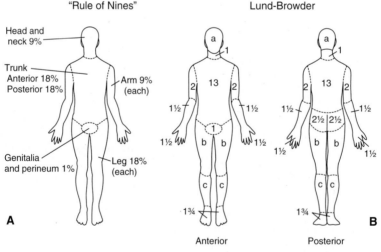

Relative percentage of body surface areas (% BSA) affected by growth

	0 yr	1 yr	5 yr	10 yr	15 yr
a— ½ of head	9½	8½	6½	5½	4½
b— ½ of 1 thigh	2¾	3¾	4	4¼	4½
c— ½ of 1 lower leg	2½	2½	2¾	3	3¼

Figure 21.3 A. Rule of nines. **B.** Lund and Browder scale. (From Irwin, R. S., Lilly, C. & Rippe, J. M. (2013). *Irwin and Rippe's manual of intensive care medicine* (6th ed.). Philadelphia, PA: Lippincott Williams & Wilkins.)

consists of a two-dimensional figure of a human body, front and back. The figure is divided into sections, each of which represents a defined percentage of the total body surface. The evaluator documents the injury on the diagram, estimates the amount of each section the injury occupies, and manually adds these numbers to determine the TBSA. The Lund and Brower scale adjusts for patients of different ages (Williams et al., 2013). This evaluation of TBSA can be time consuming and has limited accuracy.

The rule of nines (Fig. 21.3) is a quick method that may be used to estimate extent of burn. It divides the body surface into areas representing 9% or multiples of 9%. This method is also susceptible to user error and often overestimates the percentage of TBSA (Sheng et al., 2014).

The rule of palms is defined as the surface of the patient's palm that is roughly 1% of their TBSA (Sheng et al., 2014). Similar to the other methods, the rule of palms also has validity concerns. This method can result in an overestimate of the TBSA of 10% to 20% (Amirsheybani et al., 2001).

An accurate assessment of the TBSA is critical to determining care and resuscitation methods for persons that have sustained burns. As such, several computer-based methods have been developed and researched. Studies have shown that the computer-based methods can be up to 99.9% accurate in determining TBSA (Sheng et al., 2014). Mobile systems for TBSA evaluation and remote assessment have also been developed as a means to provide telehealth and impact the quality of the treatment in burns (Parvizi et al., 2014).

MEDICAL MANAGEMENT

Major burn injuries are considered one of the most severe examples of trauma and often require specialized care not available at all hospitals (Bezuhly & Fish, 2012). Since 2006, the American Burn Association identified criteria (Table 21.1) for burn injuries that should be transferred to a hospital with a designated burn/trauma unit, capable of providing the specialized care required by significant burn injuries.

■ Inhalation Injuries

Treatment of inhalation injury is aimed at maintaining adequate oxygenation through the administration of humidified oxygen by mask to maintain an oxygen saturation level >90%. Additionally, bronchial hygiene therapy, chest physiotherapy, early ambulation, and airway suctioning are used as part of inhalation injury treatment protocols (Mlcak et al., 2007). Bronchoscopies are also used in severe inhalation injuries and have been found to be effective in decreasing the duration of mechanical ventilation compared to patients who did not have a bronchoscopy (Carr, Phillips, & Bowling, 2009). Intubation and ventilator support may be indicated in the presence of severe respiratory obstruction or restrictive defects. In the presence of restrictive eschar (dark, crusty, dead skin) on the chest or abdomen, the patient's respiratory status may become compromised and the patient may require an escharotomy. Escharotomies are incisions through the eschar down to viable tissue to release the restriction

---

TABLE **21.1** **American Burn Association Criteria for Burn Center Referral**

Partial-thickness burns >10% TBSA

Burns involving the face, hands, feet, genitalia, perineum, and major joints

Full-thickness burns in any age group

Electrical burns, including lightning

Chemical burns

Inhalation injury

Burn injuries in patients with complicating preexisting medical conditions

Burns with concomitant additional trauma in which burn injury poses the greatest risk of morbidity or mortality

Burned children in hospitals without qualified personnel or equipment

Burn injury in patients requiring special social, emotional, or long-term intervention

and allow for expansion of the chest wall during inspiration and expiration (Kupas & Miller, 2010).

Management of carbon monoxide toxicity includes administration of oxygen via a facemask or artificial airway at 100% oxygen. Hyperbaric oxygen is also used as a treatment mechanism, but it is difficult to monitor a patient and provide initial burn care while in the hyperbaric chamber (Dries & Endorf, 2013). Cyanide toxicity is managed with aggressive treatment to support cardiovascular function and may include the utilization of cyanide antidotes (Dries & Endorf, 2013).

■ Fluid Resuscitation

Early aggressive **fluid resuscitation**, which is the administration of intravenous fluid, is required for stabilization. The fluid replacement of choice is crystalloid, or lactated Ringer solution. Ringer solution contains sodium, chloride, calcium, potassium, and lactate (Rowan et al., 2015). The goal of fluid resuscitation is to maintain the intravascular volume in sufficient amounts to ensure adequate perfusion and oxygenation to all tissues and organs with the least amount of fluid needed.

Several fluid resuscitation practices are used. A survey found that the Parkland formula is the most commonly used method (69.3% of respondents), followed by the Galveston (8.9%), Brooke (6.9%), and Warden hypertonic formulas (5.9%) (Greenhalgh, 2010). These formulas calculate the predicted fluid needs of patients based on their burn size and weight over the course of the first 24 hours. According to the Baxter (Parkland) formula, the patient should receive 4 mL/kg body weight/% burn, as a volume of fluid needed for the initial 24-hour fluid resuscitation. Adequate assessment of the effectiveness of fluid resuscitation is important, as excessive fluid overloading can cause the phenomenon known as **fluid creep**. It is important to avoid fluid overloading because this may be lead to compartment syndrome. Compartment syndrome is internal edema within a part of the body or often an extremity that can decrease circulation to the structure and thus putting them at risk. To avoid fluid overloading, burn resuscitation is commonly monitored by urine output. Hourly urine output in adults should be 30 mL/hour and 1 to 1.5 mL/kg/h in pediatrics (Pukar, Rajshakha, Mewada, & Lakhani, 2015).

Delayed or inadequate fluid replacement results in hypovolemia, tissue hypoperfusion, shock, and multiple organ failure. Inadequate fluid resuscitation can lead to hypovolemia and renal failure. Once fluid resuscitation is initiated, tissue edema in or directly surrounding the burned area may occur. If circumferential burn wounds are present on the extremities, distal areas should be checked frequently for compromised blood supply.

■ Nutritional Support

Nutritional support is needed to meet the resulting increase in basal energy expenditure due to hypermetabolism. Multiple formulas are available to determine the required caloric needs. Most patients cannot consume enough calories through eating and require nutritional support via the enteral route (nasogastric feedings). Early initiation of nutritional support via enteral feedings will help reduce the risk of infection and mortality (Williams et al., 2009).

BURN WOUND MANAGEMENT

Burn wound management involves the surgical debridement of nonviable skin and wound coverage in the form of skin grafts. **Debridement** is the cleansing and removal of nonadherent and nonviable tissue. Eschar, the dead tissue that sheds from healthy tissue, facilitates bacterial access and acts as the common denominator for burn sepsis. Daily cleansing and debridement of the burn wound is necessary to decrease the potential for burn wound sepsis, to facilitate healing, and to prepare the wound for grafting if this procedure is needed to achieve wound closure.

Debridement is a painful procedure, and it is important to make sure the patient has been medicated with analgesics and/or sedative medication prior to starting the dressing change. Commonly used analgesics include morphine, fentanyl, or codeine. A common drug given to sedate the patient is ketamine. Anxiolytics, such as diazepam or midazolam, are drugs given to control anxiety. The pain experienced at dressing changes can make a person feel anxious or stressed (Woo, 2010). Anxiety can influence pain perception. The use of anxiolytics can be beneficial in reducing anticipatory anxiety regarding future dressing changes. It has been found that anxiety and pain can impact the patient and delay the healing process (Upton & Andrews, 2014). Research is being done to examine interventions that can minimize pain during dressing changes. Nonpharmaceutical interventions utilized include virtual reality, massage therapy, sensory focusing, guided imagery, relaxation techniques, and music therapy.

Hydrotherapy is a form of wound cleansing in which water is used as a means of decontamination of the burn site. There are concerns with the risk of infection during the use of hydrotherapy as the patient's wounds are typically open and deep. Due to this concern, the prevalence of hydrotherapy use at burn centers has decreased since 1990 (83% vs. 95%), yet continues to be used at the majority of centers (Davison, Loiselle, & Nickerson, 2010). Showering methods are being a more common alternative to hydrotherapy (Davison et al., 2010). Showering methods and hydrotherapy assist in cleaning wounds, removing topical creams, and facilitating dressing change. A mild soap, soft washcloth, tweezers, and scissors are tools utilized to aid in debridement. To decrease the potential for hypothermia, time in the bath is limited and the temperature of the room should be kept at 85°F or higher (29°C) (Herdon, 2012).

Once the wound has been cleansed, nonadhesion, absorbent, and antimicrobial dressing should be applied. The burn dressings act as a barrier to the environment to prevent against infection and can assist in the management of wound fluids. Dressing changes are commonly performed twice weekly or on alternate days (Selig et al., 2012). If outer bandages become saturated with drainage, however, it is necessary to replace them with dry outer bandages to prevent the wicking of bacteria down to the surface of the wound.

Topical dressings are used to provide protection from contamination and from physical damage, allow gas exchange and moisture retention, and provide comfort (Rowan et al., 2015). There are several topical agents one can choose from that can encourage a moist but not wet environment to promote epithelialization and maintain moisture retention (Warner, Coffee, & Yowler, 2014). Use of silver-containing compounds has become increasingly popular (Warner et al., 2014). Silver-containing topical agents have antimicrobial properties and have been found to reduce wound pain (Abboud et al., 2014). Silver toxicity, resistance, and skin discoloration are concerns with the use of silver agents, but more research is needed to determine the true impact (Sterling, 2014). One antimicrobial agent commonly used is silver sulfadiazine 1% (Silvadene). Silvadene is a broad-spectrum antimicrobial agent effective against gram-positive and gram-negative bacteria with some antifungal activity. Silvadene does not penetrate burn eschar. It controls bacterial growth only on the surface of the wound, has few side effects, and is usually well tolerated by the patient.

The standard of care for wound management has included early excision and grafting (Rowan et al., 2015). Research has shown that excision within 24 to 48 hours reduces blood loss, indication, length of hospital stay, and mortality (Saaiq, Zaib, & Ahmad, 2012). Additionally, timely closure of wounds can prevent dehydration and assist in reducing the risk of infection (Mahjour et al., 2015). Grafting priorities are influenced by location and size of the burn. If the patient requires long-term intravenous fluid administration, skin grafting may be needed on the chest to allow for insertion of a central line. Hands, because of their functional importance, are given grafting priority. Faces and ears have a dense cross section of dermal appendages and are given additional time to ascertain if healing will occur without surgical intervention (Kao & Garner, 2000).

If the patient does not have available donor sites, the burn wound can be excised down to viable tissue and temporarily closed through the application of an **allograft**, xenograft, or skin substitute. An allograft is donor skin taken from another living or deceased person. The body will predictably reject the allograft from the wound bed 7 to 12 days after placement due to immunologic incompatibility between the burn victim and the cadaver donor (Leto Barone et al., 2015). These temporary means of wound closure provide the time needed to achieve a permanent method for closing the wound.

In full-thickness injuries, the risk of bacterial entrance and fluid and heat loss through the wound continues until the wound is closed either temporarily or permanently. Split-thickness skin grafts from an uninjured donor site of the patient (**autograft**) provide quick and permanent closure of the wound (Rowan et al., 2015). An autograft is the surgical transplantation of the patient's own skin from one area to another. Donor skin is taken from areas of unburned skin. The harvested skin is 0.008 to 0.012 in. in thickness. This leaves a wound, referred to as a donor site, that takes about 7 to 10 days to heal. Once healed, donor sites can be reharvested but will take longer to heal. Burn eschar is excised down to viable tissue, and bleeding is controlled prior to placement of the skin graft.

A split-thickness skin autograft can be applied as a mesh graft or a sheet graft. A mesh graft is a graft that has had small holes placed evenly throughout the graft, which allows it to be expanded (2:1, 3:1). Use of a mesh graft allows more area to be covered than the actual size of the donor skin taken. The scar from a mesh graft often has a crosshatch appearance. Because of this, mesh grafts are avoided in areas where there are concerns about the appearance of the scar, such as on the face or hands. Split-thickness grafts can be applied as a sheet graft in areas with aesthetic concerns. A sheet graft is a graft in which the donor skin has been laid intact over the area to be grafted. Sheet grafts are traditionally used in burn wounds of up to 20% TBSA to limit the potential cosmetic impact (Nikkhah, Booth, Tay, Gilbert, & Dheansa, 2015). While sheet grafts are preferred because of cosmetic reasons, limited availability of donor sites in large burn injuries limits their use.

In large burns with limited availability of donor sites, cultured epithelium can be used to achieve wound closure. A biopsy of unburned skin is taken and sent to a laboratory that can grow cultured epithelium. It takes 3 to 4 weeks for cultured epithelium to be available for grafting. The resulting grafts can be fragile and sensitive to infection. Cultured epithelium grafts can also be expensive, and they require a complex application process. These cultured epithelium grafts are often reserved for patients with 50% or greater TBSA burns (Nguyen, Potokar, & Price, 2010). Epidermal substitutes are also commercially available (e.g., Alloderm, Biobrane) and can be used to replace the dermis or epidermis. These substitutes can be only a few cell layers thick and do not contain all the typical components of human dermis (Fang, Lineaweaver, Sailes, Kisner, & Zhang, 2014). Use of stem cells to enhance wound healing is an emerging area of research in the field of burn management.

Immediately after grafting, with either an autograft or cultured epithelium, the graft is fragile and susceptible to loss. Factors that can cause graft failure include shearing/motion and increased edema (Lorello, Peck, Albrecht, Richey, & Pressman, 2014). To prevent loss of graft, the grafted area is often immobilized in a functional position and remains in that position until there is the establishment of circulation to the grafted area (Lorello et al., 2014). If grafts are placed on the chest or back, the bandages are sutured to the body to decrease the risk of shearing when repositioning the patient. Extremities are elevated to prevent/minimize edema formation. Immobilization time is variable, and each physician will have his or her own preference. ROM to the grafted area is avoided until the graft is stable, which is usually about 4 to 6 days after surgery.

IMPACT ON OCCUPATIONAL PERFORMANCE

A burn injury is a devastating injury that may have a significant impact on occupational performance immediately and long after the wound is healed. The impact of a burn injury on an individual's occupational performance is influenced by the size, location, and depth of the burn injury. A burn injury affects a number of client factors and can profoundly impact an individual's ability to independently perform ADLs, instrumental activities of daily living (IADLs), education pursuits, work, play, leisure, and/or social participation activities. Burn injuries that have the greatest potential to impact occupational performance include deep partial-thickness or full-thickness burns that result in more severe scar formation, contractures, and joint restrictions and burns that involve major joints and account for a high TBSA.

During the initial evaluation, it is important to complete a thorough evaluation as soon as possible. Several client factors and performance skills should be critically evaluated so that the most effective treatment plan can be developed to ensure the optimal occupational performance for the client.

■ Client Factors

A significant deficit experienced after a burn injury is decreased joint mobility and joint function. This includes the patient's passive and active ROM to any joints that may have been involved in a burn injury in addition to surrounding joints. During the emergency phase and fluid resuscitation, edema formation is expected and may be profound in patients. The edema formation will impact joint function and mobility leading to difficulties with ADLs and functional activities. Joint mobility and function are also impacted due to the formation of scarring and contractures. Scars that cross a joint may often lead to reduced ROM in that joint. It has been found that as little as a 10% reduction in joint ROM will significantly impair joint function (Fearmonti et al., 2011).

Muscle power and muscle endurance are client factors that are also commonly impacted after a burn injury. Burn survivors often experience long periods of immobilization during the acute phase of the medical management. Additionally, the body experiences many physiological responses as it heals from a burn injury. Both the prolonged periods of immobilization and the body's physiological responses can reduce a person's muscle endurance and muscle power. Muscle power and endurance may also be limited due to scar formation and limited joint ROM. If minimal joint range is available or the joint's mobility is limited due to scar formation, the muscle power exerted by the joint may be limited. Limited muscle endurance and power can significantly impact many facets of one's occupational performance. Research suggests that participation in structured progressive resistance exercise and cardiopulmonary endurance programs can aid in rapid restoration of functional independence (Paratz, Stockton, Plaza, Muller, & Boots, 2012).

Another client factor that is important to evaluate with this population is mental functions. Due to the traumatic and catastrophic nature of a burn injury, burn survivors may suffer symptoms of posttraumatic stress disorder, depression, and body image and self-image dysmorphia. A study of hospitalized burn patients found 55% of patients suffered from at least one mental disorder at a 6-month follow-up (Palmu, Suominen, Vuola, & Isometsä, 2011). The specific mental functions of "emotional" and "experience of self and time" are often overshadowed in persons who sustain burn injuries as medical personnel are focusing on survival. Support and interventions focused on loss, grief, acceptance of body image and self-image, posttraumatic stress disorder, anxiety, and depression should be provided. These psychosocial mental function-focused interventions are necessary to achieve a burn survivor's highest level of occupational performance. Palmu, Partonen, Suominen, Vuola, and Isometsä (2015) found that burn survivors' level of functioning was predicted strongly and consistently by mental disorders, most specifically depression.

It is important to recognize and assist both patients and families in dealing with the psychological and psychosocial impact of a major burn injury. Burn support groups can be helpful in assisting patients and families in dealing with the lifelong disfigurement and dysfunction that may result from a major burn injury. Having patients meet with a burn survivor can help them realize what challenges they may face and ways to overcome these challenges. Family members may experience many emotions such as fear, guilt, or sadness. If these emotions are not addressed, family members may feel the need to "take care of their loved one" and to do things for the patient that he or she needs to do independently. Having family members meet with another burn survivor and their families will help prepare them for the challenges ahead and assist them to deal with their emotions. This preparation will enable the family to provide the patient both the support and independence they will need to achieve the best outcome.

It is critical that early interventions, comprehensive home programs and patient and family education, and discharge recommendations are provided to patients to address and prevent a significant impact on client factors to limit the impact on a person's occupational performance.

CASE STUDY

Lyla, a 5-year-old girl, is playing outside when her father arrives home. He is having difficulty with his car, which is overheating. Unaware that Lyla has come over to watch him work on the car, he removes the radiator cap. Hot radiator fluid and steam strikes Lyla, and she sustains a 32% mixed partial- and full-thickness burn injury to her face, neck, chest, and scattered area on her bilateral arms.

During the emergency phase, she required fluid resuscitation and intubation to maintain her airway during the initial fluid shift and resulting swelling. She was extubated on postburn day 3 and has had no further problems with her airway. Three weeks have passed, and Lyla has had two surgeries. During the first surgery, mesh grafts were placed on her chest and arms. During the last surgical procedure, a sheet graft was placed on her neck. Her grafts are intact and healing well, but scattered open areas remain at the margins of the grafts. Lyla has donor sites on her bilateral thighs and buttock, which are healing without difficulty.

Neuromuscular components of ROM, strength, and soft tissue integrity have all been affected by the burn injury Lyla sustained. She has participated in ROM exercises since she was extubated. ROM exercises were halted for a few days, after the grafting procedures, to facilitate adherence of the graft. Currently, Lyla has some restriction of ROM to bilateral axillary areas and is at risk for hypertrophic scarring. While she currently does not demonstrate any restriction of neck ROM, she is at great risk for developing contractures in this area. ADLs and play or leisure activities are the occupational performance areas that have been affected. Currently, Lyla has few limitations on ROM to most joints, but because of the significant pain and anxiety she experiences during ROM, she is hesitant and resistant to movement. Lyla's parents express a great deal of difficulty with the discomfort that Lyla has experienced during therapy and are hesitant to make her do things that may cause pain. Lyla's father expresses a lot of guilt surrounding the circumstances that caused the burn injury.

CASE STUDY 2

Rahul is a 45-year-old male who was employed as an electrician. He was working outdoors with a coworker on a nonfunctional power box when it exploded, and he was engulfed in flames that caused third-degree burns to 75% of his body. He sustained partial- and full-thickness burns to his head, neck, chest, abdomen, bilateral upper extremities, genital and perineal area, and bilateral upper legs. His ankles and feet were spared as they were protected by his work boots. During the explosion, Rahul also sustained inhalation injuries.

Rahul was taken to an urban, local burn facility and remained in the burn ICU for more than 3 months. During this time in the burn ICU, he received early aggressive fluid resuscitation. Due to excessive fluid overloading, he experienced fluid creep. The fluid creep led to abdominal compartment syndrome and required an emergency fasciotomy to release the excessive pressure. In addition, Rahul was intubated and received ventilator support due to severe respiratory obstruction from the inhalation injury. Rahul underwent over 20 grafting procedures to assist with management of his burn injuries. After 3 months, he was transferred to a local rehabilitation hospital.

At the rehabilitation facility, he presented with extremely low endurance, significant pain, and symptoms of depression, which limited his ability to participate in the required 3 hours of therapy per day. Due to his prolonged period of decreased mobility in the ICU and poor participation at the rehabilitation facility, Rahul began to demonstrate significant limitations in his head, neck, and bilateral upper extremity ROM. Contractures and hypertrophic scarring were present in the bilateral axilla and anterior neck. Rahul also presented with webbing of the fingers on his left hand. He experienced persistent open areas on the dorsum of the hands, which limited his ability to use them functionally. Rahul was dependent to maximal assistance with all ADLs.

Rahul is married and has two children aged 5 and 8 years. His facial burns are frightening to his children, and his depression has begun to impact his marriage. Rahul has begun to pull away from his family and requested that they no longer visit him at the rehabilitation center. Because Rahul was injured at work, he is receiving worker's compensation benefits and plans to stay at the rehabilitation facility for approximately 12 weeks.

RECOMMENDED LEARNING RESOURCES

Herndon, D. N. (Ed.) (2012). *Total burn care* (4th ed.). London: WB Saunders. Associated online support at: www.totalburn-care.com

American Burn Association
311 S. Wacker Drive, Suite 4150 Chicago, IL 60606
Tel: 312-642-9260
Fax: 312-642-9130
E-Mail: info@americanburn.org
www.ameriburn.org

Shriners Burn Institutes
2900 Rocky Point Dr
Tampa, FL 33607-1460
Tel: 813-281-0300
http://www.shrinershospitalsforchildren.org/care/burn-care

The Phoenix Society for Burn Survivors, Inc
1835 R W Berends Dr SW
Grand Rapids, MI 49519-4955
Tel: 800-888-2876 or 616-458-2773
Fax: 616-458-2831
www.phoenix-society.org
E-Mail: info@phoenix-society.org

Burn Summer Camps for Kids
(Information available at Kids Camps)
909 N. Sepulveda Blvd., 11th Floor
El Segundo, CA 90245
Tel: 877-242-9330
Fax: 310-280-5177
www.kidscamps.com/special_needs/burn.html

Children's Burn Foundation
5000 Van Nuys Boulevard, Suite 450
Sherman Oaks, CA 91403
Tel: 818-907-2822
Fax: 818-501-4005
Toll free: 800-949-8898
E-Mail: info@childburn.org
www.childburn.org

International Burn Foundation
6915 Ebenezer Church Road
Hillsborough, NC 27278
Tel: 919-471-4714
E-Mail: internationalburn@gmail.com
www.internationalburnfoundation.org

REFERENCES

Abboud, E. C., Legare, T. B., Settle, J. C., Boubekri, A. M., Barillo, D. J., Marcet, J. E., & Sanchez, J. E. (2014). Do silver-based wound dressings reduce pain? A prospective study and review of the literature. *Burns, 40*(Suppl. 1), S40–S47. http://dx.doi.org/10.1016/j.burns.2014.09.012

Abdullahi, A., & Jeschke, M. G. (2015). Enteral nutrition support in burns. *Diet and nutrition in critical care*, 1539–1549. New York: Springer. http://dx.doi.org/10.1007/978-1-4614-7836-2_110

American Burn Association. (2015) *Burn incidence and treatment in the United States: 2015.* Retrieved from http://www.ameriburn.org/resources_factsheet.php

Amirsheybani, H. R., Crecelius, G. M., Timothy, N. H., Pfeiffer, M., Saggers, G. C., & Manders, E. K. (2001). The natural history of the growth of the hand: I. Hand area as a percentage of body surface area. *Plastic and Reconstructive Surgery, 107*(3), 726–733. http://dx.doi.org/10.1097/00006534-200103000-00012

Atiyeh, B. S., Dibo, S. A., Ibrahim, A. E., & Zgheib, E. R. (2012). Acute burn resuscitation and fluid creep: It is time for colloid rehabilitation. *Annals of Burns and Fire Disasters, 25*(2), 59–65.

Barillo, D. J. (2009). Diagnosis and treatment of cyanide toxicity. *Journal of Burn Care & Research, 30*(1), 148–152. http://dx.doi.org/10.1097/BCR.0b013e3181923b91

Bezuhly, M., & Fish, J. S. (2012). Acute burn care. *Plastic and Reconstructive Surgery, 130*(2), 349–358e. http://dx.doi.org/10.1097/PRS.0b013e318258d530

Carr, J. A., Phillips, B. D., & Bowling, W. M. (2009). The utility of bronchoscopy after inhalation injury complicated by pneumonia in burn patients: Results from the National Burn Repository. *Journal of Burn Care & Research, 30*(6), 967–974. http://dx.doi.org/10.1097/BCR.0b013e3181bfb77b

Chaudhari, K. R., Upadhyay, M. C., Bambhaniya, A. B., & Patel, J. B. (2015) Profile of deaths due to burns at tertiary care center with special emphasis on septicemia: A one year retrospective study. *International Journal of Health Sciences and Research (IJHSR), 5*(8), 82–88.

Church, D., Elsayed, S., Reid, O., Winston, B., & Lindsay, R. (2006). Burn wound infections. *Clinical Microbiology Reviews, 19*(2), 403–434. http://dx.doi.org/10.1128/CMR.19.2.403-434.2006

Davison, P. G., Loiselle, F. B., & Nickerson, D. (2010). Survey on current hydrotherapy use among North American burn centers. *Journal of Burn Care & Research*, *31*(3), 393–399. http://dx.doi.org/10.1097/BCR.0b013e3181db5215

Dries, D. J., & Endorf, F. W. (2013). Inhalation injury: Epidemiology, pathology, treatment strategies. *Scandinavian Journal of Trauma, Resuscitation and Emergency Medicine*, *21*, 31. http://dx.doi.org/10.1186/1757-7241-21-31

Ehanire, T., Vissoci, J. R., Slaughter, K., Coêlho, R., Bond, J., Rodrigues, C., … Levinson, H. (2013). A systematic review of the psychometric properties of self-reported scales assessing burn contractures reveals the need for a new tool to measure contracture outcomes. *Wound Repair and Regeneration*, *21*(4), 520–529. http://dx.doi.org/10.1111/wrr.12058

Fang, T., Lineaweaver, W. C., Sailes, F. C., Kisner, C., & Zhang, F. (2014). Clinical application of cultured epithelial autografts on acellular dermal matrices in the treatment of extended burn injuries. *Annals of Plastic Surgery*, *73*(5), 509–515. http://dx.doi.org/10.1097/SAP.0b013e3182840883

Fearmonti, R. M., Bond, J. E., Erdmann, D., Levin, L. S., Pizzo, S. V., & Levinson, H. (2011). The modified patient and observer scar assessment scale: A novel approach to defining pathologic and nonpathologic scarring. *Plastic and Reconstructive Surgery*, *127*(1), 242–247. http://dx.doi.org/10.1097/PRS.0b013e3181f959e8

Greenhalgh, D. G. (2010). Burn resuscitation: The results of the isbi/aba survey. *Burns*, *36*(2), 176–182. http://dx.doi.org/10.1016/j.burns.2009.09.004

Greenhalgh, D. G., Saffle, J. R., Holmes, J. H., Gamelli, R. L., Palmieri, T. L., Horton, J. W., … Latenser, B. A.; American Burn Association Consensus Conference on Burn Sepsis and Infection Group. (2007). American Burn Association consensus conference to define sepsis and infection in burns. *Journal of Burn Care & Research*, *28*(6), 776–790. http://dx.doi.org/10.1097/BCR.0b013e3181599bc9

Heppt, M. V., Breuninger, H., Reinholz, M., Feller Heppt, G., Ruzicka, T., & Gauglitz, G. (2015). Current strategies in the treatment of scars and keloids. *Facial Plastic Surgery*, *31*(4), 386–395. http://dx.doi.org/10.1055/s-0035-1563694

Herdon, D. N. (2012). *Total burn care* (4th ed.). Edinburgh: Saunders Elsevier.

James, M. F. (2012). Place of the colloids in fluid resuscitation of the traumatized patient. *Current Opinion in Anaesthesiology*, *25*(2), 248–252. http://dx.doi.org/10.1097/ACO.0b013e32834fcede

Kao, C. C., & Garner, W. L. (2000). Acute burns. *Plastic and Reconstructive Surgery*, *105*(7),

2482–2492; quiz 2493; discussion 2494. http://dx.doi.org/10.1097/00006534-200006000-00028

Kowalske, K. J. (2011). Burn wound care. *Physical Medicine and Rehabilitation Clinics of North America*, *22*(2), 213–227. http://dx.doi.org/10.1016/j.pmr.2011.03.004

Kupas, D. F., & Miller, D. (2010). Out-of-hospital chest escharotomy: A case series and procedure review. *Prehospital Emergency Care*, *14*(3), 349–354. http://dx.doi.org/10.3109/10903121003770670

Latenser, B. A., & Kowal-Vern, A. (2002). Pediatric burn rehabilitation. *Pediatric Rehabilitation*, *5*, 3–10.

Lavrentieva, A. (2016). Critical care of burn patients. New approaches to old problems. *Burns*, *42*, 13–19.

Leto Barone, A., Mastroianni, M., Farkash, E. A., Mallard, C., Albritton, A., Torabi, R., … Cetrulo, C. L. (2015). Genetically modified porcine split-thickness skin grafts as an alternative to allograft for provision of temporary wound coverage: Preliminary characterization. *Burns*, *41*(3), 565–574. http://dx.doi.org/10.1016/j.burns.2014.09.003

Lloyd, E. C., Rodgers, B. C., Michener, M., & Williams, M. S. (2012). Outpatient burns: Prevention and care. *American Family Physician*, *85*(1), 25–32.

Lorello, D. J., Peck, M., Albrecht, M., Richey, K. J., & Pressman, M. A. (2014). Results of a prospective randomized controlled trial of early ambulation for patients with lower extremity autografts. *Journal of Burn Care & Research*, *35*(5), 431–436. http://dx.doi.org/10.1097/bcr.0000000000000014

Mahjour, S. B., Fu, X., Yang, X., Fong, J., Sefat, F., & Wang, H. (2015). Rapid creation of skin substitutes from human skin cells and biomimetic nanofibers for acute full-thickness wound repair. *Burns*, *41*(8), 1764–1774. http://dx.doi.org/10.1016/j.burns.2015.06.011

McGraft, J., & Uitto, J. (2010). Anatomy and organization of human skin. In T. Burns, C. Breathnac, N. Cox, & C. Griffiths (Eds.), *Rooks textbook of dermatology* (8th ed.). Oxford, UK: Wiley-Blackwell.

Mlcak, R. P., Suman, O. E., & Herndon, D. N. (2007). Respiratory management of inhalation injury. *Burns*, *33*(1), 2–13. http://dx.doi.org/10.1016/j.burns.2006.07.007

Morgan, E. D., Bledsoe, S. C., & Barker, J. (2000). Ambulatory management of burns. *American Family Physician*, *62*(9), 2015–2029.

Nguyen, D. Q., Potokar, T. S., & Price, P. (2010). An objective long-term evaluation of integra (a dermal skin substitute) and split thickness skin grafts, in acute burns and reconstructive surgery.

Burns, 36(1), 23–28. http://dx.doi.org/10.1016/j.burns.2009.07.011

Niedzielski, L. S., & Chapman, M. T. (2015). Changes in burn scar contracture: Utilization of a severity scale and predictor of return to duty for service members. *Journal of Burn Care & Research, 36*(3), e212–e219. http://dx.doi.org/10.1097/BCR.0000000000000148

Nikkhah, D., Booth, S., Tay, S., Gilbert, P., & Dheansa, B. (2015). Comparing outcomes of sheet grafting with 1:1 mesh grafting in patients with thermal burns: A randomized trial. *Burns, 41*(2), 257–264. http://dx.doi.org/10.1016/j.burns.2014.07.023

Palmu, R., Partonen, T., Suominen, K., Vuola, J., & Isometsä, E. (2015). Functioning, disability, and social adaptation 6 months after burn injury. *Journal of Burn Care & Research.* Advanced online publication, *41*(6), 1152–60. http://dx.doi.org/10.1097/BCR.0000000000000258

Palmu, R., Suominen, K., Vuola, J., & Isometsä, E. (2011). Mental disorders after burn injury: A prospective study. *Burns, 37*(4), 601–609. http://dx.doi.org/10.1016/j.burns.2010.06.007

Paratz, J. D., Stockton, K., Plaza, A., Muller, M., & Boots, R. J. (2012). Intensive exercise after thermal injury improves physical, functional, and psychological outcomes. *Journal of Trauma and Acute Care Surgery, 73*(1), 186–194. http://dx.doi.org/10.1097/TA.0b013e31824baa52

Parihar, A., Parihar, M. S., Milner, S., & Bhat, S. (2008). Oxidative stress and anti-oxidative mobilization in burn injury. *Burns, 34*(1), 6–17. http://dx.doi.org/10.1016/j.burns.2007.04.009

Parvizi, D., Giretzlehner, M., Dirnberger, J., Owen, R., Haller, H. L., Schintler, M. V., ... Kamolz, L. P. (2014). The use of telemedicine in burn care: Development of a mobile system for tbsa documentation and remote assessment. *Annals of Burns and Fire Disasters, 27*(2), 94–100.

Pukar, M., Rajshakha, A., Mewada, S., & Lakhani, D. (2015). Outcome of heliotherapy and modified Parkland's formula for fluid resuscitation in management of moderate degree of burns: A single centre observational study. *IJSS, 1*(3), 8.

Rowan, M. P., Cancio, L. C., Elster, E. A., Burmeister, D. M., Rose, L. F., Natesan, S., ... Chung, K. K. (2015). Burn wound healing and treatment: Review and advancements. *Critical Care, 19*, 243. http://dx.doi.org/10.1186/s13054-015-0961-2

Saaiq, M., Zaib, S., & Ahmad, S. (2012). Early excision and grafting versus delayed excision and grafting of deep thermal burns up to 40% total body surface area: A comparison of outcome. *Annals of Burns and Fire Disasters, 25*(3), 143–147.

Sahin, I., Eski, M., Acikel, C., Kapaj, R., Alhan, D., & Isik, S. (2012). The role of negative pressure wound therapy in the treatment of fourth-degree burns. Trends and new horizons. *Annals of Burns and Fire Disasters, 25*(2), 92–97.

Selig, H. F., Lumenta, D. B., Giretzlehner, M., Jeschke, M. G., Upton, D., & Kamolz, L. P. (2012). The properties of an "ideal" burn wound dressing—What do we need in daily clinical practice? Results of a worldwide online survey among burn care specialists. *Burns, 38*(7), 960–966. http://dx.doi.org/10.1016/j.burns.2012.04.007

Sheng, W., Zeng, D., Wan, Y., Yao, L., Tang, H., & Xia, Z. (2014). Burncalc assessment study of computer-aided individual three-dimensional burn area calculation. *Journal of Translational Medicine, 12*, 242. http://dx.doi.org/10.1186/s12967-014-0242-x

Sterling, J. P. (2014). Silver-resistance, allergy, and blue skin: Truth or urban legend?. *Burns, 40*(Suppl. 1), S19–S23. http://dx.doi.org/10.1016/j.burns.2014.10.007

Upton, D., & Andrews, A. (2014). The impact of stress at dressing change in patients with burns: A review of the literature on pain and itching. *Wounds, 26*(3), 77–82.

Veeravagu, A., Yoon, B. C., Jiang, B., Carvalho, C. M., Rincon, F., Maltenfort, M., ... Ratliff, J. K. (2015). National trends in burn and inhalation injury in burn patients: Results of analysis of the nationwide inpatient sample database. *Journal of Burn Care & Research, 36*(2), 258–265. http://dx.doi.org/10.1097/BCR.0000000000000064

Viera, M. H., Vivas, A. C., & Berman, B. (2012). Update on keloid management: Clinical and basic science advances. *Advances in Wound Care, 1*(5), 200–206. http://dx.doi.org/10.1089/wound.2011.0313

Warner, P. M., Coffee, T. L., & Yowler, C. J. (2014). Outpatient burn management. *The Surgical Clinics of North America, 94*(4), 879–892. http://dx.doi.org/10.1016/j.suc.2014.05.009

Williams, F. N., Jeschke, M. G., Chinkes, D. L., Suman, O. E., Branski, L. K., & Herndon, D. N. (2009). Modulation of the hypermetabolic response to trauma: Temperature, nutrition, and drugs. *Journal of the American College of Surgeons, 208*(4), 489–502. http://dx.doi.org/10.1016/j.jamcollsurg.2009.01.022

Williams, J. F., King, B. T., Aden, J. K., Serio Melvin, M., Chung, K., Fenrich, C. A., ... Cancio, L. C. (2013). Comparison of traditional burn wound mapping with a computerized program. *Journal of Burn Care & Research, 34*(1), e29–e35. http://dx.doi.org/10.1097/BCR.0b013e3182676e07

Woo, K. Y. (2010). Wound-related pain: Anxiety, stress and wound healing. *Wounds UK, 6*(4), 92–98.

22

Progressive Neurodegenerative Disorders

Diane Powers Dirette

Shortly after the birth of her second child, Joan started getting the sensation of pins and needles in her hands and feet. Within a couple of months, she noticed some numbness and weakness in her arms and legs. She was having difficulty walking for long distances and began to worry that she might drop her 2-year-old son or even her newborn. When the children napped in the afternoon, she found herself slumped on the couch for a much-needed rest. Convinced that this was just part of her postpartum recovery, Joan did not inform her doctor of this difficulty. However, when she found herself struggling one day to focus on the words of her son's bedtime story, she decided to seek medical advice.

Over time, Joan found out that she had a progressive neurodegenerative disorder (PND) called multiple sclerosis (MS). PNDs are a group of diseases that affect various areas of the central nervous system (CNS), are chronic in nature, and cause a deterioration of function over time. This chapter discusses three of the most common PNDs: MS, Parkinson's disease (PD), and amyotrophic lateral sclerosis (ALS).

There is little known about the underlying etiology and there is no known cause of any of these three PNDs, but research indicates that the etiology is a combination of interrelated factors (Armon, Kurland, Beard, O'Brien, & Mulder, 1991; Kenealy, Pericak-Vance, & Haines, 2003). These include genetic predisposition, viruses, antigens, infectious diseases, and environmental factors. A genetic predisposition is suspected because these diseases are more prevalent among families and certain racial groups. Viruses, antigens, or infectious diseases and their resulting autoimmune response also may be involved as a cause of these PNDs (Nylander & Hafler, 2012). Specific viruses have not been isolated, but particular interest has focused on a viral subgroup called retroviruses. What causes them is unknown, and they can remain silent for years before the onset of a disease. Environmental factors, including exposure to such toxins as lead or pesticides, have also been associated with a higher incidence of PND (Armon et al., 1991; Kamel et al., 2006). None of these factors, however, have been isolated as the single cause of any of the PNDs.

MULTIPLE SCLEROSIS

■ Description and Definitions

MS is a debilitating immunological and neurodegenerative disease in which the genetically susceptible person's own immune system attacks the **myelin sheath** that surrounds the brain, spinal cord, and optic nerve (Kalb, 1996; Kenealy et al., 2003; Nylander & Hafler, 2012). This process is called **demyelination**. MS is characterized by chronic inflammation and diffuse demyelination not only in the white matter but also in the gray matter and the axons (Compston & Coles, 2002). Demyelination of the neurons in the CNS results in scar tissue formation or **plaques** that reduce the axons' ability to conduct impulses (Kenealy et al., 2003). The location of demyelination varies from person to person. The visual, motor, sensory, cognitive, psychological, and bowel and bladder systems can be affected. See Figure 22.1.

■ Etiology

Why the attack on the myelin sheath begins is unknown because the exact cause of MS is unknown. It is hypothesized to be a combination of genetic susceptibility and environmental factors, such as a virus or infection (Compston & Coles, 2008; Murray, 2002). The latest evidence regarding MS suggests that a viral infection triggers the immune system to wage an attack on the nerve cells of people who are genetically susceptible (Hanson & Cafruny, 2002). MS is polygenetic and although it does not follow an obvious pattern of inheritance (Wakerley, Nicholas, & Malik, 2012), it has a familial recurrence rate of 20% and is more common in first-degree relatives versus more distant relatives (Compston & Coles, 2008). Recent research has identified some potential specific genetic associations with the HLA gene on chromosome 6, and certain leukocyte antigen types (DR15 and DQ6) may play an important role in the abnormal response of the T cells (Wakerley et al., 2012). Other factors that

may contribute to the cause of MS include smoking (Hernan, Olek, & Ascherio, 2001), a lack of ultraviolet light exposure resulting in vitamin D deficiency (Berlanga-Taylor, Disanto, Ebers, & Ramagopalan, 2011), heavy metal toxins in the environment (Noonan et al., 2010), and a history of viral infections such as mononucleosis and Epstein-Barr virus (Compston & Coles, 2008; Wakerley et al., 2012).

■ Incidence and Prevalence

MS is the most common nontraumatic neurodegenerative disorder among adults under 40 years of age (Carrithers, 2014). It affects approximately

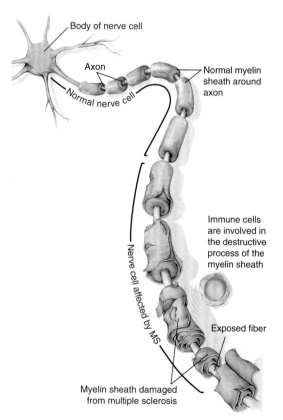

Figure 22.1 Nerve cell in multiple sclerosis. (From Anatomical Chart Co.)

1% of the population of the United States, and there is evidence that those numbers are increasing (Kalb, 1996; Kenealy et al., 2003; Noonan, Kathman, & White, 2002b). Currently, an estimated 400,000 people in the United States have MS (Harrison, 2014) and 100 per 100,000 in the United Kingdom. The distribution of prevalence varies geographically. The closer a person lives to the equator, the less likely he or she is to have MS (Matthews, 1993; Noonan et al., 2010). For example, in the southern United States, the rate of incidence is 20 to 39 for every 100,000 persons. In the northern United States and Canada, the rate is more than 40 out of every 100,000 persons (Matthews, 1993). If a person migrates from a location near the equator prior to age 15, the incidence of MS is reduced, which contributes to the theory of a possible childhood infection having a role in the onset (Hanson & Cafruny, 2002) or of the influence of limited exposure to ultraviolet light (Noonan et al., 2010).

The incidence of MS also varies according to gender. MS affects females more often than males at a ratio of between 2 and 3 females for every 1 male with the disease (Hanson & Cafruny, 2002; Harrison, 2014). The current trend supports an increasing prevalence among women with approximately 125 per 100,000 women and 40 per 100,000 men in the United States (Noonan et al., 2002b; Wakerley et al., 2012).

In general, MS has a global distribution with the frequency increasing as the distance from the equator increases and it occurs more frequently among people of European ancestry than other white racial groups (Compston & Coles, 2008). Even within northern countries, there is a distribution of increasing incidence in the northern parts of the countries (Wakerley et al., 2012). People of Scandinavian and Scottish descent are most susceptible to MS. It is twice as common among Caucasians as other races and it is rare among people of Mongolian, Japanese, Chinese, Native American, Eskimo, African Black and Aborigine descent (Hanson & Cafruny, 2002; Wakerley et al., 2012). If a person migrates from a low-risk region to a high-risk region before 15 years of age, the low risk associated with the person's region of birth remains (Compston & Coles, 2008).

Studies of offspring, twins, siblings, and adopted children demonstrate that the closer a relation genetically, the more likely a person is to have MS (Compston & Coles, 2008; Neilsen et al., 2005). The incidence of MS decreases as biological relationship decreases. If a person has MS, the identical twin, full siblings, half siblings, and offspring have increased risk of also having MS in that order (Compston & Coles, 2008; Kenealy et al., 2003). In adoption studies, increased risk was only noted in biological relatives (Compston & Coles, 2008).

■ Signs and Symptoms

Because MS can affect nearly any part of the CNS, the signs and symptoms of MS can vary greatly (Harrison, 2014). In general, the motor, sensory, visual, and autonomic systems are affected by MS. Some specific symptoms of MS include visual deficits such as diplopia (double vision) or unilateral optic neuritis, sensory disturbances such as dysesthesia or paresthesia, urinary incontinence or retention, erectile dysfunction, muscle weakness, gross and fine motor incoordination, pain, weakness, spasticity, fatigue, ataxia, dysphagia, dysarthria, vestibular dysfunction, and cognitive or emotional disturbances (Compston & Coles, 2008; Wakerley et al., 2012). Each person with MS has symptoms that result from lesions in specific areas of the CNS. The types of symptoms, their intensity, and their effects on the person's functional status are highly individualized (Delisa, Hammond, Mikulic, & Miller, 1985). Table 22.1 includes a summary of common signs and symptoms associated with the various lesion sites.

Visual disturbances often are among the earliest signs of MS (Rocca, Messina, & Filippi, 2013). They usually appear as a partial loss of vision (scotoma), double or blurred vision, or ocular pain (Harrison, 2014). Sudden loss of vision with pain in or behind the eye is caused by optic neuritis. These early symptoms may subside after 3 to 6 weeks without any residual deficit. For others, visual loss may be insidious and painless. Nonetheless, nearly 80% of all persons who have MS have some loss of visual acuity. Oculomotor control may also be affected due to lesions of the supranuclear connection to the oculomotor nuclei in the brainstem. As a result, the person loses horizontal eye movement either unilaterally or bilaterally.

The individual with MS can experience a variety of other sensory disturbances such as numbness; impairment of vibratory, proprioceptive, pain, touch, and temperature sensation; and distortion of superficial sensation. Because of

TABLE 22.1	Common Symptoms, Signs, and Medical Management of Multiple Sclerosis		
Lesion Site	**Symptom**	**Sign**	**Medication**
Cerebrum	Cognitive impairment Hemisensory and motor Affective	Impaired attention, memory, and executive functions Upper motor neuron signs Depression or euphoria	Donepezil, rivastigmine, and galantamine Citalopram, venlafaxine, and amitriptyline
Optic nerve	Loss of vision	Scotoma, reduced visual acuity, color blindness, and ocular pain	
Cerebellum	Tremor Dysarthria Incoordination and poor balance	Postural and limb insta-bility during movement Poor articulation Clumsiness, ataxic movements, and falls	Clonazepam, primidone, beta-blockers
Brainstem	Loss of vision Vertigo Dysarthria Pseudobulbar palsy	Nystagmus, reduced oculomotor control Decreased balance Impaired swallowing Impaired speech and emotional lability	Anticholinergic drugs Tricyclic antidepressant drugs
Spinal cord	Impaired muscle tone Bowel and bladder dysfunction Erectile dysfunction	Spasticity, weakness, stiffness, and painful spasms Incontinence and constipation Impotence	Baclofen, dantrolene, diaz-epam, tizanidine, cannabis extract, botulinum toxin Oxybutynin, tolterodine, intravesical, botulinum toxin, laxatives Sildenafil
Other	Fatigue Pain Dysregulation of temperature	Unexplained lethargy, exercise intolerance Complaints of pain in various body regions Hypersensitivity to heat	Amantadine, modafinil Amitriptyline, pregaba-lin, gabapentin, cannabis extract

Adapted from Compston, A., & Coles, A. (2008). Multiple sclerosis. *The Lancet, 372*, 1502–1517.

these sensory losses, the person also may lose various perceptual skills such as stereognosis, kinesthesia, and body scheme (Umphred, 1990).

Fatigue is the most common complaint and is often identified as the most debilitating symptom (Filippi et al., 2002). Increased energy is required for nerves to conduct their impulses in a demye-linated nervous system, making it difficult for the individual to initiate movement and perform sus-tained activities. The individual also may experi-ence muscle weakness. As the disease progresses, the person requires more frequent rest periods between activities, and decreased levels of activ-ity lead to further debilitation.

Approximately 40% to 70% of individuals with MS experience some change in their cog-nitive ability (Rocca et al., 2013). Short-term memory, attention, processing speed, visuospa-tial abilities, verbal fluency, and executive func-tions have all been identified as deficit areas related to MS (Bobholz & Rao, 2003; Lyros, Messinis, Papageorgiou, & Papathanosopoulos, 2010). As with all aspects of MS, there is con-siderable variability among individuals with the disease depending on the area of the brain affected (Bobholz & Rao, 2003). An emotional component to this disease results in some indi-viduals having bouts of depression, euphoria, or lability caused by lesions in the frontal lobes of the brain (Feinstein, 2006).

Course and Prognosis

MS is the most common PND found in young adults and is usually diagnosed between the ages of 20 and 40 years (Matthews, 1993). Peak age of onset is about 30 years, and it is rarely seen in children or diagnosed in adults older than age 60 (Wakerley et al., 2012). The clinical course of this disease is variable among individuals, but it can be roughly organized into four types or patterns including benign, relapsing-remitting-nonprogressive, relapsing-remitting-progressive, and primary progressive.

The first type of MS is **benign**, in which the person experiences one or two episodes of neurological deficits with no residual impairments. This person's chance of remaining symptom free increases with each nonsymptomatic year. The next pattern of progression is **relapsing-remitting-nonprogressive**. In this pattern, the person returns to the previous level of function after each exacerbation with no residual deficits. With the third type, **relapsing-remitting-progressive**, however, the person has some residual impairment with each remission. The course of this type is unpredictable with varied patterns of exacerbation and remission. Finally, there is the **primary progressive** pattern, which involves a steady decline in function without remissions and exacerbations. Approximately 65% to 85% of people have one of the relapsing-remitting forms of MS in which they experience neurological symptoms followed by complete or partial recovery (Hanson & Cafruny, 2002; Harrison, 2014), but about 25% of these individuals will develop a progressive form of MS in which they do not experience remissions (Wakerley et al., 2012). Approximately 10% to 20% experience the primary progressive pattern of decline in function without periods of remission of symptoms from the outset (Compston & Coles, 2008; Harrison, 2014; Noonan et al., 2010; Nylander & Hafler, 2012).

The course of MS varies not only among the subtypes but also among individuals. In general, progression of symptoms begins around 40 years of age and the clinical course evolves over several decades (Compston & Coles, 2008). Ten years after the disease onset, about 10% will be wheelchair bound and about 50% will be unable to work (Wakerley et al., 2012).

The median time from disease onset to death is around 30 years (Compston & Coles, 2008).

This prognosis, however, depends on the time of onset. People diagnosed with MS in their 20s have a prognosis of approximately 46 to 60 years, whereas people diagnosed with MS in their 60s have a prognosis of approximately 13 to 22 years (Hurwitz, 2011).

Diagnosis

The diagnosis of MS involves excluding alternate neurological conditions that share the symptomatology of MS such as systemic lupus erythematosus, neuromyelitis optica, acute disseminated encephalomyelitis, and neurosarcoidosis (Kenealy et al., 2003; Rocca et al., 2013; Wakerley et al., 2012). Because there are no specific MS biomarkers, the physician will use a full assessment of clinical symptoms combined with testing to aid in diagnosis (Harrison, 2014). The McDonald criteria combine the assessment of these clinical symptoms with the outcome of magnetic resonance imaging (MRI) and cerebral spinal fluid (CSF) analysis to make a definitive diagnosis of MS (Harrison, 2014; Wakerley et al., 2012). According to these criteria, there are three combinations of clinical symptoms and test results that can provide the diagnosis of MS. The first criterion is two or more relapses of clinical symptoms and evidence of two or more objective lesions. The second criterion that may be used includes one relapse and evidence of one objective lesion, plus a positive CSF with 2+ lesions as demonstrated on MRI or a further relapse. The last criterion includes insidious neurological progression suggestive of MS plus a positive CSF and MRI evidence of 9+ lesions in the brain, 2+ lesions in the spinal cord, or 4 to 8 lesions in the brain and one lesion in the spinal cord.

Medical/Surgical Management

Surgical intervention is not part of the routine care given for MS. There are some medications, however, currently available to provide some overall disease modification, and several medications are used to alleviate the myriad symptoms caused by MS (Carrithers, 2014). Disease-modifying drugs such as interferon β-1b, glatiramer acetate, azathioprine, and fingolimod show some potential to provide a reduction in relapses in the progression of MS (Carrithers, 2014; Harrison, 2014; Lyros et al., 2010; Wakerley et al., 2012). Second-line disease-modifying treatments that promote antibodies include natalizumab, rituximab, and alemtuzumab (Carrithers, 2014). Possible future treatments include antiviral medications, vaccinations, transplantation of Schwann cells, cell lines or stem cells, and/or gene therapy (Noseworthy, 2003). Other antibody treatments, such as anti-LINGO-1, are being tested for the potential to regenerate myelin (Ledford, 2015). Teriflunomide to inhibit rapidly dividing T cells and alemtuzumab to kill T cells show some promise in the reduction of relapses (Wakerley et al., 2012).

There are several medications prescribed to manage the symptoms of MS. See Table 14.1 for a complete list. Beta-blockers may be prescribed to treat spasticity. Anticholinergic drugs are used to treat difficulty swallowing. Several different antidepressant drugs may be prescribed to treat changes in affect. Various painkillers may be prescribed and steroids may be used to reduce nerve inflammation (Harrison, 2014). Cannabis extract has been used to treat both pain and spasticity (Wakerley et al., 2012). Acetylcholinesterase inhibitors such as donepezil, rivastigmine, and galantamine, which were developed for the treatment of Alzheimer's disease, have shown some promise for alleviating cognitive symptoms such as attention, information processing, and memory/learning (Bobholz & Rao, 2003; Lyros et al., 2010).

Nonpharmacological interventions that have been found to alleviate some symptoms of MS include cognitive rehabilitation, occupational therapy, physical therapy, psychotherapy, and early nursing education (Bobholz & Rao, 2003; Harrison, 2014; Lyros et al., 2010; Wassem & Dudley, 2003). Lifestyle changes, such as a healthy diet and adequate sleep, may be helpful (Harrison, 2014). Low-impact exercise with a gradual increase in intensity, duration, and frequency was also found to be effective for reducing fatigue in adults with MS (Neill, Belan, & Reid, 2006). Bone marrow transplants intended to reset the immune system have also shown promise for reducing relapses, but because of the neurodegenerative aspect of MS, this treatment has not been able to thwart the disease progression (Wakerley et al., 2012).

PARKINSON'S DISEASE

■ Description and Definitions

Parkinson's disease (PD) is a PND characterized by death of dopaminergic neurons in the **substantia nigra** pars compacta and the presence of Lewy bodies (Kalia & Lang, 2015; Zhang, Dawson, & Dawson, 2000). The substantia nigra, which is located in the basal ganglia, produces **dopamine**, a neurotransmitter, and transports it to the dorsal striatum (see Fig. 22.2). The decrease in dopamine leads to deficits in the speed and quality of motor

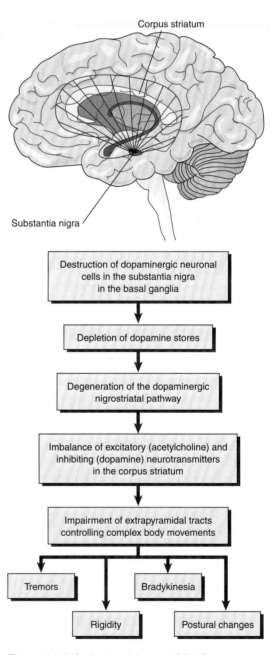

Figure 22.2 Pathophysiology of PD. (From Smeltzer, S. C., Bare, G. B., Hinkle, J. L. (2008). *Brunner & Suddarth's textbook of medical surgical nursing* (11th ed.). Philadelphia, PA: Lippincott Williams & Wilkins.)

movements, postural stability, cognitive skills, and affective expression (DeLong, 2000; Duvoisin & Sage, 1996). In addition to dopaminergic denervation, there is also evidence of serotonergic loss as well (Politis & Niccolini, 2015). The progression of serotonergic denervation, however, happens at a slower pace.

Neuronal degeneration progresses beyond the substantia nigra and the brainstem and can affect other neurotrasmitter systems (Zhang et al., 2000). **Lewy body pathology** is a process in which proteins abnormally fold and form intracellular inclusions within the cell body and neurons (Kalia & Lang, 2015). The progression of Lewy body pathology stereotypically progresses through six stages over time and throughout the CNS beginning with the peripheral nervous system and progressing through the pons, spinal cord gray matter, midbrain, basal forebrain, limbic system, thalamus, and temporal cortex before affecting multiple cortical regions of the brain (see Table 22.2) (Braak et al., 2003). Neuroinflammation is another typical feature of PD (Kalia & Lang, 2015).

There are variations in the clinical and pathological presentation of PD, and there is overlap with other parkinsonian disorders (Albanese, 2003). Two subtypes of PD have been proposed that include **tremor-dominant PD** with relative absence of other motor symptoms and **nontremor-dominant PD** with akinetic-rigid syndrome and postural instability gait disorder (Kalia & Lang, 2015).

■ Etiology

The underlying cause of PD is unknown although there is some evidence that implicates an interaction of genetic and environmental factors (Kalia & Lang, 2015; Kamel et al., 2006). Two types of PD include **familial** PD in which there is a genetic association and the more common type called

sporadic PD. Several genetic factors, such as linkages to chromosomes 2 and 4, have been identified in familial PD (Macphee & Stewart, 2012; Zhang et al., 2000). As many as 43% of people with familial PD have an affected relative, and a predisposition for developing PD was found to significantly more common in monozygotic twins versus dizygotic twins (Macphee & Stewart, 2012). The involvement of genetic factors in sporadic PD has not been fully established, but increasing evidence points to an interaction with environmental factors (Kalia & Lang, 2015; Kamel et al., 2006).

The environmental factors that have been associated with PD include dietary intake, exposure to environmental elements, and a history of head trauma. Diet may not be a primary cause of PD, but many studies have found an association between diet and the risk for PD suggesting a role in the susceptibility to the disease (Gao et al., 2008). Some examples include the following: exposure to iron sources and intake of too much iron supplement was associated with increased risk of PD (Logroscino, Gao, Chen, Wing, & Ascherio, 2008), increased dairy consumption was associated with increased risk of PD in men (Chen et al., 2007), and higher total blood cholesterol levels were associated with decreased risk of PD in women (de Lau, Koudstaal, Hofman, & Breteler, 2006). The use of beta-blockers and antipsychotics also has been found to enhance the risk of PD as does the consumption of well water (Kalia & Lang, 2015).

Exposure to various environmental elements is also a risk factor for developing PD. Several studies have found that living in rural areas, drinking well water, having an agricultural occupation, and being exposed to pesticides can each increase a person's risk for PD (Kalia & Lang, 2015; Kamel et al., 2006; McCormack, Thiruchelvam, Mannig-Bog, Thiffault, Langston, 2002; Priyadarshi, Khuder, Schaub, & Priyadarshi, 2001).

TABLE 22.2 Braak Model of Lewy Pathology in PD	
Stage 1	Peripheral nervous system, olfactory system, medulla
Stage 2	Pons, spinal cord gray matter
Stage 3	Pons, midbrain, basal forebrain, limbic system
Stage 4	Limbic system, thalamus, temporal cortex
Stages 5 and 6	Multiple cortical regions (insular cortex, association cortical areas, primary cortical areas)

■ Incidence and Prevalence

Parkinson's disease (PD) is the second most common neurodegenerative disorder (Kalia & Lang, 2015; Zhang, Dawson, & Dawson, 2000). Worldwide, the prevalence of PD is estimated at 1% of the population above the age of 60 years, with estimates as high as one million cases in the United States (Connolly & Lang, 2014; Kamel et al., 2006). The prevalence and incidence increase greatly with age to around 2% in the population over 80 years of age (Macphee & Stewart, 2012). Because of the aging of the world's population, the prevalence of PD is expected to continue to increase. PD is more prevalent in Europe, North America, and South America compared to African, Asian, and Arabic countries (Kalia & Lang, 2015).

The incidence of PD ranges from 10 to 18 per 100,000 people per year (Kalia & Lang, 2015). PD affects males slightly more than females with a 3:2 ratio and varies among races. In the United States, the incidence is greatest among people who are Hispanic, followed by Caucasians, Asians, and African Americans in descending order (Kalia & Lang, 2015). PD is more common in urban counties than in rural counties and is more concentrated in the Midwestern and Northeastern United States (Willis et al., 2010).

■ Signs and Symptoms

There are motor, cognitive, psychiatric, and autonomic symptoms associated with PD. The primary motor symptoms are resting tremor, muscle rigidity, and bradykinesia (Albanese, 2003; Connolly & Lang, 2014) (see Table 22.3). The most obvious and familiar of these symptoms is tremor, which is usually noted initially in the hand on one side and sometimes in the foot. In the hand, the movement is frequently described as "pill-rolling." The tremors are usually variable, and they disappear when the person is asleep or calmly resting and they increase under stress or intense mental activity (Duvoisin & Sage, 1996). Infrequent eye blinking is often an early sign of PD followed by progressive loss of facial expression. Other early nonmotor symptoms include hyposmia (reduced olfactory sense), fatigue, depression, rapid eye movement (REM), sleep behavior disorder, and constipation (Connolly & Lang, 2014).

Secondary symptoms of PD include gait disturbances referred to as a "festinating gait" (short-stepped or shuffling with reduced arm swing), dexterity and coordination difficulties, involuntary immobilization, micrographia (small handwriting), cognitive impairments (visuospatial, memory, and frontal lobe functions), sensory loss, muffled speech (Liu et al., 2015), frequent swallowing, postural instability, poor balance, oculomotor impairments, reduced perception of and expression of emotions, sleep disturbances (Politis & Niccolini, 2015; Yu, Tan, & Wu, 2015), reduced bowel and bladder function, painful cramping, sexual dysfunction, low blood pressure, seborrhea, depression or anxiety, and fatigue (Breitenstein, Van Lancker, Daum, & Waters, 2001; Carbon & Marie, 2003; Chen, Schernhammer, Schwarzschild, & Ascherio, 2006; Rearick, Stelmach, Leis, & Santello, 2002). This array of symptoms varies among people with PD. It is highly unlikely that any person with PD would develop all of the symptoms listed above. Some people may not experience a specific symptom, whereas for another person, that symptom might be a major complaint. For example, some people may experience cognitive deficits, such as executive functions impairment, as the initial symptoms, while others may never demonstrate any cognitive decline.

■ Course and Prognosis

PD is usually first diagnosed when a person is older than 50 years with the average onset age at about 60 years. It rarely affects people younger than age 40 (Duvoisin & Sage, 1996; Macphee & Stewart, 2012). As with MS, the progression of PD differs with each person. In general, PD is a slow, progressive disorder (Macphee & Stewart, 2012). The three phases of the disease include the **preclinical period** when neurons have begun to degenerate, but no symptoms are yet evident (Albanese, 2003; Macphee & Stewart, 2012). In this first phase, there may be some peripheral neuroinflammation that can be found with medical testing, but the implications of this are still being researched (Chen, O'Reilly, Schwarzschild, & Ascherio, 2008). The second phase of PD is the **prodromal period** that can last months or even years. During this phase, generalized symptoms such as depression, anxiety, constipation, REM, behavior disorder, and fatigue may appear (Kalia & Lang, 2015; Macphee & Stewart, 2012). The third phase is the **symptomatic period** when the classic motor PD symptoms are evident followed by progressive nonmotor symptoms (Albanese, 2003; Kalia & Lang, 2015; Macphee & Stewart,

TABLE 22.3	Primary and Secondary Symptoms, Signs, and Medical Management of PD	
Symptom	**Signs**	**Medication**
Tremor	Resting tremor, pill-rolling	Levodopa, dopamine agonists, monoamine oxidase type B inhibitors, propranolol, trihexyphenidyl, benztropine, clozapine
Rigidity	Cogwheel resistance	Levodopa, dopamine agonists, monoamine oxidase type B inhibitors
Bradykinesia and involuntary immobilization	Slowness or frozen movement	Levodopa, dopamine agonists, monoamine oxidase type B inhibitors
Postural and balance changes	Stooped, unsteady posture, instability, falls	Levodopa, dopamine agonists, monoamine oxidase type B inhibitors
Gait disturbances	Shuffle, reduced reflexes, and arm swing	Amantadine
Impaired coordination	Reduced dexterity	Levodopa, dopamine agonists, monoamine oxidase type B inhibitors
Cognitive dysfunction	Memory and executive function loss, dementia	Rivastigmine
Psychiatric changes	Depression, anxiety, psychosis	Pramipexole, venlafaxine, nortriptyline, clozapine, quetiapine
Speech difficulties	Soft, monotone, rapid	
Swallowing difficulties	Drooling	
Oculomotor impairments	Deficits in fixation, scanning, tracking	
Reduced facial expression	Infrequent eye blink, loss of facial movement	
Sleep disturbances	Abnormal or disruptive behaviors (verbal and physical) during REM sleep	Clonazepam, melatonin
Reduced bowel and bladder function	Urinary urgency, constipation, and incontinence	Polyethylene glycol, lubiprostone, domperidone
Fatigue	Excessive daytime sleepiness	Methylphenidate, modafinil
Sensory disturbances	Numbness, tingling, burning sensations, loss of smell	
Seborrhea	Oily skin, dandruff	
Orthostatic hypotension	Low blood pressure, postural light-headedness	

2012). According to a clinical scale by Hoehn and Yahr, the third phase can be divided into five stages, as follows.

Stage I: Signs of PD are strictly one-sided, affecting one side of the body only.
Stage II: Signs of PD are bilateral and balance is not impaired.

Stage III: Signs of PD are bilateral and balance is impaired.
Stage IV: PD is functionally disabling.
Stage V: The person is confined to bed or a wheelchair.

Although there is a general progressive worsening of symptoms, the progression through these stages is variable for each person. Usually, a person will have PD for 15 to 20 years before entering the most severe stages (Kalia & Lang, 2015). Some people may be in the first asymptomatic, preclinical phase and remain there until death (Albanese, 2003). There are also fluctuations within each stage. The loss of function is not a linear progression. Each person experiences some periods of improvement scattered throughout the progressive loss of function. Because of advances in medical treatment, life expectancy is not significantly affected by a diagnosis of PD.

■ Diagnosis

Historically, a definitive diagnosis of PD could only be made postmortem and there are still no diagnostic tests that allow for a definitive diagnosis in the early stages (Albanese, 2003; Kalia & Lang, 2015). Therefore, a person may initially be given a diagnosis of probable PD. To determine a diagnosis of PD, the physician observes the current clinical symptoms, eliminates other neurodegenerative diseases as the cause of those symptoms, and evaluates the person's response to medications used to treat PD (Macphee & Stewart, 2012). The main clinical symptoms that denote PD are bradykinesia plus rigidity and resting tremor (Kalia & Lang, 2015). Additional clinical assessment may include standard tests for olfactory function and REM sleep behavior disorder.

Recent advancements in the development of medical diagnostic tools have aided in a more definitive diagnosis as the disease progresses. Positron emission tomography (PET) and single photon emission computed tomography (SPECT) can be used to assess the density of presynaptic dopaminergic terminals within the striatum (Kalia & Lang, 2015), and genetic testing may be used to determine familial PD (Merims & Freedman, 2008). Positive genetic test results without the presence of symptoms, however, do not indicate a definitive diagnosis of PD (Kalia & Lang, 2015).

■ Medical/Surgical Management

There are no medications that inhibit the progression of PD. The medications usually prescribed to treat the primary motor symptoms of PD aim to increase the concentrations and uptake of dopamine. These medications include levodopa, dopamine agonists, and monoamine oxidase type B inhibitors (Connolly & Lang, 2014; Kalia & Lang, 2015). Specific medications in these categories may include levodopa-carbidopa, levodopa-benserazide, piribedil, ropinirole, bromocriptine, and rasagiline. There are many side effects associated with long-term use of these medications, and those include motor and nonmotor fluctuations, nausea and loss of appetite, dyskinesia, impulsive and compulsive behaviors, hallucinations, and psychosis (Connolly & Lang, 2014; Kalia & Lang, 2015).

There are several surgical procedures that have been developed to treat the symptoms of PD. These procedures include thalamotomy, pallidotomy, deep brain stimulation, and continuous device-aided drug delivery (DeLong, 2000; Katzenschlager, 2014; Merims & Freedman, 2008). Thalamotomy is a surgical procedure in which heat via an electrode or gamma-knife radiosurgery is used to destroy part of the thalamus. The thalamus is an area of the brain involved in movement. A thalamotomy can reduce tremors associated with PD and may sustain the improvement for over 10 years. A pallidotomy is a surgical procedure in which heat via an electrode or gamma-knife radiosurgery is used to destroy part of the globus pallidus. The globus pallidus is also an area of the brain involved in movement. A pallidotomy can reduce tremors, shuffling gait, flat affect, rigidity, and slowness of movement. These symptoms may be dramatically reduced following this procedure, and the effects may last for at least 5 years. Deep brain stimulation (neurostimulation) is the implantation of a type of "brain pacemaker" that delivers electrical impulses to the subthalamic nucleus, the internal globus pallidus, or the thalamus to reduce tremors associated with PD. The potential side effects of this procedure include depression, slurred speech, tingling in the head and hands, and problems with balance. The generator usually needs to be replaced every 3 to 5 years. Continuous device-aided drug delivery involves implanting a subcutaneous or gastrostomy pump to provide continuous delivery of levodopa (Katzenschlager, 2014).

Other medical management techniques that are being explored are gene therapy to replace enzymes involved in dopamine synthesis or to enhance the survival of dopamine neurons (Bohn, 2000), the use of growth factors pumped directly into dopamine-deficient areas of the brain (Mayor, 2002), and stem cell or fetal cell transplantation to generate dopamine-producing cells in the substantia nigra (Bega & Krainc, 2014;

Merims & Freedman, 2008; Politis & Lindvall, 2012). While the stem cell or fetal cell transplants have shown promise for long-term motor improvements, the use of this treatment has been limited by problems with tissue availability and standardization of grafts (Bega & Krainc, 2014; Politis & Lindvall, 2012).

AMYOTROPHIC LATERAL SCLEROSIS

■ Description and Definitions

ALS, also known as Lou Gehrig disease, is a fatal, progressive, degenerative motor neuron disease in which scars form on the upper **motor neurons** in the corticospinal pathways and the functionally linked lower motor neurons in the motor nuclei of the brainstem and the anterior horn cells of the spinal cord (Douaud, Filippini, Knigh, Talvot, & Turner, 2011; Przedborski, Mitsumoto, & Rowland, 2003; Weydt, Weiss, Moller, & Carter, 2002). Neurodegeneration is also found in the corpus callosum, extramotor cerebral regions, and the frontotemporal lobes (Douaud et al., 2011). The actual mechanism of neurodegeneration remains a mystery, but significant progress has been made with the identification of several genetic mutations including mutation in the superoxide dismutase 1 gene seen mostly in the familial type of ALS (Kuehn, 2011). There is speculation that cytosolic and mitochondrial pathway dysfunction results in the buildup of proteins that lead to motor neuron death (Shaw, Al-Chalabi, & Neigh, 2001). There is also evidence of an inflammatory component in the mechanisms of the disease process (Weydt et al., 2002). See Figure 22.3.

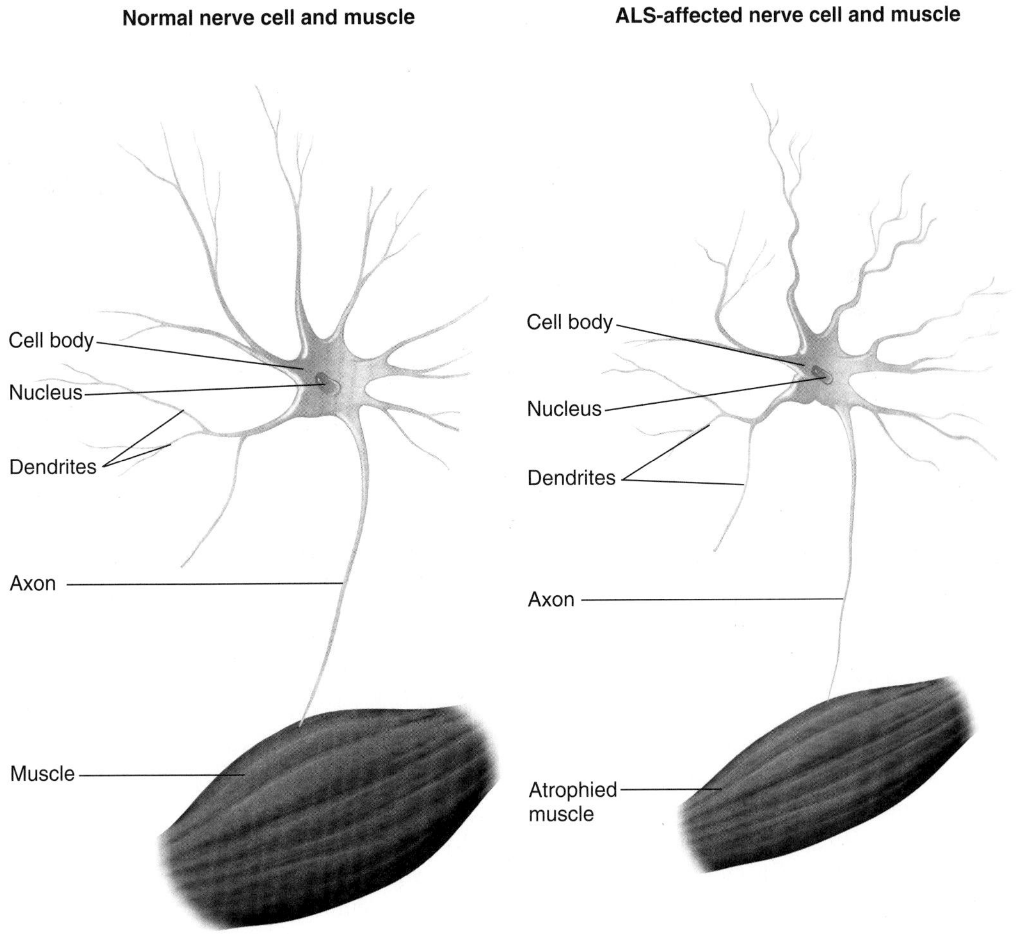

Normal nerve cell and muscle

Cell body

Nucleus

Dendrites

Axon

Muscle

ALS-affected nerve cell and muscle

Cell body

Nucleus

Dendrites

Axon

Atrophied muscle

Figure 22.3 Motor neuron changes in amyotrophic lateral sclerosis (ALS). (From Anatomical Chart Co.)

There are two types of ALS: sporadic and familial. Sporadic ALS does not have a known genetic link whereas familial ALS does. Sporadic ALS accounts for 90% of cases while the remaining 10% are the familial type (Gupta, Prabhakar, Sharma, & Anand, 2012).

Etiology

There is no known cause of ALS, but it is speculated that several disorders with several causes lead to this motor neuron disease (Weydt et al., 2002). The two types of ALS, familial and sporadic, may have different causes. Only 10% of cases are familial (Zoccolella, Santamato, & Lamberti, 2009). Researchers have discovered a genetic mutation as one cause for familial ALS (Kuehn, 2011; Shaw et al., 2001). There is also evidence of genetic causes using familial patterns of susceptibility. Family history of a first- or second-degree relative with ALS is a significant risk factor for the disease.

In most cases, however, ALS occurs sporadically and is presumed to be acquired. There is no known cause of sporadic ALS, but there is some speculation regarding viral, retroviral, and environmental causes (Shaw et al., 2001). There is also some evidence of genetic susceptibility with higher rates of ALS among relatives of people with other common neurodegenerative disorders (Kiernan et al., 2011). Other identified risk factors associated with sporadic ALS include occupational exposure such as chemicals or electromagnetic fields (Weisskopf et al., 2005), lead exposure (Kamel et al., 2003), military service (Mehta et al., 2014), cigarette smoking (Gupta et al., 2012; Weisskopf et al., 2004), alcohol use (Gupta et al., 2012), physical activity, trauma (Mehta et al., 2014), and dietary consumption with increased fat and glutamate intake associated with increased risk and fiber intake with reduced risk (Nelson, Matkin, Longstreth, & McGuire, 2000). Recent research has found that rural residence alone is not a risk factor for ALS, but participation in agricultural activities, such as farming, has a significant association with developing the bulbar form of ALS possibly due to exposure to agricultural chemicals (Furby, Beauvais, Kolev, Rivain, & Sebille, 2009). Some of the aforementioned risk factors may also be related to the familial type of ALS as environmental exposure may be combined with genetic susceptibility (Kamel et al., 2003).

Incidence and Prevalence

Worldwide, ALS affects white males who are older than 60 years more than any other group (Mehta et al., 2014). The prevalence rate of people with ALS is estimated to be 5.4 per 100,000 people in Europe (Chiò et al., 2013) with worldwide numbers difficult to track (Kiernan et al., 2011). Recent prevalence numbers for the United States indicate a prevalence of 3.9 cases per 100,000 persons (Mehta et al., 2014). Some estimates state that as many as 30,000 Americans are diagnosed with ALS annually (Weisskopf et al., 2004). Sporadic ALS affects males more often than females with a ratio of 1.7:1 and an overall lifetime risk of 1:350 for men and 1:400 for women (Kiernan et al., 2011; McCombe & Henderson, 2010; Mehta et al., 2014; Shaw et al., 2001), but there is evidence that this gender difference is decreasing over time (Noonan, Hilsdon, White, Wong, & Zack, 2002a). The incidence among males and females for familial ALS is relatively the same (Kiernan et al., 2011). Ongoing investigation indicates the possibility of increasing prevalence of ALS in the United States (Noonan et al., 2002a) and worldwide (Przedborski et al., 2003). Reduced frequency of ALS has been noted among people of Hispanic origins (Kiernan et al., 2011; Mehta et al., 2014). The age groups with the lowest ALS frequency are ages 18 to 39 years and ages >80 years (Mehta et al., 2014).

Signs and Symptoms

The most common initial symptom of ALS is weakness of the small muscles of the hand or an asymmetrical foot drop (Beresford, 1995). Night cramps, particularly in the calf muscles, also may be present. Progressive loss of muscle movement, spasticity, difficulty speaking and swallowing, loss of emotional control, and reduced body temperature regulation are common (Beresford, 1995). Although often overlooked, there is now evidence of significant cognitive deficits such as reduced executive functions and changes in language abilities or personality related to frontotemporal involvement (Kiernan et al., 2011). The progressive neurodegeneration of the CNS eventually leads to respiratory failure.

The signs and symptoms of ALS are progressive, most commonly in a distal to proximal pattern. The symptoms can be divided into three areas, including lower motor neuron, corticospinal

TABLE 22.4 Signs and Symptoms of Amyotrophic Lateral Sclerosis

Lower Motor Neuron	Corticospinal Tract	Corticobulbar Tract
Focal and multifocal weakness	Spasticity Hyperreactive reflexes	Dysphagia (difficulty swallowing)
Atrophy (progressive; distal to proximal)	Dysphagia (difficulty swallowing)	Dysarthria (impaired quality of speech production)
Muscle cramping Muscle twitching	Dysarthria (impaired quality of speech production)	

tract, and corticobulbar tract dysfunction (see Table 22.4). The lower motor neuron dysfunction symptoms include focal and multifocal weakness, atrophy, cramps, and muscle twitching. Muscle spasticity, weakness, and hyperresponsive reflexes are associated with corticospinal tract dysfunction (Kiernan et al., 2011; Nelson et al., 2000). Slow, labored, and distorted speech, often with a nasal quality, hyperactive gag reflex, tongue atrophy, and dysphasia, are seen with bulbar lower motor neuron involvement (Kiernan et al., 2011; Beresford, 1995).

Course and Prognosis

The age of onset of ALS occurs between 16 and 77 years, but it is usually diagnosed when a person is between the ages of 55 and 75 years (Noonan et al., 2002a). The peak age of onset is 58 to 63 years for sporadic ALS and 47 to 52 years for familial ALS (Kiernan et al., 2011). The course of ALS is usually progressive and rapid. The duration of survival after diagnosis is usually 1 to 5 years, with a mean survival of 3 years (Beresford, 1995; Weisskopf et al., 2004). Nearly 50% of people die within 30 months from the onset of symptoms (Kiernan et al., 2011). Life expectancy is dependent on the type of ALS (sporadic or familial), rate of disease progression, early presence of respiratory failure, and nutritional status (Kiernan et al., 2011). The younger a person is and the more mild the symptoms at the time of diagnosis, the longer the course. There is some evidence of a "resistance in ALS," in which a person may demonstrate improvements and live longer than 10 years. This is seen in approximately 10% to 16% of people with ALS (Mitsumoto Hanson, & Chad, 1988). Death is usually from respiratory failure, often precipitated by pneumonia (Kiernan et al., 2011; Weydt et al., 2002).

Diagnosis

It is difficult to diagnose ALS in the early stages because the symptoms are similar to many other neuromuscular disorders (Gupta et al., 2012). A definitive diagnosis requires a complete neurological examination with electrophysiological and radiological testing, which can take several months and delay much-needed intervention (Gupta et al., 2012). As with the other PNDs, there is not a specific diagnostic test for ALS and the physician must piece together clinical symptoms, electromyogram (EMG) results, and tests to exclude other causes of the clinical presentation (Beresford, 1995; Kiernan et al., 2011). The EMG findings will include motor denervation and fasciculation (twitching) with intact sensory responses. Although MRI of the CNS is usually used to rule out other causes of the symptoms (Kiernan et al., 2011), some recent successful identification of ALS has been found by combining structural and functional MRI results to identify cerebral network connectivity failure (Douaud et al., 2011). Blood tests are usually normal. Cerebrospinal fluid is often normal but may show raised protein levels.

Medical/Surgical Management

The medical treatments that are currently available do little to alter the fatal course of ALS (Weydt et al., 2002). Riluzole is the only medication that has been approved by the U.S. Food and Drug Administration to treat ALS (Mehta et al., 2014). There is evidence that riluzole helps people stay in the milder stages for a longer time and it is the only medication that increases survival, although for only a modest amount of time (3 to 6 months) (Kiernan et al., 2011; Zoccolella et al.,

2009). Riluzole, however, does not provide significant relief from the symptoms of ALS (Mehta et al., 2014). The medications prescribed to treat the symptoms of ALS include antispasmodic medications, nonsteroidal anti-inflammatory medications, and antibiotics. Several medications to treat ALS are in the clinical phases of development (Bucchia et al., 2015). The most promising of these experimental medications is dexpramipexole, which is used to protect motor neurons and is currently approved for use with people who have PD (Bucchia et al., 2015). Neural stem cell therapy is also being explored as a means to replace motor neurons (Bucchia et al., 2015).

Gastrostomy and noninvasive positive-pressure ventilation have been shown to increase both quality and possibly length of life (Przedborski et al., 2003). Nebulizers with N-acetylcysteine may be used to thin saliva, and low-dose radiation and botulinum toxin injections into the salivary glands are sometimes used to treat drooling (Kiernan et al., 2011).

There is some evidence that attending a clinic staffed by a multidisciplinary team (including neurologists; specialist nurses; physical, occupational, and speech therapists; and a pulmonologist, nutritionist, psychologist, and social worker) is effective for improving quality and length of life (Kiernan et al., 2011; Traynor, Alexander, Corr, Frost, & Hardiman, 2003). Palliative care may also be very important for people with ALS and their families. It has been estimated that 62.4% die in a hospice-supported environment (Przedborski et al., 2003).

IMPACT OF CONDITIONS ON OCCUPATIONAL PERFORMANCE

Each of these PNDs is progressive and can affect all occupations, client factors, performance skills, and performance patterns. The extent of this effect depends on the stage and severity of the disease. In each case, a person may have any combination of the deficits listed.

■ Activities of Daily Living

Self-care skills are affected by changes in the person's sensorimotor skills. Changes are usually noted in gross and fine motor coordination, postural control, muscle tone, endurance, and sensation (except in ALS). Loss of independence in bathing, dressing, personal device care, and toilet hygiene may occur. Toileting can become problematic for persons with MS or PD because of the loss of bladder and bowel control. The individual may experience any combination of the complications noted earlier in this chapter.

Eating may be difficult, either because the person loses the strength and coordination to self-feed or because of chewing or swallowing difficulties (dysphagia). The latter is caused by weakness or incoordination of the pharyngeal musculature, which also can make it difficult for an individual to ingest oral medications.

Functional mobility is another critical concern. Neuromuscular and motor problems make ambulation difficult or impossible, either independently or with assistive devices, even in an electrically propelled wheelchair. Acquiring alternate methods of mobility requires the ability to adapt. The person must be able to change motor patterns, requiring concurrent new and varied perceptual and cognitive strategies. At the same time, the individual is challenged psychologically to make the necessary adjustments to new and different types of mobility. As the person's function decreases, issues of home and work accessibility must be considered, and the necessary adaptations must be made to maintain performance in activities of daily living.

■ Instrumental Activities of Daily Living

Deficits in neuromusculoskeletal and movement-related functions and motor skills due to PNDs usually lead to reduced ability to perform all instrumental activities of daily living. In addition to neuromusculoskeletal losses, reduced sensory, cognitive, and perceptual functions (Kiernan et al., 2011) may also interfere with independence in this area. In the early stages of these diseases, adaptations need to be made to afford the person the opportunity to maintain function for as long as possible. Most of these tasks, however, eventually need to be delegated to other members of the household, further creating issues of dependence and loss of role function.

A normal activity for many persons, including those with PND, is the care of others, including a spouse or significant other, children, or older, dependent adults. The individual with a PND may have increasing difficulty fulfilling this role. In fact, he or she may have to rely on these care receivers to provide support and care, creating a major role reversal. These changes in responsibilities can be very stressful for all concerned; they challenge everyone's ability to maintain the integrity of relationships.

■ Education

Because of the age of onset for these PNDs, many people will not be involved in formal educational activities. Those who are may gradually experience a reduced ability to physically participate due to decline in underlying neuromusculoskeletal and movement-related functions and motor skills. Deficits in cognitive and perceptual functions may further limit learning ability. Adaptations such as computer-based courses for formal and informal education may be a viable option.

■ Work

All client factors have the potential to affect work activities. Work is a crucial area of occupational performance and, for many adults, is an important part of self-identity. As motor skills decline, the ability to perform specific work tasks also declines. "Invisible symptoms" such as fatigue, weak or blurred vision, and difficulties with bladder control often confound the issue. Coworkers may not understand why someone who does not look ill cannot work. Again, this affects the person psychologically, with changes in societal roles and self-concept. This is particularly true for an individual whose job requires a high degree of physical stamina and skill. For example, assembly workers or truck drivers may lose their jobs fairly early in the course of these diseases. An individual who has been the breadwinner of the family and whose identity is closely tied to physical strength and endurance may have serious adjustment problems. Cognitive deficits also may make it difficult for the person to function and continue to find satisfaction in work.

■ Play and Leisure

Many leisure activities can be affected by the changes that result from PNDs. Fatigue and reduced exercise capacity are common (Kiernan et al., 2011). Alternative leisure activities must be explored as more and more performance deficits occur. A balance between work and play should be maintained as long as possible. However, if the person can no longer engage in usual work and daily living activities, it is even more critical to have meaningful and fulfilling leisure pursuits. These activities will grow in importance as a means of self-actualization and satisfaction.

■ Social Participation

Communication, mobility, sexual dysfunction, and eating problems may all affect the person's normal socialization with individuals or groups. Dysarthria or imperfect articulation is caused by a lack of control of the tongue and other oral muscles essential to speech. This problem can affect the person's ability to communicate thoughts, needs, and desires and can limit social interaction (Kiernan et al., 2011). The individual may lose upper extremity function, making it difficult to compensate for speaking problems with written communication.

Sexual dysfunction may also be present. Because of depression and diminished self-concept, the person may no longer feel attractive, which causes problems in sexual expression. Also, loss of specific motor and sensory function can affect physical performance.

Because of the unpredictable nature of the course of each PND, potential dependency issues are ongoing problems. This may lead to secondary psychosocial issues caused by these lifestyle changes. PNDs require an initial social-psychological adjustment as well as continual readjustment because of erratic progression of symptoms. A person who was active and outgoing may have a diminished self-concept because of the inability to engage in activities that were once of interest and value. The result is a variety of role changes in the family or society.

Role expectations, which exist in every social situation, are ways of behaving or reacting that fit with one's self-image and the expectations of others. These include attitudes, activities, and patterns of decision making, expression of feelings, and meeting the needs of significant others. Some individuals with loss of bladder control may avoid going out in public. Mothers may be unable to care for their children. Some may come to see themselves as no longer useful or attractive to others. Marriages may break up under the strain of living with PNDs. Occasionally, individuals with PNDs threaten suicide. An individual with a PND must think seriously about current role expectations and how these might be threatened by the PND.

CASE STUDY

Jennifer is a 38-year-old woman who was diagnosed with MS 5 years before this hospital admission. She was admitted because she noticed a progressive deterioration of function during the past 6 months. The main problems she identifies are an increase in fatigue, difficulty with bowel and bladder function, and several falls. She complains of feeling moody and forgetting information.

She is married and has two children, an 11-year-old girl and a 5-year-old boy. She is self-employed as a graphic designer, which requires her to spend many hours typing on the computer and talking via phone and face-to-face with clients. Her husband works full time as a school counselor and has been very supportive. At the time of admission, he seemed overwhelmed.

Jennifer tries to do her morning self-care but is finding it more difficult and frustrating. Getting dressed is particularly fatiguing, and she admits that at times, she goes to bed fully dressed to avoid having to get dressed in the morning. She has been using a manual wheelchair off and on for the past 2 years.

Her daughter is currently helping with the laundry, cooking, and simple cleaning. Jennifer states that she has problems doing household tasks because she must hold onto something stable before reaching for, or lifting, an object. She currently enjoys no leisure activities. At one time, she liked to knit, but it has become too frustrating to be pleasurable.

Jennifer complains of bladder urgency but often cannot void. She also has a mild dysarthria, spasticity of the lower extremities, weakness of the upper extremities (able to move against gravity withstanding minimal resistance), poor sitting balance, poor fine and gross motor coordination, blurred vision, and loss of stereognosis and light touch. When the occupational therapist spoke with her, it became apparent that she did not comprehend the nature and course of MS. She is feeling frustrated and depressed about her recent decline of function. Jennifer recently began receiving interferon β-1b treatment. She is currently taking Tylenol, Senokot, Metamucil, Colace, heparin, and multivitamins and is using Dulcolax suppositories.

CASE STUDY 2

Cal is a 72-year-old man with stage III PD. He has recently experienced a severe loss of balance and functional mobility. He reports difficulty moving quickly and gracefully. He also complains of poor handwriting, problems sleeping, and numbness in both hands.

Cal is a single, retired accountant who lives independently in a two-story home. His bedroom and bathroom are on the second floor. There are four steps to enter the home. He has no children. He has one sister who lives within walking distance of his home. She, however, is suffering from arthritis and has difficulty offering much assistance.

Cal has been caring for himself thus far, but his sister reports she is concerned about his safety, especially with activities such as cooking

and bathing. She reports that he has fallen on several occasions recently and spends most of his time sitting in his chair in his living room. His sister brings him meals as often as possible, but is unable to bring meals in the morning or during bad weather. Her children live out of state and are only able to offer assistance to him during occasional visits when they try to do some of the major household chores such as painting, repairs, and cleaning.

Cal was once interested in music and art. He played the piano and painted with watercolors. He reports that he has not participated in these leisure activities for "a long time." He also played tennis on a regular basis at the local club. He is still a member of the club but has not been there in more than a year.

Cal is reportedly self-conscious of his illness and, therefore, does not like to go out in public very much. His sister, who has always been very close to her brother, expresses concern about his "depression and lack of motivation." She states that she has tried on several occasions to get him to go to local musical concerts or museums, but she feels he is just too depressed. He is currently taking levodopa-carbidopa. His sister, however, reports that he does not consistently take his medication because it "makes him feel sick."

CASE STUDY 3

Tomas is a 48-year-old man who has recently been diagnosed with ALS. Six months before being referred to O.T. services, he began to experience some weakness in his hands and he began dropping objects, such as tools. He reports loss of strength in his arms and legs. The weakness in his legs has become so severe that he now uses a borrowed wheelchair part of the time. He complains of difficulty sleeping due to cramps in his legs. He also reports that he has lost almost 20 lb in the last 6 or 8 months.

Tomas is married and has two sons, ages 6 and 4. He independently owns and operates a lawnmower shop at which he sells and repairs lawnmowers. He reports significant difficulty performing the repair parts of his job because of weakness in his hands and arms. Most of the repairs have become backed up in the shop and he is considering hiring assistance or sending the work to another shop. His wife is employed full-time as a legal secretary. She has helped with the business as much as possible by completing some of the bookkeeping after hours. She is very busy caring for their boys and trying to maintain the household. She appears to be very supportive of Tomas, but also seems very burdened by her responsibilities.

Tomas has many interests in sports and outdoor activities. He has been racing in "Iron Man" triathlons and marathons for the last several years. He was a high school track and cross-country star. He enjoys biking and camping. Every summer, he and his family take a 2-week trip to a remote location where they hike and camp. He is also supportive of his sons' sports events and enjoys teaching them various sports. Last year, he was a soccer coach for his oldest boy's team.

The course and prognosis of ALS have been explained to Tomas and his wife, and they have reportedly been discussing future plans. They are, however, "hoping for a miracle." At this time, he is taking riluzole and pain relievers to reduce the pain from the cramping in his legs.

RECOMMENDED LEARNING RESOURCES

Multiple Sclerosis

National Multiple Sclerosis Society
http://www.nmss.org/

The Multiple Sclerosis Foundation
http://www.msfacts.org/

The Multiple Sclerosis Association of America
http://www.msaa.com/

Parkinson Disease

National Parkinson Foundation
http://parkinson.org/

Parkinson's Disease Foundation, Inc.
http://pdf.org/

The American Parkinson Disease Association, Inc.
http://www.apdaparkinson.com/

Amyotrophic Lateral Sclerosis

The ALS Association
http://www.alsa.org/

World Federation of Neurology Amyotrophic Lateral Sclerosis
http://www.wfnals.org/

REFERENCES

Albanese, A. (2003). Diagnostic criteria for Parkinson's disease. *Neurological Science, 24*, S23–S26.

Armon, C., Kurland, L. T., Beard, C. M., O'Brien, P. C., & Mulder, D. W. (1991). Psychologic and adaptational difficulties anteceding amyotrophic lateral sclerosis: Rochester, Minnesota, 1925–1987. *Neuroepidemiology, 10*(3), 132–137.

Bega, D., & Krainc, D. (2014). Long-term clinical outcomes after fetal cell transplantation in Parkinson disease: Implications for the future of cell therapy. *The Journal of the American Medical Association, 71*(1). Retrieved from http://dx.doi.org/10.1001/jamaneurol.2013.4749

Beresford, S. (1995). *Motor neurone disease (amyotrophic lateral sclerosis).* London, UK: Chapman & Hall.

Berlanga-Taylor, A. J., Disanto, G., Ebers, G. C., & Ramagopalan, S. V. (2011). Vitamin D-gene interactions in multiple sclerosis. *Journal of the Neurological Sciences, 311*, 32–36. Retrieved from http://dx.doi.org/10.1016/j.jns.2011.08.014

Bobholz, J. A., & Rao, S. M. (2003). Cognitive dysfunction in multiple sclerosis: A review of recent developments. *Current Opinions in Neurology, 16*, 283–288.

Bohn, M. C. (2000). Parkinson's disease: A neurodegenerative disease particularly amenable to gene therapy. *Molecular Therapy, 1*(6), 494–496.

Braak, H, Del Tredici, K., Rub, U., de Vos, R. A. I., Jansen Steur, E. N. H., & Braak, E. (2003). Staging of brain pathology related to sporadic Parkinson's disease. *Neurobiological Aging, 24*, 197–211.

Breitenstein, C., Van Lancker, D., Daum, I., & Waters, C. H. (2001). Impaired perception of vocal emotions in Parkinson's Disease: Influence of speech time processing and executive functioning. *Brain and Cognition, 45*, 277–314.

Bucchia, M., Ramirez, A., Parente, V., Simone, C., Nizzardo, M., Magri, F., … Corti, S. (2015). Therapeutic development in amyotrophic lateral sclerosis. *Clinical Therapeutics, 37*(3), 668–680. Retrieved from http://dx.doi.org/10.1016/j.clinthera.2014.12.020

Carbon, M., & Marie, R. (2003). Functional imaging of cognition in Parkinson's disease. *Current Opinions in Neurology, 16*, 475–480.

Carrithers, M. D. (2014). Update on disease-modifying treatments for multiple sclerosis. *Clinical Therapeutics, 36*(12), 1938–1945.

Chen, H., O'Reilly, E., McCullough, M. L., Rodriguez, C., Schwarzschild, M. A., Calle, E. E., … Ascherio, A. (2007). Consumption of dairy products and risk of Parkinson's disease. *American Journal of Epidemiology, 165*(9), 998–1006.

Chen, H., O'Reilly, E., Schwarzschild, M. A., & Ascherio, A. (2008). Peripheral inflammatory biomarkers and risk of Parkinson's Disease. *American Journal of Epidemiology, 167*(1), 90–95.

Chen, H., Schernhammer, E., Schwarzschild, M. A., & Ascherio, A. (2006). A prospective study of night shift work, sleep duration and risk of Parkinson's Disease. *American Journal of Epidemiology, 163*(8), 726–730.

Chiò, A., Logroscino, G., Traynor, B. J., Collins, J., Simeone, J. C., Goldstein, L. A., & White, L. A. (2013). Global epidemiology of amyotrophic lateral sclerosis: A systematic review of the published literature. *Neuroepidemiology, 41*(2), 118–130. Retrieved from http://dx.doi.org/10.1159/000351153

Compston, A., & Coles, A. (2002). Multiple sclerosis. *Lancet, 359*, 1221–1231.

Compston, A., & Coles, A. (2008). Multiple sclerosis. *The Lancet, 372*, 1502–1517.

Connolly, B. S., & Lang, A. E. (2014). Pharmacological treatment of Parkinson disease: A review. *The Journal of the American Medical Association, 311*(16), 1670–1683. Retrieved from http://dx.doi.org/10.1001/jama.2014.3654

de Lau, L. M. L., Koudstaal, P. J., Hofman, A., & Breteler, M. B. (2006). Serum cholesterol levels and the risk of Parkinson's disease. *American Journal of Epidemiology, 164*(10), 998–1002.

Delisa, J. A., Hammond, M. C., Mikulic, M. A., & Miller, R. M. (1985). Multiple sclerosis: Part 1. Common physical disabilities and rehabilitation. *American Family Physician, 32*(4), 157–163.

DeLong, M. (2000). Parkinson's disease. *Neurobiology of Disease, 7*, 559–560.

Douaud, G., Filippini, N., Knight, S., Talbot, K., & Turner, M. R. (2011). Integration of structural and functional magnetic resonance imaging in amyotrophic lateral sclerosis. *Brain, 134*(12), 3470–3479. Retrieved from http://dx.doi.org/10.1093/brain/awr279

Duvoisin, R. C., & Sage, J. (1996). *Parkinson's disease: A guide for patient and family.* Philadelphia, PA: Lippincott-Raven.

Feinstein, A. (2006). Mood disorders in multiple sclerosis and the effects on cognition. *Journal of the Neurological Sciences, 245*, 63–66.

Filippi, M., Rocca, M. A., Colombo, B., Falini, A., Codella, M., Scotti, G., & Comi, G. (2002). Functional magnetic resonance imaging correlates of fatigue in multiple sclerosis. *NeuroImage, 15*, 559–567.

Furby, A., Beauvais, K., Kolev, I., Rivain, J.-G., & Sébille, V. (2009). Rural environment and risk factors of amyotrophic lateral sclerosis: A case-control study. *Journal of Neurology*, *257*(5), 792–798. Retrieved from http://dx.doi.org/10.1007/s00415-009-5419-5

Gao, X., Chen, H., Choi, H. K., Curhan, G., Schwarzschild, M. A., & Ascherio, A. (2008). Diet, urate, and Parkinson's disease in men. *American Journal of Epidemiology*, *167*(7), 831–838.

Gupta, P. K., Prabhakar, S., Sharma, S., & Anand, A. (2012). A predictive model for amyotrophic lateral sclerosis (ALS) diagnosis. *Journal of the Neurological Sciences*, *312*, 68–72. Retrieved from http://dx.doi.org/10.1016/j.jns.2011.08.021

Hanson, L. J., & Cafruny, W. A. (2002). Current concepts in multiple sclerosis: Part 1. *South Dakota Journal of Medicine*, *55*(10), 433–436.

Harrison, D. M. (2014). In the clinic: Multiple sclerosis. *Annals of Internal Medicine*, *160*(7). Retrieved from http://dx.doi.org/10.7326/0003-4819-160-7-201404010-01004

Hernan, M. A., Olek, M. J., & Ascherio, A. (2001). Cigarette smoking and incidence of multiple sclerosis. *American Journal of Epidemiology*, *154*(1), 69–74.

Hurwitz, B. J. (2011). Analysis of current multiple sclerosis registries. *Neurology*, *76*, S7–S13.

Kalb, R. C. (1996). *Multiple sclerosis: The questions you have, the answers you need*. New York, NY: Demos Vermande.

Kalia, L. V., & Lang, A. E. (2015). Parkinson's disease. *The Lancet*, *386*, 896–912. Retrieved from http://dx.doi.org/10.1016/S0140-6736(14)61393-3

Kamel, F., Umbach, D. M., Lehman, T. A., Park, L. P., Munsat, T. L., Shefner, J. M., … Taylor, J.A. (2003). Amyotrophic lateral sclerosis, lead and genetic susceptibility: Polymorphisms in the aminolevulinic acid dehydratase and vitamin D receptor genes. *Environmental Health Perspectives*, *111*(10), 1335–1339.

Kamel, F., Tanner, C. M., Umbach, D. M., Hoppin, J. A., Alavanja, M. C. R., Blair, A., … Sandler, D. P. (2006). Pesticide exposure and self-reported Parkinson's disease in the agricultural health study. *American Journal of Epidemiology*, *165*, 364–374.

Katzenschlager, R. (2014). Parkinson's disease: Recent advances. *Journal of Neurology*, *261*(5), 1031–1036. Retrieved from http://dx.doi.org/10.1007/s00415-014-7308-9

Kenealy, S. J., Pericak-Vance, M. S., & Haines, J. L. (2003). The genetic epidemiology of multiple sclerosis. *Journal of Neuroimmunology*, *143*, 7–12.

Kiernan, M. C., Vucic, S., Cheah, B. C., Turner, M. R., Eisen, A., Hardiman, O., … Zoing, M. C. (2011). Amyotrophic lateral sclerosis. *The Lancet*, *377*, 942–955. Retrieved from http://dx.doi.org/10.1016/S0140-6736(10)61156-7

Kuehn, B. M. (2011). New model system offers clues to ALS. *Journal of the American Medical Association*, *306*(14), 1534.

Ledford, H. (2015). Drug that boosts nerve signals offers hope for multiple sclerosis. *Nature*, *520*. Retrieved from http://dx.doi.org/10.1038/520417a

Liu, L., Luo, X.-G., Dy, C.-L., Ren, Y., Feng, Y., Yu, H.-M, … He, Z.-Y. (2015). Characteristics of language impairment in Parkinson's disease and its influencing factors. *Translational Neurodegeneration*, *4*(1), 2.

Logroscino, G., Gao, X., Chen, H., Wing, A., & Ascherio, A. (2008). Dietary iron intake and risk of Parkinson's disease. *American Journal of Epidemiology*, *168*(12), 1381–1388.

Lyros, E., Messinis, L., Papageorgiou, S. G., & Papathanosopoulos, P. (2010). Cognitive dysfunction in multiple sclerosis: The effects of pharmacological interventions. *International Review of Psychiatry*, *22*(1), 35–42.

Macphee, G. J. A., & Stewart, D.A. (2012). Parkinson's disease—pathology, aetiology and diagnosis. *Reviews in Clinical Gerontology*, *22*(3), 165–178. Retrieved from http://dx.doi.org/10.1017/S095925981200007x

Matthews, B. (1993). *Multiple sclerosis: The facts* (3rd ed.). Oxford, UK: Oxford University Press.

Mayor, S. (2002). New treatment improves symptoms of Parkinson's disease. *British Medical Journal*, *324*(7344), 997.

McCombe, P. A., & Henderson, R. D. (2010). Effects of gender in amyotrophic lateral sclerosis. *Gender Medicine*, *7*(6), 557–570. Retrieved from http://dx.doi.org/10.1016/j.genm.2010.11.010

McCormack, A. L., Thiruchelvam, M., Mannig-Bog, A. B., Thiffault, C., Langston, J. W., Cory-Slechta, D. A., & Di Monte, D. A. (2002). Environmental risk factors and Parkinson's disease: Selective degeneration of nigral dopaminergic neurons caused by the herbicide paraquat. *Neurobiology of Disease*, *10*, 119–127.

Mehta, P., Antao, V., Kaye, W., Sanchez, M., Williamson, D., Bryan, L., … Horton, K. (2014). Prevalence of amyotrophic lateral sclerosis—United States, 2010-2011. *Morbidity and Mortality Weekly Report*, *63*(7), 1–14.

Merims, D., & Freedman, M. (2008). Cognitive and behavioural impairment in Parkinson's disease. *International review of Psychiatry*, *20*(4), 364–373.

Mitsumoto, H., Hanson, M. R., & Chad, D. A. (1988). Amyotrophic lateral sclerosis: Recent advances in pathogenesis and therapeutic trials. *Arch Neurol*, *45*, 189–202.

Murray, J. (2002). Infection as a cause of multiple sclerosis. *British Medical Journal*, *325*(7373), 1128.

Neill, J., Belan, I., & Reid, K. (2006). Effectiveness of non-pharmacological interventions for fatigue in adults with multiple sclerosis, rheumatoid arthritis, or systemic lupus erythematosus: A systemic review. *Integrative Literature Reviews and Meta-analyses, 56*(6), 617–635.

Neilsen, N. M., Westergaard, T., Rostgaard, K., Frisck, M., Hjalgrim, H., Wohlfahrt, J., ... Melbye, M. (2005). Familial risk of multiple sclerosis: A nationwide cohort study. *American Journal of Epidemiology, 162*(8), 774–778.

Nelson, L. M., Matkin, C., Longstreth, W. T. Jr., & McGuire, V. (2000). Population-based case-control study of amyotrophic lateral sclerosis in western Washington state. II. Diet.. *American Journal of Epidemiology, 151*(2), 164–173.

Noonan, C. W., Hilsdon, R., White, M. C., Wong, L.-Y., & Zack, M. (2002a). Continuing trend of increased motor neuron disease mortality in the United States. *Epidemiology, 13*, S202.

Noonan, C. W., Kathman, S. J., & White, M. C. (2002b). Prevalence estimates for MS in the United States and evidence for an increasing trend for women. *Neurology, 58*, 136–138.

Noonan, C. W., Williamson, D. M., Henry, J. P., Indian, R., Lynch, S. G., Neuberger, J.S., ... Marrie, R. A. (2010). The prevalence of multiple sclerosis in 3 US communities. *Preventing Chronic Disease, 7*(1). Retrieved from http://www.cdc.gov/pcd/Issues/2010

Noseworthy, J. H. (2003). Management of multiple sclerosis: Current trials and future options. *Current Opinion in Neurology, 16*, 289–297.

Nylander, A., & Hafler, D. A. (2012). Multiple sclerosis. *Journal of Clinical Investigation, 122*(4), 1180–1186.

Politis, M., & Niccolini, F. (2015). Serotonin in Parkinson's disease. *Behavioural Brain Research, 277*(15), 136–145. Retrieved from http://dx.doi.org/10.1016/j.bbr.2014.07.037

Politis, M., & Lindvall, O. (2012). Clinical application of stem cell therapy in Parkinson's disease. *BMC Medicine, 10*(1). Retrieved from http://dx.doi.org/10.1186/1741-7015-10-1

Priyadarshi, A., Khuder, S. A., Schaub, E. A., & Priyadarshi, S. S. (2001). Environmental risk factors and Parkinson's disease: A metaanalysis. *Environmental Research Section A, 86*, 122–127.

Przedborski, S., Mitsumoto, H., & Rowland, L. P. (2003). Recent advances in amyotrophic lateral sclerosis research. *Current Neurology and Neuroscience Reports, 3*, 70–77.

Rearick, M. P., Stelmach, G. E., Leis, B., & Santello, M. (2002). Coordination and control of forces during multifingered grasping in Parkinson's disease. *Experimental Eurology, 177*, 428–442.

Rocca, M. A., Messina, R., & Filippi, M. (2013). Multiple sclerosis imaging: Recent advances. *Journal of Neurology, 260*(3), 929–935. Retrieved from http:///dx.doi.org/10.1007/s00415-012-6788-8

Shaw, C. E., Al-Chalabi, A., & Neigh, N. (2001). Progress in pathogenesis of amyotrophic lateral sclerosis. *Current Neurology and Neuroscience Reports, 1*, 69–76.

Traynor, B. J., Alexander, M., Corr, B., Frost, E., & Hardiman, O. (2003). Effect of a multidisciplinary amyotrophic lateral sclerosis (ALS) clinic on ALS survival: A population based study, 1996-2000. *J Neurol Neurosurg Psychiatry, 74*, 1258–1261.

Umphred, D. A. (1990). *Neurological Rehabilitation* (2nd ed.). St Louis, MO: CV Mosby.

Wakerley, B., Nicholas, R., & Malik, O. (2012). Multiple sclerosis. *Medicine, 40*(10), 523–528.

Wassem, R., & Dudley, W. (2003). Symptom management and adjustment of patients with multiple sclerosis: A 4-year longitudinal intervention study. *Clinical Nursing Research, 12*(1), 102–117.

Weisskopf, M. G., McCullough, M. L., Calle, E. E., Thun, M. J., Cudkowicz, M., & Ascherio, A. (2004). Prospective study of cigarette smoking and amyotrophic lateral sclerosis. *American Journal of Epidemiology, 160*(1), 26–33.

Weisskopf, M. G., McCullough, M. L., Morozova, N., Calle, E. E., Thun M. J., & Ascherio, A. (2005). Prospective study of occupation and amyotrophic lateral sclerosis mortality. *American Journal of Epidemiology, 162*(12), 1146–1152.

Weydt, P., Weiss, M. D., Moller, T., & Carter, G. T. (2002). Neuro-inflammation as a therapeutic target in amyotrophic lateral sclerosis. *Current Opinion in Investigative Drugs, 3*(12), 1720–1724.

Willis, A. W., Evanoff, B. A., Lian, M., Criswell, S. R., & Racette, B. A. (2010). Geographic and ethnic variation in Parkinson disease: A population-based study of US Medicare beneficiaries. *Neuroepidemiology, 34*(3), 143–151. Retrieved from http://dx.doi.org/10.1159/000275491

Yu, R.-L., Tan, C.-H., & Wu, R.-M. (2015). The impact of nocturnal disturbances on daily quality of life in patients with Parkinson's disease. *Neuropsychiatric Disease and Treatment, 11*, 2005–2012. Retrieved from http://dx.doi.org/10.2147/NDT.S85483

Zhang, Y., Dawson, V. L., & Dawson, T. M. (2000). Oxidative stress and genetics in the pathogenesis of Parkinson's disease. *Neurobiology of Disease, 7*, 240–250.

Zoccolella, S., Santamato, A., & Lamberti, P. (2009). Current and emerging treatments for amyotrophic lateral sclerosis. *Neuropsychiatric Disease and Treatment, 5*, 577–595.

Rheumatic Diseases

Timothy M. Mullen

KEY TERMS

Boutonniere deformity
Chondropenia
Crepitus
Disease-modifying
   antirheumatic drug
   (DMARD)
Energy conservation
Fibromyalgia
Gout
Guarding
Hyperuricemia
Joint protection
Juvenile rheumatoid
   arthritis
Osteoarthritis
Pannus
Rheumatoid arthritis
Systemic lupus
   erythematosus
Swan-neck deformity

G race Kennedy is a very pleasant 68-year-old retired woman living in a rural community. She is recently widowed and is finding more difficulty maintaining her independence. Grace belongs to a very supportive parish whose members have supported many of her instrumental activities of daily living (IADLs), including shopping, meal preparation, housework, laundry, and paying bills. Her adult children live several hours away and spend as many weekends with her as possible to support her bathing and other hygiene activities of daily living. Grace recounts gradually losing the ability to grasp and pinch small objects and progressing to larger objects. Opening jars, functioning zippers, and fastening buttons eventually became impossible. From there, gross motor challenges become apparent. Transitions in and out of bed, from a chair and off, and on the toilet were slow and full of effort. She began to feel helpless and thought she would lose her independence.

Seeing the apparent decline of independence, Grace's children intervened and arranged for an in-home occupational therapy assessment. The occupational therapist (OT) spent considerable time evaluating Grace's needs and focusing on her preferences. The OT also had Grace demonstrate all IADLs and activities of daily living (ADLs) required for her to live independently. Subsequently, the OT had a meeting with Grace and her family and made several recommendations to optimize her ability to stay at home. The meeting focused on what could be adapted to maintain independence and what could be outsourced. Grace had no strong desire to maintain some basic IADLs; therefore, the family agreed to look into a service to provide housekeeping, meal preparation, and grocery shopping. The OT then demonstrated several assistive devices that could aid in writing, pulling zippers, gripping, and opening objects. The concept was to make items larger and lighter so manipulations were easier and more sustainable. The OT further recommended devices and grab bars to facilitate transitions.

DESCRIPTIONS AND DEFINITIONS

Rheumatic disease is an umbrella category of over 100 different individual diagnoses identified by the pathology of normal muscle, joint, nerve, and connective tissue mechanics. The root definition rheuma in Latin means discharge of mucous membranes because in early days, it was thought to be the origin of all aches and pains associated with muscles and joints. The science of rheumatology has greatly advanced since the early days of medicine (American Heritage Dictionary). It is now well known that rheumatic diseases range from autoimmune responses to wear-and-tear–type pathologies. The more common diagnoses include rheumatoid arthritis (RA) (Garrod 1890, 2001), osteoarthritis (OA), fibromyalgia, gout, and systemic lupus erythematosus.

■ Rheumatoid Arthritis

In the year 1800, a 28-year-old resident physician from France, Augustin Jacob Landré-Beauvais, described in his dissertation what modern medicine now calls **rheumatoid arthritis** (Landré-Beauvais, 2001). He began to differentiate the symptoms and characteristics from gout. It was not until 1859 that an English physician named Alfred Garrod identified the presence of excessive uric acid in the blood of patients with gout but the absence of this characteristic in those with other forms of arthritis. In 1890, Archibald Garrod, son of Alfred, first coined the diagnosis "rheumatoid arthritis" in his book *Treatise on Rheumatism and Rheumatoid Arthritis.*

Based on modern definitions, scientists studying paleopathology now study eight specific characteristics of skeletons related to RA. These characteristics include subchondral cysts; erosions/periarticular sinuses in affected joints; rebuilding and/or presence of osteophytes; severe periarticular bone fragmentation or sinuses; ulnar deviation of the metacarpophalangeal (MCP) joints; traces in cartilage-supporting bone tissues of a multiarticular joint, as evidence of the disease's effect on all the articular facets of the joint (distinguishing it from OA); osseous ankylosis of joints (especially carpal and metacarpal); eburnation; and multiple joints that are bilaterally affected (Entezami, Fox, Clapham, & Chung, 2011). Common locations and symptoms of RA are depicted in Figure 23.1.

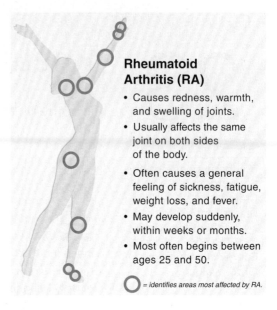

Rheumatoid Arthritis (RA)

- Causes redness, warmth, and swelling of joints.
- Usually affects the same joint on both sides of the body.
- Often causes a general feeling of sickness, fatigue, weight loss, and fever.
- May develop suddenly, within weeks or months.
- Most often begins between ages 25 and 50.

○ = identifies areas most affected by RA.

Figure 23.1 Common locations and symptoms of RA. (From Anatomical Chart Company.)

Societal costs associated with RA are significant. It has been determined that annual costs are $39.2 billion. This can be broken down into direct, indirect, and intangible costs. The direct costs total $19.3 billion, with the burden shared across employers (33%), patients (28%), the government (20%), and caregivers (19%). Intangible costs consist of premature mortality ($9.6 billion) and quality of life deterioration ($10.3 billion) (Birnbaum et al., 2010).

■ Osteoarthritis

Degenerative joint disease, more commonly called **osteoarthritis**, is, as the name indicates, inflammation of the bone and joints (*The American Heritage Science Dictionary, 2015*). Hippocrates described general incidence of joint pain but not in detail. It was not until British physician William Musgrave first detailed OA and its effects in 1715 in his published work *De arthritide symptomatica* (Cameron, 1998). Since, OA has been subdivided into primary and secondary forms. Primary OA consists of the typical wear and tear associated with eroding the joint cartilage over time. Secondary OA involved an injury or insult to the joint, such as a fracture, that leads to premature erosion of the joint cartilage. Common locations and symptoms of OA are depicted in Figure 23.2.

Osteoarthritis (OA)

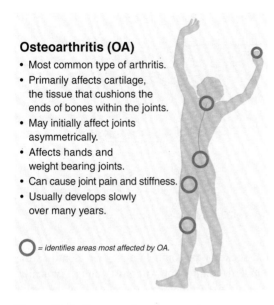

- Most common type of arthritis.
- Primarily affects cartilage, the tissue that cushions the ends of bones within the joints.
- May initially affect joints asymmetrically.
- Affects hands and weight bearing joints.
- Can cause joint pain and stiffness.
- Usually develops slowly over many years.

○ = identifies areas most affected by OA.

Figure 23.2 Common locations and symptoms of OA. (From Anatomical Chart Company.)

Societal costs can be broken down into direct and indirect costs. It is estimated that combined, these costs average over $5700 per person annually (Maetzel, Li, Pencharz, Tomlinson, & Bombardier, 2004). Thirteen point two billion dollars alone can be assigned to costs associated with employment (Buckwalter, Saltzman, & Brown, 2004). Absenteeism costs society approximately $10.3 billion (Kotlarz, Gunnarsson, Fang, & Rizzo, 2010). Murphy and Helmick estimate that hospitalization costs for total knee and total hip arthroplasties combined cost $42.2 billion in 2009 (Murphy & Helmick, 2012).

■ Fibromyalgia

Scottish surgeon, William Balfour, first described the symptoms of **fibromyalgia** in 1816. In 1904, the work by a pathologist Ralph Stockman presented inflammatory changes in the intramuscular septa on patient biopsies, and separately, Sir William Gowers coined the term fibrositis to describe tender points in patients with low back pain. The modern definition evolved in 1972 when physician Hugh Smythe detailed fibromyalgia as widespread pain and tender points (Inanici & Yunus, 2004). Common locations of tenderness with fibromyalgia are depicted in Figure 23.3.

Silverman et al. studied the economic burden associated with fibromyalgia and often found it accompanied RA. They quantified the direct costs of fibromyalgia as nearly $11,000 annually per patient but nearly doubled at $19,395 when both diagnoses were present. Indirect costs, such as work absence, are significant for this disease (Silverman et al., 2009).

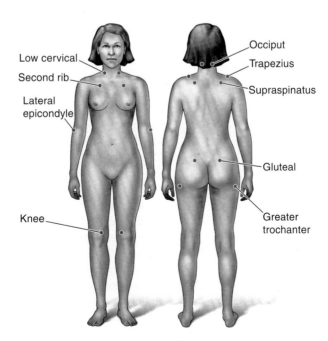

Low cervical
Second rib
Lateral epicondyle
Knee

Occiput
Trapezius
Supraspinatus
Gluteal
Greater trochanter

Figure 23.3 Common locations of tenderness with fibromyalgia.

■ Gout

In 2640 BC, the Egyptians were the first to describe podagra, what modern medicine calls **gout**. Later, Hippocrates wrote about the disease as the "unwalkable disease" because of its primary impact on the first metatarsophalangeal joint. Throughout history, it was associated with an excessive lifestyle of rich foods and alcohol consumption and often referred to as the "disease of kings." In medieval times, it was believed that this excess would cause a "drop" or flow into the joint; therefore, the Latin derivative of drop or gutta was applied and the origination of gout (Nuki & Simkin, 2006). Common locations of gout include the first metatarsal phalangeal joint, the interphalangeal joints of the hands and the elbows.

It has been estimated that annual costs directly attributable to gout alone exceed $4 billion. In addition, indirect costs have an added societal burden related to lost wages and productivity due to absenteeism totaling $2.6 billion. While not quantified, the indirect costs to caregivers and other indirect costs are also substantial (Wertheimer, Morlock, & Becker, 2013).

■ Systemic Lupus Erythematosus

Systemic lupus erythematosus was first described by Hippocrates through his work on cutaneous ulcers. The word lupus in Latin means wolf and was applied to these patients as a descriptor by Rogerious in the thirteenth century to describe his patients whose facial lesions bore a strong resemblance to a wolf's bite (Boltzer, 1983). It wasn't until 1833 when Biett began to clarify the categories and descriptions of lupus erythematosus. In 1872, Kaposi's work clarified the variations into discoid and systemic forms leading to the modern definition of systemic lupus erythematosus (Smith & Cyr, 1988). Systemic lupus erythematosus tends to impact similar joints associated with RA.

Systemic lupus erythematosus also is a significant burden on society. Direct and indirect costs per patient range from $4,453 to $52,415 (Meacock, Dale, & Harrison, 2013).

ETIOLOGY

Healthy articular joint anatomy and function is the foundation for understanding pathology associated with rheumatic diseases. The healthy joint has a smooth well-lubricated articular surface whether it is a hinge joint, pivot joint, or ball

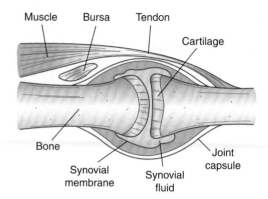

Figure 23.4 Normal, healthy joint.

and socket–type joint. Figure 23.4 identifies the standard components of most joints. Typically, the soft tissue includes muscles, tendons, joint capsule, and ligaments, which provide the mobility and stability of the joints. The cartilaginous joint surface and synovial fluid provide the necessary lubrication and durability for high-repetition load bearing. The combined structure is smooth, stable, and efficient.

It is apparent with RA that a combination of genetic and environmental factors leads to autoimmune reactions within the body (Gibofsky, 2012). If left untreated, these reactions result in the formation of synovitis and tenosynovitis, which often lead to joint damage and ligament laxity, which can subsequently create muscle imbalance (Horsten & Ursum, 2010). The infiltration of infectious agents into the synovial tissues triggers a chronic inflammatory process, and ensuing immune reaction leads to cell degradation of cartilage and bone tissue (Baecklund, Askling, Rosenquist, Ekbom, & Klareskog, 2004). Depicted in Figure 23.5 is the typical appearance of a hand with RA. The swelling around the joints is often quite visible. **Pannus** is formed from the synovial lining, which is a substance that causes the soft tissue destruction. Subsequently, the cartilage and bone erode creating a narrowed joint space and joint instability. Figures 23.6 and 23.7 describe and depict the cellular response to the disease state.

OA, often synonymous with degenerative joint disease, has polygenic hereditary component as well as an environmental component. New research is linking genes to the development of synovial joints and may be able to predict onset and specific joint involvement (Sandell, 2012). Aging and other environmental factors can also lead to OA following

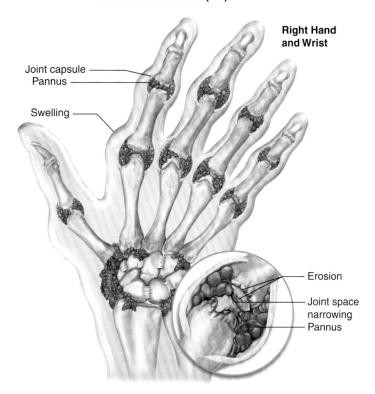

Figure 23.5 Typical impact of rheumatoid arthritis in the hand. (From Anatomical Chart Company.)

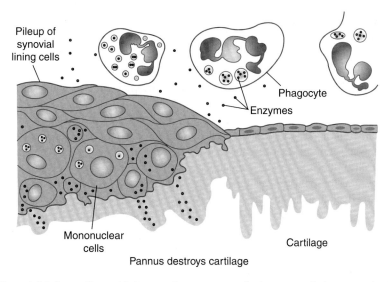

Figure 23.6 Synovial lining cells multiply, creating a mass called pannus. Substances in this mass further damage the underlying cartilage, which softens, weakens, and ultimately is destroyed. The waste products of cartilage cell destruction further stimulate the inflammatory process. New phagocytes rush to the area to clean up the debris. Some lymphocytes and other mononuclear cells are mistakenly rendered capable of attacking cartilage. Lysosomal enzymes and collagenase are released, thus perpetuating the abnormal process. (Reprinted with permission from the Arthritis Foundation. (1988). *The AHPA Arthritis Teaching Slide Collection* (2nd ed.).)

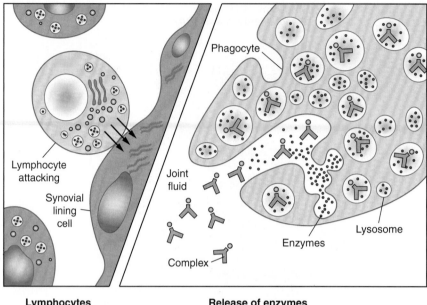

**Lymphocytes
attack-synovium**   **Release of enzymes**

Figure 23.7 In the development of inflammatory rheumatic diseases, the normal protective process of inflammation goes awry. Lymphocytes can no longer distinguish between antigens and healthy tissue, and they secrete substances that cause the synovial lining to become inflamed. Phagocytes become overloaded with immune complexes and release lysosomal enzymes into the joint fluid. The enzymes then attach to the cells of the joint lining, eventually destroying them. (Reprinted with permission from the Arthritis Foundation. (1988). *The AHPA Arthritis Teaching Slide Collection* (2nd ed.).)

period of **chondropenia** or a loss of cartilage faster than the rate of self-repair (Lohmander, Saxne, & Heinegard, 1994). Acute injury, mechanical stress, and even immobilization can lead to elevated levels of degradative enzymes in synovial fluid that remain present for years following the insult (Dahlberg, Friden, Roos, Lark, & Lohmander, 1994; Ghosh, Sutherland, Taylor, Pettit, & Bellenger, 1983). The extent determines whether the process becomes progressive or not (Dahlberg et al., 1994). Figure 23.8 depicts chondropenia at the cellular level leading to OA. Figure 23.9 is a depiction of cartilage degradation typical of knee OA.

Disabling pain and tenderness that impact muscles, tendons, and joints are commonly associated with fibromyalgia. While the incidence is rapidly increasing, the etiology remains unclear (Jahan, Nanji, Qidwai, & Qasim, 2012). It is theorized that genetic, immunological, and hormonal factors may play an important role, but it is still uncertain (Bellato et al., 2012). Unlike typical rheumatic diseases, fibromyalgia is not characterized by joint inflammation.

Gout is a common inflammatory arthritis caused by crystallization of uric acid within the affected joints. Long associated with diet high in purines, it can give rise to elevations in blood uric acid. When synthesis and excretion cannot balance with dietary intake, **hyperuricemia** results. Hyperuricemia can also be attributed to insulin resistance syndrome, hypertension, nephropathy, and similar conditions. Chronic elevation of urate levels can lead to permeation and crystallization within the joint (Choi, Mount, & Reginato, 2005). In Figure 23.10, the urate crystals are depicted within a knee joint and the erosive impact it can have on cartilage.

Systemic lupus erythematosus remains an autoimmune disorder without certain etiology. Many studies have been performed to identify the potential trigger of the autoimmune response including allergies, infections, and exposure to certain agents, but nothing is conclusive. The impact on joints is very similar to that of RA (Harvey, Shulman, Tumulty, Conley, & Schoenrich, 1954).

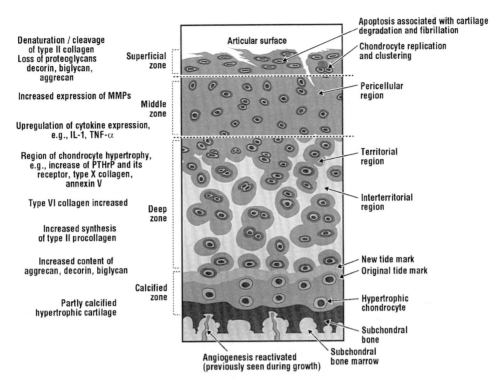

Denaturation / cleavage
of type II collagen
Loss of proteoglycans
decorin, biglycan,
aggrecan

Increased expression of MMPs

Upregulation of cytokine expression,
e.g., IL-1, TNF-α

Region of chondrocyte hypertrophy,
e.g., increase of PTHrP and its
receptor, type X collagen,
annexin V

Type VI collagen increased

Increased synthesis
of type II procollagen

Increased content of
aggrecan, decorin, biglycan

Partly calcified
hypertrophic cartilage

Superficial zone
Middle zone
Deep zone
Calcified zone

Articular surface

Apoptosis associated with cartilage
degradation and fibrillation
Chondrocyte replication
and clustering
Pericellular
region
Territorial
region
Interterritorial
region
New tide mark
Original tide mark
Hypertrophic
chondrocyte
Subchondral
bone
Subchondral
bone marrow

Angiogenesis reactivated
(previously seen during growth)

Figure 23.8 Chondropenia at a cellular level leading to osteoarthritis. (From Moskowitz, R. W., Altman, R. D., Buckwalter, J. A., Goldberg, V. M., & Hochberg, M. C. (2006). *Osteoarthritis* (4th ed.). Philadelphia, PA: Wolters Kluwer.)

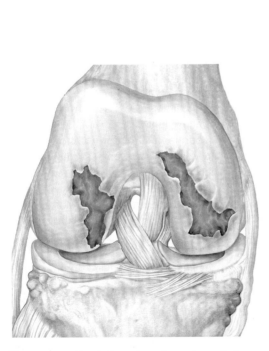

Figure 23.9 Depiction of cartilage degradation typical of knee osteoarthritis. (From Anatomical Chart Company.)

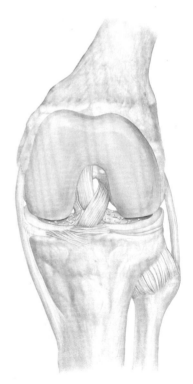

Figure 23.10 Erosive impact of urate crystals on the cartilage of a knee joint. (From Anatomical Chart Company.)

INCIDENCE AND PREVALENCE

Rheumatic diseases lead to significant disability worldwide; arthritis is the leading cause of disability in the United States (Bolen et al., 2010). RA has been reported to affect approximately 1% of the world population (Gibofsky, 2012). While the prevalence of RA increases with age, it can occur at any age. Most commonly, it will be diagnosed between the ages of 40 and 70 years (Helmick, et al., 2008). Studies show RA equally impacts all races, ethnic groups, and gender (Escalante & del Ricon, 2001). In order to be considered **juvenile rheumatoid arthritis**, the onset must occur prior to the age of 16, with involvement of one or more joints for at least 6 weeks (Gewanter, Rohnmann, & Baum, 2005). Typical onset occurs between ages 1 and 6, with no gender bias. Children may have the diagnoses with or without the presence of rheumatoid factor in their blood. Those with a presence have a higher likelihood of greater disease severity (Colbert, 2010).

While RA has a significant impact on the world, OA is far more prevalent. Studies indicate that 10% to 15% of the world population has the disease. Approximately 27 million people in the United States alone are impacted with OA, with expected exponential growth due to our aging population and the increased incidence of obesity (Neogi & Zhang, 2013). Studies show the impact varies by gender and race depending on the involved joint. The knee remains the most common site for OA, and it is estimated to impact 47% of women and 40% of men during their lifetime. Similarly, for hand OA, it is estimated that 9.7% of women and 4% of men will be affected. A recent study identified that African American men had a 32.3% incidence of hip OA while 23.8% of Caucasian men had hip OA. Chinese women were more likely to develop knee OA over Caucasian women (46.6% compared to 34.8%), while Caucasians had a higher incidence of hand and hip OA (47% compared to 85% for hip OA and 0.8% compared to 4.5% for hand OA) (Neogi & Zhang, 2013).

Fibromyalgia can often accompany OA and RA, and in fact, it is one of the more common diagnoses referred to a rheumatologist. Studies indicate prevalence worldwide ranges from 1% to 4.7%. Fibromyalgia is more common in women than men, and the incidence increases with age (Jones, Atzeni, Beasley, Flüß, Sarzi-Puttini, & Macfarlane, 2015). It has been reported that the prevalence in the United States is 0.5% in men and 3.4% in women (Vincent et al., 2013).

The most common form of inflammatory arthritis is gout. Gout has been reported to affect 1% to 4% of the world population (Helmick et al., 2008; Lawrence et al., 2008). In the United States, it has been reported that 8.3 million people are affected by gout. Men and African Americans are significantly more likely to be affected (Singh, 2013).

Several studies report the proportion of the population with systemic lupus erythematosus is increasing while the frequency of new cases is decreasing. Internationally, Northern Ireland has the highest prevalence of systemic lupus erythematosus while people of Black Caribbean descent have the highest incidence and prevalence. Females are six times more likely to be affected by systemic lupus erythematosus than are males (Rees et al., 2014).

SIGNS AND SYMPTOMS

RA is quite variable in its onset and progression by individual. While some experience sudden onset of symptoms, some experience a gradual onset, some experience exacerbations and remissions, some experience mild symptoms, and some experience severe symptoms. RA can affect one joint or have polyarticular involvement. It can affect joints symmetrically or asymmetrically. Most frequently, RA is polyarticular with the initial signs being that of fatigue and generalized weakness (Kasper et al., 2012).

The inflammatory process is the primary source of the signs and symptoms. Table 23.1 depicts the most common presentation for each stage of the inflammatory joint disease process ranging from acute to chronic-inactive. Following fatigue and generalized weakness is often the loss of range of motion. Joint edema may impede normal joint articulation in early stages. Joint **guarding** or self-bracing is also a frequent response in those with RA and Juvenile Rheumatoid Arthritis (JRA) due to pain associated with movement. Limiting range of motion may in turn lead to adhesions, which mechanically limit joint movement (Gewanter et al., 2005). As the disease progresses, contractures may develop, joint erosions progress, and subluxation, ankylosis, or dislocation may ensue. Typically, RA affects the smaller joints with higher synovium to cartilage ratio (Matschke,

TABLE 23.1	Signs and Symptoms by Stage of the Inflammatory Disease Process	
Stages	**Objective Signs**	**Subjective Symptoms**
Acute	Limited range of motion	Pain at rest and movement most severe
	Fever	Inflammation most severe
	Decreased muscle strength	Hot, red joints
	Possible cold, sweaty hands	Decreased function
	Overall stiffness	Tingling and numbness in hands and feet
	Gel phenomenon most prominent	
	Weight loss	
	Decreased appetite	
Subacute	Decreased range of motion	Pain and tenderness at rest and movement decreases
	Poor endurance	
	Mild fever	Joints warm and pink
	Decreased muscle strength	Inflammation subsiding
	Morning stiffness	Decreased function
	Gel phenomenon	Tingling and numbness in hands and feet
	Weight loss	
	Decreased appetite	
Chronic-active	Decreased range of motion	Pain and tenderness at rest minimal
	Fever has subsided.	Pain on motion decreases
	Muscle strength decreased	Inflammation low grade
	Endurance low	Increased activity noted, owing to adjustment to pain
Chronic-inactive	Limited range of motion	Pain at motion caused by stiffness from disuse during previous stages and instability of joint
	Muscle atrophy	
	Decreased endurance from limited activity in previous stages	No inflammation
	Residuals seen from above stages	Residuals seen from above stages
	Potential contracture	Functioning may be decreased due to pain

Murphy, Lemmy, Maddison, & Thom, 2009). The MCP and proximal interphalangeal joints are most severely impacted by RA (Fouque-Aubert, Chapurlat, Miossec, & Delmas, 2010). A **swan-neck deformity** results when the volar plate of the Proximal interphalangeal joint (PIP) joint elongates and allows the extensors to force the PIP joint into hyperextension, which causes an imbalance, and the Distal interphalangeal joint (DIP) joint subsequently moves into flexion. A **boutonniere deformity** results when the central slip of the extensor tendon erodes from its attachment on the middle phalanx. The inability to extend the PIP joint allows the lateral bands to migrate, creating PIP flexion and DIP hyperextension. The anatomy of this injury has the appearance of a buttonhole, which gives rise to its name. When either of these deformities remains uncorrected for a long period of time, it becomes contracted or fixed. Figure 23.11 depicts a typical presentation of a rheumatoid hand with an index finger boutonniere deformity as well as middle and ring finger swan-neck deformity. Figure 23.12 is a diagram of each of the deformities that frequently develop.

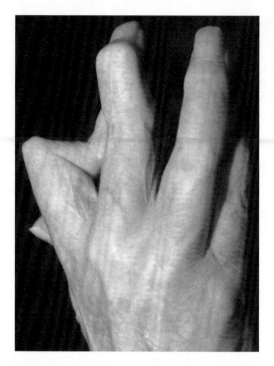

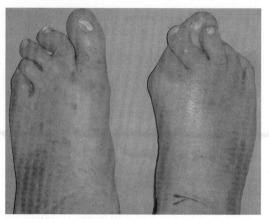

Figure 23.13 Typical presentation of feet in an individual with RA. (From St. Clair, E. W., Pisetsky, D. S., Haynes, B. F. (2004). *Rheumatoid arthritis*. Philadelphia, PA: Wolters Kluwer.)

Figure 23.11 Rheumatoid hand with an index finger boutonniere deformity and middle and ring finger swan-neck deformities. (From St. Clair, E. W., Pisetsky, D. S., & Haynes, B. F. (2004). *Rheumatoid arthritis*. Philadelphia, PA: Wolters Kluwer.)

While less common, the small joints of the feet are impacted in a similar fashion. Figure 23.13 depicts a common presentation of the toes of an individual with RA.

In the progression of the disease, the soft tissue allows for deformity of small joints as previously discussed, but the erosive properties continue on the bony structure until they become dislocated and perhaps ankylosed.

Figure 23.14 shows a picture of the typical zig-zag deformity found in the hands of a person with severe RA. The prolonged inflammation surrounding the joint, tendons, and ligaments degrades the structures to the point of laxity, imbalance, and erosion. The typical pattern of imbalance allows significant radial deviation of the radiocarpal joint as well as ulnar deviation of the MCP joints of the index through small fingers. This disease is truly erosive on bony structures.

While it is less common in other areas of the body, it is still quite significant. The presentation often begins with pain and tenderness and localized inflammation. Prolonged presence can lead to tendonitis, tenosynovitis, joint capsule inflammation,

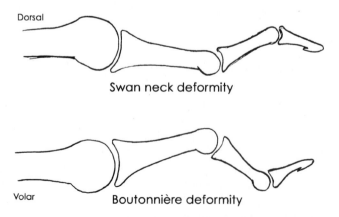

Dorsal

Swan neck deformity

Volar   **Boutonnière deformity**

Figure 23.12 Diagram of a swan-neck and boutonniere deformity. (From St. Clair, E. W., Pisetsky, D. S., Haynes, B. F. (2004). *Rheumatoid arthritis*. Philadelphia, PA: Wolters Kluwer.)

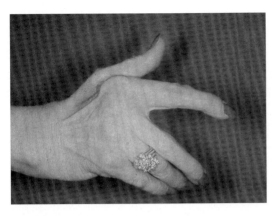

Figure 23.14 Zigzag deformity: radial deviation of the wrist and ulnar deviation of the MCP joints. (From Thorne, C. H., Gurtner, G. C., Chung, K., Gosain, A., Mehrara, B., Rubin, P., & Spear, S. L. (2013). *Grabb and Smith's plastic surgery* (7th ed.).)

and joint degradation. Following pain and tenderness, it is common to observe reduced range of motion. The elbow and forearm can be susceptible to limitations in flexion, extension, pronation, and supination. It can also impact the shoulder with the intricate ball and socket joint structure, which allows the performance of complex ADLs. If the cervical spine is involved, specifically C1 and C2, the presentation includes headaches with pain and loss of motion and may produce life-threatening conditions (Niere & Jerak, 2004). Figures 23.15 and 23.16 characterize cervical degeneration for RA.

If the lower cervical spine is involved, resulting in nerve root compression, the signs may

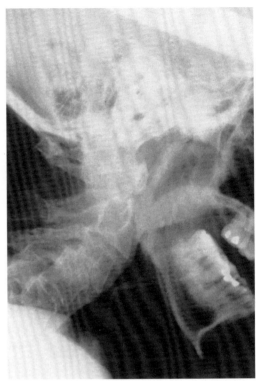

Figure 23.16 Cervical subluxations.

include numbness in the extremities and muscle weakness with varying severity.

As RA progresses untreated, individuals may develop an abnormal gait pattern resulting from hip involvement (Williams, Brand, Hill, Hunt, & Moran, 2010) (Fig. 23.17). As hip involvement advances, typical ADLs begin to become more difficult including climbing stairs, sitting, donning and doffing garments, and positioning during sexual activity (Josefsson & Gard, 2010). RA manifestation in the knee is very similar to that in the hip including pain and localized edema, often presenting as a limp and progressing to loss of motion and difficulty with ADLs.

Often confused with RA because of similar presentation, OA primarily impacts the knees, hips, hands, and spine. Typically, pain will first appear localized to a particular joint. Visible and palpable edema will appear next, often accompanied with point tenderness about the joint involved. Individuals with OA will typically describe significant joint stiffness following any prolonged period of inactivity including sitting or lying down to sleep. It is also common for individuals to complain of postactivity flare-ups of edema and pain.

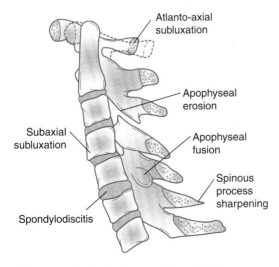

Atlanto-axial subluxation

Apophyseal erosion

Apophyseal fusion

Spinous process sharpening

Subaxial subluxation

Spondylodiscitis

Figure 23.15 Neck abnormalities in RA.

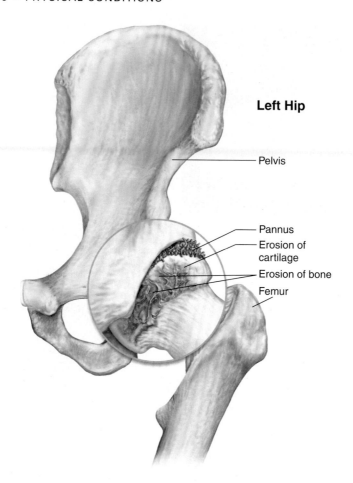

Left Hip

Pelvis

Pannus

Erosion of
cartilage

Erosion of bone

Femur

Figure 23.17 Erosive nature of RA on a hip joint. (From Anatomical Chart Company.)

Upon examination, more advanced cases of OA will present with **crepitus** during range of motion, which is the crunching feeling or sound coming from the articular surface (Hochberg et al., 1995). As with other rheumatic disease, individuals with OA often guard motion and avoid use of the painful joint leading to a more rapid development of muscle weakness and increase feeling of fatigue.

Fibromyalgia can exist in conjunction with other rheumatic disease or independent of them. It is a very complicated condition that is characterized by chronic widespread pain, point tenderness, headaches, fatigue, poor sleep, lower abdomen cramps, and depression. Severity and presence of other comorbid factors are significant to the presentation of fibromyalgia (Vincent et al., 2013). Presentation can occur unilaterally or bilaterally and most commonly affect the neck, buttocks, shoulders, arms, the upper back, and the chest. Symptoms can be chronic or episodic typically tied to some type of physical or psychological stressor (Jahan et al., 2012).

Gout presents clinically very similar to RA with its typical joint destructive properties beginning with inflammation. The symptoms of gout are usually more intermittent than progressive but, if left untreated, can be quite destructive. Individuals typically complain of joint-specific pain first that is accompanied by edema, erythema, and increased localized temperature. This will subsequently lead to stiffness. Most commonly, the big toe will be affected bilaterally or unilaterally. Gout may manifest in other parts of the feet and ankles, knees, wrist, hands, and elbows (Hall, Barry, Dawber, & McNamara, 1967). The images in Figure 23.18 (left and right) show the characteristic localized edema and erythema associated with gout of the big toe and a digit, respectively. The onset is often quite rapid.

One common symptom of all chronic rheumatic diseases is depression. Research suggests that there is a direct correlation with severity of pain and fatigue and the tendency to experience

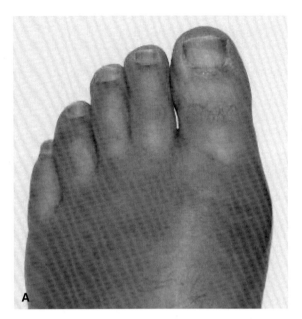
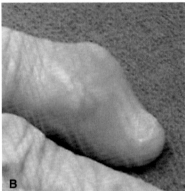

Figure 23.18 Localized **(A)** edema and **(B)** erythema associated with gout. (Courtesy of Tim Mullen.)

depression. Furthermore, as participation in ADLs diminishes in line with disease progression, the more likely an individual is to experience depression (Wolfe & Michaud, 2009).

COURSE AND PROGNOSIS

The physical manifestations and individual responses to RA present across a wide spectrum. Surveys suggest that the onset is typically insidious and function declines with severity (Adams, Burridge, Mullee, Hammond, & Cooper, 2004). While 20% of adults diagnosed with RA may go into remission in the first year, the majority will develop a chronic progressive disease (Goronzy et al., 2004). In contrast, people diagnosed with JRA have a 70% to 90% likelihood of making a satisfactory recovery with only a small chance of recurrence as an adult (Gewanter et al., 2005). While remission is possible, research has identified the following prognostic indicators: (a) number and length of remission, (b) levels of rheumatoid factor, (c) presence of subcutaneous nodules, (d) extent of bone erosion seen radiographically at the initial evaluation, and (e) sustained disease activity for more than 1 year. Additionally, women diagnosed prior to age 50 had a worst prognosis for developing a severe and chronic form of RA (Iikuni et al., 2009).

Table 23.2 identifies the criteria necessary to be considered in remission from RA.

The course and progression of OA widely vary based on whether the onset was insidious or traumatic. The degenerative process has previously been described and is progressive in nature. Research suggests the rate of progression may be slower when the baseline is more severe than when the disease is mild. Progression has also found to be faster in joints more distal when compared to proximal joints (Hochberg, 1996). Comorbidities also play a significant role in disease progression. The greater the body mass index, the more rapid the progression (Neogi & Zhang, 2013). Presence of Heberden's nodes correlated with progression of cartilage loss when monitoring x-ray images longitudinally. When osteophytes and sclerosis are present on baseline radiographs compared to radiographs when only osteophytes were present, there was a greater progression of joint degeneration including narrowing of the joint space, increased angular deformity, as well as worsening symptoms. Interestingly, there is not always a significant correlation between progressing radiographs and worsening symptoms (Hochberg, 1996). This all leads to a widely varying presentation of OA. With modern treatments, symptoms can be reduced and progression can be impeded. Joint replacement surgeries can eliminate localized OA and dramatically improve the prognosis.

TABLE 23.2 Criteria for Remission in Rheumatoid Arthritis

Five or more of the following requirements must be fulfilled for at least 2 consecutive months:

1. Duration of morning stiffness not exceeding # minutes
2. No fatigue
3. No joint pain (by history)
4. No joint tenderness or pain on motion
5. No soft tissue swelling in joints of tendon sheaths
6. Erythrocyte sedimentation rate (Westergren method) <30 mm/h for a female or 20 mm/h for a male

These criteria are intended to describe either spontaneous remission or drug-induced disease suppression, which stimulates spontaneous remission. To be considered for this designation, a patient must have met the American Rheumatism Association criteria for definite or classic rheumatoid arthritis at some time in the past. No alternative explanation may be involved to account for the failure to meet a particular requirement. For instance, in the presence of knee pain that might be related to degenerative arthritis, a point for "no joint pain" may not be awarded.

Contrary to the progressive nature of other rheumatic disease, fibromyalgia is not progressive and does not impact morbidity rates. The onset varies widely based on comorbidities. Fibromyalgia can begin as a widespread effect or manifest unilaterally and progress bilaterally. Multiple etiological factors make it difficult to identify and treat. Current research is focusing on psychosocial management and biochemical, metabolic, and immunoregulatory abnormalities. Until more is understood about the disease itself, the prognosis is difficult to determine (Jahan et al., 2012).

Gout has episodic and chronic components. Typical acute attacks have been previously prescribed and, if left untreated, can be very progressive and destructive to joints. If diagnosed and treated early, long-term effects can be eliminated. The American College of Rheumatology (ACR) recently put out guidelines suggesting dietary recommendations as well as pharmaceutical recommendations. They also stressed the importance of identifying all related comorbidities to determine potential secondary causes for the hyperuricemia. Their dietary recommendations included lists of foods to avoid, limit, and encourage. Because of the episodic nature of gout, it is suggested that these dietary standards be maintained as a means of preventing or limiting the potential return of symptoms (Khanna et al., 2012).

As any of the rheumatic diseases progress, function declines in work, play, and leisure. The lack of ADL independence will cause a faster decline. There is no known cure for these diseases; however, early diagnosis and subsequent treatment offer the best outcomes. Modern treatments can delay or prevent the destructive nature of these diseases; provide functional, emotional, and social supports to facilitate independence; and enhance quality of life.

DIAGNOSIS

A comprehensive history of symptoms and detailed timeline of the disorder provide necessary details for identification and diagnosis. Unfortunately, individuals will self-manage for 2 to 4 years prior to seeking medical intervention (Kumar et al., 2007). As previously indicated, differentiation between RA and other rheumatic diseases can pose significant difficulty. In order to support differential diagnosis, criteria were created to aid physicians (Symmons, 2007). See Table 23.3.

As indicated in the table, a detailed physical examination, blood analysis, radiographic analysis, and tissue/fluid biopsy will be required to aid in the diagnosis of RA.

OA has degenerative and acute onsets. If an insult to the joint occurs, an individual is likely

TABLE 23.3 Diagnostic Criteria for Rheumatoid Arthritis

1. Morning stiffness	Morning stiffness in and around the joints lasting at least 1 h before maximal improvement
2. Arthritis of three or more joint areas	At least three joint areas at the same time have had soft tissue swelling or fluid observed by a physician. The 14 possible areas are right or left PIP, MCP, wrist, elbow, knee, ankle, and MTP joints.
3. Arthritis of hand joints	At least one area swollen in a wrist, MCP, or PIP joint
4. Symmetric arthritis	Simultaneous involvement of the same joint areas on both sides of the body (bilateral involvement of PIPs, MCPs, or MTPs is acceptable without absolute symmetry)
5. Rheumatoid nodules	Subcutaneous nodules over bony prominences or extensor surfaces or in juxta-articular regions, observed by a physician
6. Serum rheumatoid factor	Demonstration of abnormal amounts of serum RF by any method for which the result has been positive in 5% of normal subjects
7. Radiographic changes	Radiographic changes typical of RA on posteroanterior hand and wrist radiographs, which must include erosions or unequivocal bony decalcification localized in the involved joints

aware. The initial injury typically heals and normal activity resumes, yet persistent pain can linger. Radiographic evaluation will aid in the diagnosis. If the onset is insidious from overuse or biological factors, diagnosis may be more difficult without the use of radiographic imaging. Detailed history and physical examination are also important. Research has shown that habitual vigorous exercise increases the incidence of OA. Certain sports and occupations have been linked to soft tissue damage within a joint leading to OA. The best indicator for knee OA is malalignment as seen in radiographs. If an individual has a leg length discrepancy of at least 2 cm, they have a higher likelihood of incidence of OA. Finally, if the shape of the bone or joint departs from normal anatomy, biomechanical loads can be imbalanced leading to increased joint wear leading to OA (Neogi & Zhang, 2013).

Diagnosing fibromyalgia is inherently more challenging because there are no laboratory or radiographic analyses that can make a confirmation. History and physical examination are essential (Bellato et al., 2012). In an effort to aid diagnosis of fibromyalgia, the following criteria were created. In order to be considered fibromyalgia, an individual must have a Widespread Pain Index (WPI) score greater or equal to seven and a symptom severity scale score greater or equal to five or a WPI score between three and six and a symptom severity scale score greater or equal to 9. In addition, these symptoms must be present at these levels for a minimum of 3 months. Finally, the individual must not have any other disorder that could be causing the symptoms primarily or secondarily. The WPI focuses on frequency and location of pain and tenderness and the symptom severity scale focuses on level of fatigue and cognitive involvement in the symptoms (Wolfe et al., 2010).

Gout can be diagnosed through history and physical examination and confirmed with blood work and laboratory analysis. If the disease has progressed or has chronic episodes of flare-ups, it may be important to have radiographic evaluation to determine if any joint erosion has occurred. Advanced imaging such as CT scans may be more sensitive for detecting early changes when compared to standard radiography. It is important to be aware of the frequency of symptoms as well as the number of joints involved (Khanna, 2012).

MEDICAL/SURGICAL MANAGEMENT

Significant advances in pharmaceutical agents have enhanced the medical management of RA exponentially. Physicians typically focus on managing six factors including relief of pain and joint stiffness; reduction of edema; preservation of normal joint function, musculature, and soft tissue support structures; minimization of the unintended consequences of the medication; promotion of normal growth and development; and maintenance of ADL independence. If early diagnosis can occur and proper interventions can be initiated within the first 2 years, disease progress may be halted and in some cases reversed (Finckh et al., 2009).

The ACR collaboratively with the European League Against Rheumatism developed medication criteria. Research shows synthetic **disease-modifying antirheumatic drugs (DMARDs)** should be the first medication introduced as it has the best chance to achieve low disease activity or remission. Individuals should be regularly monitored for treatment modification for maximum efficacy. Methotrexate is the primary synthetic DMARD that has proven to be highly effective. If methotrexate is not tolerated or contraindications exist, injectable gold, sulfasalazine and leflunomide can also be considered. Additionally, DMARDs can be used alone or as a combination therapy for possible added benefit if the course of the disease does not seem to be altering. Combination therapy can also include glucocorticosteroids (GCs). GCs can supplement the DMARDs and also have excellent anti-inflammatory properties. If treatment targets are not being met or if there are poor prognostic indicators present, a biological DMARD can be added to the treatment. While synthetic DMARDs target the T cells to control the inflammatory process, biologic DMARDs focus directly on the intracellular inflammatory process. Often, biological medications include tumor necrosis factor (TNF) inhibitor as some individuals have better responses with and some have better responses without these inhibitors. Research is lacking on how to taper use of these costly medications if remission is achieved (Smolen et al., 2010).

Similarly, the treatment of OA is focused on inflammation reduction. Nonsteroidal anti-inflammatory drugs (NSAIDs) are widely used because they are effective at managing both inflammation and pain. Most NSAIDs are nonselective and act by inhibiting cyclooxygenase (COX) enzymes. Newer medications have become selective due to gastrointestinal (GI) complications found in early medications. These

are known as coxibs and target just the COX-2 enzymes. Further advancement discovered that protecting prostaglandins in the GI tract was key to tolerating these medications for acute and chronic symptoms. These medications are COX-inhibiting nitric oxide donors (CINODs) and have proven to be very effective for pain modulation and inflammation reduction while maintaining GI safety (Schnitzer, Kivitz, Lipetz, Sanders, & Hee, 2005).

For the treatment of fibromyalgia, NSAIDs and opioids are typically initiated to manage the pain and improve physical function prior to diagnosis confirmation. These medications have limited benefit. Research suggests the most effective treatment includes antidepressants and neuromodulating antiepileptic medications. Pregabalin, duloxetine, and milnacipran are the only medications approved for the treatment of fibromyalgia (Bellato et al., 2012). Research is now focusing on the stress adaptation response along the hypothalamic-pituitary axis and aberrant pain processing (Jahan et al., 2012).

NSAIDs are often used as a frontline treatment for gout, but the development of xanthine oxidase inhibitors (XOI) to treat hyperuricemia revolutionized outcomes. These medications act to reduce urate levels and can reverse the development of tophaceous deposits (Nuki & Simkin, 2006). Recently, the ACR put together guidelines for the management of gout. At the time of diagnoses, the individual is directed to adopt new dietary standards previously discussed and evaluated for all possible causes of hyperuricemia with a comorbidity checklist, current medications are reviewed to make sure that is not the cause, and finally, upon history and physical examination, if the individual has been found to have frequent presentations and/or have palpable tophi, a urate-lowering treatment plan must be initiated. XOI treatment is initiated, typically allopurinol or febuxostat. The treatment plan continues until targeted urate levels are achieved (Khanna, 2012).

Because of the pain involvement and chronic nature of the disease process, most rheumatic disease can have a component of depression. It is imperative to consider this in all treatment approaches within the medical model. Psychosocial factors can degrade pain tolerance, causing a worsening of the disease process. Identifying and managing these components are critical to coping with chronic pain (Backman, 2006).

■ Surgery

The management of rheumatic disease focuses primarily on medical management, environment modification, adaptive techniques and tools, and psychosocial interventions, but when those fail to prevent the erosive properties of the disease, surgical intervention is recommended. Every surgical procedure has its own inherent risks and complications. Individuals should understand these risks and complications and have reasonable expectations for the outcomes. Simple procedures dealing with synovitis issues like trigger finger and carpal tunnel surgery are extremely effective with full functional outcomes. Larger procedures, such as arthrodesis or joint replacement, fully remove the damaged bone but do not restore full function. While joint replacements often provide significant pain relief, deformity correction, and functional improvements, they may not restore every facet of previous function. It is important that individuals are prepared for the outcomes and the recovery process before entering into any surgery (Grotle et al., 2010). Common joint replacements include hip, knee, and thumb carpometacarpal, MCP, and PIP joints.

Figure 23.19 shows an x-ray of an individual following implant resection arthroplasty using a silicone implant of their MCP joints. Figure 23.20 depicts a pyrocarbon implant inserted in a PIP joint. Figure 23.21 depicts a tendon interposition arthroplasty for the thumb. The arthritic

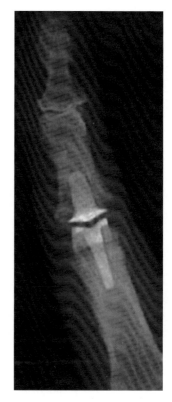

Figure 23.20 A pyrocarbon implant inserted in a PIP joint. (Courtesy of Timothy M. Mullen.)

trapezium is removed and replaced with a harvested tendon sutured to maintain the space previously occupied by the trapezium. Figure 23.22 depicts an x-ray where the hip has undergone a total hip arthroplasty.

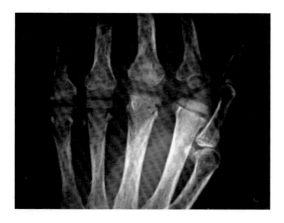

Figure 23.19 An x-ray of an individual following implant resection arthroplasty using a silicone implant of his or her MCP joints. (Courtesy of Timothy M. Mullen.)

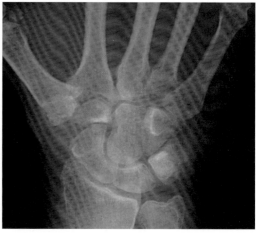

Figure 23.21 A tendon interposition arthroplasty for the thumb. (Courtesy of Timothy M. Mullen.)

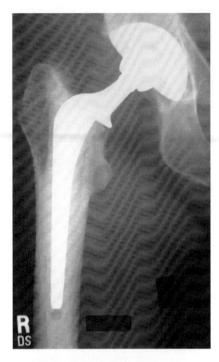

Figure 23.22 An x-ray where the hip has undergone a total hip arthroplasty. (From St. Clair, E. W., Pisetsky, D. S., Haynes, B. F. (2004). *Rheumatoid arthritis*. Philadelphia, PA: Wolters Kluwer.)

IMPACT ON OCCUPATIONAL PERFORMANCE

In 172 AD, Galen wrote, "employment is nature's best physician and essential to human happiness." The roots of occupational therapy are founded in this notion and aim to maximize occupational performance (Wright, 1947). Trombly suggests identifying all deficits in occupational performance first in order to set priorities (Trombly, 1995). When considering rheumatic diseases, occupational deficits often include fatigue, difficulty with fine motor ADLs, pain, and lifestyle changes. Quality of life must be maximized.

After all activities that make up an individual's occupational performance have been identified, it is important to categorize which of them are necessities and which are preferred. The goal is to maintain an individual's ability to engage in the preferred occupation. Employing concepts of **energy conservation** can be key to this concept. Educating proper technique and balancing rest and activity in an individualized plan are imperative to maintaining quality of life in those with disabling conditions (Furst, Gerber, Smith, Fisher, & Shulman, 1987). In coordination with energy conservation, using **joint protection** principles is also effective. Altering work methods, using orthotics, implementing assistive devices, and educating clients can reduce the impact on the involved joints and maximize independence. Some examples of joint protection include larger handles on utensils for writing and food preparation, carrying heavy objects in bags using larger joints versus holding larger items with fingers alone, and wearing resting orthotics to sleep and functional orthotics to support activities that require force like a Silver Ring Splint in someone with a swan-neck deformity. Joint protection can reduce pain and localized inflammation and help preserve the integrity of joint structures (Hammond & Freeman, 2001).

Lifestyle management must include the above interventions to mechanically deal with rheumatic disease, but managing psychosocial functioning completes the quality of life balance. Prolonged pain and feelings of hopelessness can lead to maladaptive coping techniques. Research suggests that nearly half of all individuals with RA report psychosocial issues (Bai et al., 2009).

Managing individuals with rheumatic diseases must be an interdisciplinary approach focused on the individual's medical needs, performance limitations, and psychosocial issues. Maximizing quality of life through the most advanced diagnostic and treatment approaches is fundamental to success. A diagnosis of any rheumatic disease does not have to be a terminal sentence with our modern approach.

CASE STUDY 1

James Lochlan is an 11-year-old middle school student and active in club sports and recreational activities. Lately, he has been coming home from school complaining of back pain, knee pain, and hand weakness. He takes lengthy naps and has difficulty making it to evening soccer practice. He has good days where he was able to fully participate and bad days that prevented him from active engagement. After several months, his parents took him to his pediatrician. The physician ordered lab work and made a referral to occupational therapy and a child psychologist. The lab work revealed rheumatoid factor, and James was referred to a rheumatologist for evaluation and treatment. Meanwhile, the psychologist employed modified coping techniques for the times when he was too fatigued and the OT worked out a schedule that spread out the periods of activity and inactivity and educated him and his parents on some adaptive devices and strategies to manage the times of extreme fatigue. The rheumatologist was able to establish a pharmaceutical program that allowed him to go into remission approximately 2 years after his initial diagnosis.

CASE STUDY 2

Dorothea Kapp is a 47-year-old female who considers herself to be a typical suburban mother with two teenage children. She works full-time as an elementary school teacher. She began noticing increasing tenderness in her index fingers of both hands. Within a week, the ends of her fingers were quite swollen and red and she began to notice something similar in her right big toe, to the point that she was unable to wear her shoe. She assumed it was an infection that would go away in a day or two. After 2 weeks, she was unwilling to weight-bear on her right foot and she was losing the ability to bend her index fingers. When describing her symptoms to her primary care physician, a referral was made to a rheumatologist. The rheumatologist took blood and aspirated the edematous area on her right foot and sent the samples out for laboratory evaluation. The rheumatologist referred her to occupational therapy for management. The OT was able to determine Dorothea's goals were to be able to continue teaching, cooking for her family, and caring for herself independently. The OT recommended a modified metatarsal shoe, which applied no direct pressure to the area of inflammation and had a hard sole to better disperse the pressure for weight bearing. The OT also made custom orthotic tip protectors so that if her fingers were bumped or she needed to use them for ADLs, the pressure was dispersed and the areas of tenderness were fully protected. Built-up foam handles with various inner diameters were issued for ease of manipulations of things like toothbrush, pencils, dry-erase marker, razor, and eating utensils. She was taught joint protection techniques and was encouraged to ask her family for help with some household chores. She was prescribed allopurinol, and within 4 weeks, the red, erythematic painful joints were unnoticeable and she was able to resume normal activities.

LEARNING RESOURCES

American Juvenile Arthritis Organization (AJAO)
Tel: 404-872-7100, 1-800-568-4045
www.arthritis.org

Arthritis Foundation (AF)
Tel: 404-872-7100, 800-568-4045
www.arthritis.org

The European League Against Rheumatism (EULAR)
EULAR Executive Secretariat
Seestrasse 240
8802-Kilchberg
Switzerland
Tel: +41-44-716-30-30
www.secretariat@eular.org

Higher Education and Training for People with Handicaps (HEATH)
George Washington University
HEATH Resource Center
2121 K Street NW, Suite 220
Washington, D.C. 20037
Tel: 800-544-3284
www.heath.gwu.edu

National Chronic Pain Outreach Association (NCPOA)
P.O. Box 274
Millboro, VA 24460
Tel: 540-862-9437; Fax: 540-862-9485
www.chronicpain.org

Support Groups
Contact the Arthritis Foundation for local groups across
the United States of America

Professional Organizations
American College of Rheumatology (ACR)/ Arthritis Health Professionals Association (AHPA)
1800 Century Place
Suite 250
Atlanta, GA 30345
Tel: 404-633-3777; Fax: 404-633-1870
www.acr@rheumatology.org

American Occupational Therapy Association (AOTA)
4720 Montgomery Lane
P.O. Box 31220
Bethesda, MD 20824-1220
Tel: 301-652-7711, 800-377-8555 (TDD), 1-800-SAYAOTA
www.aota.org

The American Orthopedic Society for Sports Medicine
6300 N. River Road Suite 500
Rosemont, IL 60018
Tel: 847-292-4900
www.sportsmed.org

American Podiatric Medical Association, Inc.
9312 Old Georgetown Road
Bethesda, MD 20814-1621
Tel: 1-800-FOOTCARE
www.apma.org

American Physical Therapy Association (APTA)
111 N. Fairfax Street
Alexandria, VA 22314-1488
Tel: 1-800-999-2782, 703-683-6748 (TDD)
www.apta.org

Arthritis Center
University of Missouri-Columbia
MA427 Health Sciences Center
1 Hospital Drive
Columbia, MO 65212
Tel: 314-882-8738

National Arthritis and Musculoskeletal and Skin Diseases
Information Clearinghouse (NAMSIC)
9000 Rockville Pike
PO Box AMS
Bethesda, MD 20892
Tel: 301-495-4484
www.niams.nih.gov/

AliMed Rehabilitation Products, Inc.
297 High Street
Dedham, MA 02026-9135
Tel: 1-800-255-2160
www.alimed.com

Amigo Mobility International, Inc.
6692 Dixie Highway
Bridgeport, MI 48722-9725
Tel: 1-800-248-9131
info@myamigo.com

DeRoyal/LMB, Inc.
P.O. Box 1181
San Luis Obispo, CA 93406
Tel: 1-800-541-3992

Independent Living Aids, Inc.
27 East Mall
Plainview, NY 11803
Tel: 1-800-537-2118

Invacare Corporation
899 Cleveland Street
Elyria, OH

**American Fibromyalgia Syndrome
Association, Inc**
AFSA
7371 E Tanque Verde Rd
Tucson, AZ 85715
http://www.afsafund.org/

Lupus Foundation of America, Inc.
2000 L Street, N.W., Suite 410
Washington, DC 20036
http://www.lupus.org

Scleroderma Foundation
300 Rosewood Drive, Suite 105
Danvers, MA 01923
http://www.scleroderma.org

REFERENCES

Adams, J., Burridge, J., Mullee, M., Hammond, A., & Cooper, C. (2004). Correlation between upper limb functional ability and structural hand impairment in an early rheumatoid population. *Clinical Rehabilitation*, *18*(4), 405–413. http://dx.doi.org/10.1191/0269215504cr732oa

Backman, C. L. (2006). Arthritis and pain. Psychological aspects in the management of arthritis pain. *Arthritis Research and Therapy*, 8, 221. http://dx.doi.org/10.1186/ar2083

Baecklund, E., Askling, J., Rosenquist, R., Ekbom, A., & Klareskog, L. (2004). Rheumatoid arthritis and malignant lymphomas. *Current Opinion in Rheumatology*, *16*(3), 254–261. http://dx.doi.org/10.1097/00002281-200405000-00014

Bai, M., Tomenson, B., Creed, F., Mantis, D., Tsifetaki, N., Voulgan, P. V., et al. (2009). The role of psychological distress and personality variables in the disablement process in rheumatoid arthritis. *Scandinavian Journal of Rheumatology*, *38*(6), 419–430. http://dx.doi.org/10.3109/03009740903015135

Bellato E., Marini E., Castoldi F., Barbasetti N., Mattei L., Bonasia D. E., & Blonna D. (2012). Fibromyalgia syndrome: Etiology, pathogenesis, diagnosis, and treatment. *Pain Research and Treatment*, *2012*, 426130. http://dx.doi.org/10.1155/2012/426130

Birnbaum, H., Pike, C., Kaufman, R., Marynchenko, M., Kidolezi, Y., & Cifaldi, M. (2010). Societal cost of rheumatoid arthritis patients in the US. *Current Medical Research and Opinion*, *26*(1), 77–90. http://dx.doi.org/10.1185/03007990903422307

Bolen, J., Schieb, L., Hootman, J. M., Helmick, C. G., Theis, K., Murphy, L. B., & Langmaid, G. (2010). Differences in the prevalence and impact of arthritis among racial/ethnic groups in the United States, National Health Interview Survey, 2002, 2003, and 2006. *Preventing Chronic Disease*, *7*(3), A64.

Boltzer J. W. (1983). Systemic lupus erythematosus I: Historical aspects. *Maryland State Medical Journal*, *37*, 439–441.

Buckwalter, J. A., Saltzman, C., & Brown, T. (2004). The impact of osteoarthritis: Implications for research. *Clinical Orthopedics and Related Research*, *427*, S6–S15. http://dx.doi.org/10.1097/01.blo.0000143938.30681.9d

Cameron, A. (1998). A west country polymath: William Musgrave MD FRS FRCP, of Exeter (1655–1721). *Journal of Medical Biography*, *6*(3), 166–170.

Choi, H. K., Mount, D. B., & Reginato, A. M. (2005). Pathogenesis of gout. *Annals of Internal Medicine*, *143*(7), 499–516. http://dx.doi.org/10.7326/0003-4819-143-7-200510040-00009

Colbert, R. A. (2010). Classification of juvenile spondyloarthritis: Enthesitis-related arthritis and beyond. *Nature Reviews. Rheumatology*, *6*, 477–485. http://dx.doi.org/10.1038/nrrheum.2010.103

Dahlberg, L., Friden, T., Roos, H., Lark, M. W., & Lohmander, L. S. (1994a). A longitudinal study of cartilage matrix metabolism in patients with cruciate ligament rupture-synovial fluid concentrations of aggrecan fragments, stromelysin-1 and tissue inhibitor of metalloproteinase-1. *British Journal of Rheumatology*, *33*(12), 1107–1111. http://dx.doi.org/10.1093/rheumatology/33.12.1107

Dahlberg, L., Roos, H., Saxne, T., Heinegard, D., Lark, M. W., Hoerrner, L. A., & Lohmander, L. S. (1994b). Cartilage metabolism in the injured and uninjured knee of the same patient. *Annals of the Rheumatic Diseases*, *53*, 823–827. http://dx.doi.org/10.1136/ard.53.12.823

Entezami, P., Fox, D. A., Clapham, P. J., & Chung, K. C. (2011). Historical perspective on the etiology of rheumatoid arthritis. *Hand Clinics*, *27*(1), 1–10. http://dx.doi.org/10.1016/j.hcl.2010.09.006

Escalante, A., & del Ricon, I. (2001). Epidemiology and the impact of rheumatic disorders in the United States. *Current Opinion in Rheumatology*, *13*(2), 104–110. http://dx.doi.org/10.1097/00002281-200103000-00003

Finckh, A., Bansback, N., Marra, C. A., Anis, A. H., Michaud, K., Lubin, S., … Liang, M. H. (2009). Treatment of very early rheumatoid arthritis with symptomatic therapy, disease-modifying antirheumatic drugs, or biologic agents. *Annals of Internal Medicine*, *151*(9), 612–621. http://dx.doi.org/10.7326/0003-4819-151-9-200911030-00006

For the American Heritage Dictionary Definition: Rheum. (2011). *American Heritage® Dictionary of the English Language* (5th ed.). Retrieved from http://www.thefreedictionary.com/rheum, December 20, 2015.

Fouque-Aubert, A., Chapurlat, R., Miossec, P., & Delmas, P. D. (2010). A comparative review of the different techniques to assess hand bone damage in rheumatoid arthritis. *Joint, Bone, Spine*, *77*(3), 212–217. http://dx.doi.org/10.1016/j.jbspin.2009.08.009

Furst G. P., Gerber L. H., Smith C. C., Fisher S., & Shulman, B. (1987). A program for improving energy conservation behaviors in adults with rheumatoid arthritis. *American Journal of Occupational Therapy*, *41*, 102–111. http://dx.doi.org/10.5014/ajot.41.2.102

Garrod A. E. (1890). *A treatise on rheumatism and rheumatoid arthritis*. London: Charles Griffin and Company.

Garrod, A. B. (2001). Treatise on nature of gout and rheumatic gout. London: Walton and Maberly; 1859. *Rheumatology*, *40*, 1189–1190. http://dx.doi.org/10.1093/rheumatology/40.10.1189

Gewanter, H. L., Rohnmann, K. J., & Baum, J. (2005). The prevalence of juvenile arthritis. *Arthritis & Rheumatism*, *26*(5), 599–603. http://dx.doi.org/10.1002/art.1780260504

Ghosh, P., Sutherland, J. M., Taylor, T. K., Pettit, G. D., & Bellenger, C. R. (1983). The effects of postoperative joint immobilization on articular cartilage degeneration following meniscectomy. *Journal of Surgical Research*, *35*(6), 461–473. http://dx.doi.org/10.1016/0022-4804(83)90035-5

Gibofsky, A. (2012). Overview of epidemiology, pathophysiology, and diagnosis of rheumatoid arthritis. *American Journal of Managed Care*, *18*, S295–S302.

Goronzy, J. J., Matteson, E. L., Fulbright, J. W., Warrington, K. J., Chang-Miller, A., Hunder, G.G., … Weyand, C. M. (2004). Prognostic markers of radiographic progression in early rheumatoid arthritis. *Arthritis & Rheumatism*, *50*(1), 43–54. http://dx.doi.org/10.1002/art.11445

Grotle, M., Garratt, A. M., Klokkerud, M., Lochting, I., Uhlig, T., & Hagen, K. B. (2010). What's in team rehabilitation care after arthroplasty for osteoarthritis? Results from a multi-center, longitudinal study assessing structure, process, and outcome. *Journal of the American Physical Therapy Association*, *90*(1), 121–131. http://dx.doi.org/10.2522/ptj.20080295

Hall, A. P., Barry, P. E., Dawber, T. R., & McNamara P. M. (1967). Epidemiology of gout and hyperuricemia. *The American Journal of Medicine*, *42*(1), 27–37. http://dx.doi.org/10.1016/0002-9343(67)90004-6

Hammond, A., & Freeman, K. (2001). One-year outcomes of a randomized controlled trial of an educational-behavioural joint protection programme for people with rheumatoid arthritis. *Rheumatology*, *40*(9), 1044–1051. http://dx.doi.org/10.1093/rheumatology/40.9.1044

Harvey, A. M., Shulman, L. E., Tumulty, P. A., Conley, C. L., & Schoenrich, E. H. (1954). Systemic lupus erythematosus: Review of the literature and clinical analysis of 138 cases. *Medicine*, *33*(4), 291–425. http://dx.doi.org/10.1097/00005792-195412000-00001

Helmick, C. G., Felson, D. T., Lawrence, R. C., Gabriel, S., Hirsch, R., Kwoh, C. K., … Stone, J. H. (2008). Estimates of the prevalence of arthritis and other rheumatic conditions in the United States: Part I. *Arthritis & Rheumatology*, *58*(1), 15–25. http://dx.doi.org/10.1002/art.23177

Hochberg, M. C., Altman, R. D., Brandt, K. D., Clark, B. M., Dieppe, P. A., Griffin, M. R., … Schnitzer T. J. (1995). Guidelines for the medical management of osteoarthritis. *Arthritis and Rheumatism*, *38*(11), 1535–1540. http://dx.doi.org/10.1002/art.1780381103

Iikuni, N., Sato, E., Hoshi, M., Inoue, E., Taniguchi, A., Hara, M., … Yamanaka, H. (2009). The influence of sex on patients with rheumatoid arthritis in a large observational cohort. *Journal of Rheumatology*, *36*(3), 508–511. http://dx.doi.org/10.3899/jrheum.080724

Inanici, F., & Yunus, M. B. (2004). History of fibromyalgia: Past to present. *Current Pain and Headache Reports*, *8*(5), 369–378. http://dx.doi.org/10.1007/s11916-996-0010-6

Jahan, F., Nanji, K., Qidwai, W., & Qasim, R. (2012). Fibromyalgia syndrome: An overview of pathophysiology, diagnosis and management. *Oman Medical Journal*, *27*(3), 192–195. http://dx.doi.org/10.5001/omj.2012.44

Jones, G. T., Atzeni, F., Beasley, M., Flüß, E., Sarzi-Puttini, P., & Macfarlane, G. J. (2015). The prevalence of fibromyalgia in the general population: A comparison of the American College of Rheumatology 1990, 2010, and modified 2010 classification criteria. *Arthritis & Rheumatology*, *67*(2), 568–575. http://dx.doi.org/10.1002/art.38905

Josefsson, K. A., & Gard, G. (2010). Women's experiences of sexual health when living with rheumatoid arthritis: An explorative qualitative study. *BMC Musculoskeletal Disorders*, *11*, 240–248. http://dx.doi.org/10.1186/1471-2474-11-240

Kasper, D. L., Braunwald, E., Fauci, A., Longo, D., Jameson, J. L., & Fauci, A. S. (2012). Harrison's principles of internal medicine (16th ed.). *The American Journal of Managed Care*, *18*(13), 295–302.

Khanna, D., Fitzgerald, J. D., Khanna, P. P., Bae, S., Singh, M. K., Neogi, T., … Terkeltaub, R. (2012). 2012 American college of rheumatology guidelines for management of gout. Part 1: Systematic nonpharmacologic and pharmacologic therapeutic approaches to hyperuricemia. *Arthritis Care & Research*, *64*(10), 1431–1446. http://dx.doi.org/10.1002/acr.21772

Kotlarz, H., Gunnarsson, C. L., Fang, H., & Rizzo, J. A. (2010). Osteoarthritis and absenteeism costs: Evidence from US national survey data. *Journal of Occupational and Environmental Medicine*, *52*(3), 263–268. http://dx.doi.org/10.1097/JOM.0b013e3181cf00aa

Kumar, K., Daley, E., Carruthers, D. M., Situnayake, D., Gordon, C.,Grindulis, K., … Raza, K. (2007). Delay in presentation to primary care physicians is the main reason why patients with rheumatoid arthritis are seen late by rheumatologists. *Rheumatology. 46*(9), 1438–1440.

Landré-Beauvais, A. J. (2001). The first description of rheumatoid arthritis. Unabridged text of the doctoral dissertation presented in 1800. *Joint, Bone, Spine*, *68*, 130–142.

Lawrence, R. C., Felson, D. T., Helmick, C. G., Arnold, L. M., Choi, H., Deyo, R. A., … Wolfe, F. (2008). Estimates of the prevalence of arthritis and other rheumatic conditions in the United States: Part II. *Arthritis & Rheumatology*, *58*(1), 26–35. http://dx.doi.org/10.1002/art.23176

Lohmander, L. S., Saxne, T., & Heinegard, D. K. (1994). Release of cartilage oligomeric matrix protein (COMP) into joint fluid after knee injury and in osteoarthritis. *Annals of the Rheumatic Diseases*, *53*, 8–13. http://dx.doi.org/10.1136/ard.53.1.8

Maetzel, A., Li, L.C., Pencharz, J., Tomlinson, F., & Bombardier, C. (2004). The economic burden associated with osteoarthritis, rheumatoid arthritis, and hypertension: A comparative study. *Annals of the Rheumatic Diseases*, *63*(4), 395–401. http://dx.doi.org/10.1136/ard.2003.006031

Matschke, V., Murphy, P., Lemmy, A. B., Maddison, P. J., & Thom, J. M. (2009). Muscle quality, architecture, and activation in cachetic patients with rheumatoid arthritis. *The Journal of Rheumatology*, *37*(2), 282–284. http://dx.doi.org/10.3899/jrheum.090584

Meacock, R., Dale, N., & Harrison, M. J. (2013). The humanistic and economic burden of systemic lupus erythematosus: A systematic review. *PharmacoEconomics*, *31*(1), 49–61. http://dx.doi.org/10.1007/s40273-012-0007-4

Murphy, L., & Helmick, C. G. (2012). The impact of osteoarthritis in the United States: A population-health perspective. *American Journal of Nursing*, *112*(3), S13–S19. http://dx.doi.org/10.1097/01.NAJ.0000412646.80054.21

Neogi, T., & Zhang, Y. (2013). Epidemiology of osteoarthritis. *Rheumatic Disease Clinics of North America*, *39*(1), 1–19. http://dx.doi.org/10.1016/j.rdc.2012.10.004

Niere, K., & Jerak, A. (2004). Measurement of headache frequency, intensity and duration: Comparison of patient report by questionnaire and headache diary. *Physiotherapy Research International*, *9*(4), 149–156. http://dx.doi.org/10.1002/pri.318

Nuki, G., & Simkin, P. A. (2006). A concise history of gout and hyperuricemia and their treatment. *Arthritis Research and Therapy*, *8*(1), S1. http://dx.doi.org/10.1186/ar1906

Rees, F., Doherty, M., Grainge, M., Davenport, G., Lanyon, P., & Zhang, W. (2014). The incidence and prevalence of systemic lupus erythematosus in the UK, 1999–2012. *Annals of the Rheumatic Diseases*, *75*(1), 136–41. http://dx.doi.org/10.1136/annrheumdis-2014-206334

Sandell, L. J. (2012). Etiology of osteoarthritis: Genetics and synovial joint development. *Nature Reviews Rheumatology*, *8*(2), 77–89.

Schnitzer, T. J., Kivitz, A. J., Lipetz, R. S., Sanders, N., & Hee, A. (2005). Comparison of the COX-inhibiting nitric oxide donor AZD3582 and rofecoxib in treating the signs and symptoms of osteoarthritis of the knee. *Arthritis Care & Research*, *53*(6), 827–837. http://dx.doi.org/10.1002/art.21586

Silverman, S., Dukes, E. M., Johnston, S. S., Brandenburg, N. A., Sadosky, A., & Huse, D. M. (2009). The economic burden of fibromyalgia: Comparative analysis with rheumatoid arthritis. *Current Medical Research and Opinion*, *25*(4), 829–840. http://dx.doi.org/10.1185/03007990902728456

Singh J. A. (2013). Racial and gender disparities among patients with gout. *Current Rheumatology Reports*, *15*, 307. http://dx.doi.org/10.1007/s11926-012-0307-x

Smith, C. D., & Cyr, M. (1988). The history of lupus erythematosus from hippocrates to osler. *Rheumatic Diseases Clinics of North America*, *14*(1), 1–14.

Smolen, J. S., Landewe, R., Breedveld, F. C., Dougados, M., Emery, P., Gaujoux-Viala, C., … van der Heijde, D. (2010). EULAR recommendations for the management of rheumatoid arthritis with synthetic and biological disease-modifying antirheumatic drugs. *Annals of the Rheumatic Diseases*, *69*, 964–975. http://dx.doi.org/10.1136/ard.2009.126532

Symmons, D. P. M. (2007). Classification criteria for rheumatoid arthritis—Time to abandon rheumatoid factor? *Rheumatology, 46*(5), 725–726. http://dx.doi.org/10.1093/rheumatology/kel418

Trombley, C. C. (1995). Theoretical foundations for practice. In C. A. Trombley (Ed.), *Occupational therapy for physical dysfunction* (4th ed., pp. 15–27).

Vincent, A., Lahr, B. D., Wolfe, F., Clauw, D. J., Whipple, M. O., Oh, T. H., … St. Sauver, J. (2013). Prevalence of fibromyalgia: A population-based study in olmsted county, minnesota, utilizing the rochester epidemiology project. *Arthritis Care & Research, 65*(5), 786–792. http://dx.doi.org/10.1002/acr.21896

Wertheimer, A., Morlock, R., & Becker, M. A. (2013). A revised estimate of the burden of illness of gout. *Current Therapeutic Research, 75*, 1–4. http://dx.doi.org/10.1016/j.curtheres.2013.04.003

Williams, S. B., Brand, C. A., Hill, K. D., Hunt, S. B., & Moran, H. (2010). Feasibility and outcomes of a home-based exercise program on improving balance and gait stability in women with lower-limb osteoarthritis or rheumatoid arthritis: A pilot study. *Archives of Physical Medicine and Rehabilitation, 91*(1), 106–114. http://dx.doi.org/10.1016/j.apmr.2009.08.150

Wolfe, F., Clauw, D. J., Fitzcharles, M. A., Goldenberg, D. L., Katz, R. S., Mease, P., … Yunus, M. B. (2010). The American college of rheumatology preliminary diagnostic criteria for fibromyalgia and measurement of symptom severity. *Arthritis Care & Research, 62*(5), 600–610. http://dx.doi.org/10.1002/acr.20140

Wolfe, F., & Michaud, K. (2009). Predicting depression in rheumatoid arthritis: The signal importance of pain extent and fatigue, and comorbidity. *Arthritis & Rheumatism, 61*(5), 667–673.

Wright, H. P. (1947). Occupational therapy in rheumatoid arthritis. *Canadian Medical Association Journal, 56*, 313.

24 Spinal Cord Injury

Laura V. Miller and Rosanne DiZazzo-Miller

"... of the many forms of disability which can beset mankind, a severe injury or disease of the spinal cord undoubtedly constitutes one of the most devastating calamities in human life" (Guttmann, 1976).

—SIR LUDWIG GUTTMANN, pioneer in 20th-century management of spinal cord injury

"The future lies in our own hands, and if a challenge should enter our life, it is important to remember we have tremendous strength, courage, and ability to overcome any obstacle."

—DOUGLAS HEIR, Esq., Attorney-at-Law (personal communication, December 1994)

The full impact of the preceding quotes may not strike the reader unless the whole story is known. The latter author, Doug Heir, sustained a spinal cord injury (SCI) at age 18. He dove into a pool to save a boy who appeared to be drowning. The boy was only playing, but Doug's injury resulted in tetraplegia. Decades later, Doug has become known for being many things, among them an author, US ambassador to the Soviet Union, cover athlete for Wheaties cereal, associate legal editor of the National Trial Lawyer, and a gold medalist in the 1988 Olympics in Seoul, South Korea—an impressive list of accomplishments for someone who sustained "one of the most devastating calamities in human life!"

The goals of the health care team should include empowering clients to take charge of their futures. To accomplish this, the health professional must understand the complexities of the diagnosis. This chapter explores the ramifications of spinal cord injuries, beginning with a brief overview of the central nervous system (CNS) and surrounding structures.

DESCRIPTION AND DEFINITIONS

■ Overview of CNS and Related Structures

The brain and spinal cord make up the CNS. The spinal cord receives sensory (afferent) information from the peripheral nervous system and transmits this information to higher structures (i.e., the thalamus, cerebellum, cerebral cortex) in the CNS. Descending motor (efferent) information, originating from the cortex, is also transmitted by the spinal cord back to the peripheral nervous system. The consistency of the spinal cord has been compared to a ripe banana, and it is fortunate that the spinal cord and cerebral cortex are protected by bony structures. Whereas the skull protects the brain, the vertebral column protects the spinal cord. The vertebral column is composed of 33 vertebrae, with 7 cervical vertebrae in the neck region (C1 through C7); 12 thoracic vertebrae in the chest region (T1 through T12); 5 lumbar vertebrae in the midback region (L1 through L5); 5 sacral vertebrae (S1 through S5), which are actually fused in the lower back and pelvic region; and 4 fused coccygeal vertebrae that make up the coccyx, or tail bone (Fig. 24.1). There are 31 pairs of spinal nerves, which exit from the spinal cord and branch to form the peripheral nervous system. The nerves exit through the openings formed between each two vertebrae. The spinal nerves are named according to the vertebrae above or below the point of exit. Note that spinal nerves C1 through C7 exit above the corresponding vertebrae, whereas the remaining spinal nerves (C8 through S5) exit below the corresponding vertebrae. Thus, although there are seven cervical vertebrae, there are eight cervical spinal nerves. The actual spinal cord ends just below the L1 vertebra. However, some spinal nerves continue and exit beyond the point where the spinal cord ends. Because of their visual resemblance, this bundle of nerves is referred to as the **cauda equina**, which is Latin for horse's tail (Grundy, Tromans, & Jamil, 2002). The meningeal covering of the spinal cord, which contains the cerebrospinal fluid (CSF) that bathes the structures of the CNS, also extends past the end of the spinal cord to the L4 vertebral level. The CSF-filled meningeal space between L2 and L4, referred to as the lumbar cistern, is the site where diagnostic or therapeutic lumbar punctures, that is, spinal taps, are performed, because the spinal cord is not present, yet CSF is accessible.

■ Sensory and Motor Tracts

The terms tract, pathway, lemniscus, and fasciculus all refer to bundles of nerve fibers that have a similar function and travel through the spinal cord in a particular area. It is important to know the names, locations, and functions of these tracts to understand the possible outcomes of an SCI at a given level. Figure 24.2 shows the location of major tracts within a cross section of the spinal cord.

Two basic types of nerve tissue make up the spinal cord. Gray matter is located centrally and resembles a butterfly in cross sections of the cord. Gray matter is composed of cell bodies and synapses. White matter encompasses most of the periphery of the cord and contains the ascending and descending pathways. Table 24.1 provides a more detailed description of the functions of the various sensory and motor pathways that travel through the white matter of the spinal cord. It may be helpful to remember that many pathways are named according to their origin and the location of their final synapse (e.g., spinocerebellar, corticospinal).

Each pair of spinal nerves carries specific motor and sensory information. In general, the cervical nerves (C1 through C8) carry afferent and efferent impulses for the head, neck, diaphragm, arms, and hands. The thoracic spinal nerves (T1 through T12) serve the chest and upper abdominal musculature. The lumbar spinal nerves (L1 through L5) carry information to and from the legs and a portion of the foot, and the sacral spinal nerves (S1 through S5) carry impulses for the remaining foot musculature, bowel, bladder, and the muscles involved in sexual functioning. Table 24.2 and Figure 24.3 present a more detailed outline of muscles innervated by each level of the spinal cord and a dermatomal segmentation (sensory map) of the body.

■ Reflex Arc

Most nerve impulses move up the spinal cord to the brain and back through the cord to the peripheral nerves. However, some impulses directly enter the cord through the dorsal nerve root, synapse, and exit by the ventral nerve root. This causes certain muscle functions or responses to occur without direction from the brain. A simple example of this "looping" can

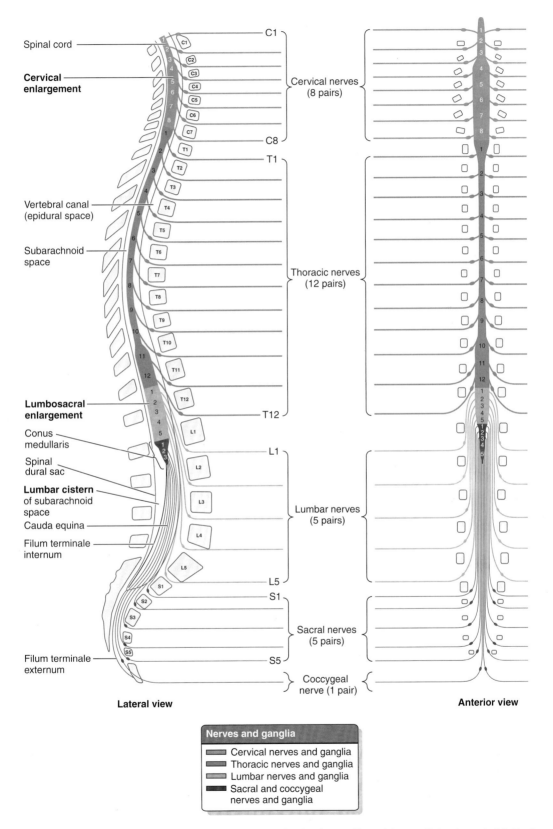

Figure 24.1 The spinal cord, spinal nerves, and vertebral column. (From Moore, K. L., Agur, A. M. R., & Dalley, A. F. (2013) *Clinically oriented anatomy* (7th ed.). Philadelphia, PA: Lippincott Williams & Wilkins.)

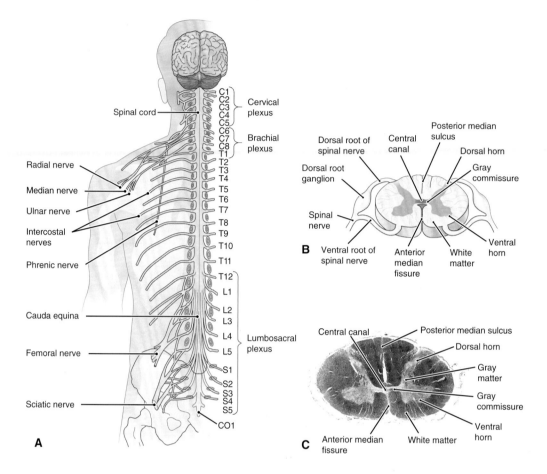

Figure 24.2 Cross section of cervical spinal cord, shown in relation to surrounding vertebral structures. (From Cohen, B. J. (2012). *Memmler's structure and function of the human body* (10th ed.). Philadelphia, PA: Lippincott Williams & Wilkins.) **A.** Spinal cord vertebral level and innervation. **B.** Spinal cord cross-section diagram. **C.** Spinal cord cross-section image

TABLE 24.1 Noninclusive Listing of Ascending and Descending Pathways	
Ascending Afferent (Sensory) Pathways	**Function**
Spinocerebellar	Nonconscious proprioception
Lateral spinothalamic	Pain, temperature
Ventral spinothalamic	Touch, pressure
Fasciculus gracilis/fasciculus cuneatus[a]	Two-point tactile discrimination, vibration, conscious proprioception, stereognosis
Spinocervicothalamic	Touch, proprioception, stereognosis, vibration
Descending Efferent (Motor) Pathways	**Function**
Lateral corticospinal	Movement to extremities
Ventral corticospinal	Movement of neck and trunk
Vestibulospinal	Equilibrium
Reticulospinal	Autonomic functions: motor respiratory functions

[a]Called the posterior column.

TABLE 24.2 Spinal Cord Innervations/Function

Spinal Cord Level	Primary Muscle Groups	Primary Movements
C1–C3	Infrahyoid muscles	Depression of hyoid
	Head/neck extension	Neck extension, flexion, rotation, and lateral flexion
	Rectus capitis (anterior and lateral)	
	Sternocleidomastoid	
	Longus colli	
	Longus capitis	
	Scalene	
	Additional Primary Muscle Groups	**Additional Primary Movements**
C4	Trapezius	Shoulder elevation, scapular adduction and depression, and independent breathing
	Upper cervical paraspinals	
	Diaphragm	
C5	Rhomboids	Scapular downward rotation
	Deltoids	Weak shoulder external rotation, flexion, and extension
	Rotator cuff muscles (partially—some nerve supply is at C6 level)	Shoulder abduction and rotation
	Biceps	Weak approximation of humeral head to glenoid fossa
	Brachialis (partially)	Elbow flexion
	Brachioradialis (partially)	
C6	Rotator cuff muscles (complete innervation)	Full shoulder rotation, adduction, flexion, and extension
	Serratus anterior (partially)	Scapular abduction
	Pectoralis (clavicular segments)	Horizontal shoulder adduction
	Total innervation of elbow flexors	Strong elbow flexion and supination
	Supinators	Wrist extension (weak)
	Extensor carpi radialis	Tenodesis action of hand
	Flexor carpi radialis	Very weak wrist flexion
C7	Latissimus dorsi	Elbow extension
	Pectoralis major (sternal portion)	Forearm pronation
	Triceps	Wrist flexion
	Pronator teres	Finger flexion (trace)
	Flexor carpi radialis	Finger extension (weak)
	Flexor digitorum superficialis	Thumb extension (weak)
	Extensor digitorum (partially)	
	Extensor pollicis longus and brevis	
C8	Flexor carpi ulnaris	Complete wrist extension, adduction, and abduction
	Extensor carpi ulnaris	Finger flexion (stronger)
	Flexor digitorum profundus and superficialis	Thumb flexion, abduction, adduction, and opposition
		Weak flexion at MCP with IP extension

TABLE **24.2** *Continued*		

Spinal Cord Level	Additional Primary Muscle Groups	Additional Primary Movements
	Flexor pollicis longus and brevis	
	Abductor pollicis longus	
	Abductor pollicis	
	Opponens pollicis	
	Lumbricals (partially)	
T1	Dorsal interossei	Finger abduction
	Palmar interossei	Finger adduction
	Abductor pollicis brevis	Thumb abduction (strong)
	Lumbricals (complete innervation)	MCP flexion with IP extension (strong)
	Erector spinae muscles (partially)	Thoracic spine extension
	Intercostal muscles (partially)	Increased respiratory function with presence of intercostals
T4–T8	Erector spinae muscles (partially)	Stronger thoracic spine extension
	Intercostal muscles (partially)	Stronger respiratory function
	Abdominal muscles (beginning at T7)	Thoracic flexion
		Weak trunk flexion
T9–T12	Lower erector spinae muscles	Strong thoracic spine extension
	Lower intercostal muscles	Trunk flexion, extension, rotation, and stability
	Abdominal muscles	
	Quadratus lumborum (partially)	Pelvic control and stability
L1–L3	Quadratus lumborum (full innervation)	Pelvic elevation
	Iliopsoas	Hip flexion
	Erector spinae (lumbar segment)	Lumbar extension
L4–L5	Lumbar erector spinae	Lumbar extension and stability
	Hip adductors	Hip adduction
	Hip rotators	Hip rotation
	Quadriceps	Knee extension
	Hamstrings (partially)	Knee flexion (weak)
	Tibialis anterior	Ankle dorsiflexion (weak)
S1–S2	Hip extensors	Hip extension
	Hip abductors	Hip abduction and stability
	Hamstrings (complete innervation)	Knee flexion
	Plantar flexors	Ankle plantar flexion
	Invertors of ankle	Ankle inversion and stability
	Evertors of ankle	Ankle eversion and stability
S2–S5	Bladder	Genitourinary functions
	Lower bowel	Bowel functions
	Genital innervations	

MCP, metacarpophalangeal; IP, interphalangeal.

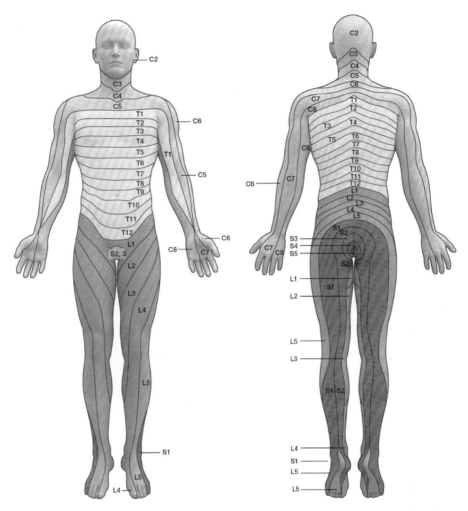

Figure 24.3 Dermatome map. (From Hoppenfeld, J. D. (2014). *Fundamentals of pain medicine.* Philadelphia, PA: Lippincott Williams & Wilkins.)

be seen in the knee-jerk reflex. If the knee is tapped with a reflex hammer, the knee will extend without any influence from the brain. The stimulation by the hammer causes afferent impulses to enter the cord, synapse, and exit, causing a contraction of the muscle fibers (Fig. 24.4). This activity is called a **reflex arc**. In people with an intact spinal cord, afferent nerve impulses also travel to the brain almost instantaneously. This allows an awareness, or "feeling," of the initial stimulation (knee tap) and subsequent response (knee jerk). This concept is important to an understanding of SCIs. It explains why some individuals with SCI continue to have reflexes but do not have voluntary control of their muscles. It also explains why others have no reflexes at all below the level of

their injury. This is discussed in much greater detail in the section on classification of injuries.

ETIOLOGY

Historically, many demographic sources attempted to count the number of people who have sustained SCIs. Since 1973, the National Spinal Cord Injury Database has been in existence, making strides in collecting comprehensive data on a national level. In 1985, the Centers for Disease Control and Prevention (CDC) began promoting surveillance mechanisms at state and national levels for the collection and reporting of these data. Prior to this time, data related to etiology and incidence of SCI in this country were inconsistently collected and

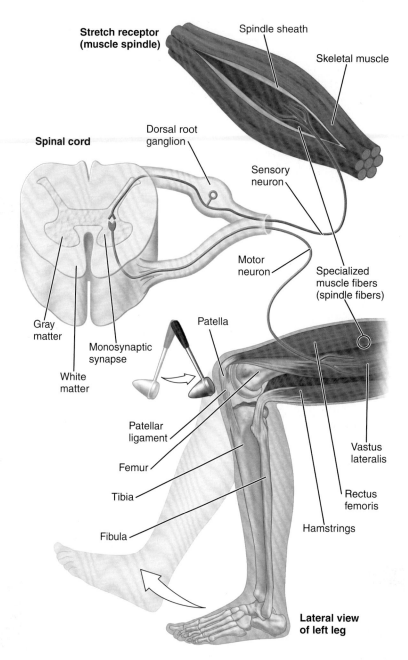

Figure 24.4 Knee-jerk reflex. (From Anderson, M. K. (2012). *Foundations of athletic training* (5th ed.). Philadelphia, PA: Lippincott Williams & Wilkins.)

lacked uniformity; advancements are continuing to be made in this area.

The leading cause of SCI in the United States is motor vehicle accidents, followed by falls and acts of violence (Fig. 24.5). Sports-related injuries account for most of the remaining SCIs, with diving being historically the most common (and preventable) cause (Table 24.3). Understanding the different contexts in which SCI occurs is critical throughout the course of occupational therapy evaluation and intervention. For example, inner-city populations in particular comprise more SCI secondary to violence than in other environmental contexts. In fact, in the United States,

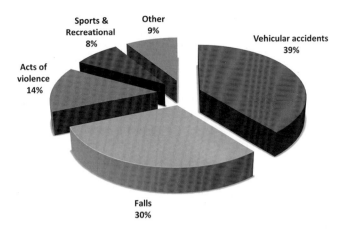

Figure 24.5 Etiologic distribution of spinal cord injury since 2015. National Spinal Cord Injury Statistical Center (NSCISC). (2015). Recent trends in causes of spinal cord injury. Birmingham, AL: University of Alabama at Birmingham. Retrieved from https://www.nscisc.uab.edu/PublicDocuments/fact_sheets/Recent%20trends%20in%20causes%20of%20SCI.pdf

gunshot wounds (GSW) are the third most common cause of SCI (Mayo Clinic, 2011; National Institute of Neurological Disorders and Stroke, 2013). Occupational therapists need to be aware of the culture of violence, environmental influences, and challenges with access to resources that are often unsupportive of individuals with SCI secondary to GSW (DiZazzo-Miller, 2015). Occupations take place throughout the dynamic union of client factors, performance skills, and performance patterns (AOTA, 2014) and are unique to each and every person with an SCI.

Analyzing the etiology of SCIs helps target prevention programs. Public awareness of the effects of using substances while operating a vehicle is certainly heightened. Tougher penalties for driving under the influence of cognitive altering substances have been enacted, and many states have adopted seat belt, child restraint, and "distracted" driving legislation. All of these efforts have the potential to reduce the leading cause of SCI. Grant monies have even been awarded to hospital-based programs that evaluate the home environments of senior citizens for

TABLE 24.3 Comparison of Select Sports-Related Spinal Cord Injuries

Sport	No. of Reported Injuries—2009	Percentage
Diving	1,676	59.4
Bicycling	328	11.6
Football	136	5.7
Snow skiing	127	4.5
Horseback riding	121	4.3
Other winter sports	115	4.1
Surfing	98	3.5
Wrestling	83	2.9
Trampoline	60	2.1
Gymnastics	48	1.7
Waterskiing	30	1.1

Developed with data from The National Spinal Cord Injury Statistical Center. 2014 Annual Statistical Report, p. 48. University of Alabama at Birmingham, 2014.

safety. Their recommendations may reduce the risk of falls—a major cause of SCI in the elderly. An innovative effort sponsored by the University of Michigan Health System involves airing public service announcements on the prevention of diving injuries before the "coming attractions trailers" at popular movies for teens during the summer months.

Although much of the literature focuses on trauma, there are many nontraumatic causes of spinal cord damage. Developmental conditions, such as **spina bifida**, which is a congenital neural tube dysfunction resulting in an incomplete closing of the vertebral column and spinal cord agenesis, may yield many of the same clinical signs as traumatic SCI. Acquired conditions, such as bacterial or viral infections, benign or malignant growths, embolisms, thromboses, and hemorrhages—even radiation or vaccinations—can also lead to damage of spinal cord tissue.

INCIDENCE AND PREVALENCE

Incidence rates for SCI in the United States are estimated at 40 cases/million population/year, excluding those who die at the scene of an accident (The National SCI Statistical Center [NSCISC], 2013). This translates to about 12,000 new cases of SCI every year. The statistics indicate that over 80% of people who sustain spinal cord injuries are male; notably, the mean age at time of injury has increased from 28.7 years in the 1970s to the present mean age of 34.7 years (NSCISC, 2014). Seasonal sports cause fluctuations in etiology and incidence statistics throughout a given year, and some urban hospitals are reporting that a disproportionate number of their SCI cases are caused by acts of violence (NSCISC, 2014). In the United States, of the spinal cord injuries reported to the national database since 2010, 63% of individuals were identified as White, 24% Black, 2% Asian, and 10% Hispanic (NSCISC, 2014). One may be tempted to conclude from these statistics that Caucasians are at higher risk for sustaining spinal cord injuries—but this would be erroneous. When compared to the composition of the general population, spinal cord injuries have a higher incidence among non-Whites—specifically among Blacks where the general population is 12% compared to 24% who acquire SCI (NSCISC, 2014).

SIGNS AND SYMPTOMS

■ Sensory Functions

The two major classifications of SCI are complete and incomplete. A complete SCI occurs with a complete transection of the cord. In this case, all ascending and descending pathways are interrupted, and there is a total loss of motor and sensory function below the level of injury. The injury also may be referred to as an upper motor neuron (UMN) injury, if the reflex arcs are intact below the level of injury but are no longer mediated by the brain. UMN lesions are characterized by (a) a loss of voluntary function below the level of the injury, (b) spastic paralysis, (c) no muscle atrophy, and (d) hyperactive reflexes (Fig. 24.6).

Complete injuries below the level of the conus medullaris (Fig. 24.1) are referred to as lower motor neuron (LMN) injuries, because the injury has affected the spinal nerves after they exit from the cord. In fact, injuries involving spinal nerves after they exit the cord at any level are referred to as LMN injuries. In these injuries, the reflex arc cannot occur, because impulses cannot enter the cord to synapse. As a result, LMN injuries are characterized by (a) a loss of voluntary function below the level of the injury, (b) flaccid paralysis, (c) muscle atrophy, and (d) absence of reflexes. UMN and LMN injuries may be complete or incomplete. There also may be a mixture of UMN and LMN signs after an incomplete lesion in the lower thoracic/upper lumbar region. The following section discusses incomplete injuries in greater detail.

■ Incomplete Injuries

If damage to the spinal cord does not cause a total transection, there will still be some degree of voluntary movement or sensation below the level of injury. This is known as an incomplete injury, which may be further categorized according to the area of the spinal cord that was damaged and the clinical signs that are present.

■ Anterior Cord Syndrome

This syndrome results from damage to the anterior spinal artery or indirect damage to anterior spinal cord tissue (Fig. 24.7). Clinical signs include loss of motor function below the level of injury and

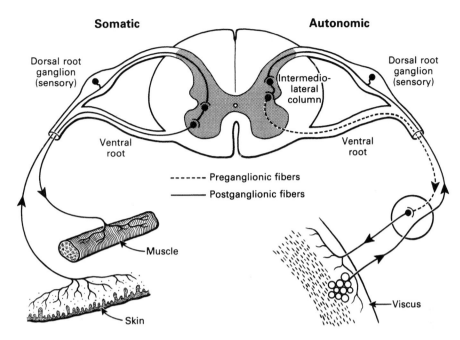

Figure 24.6 A diagrammatic representation of the reflex arc. (From Barash, P. G., Cullen, B. F., & Stoelting, R. K. (2012). *Clinical anesthesia* (5th ed.). Philadelphia, PA: Lippincott Williams & Wilkins.)

loss of thermal, pain, and tactile sensation below the level of injury. Light touch and proprioceptive awareness are generally unaffected (Hayes, Hsieh, Wolfe, Potter, & Delaney, 2000).

■ Brown-Séquard's Syndrome

This syndrome occurs when only one side of the spinal cord is damaged (Fig. 24.8). A hemisection of this nature frequently is the result of a penetrating (e.g., stab, gunshot) wound. The

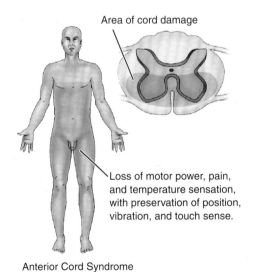

Figure 24.7 A cross section of the spinal cord illustrating the damage that causes anterior cord syndrome. The anterior artery is involved, resulting in damage to most areas, with the exception of the posterior columns. (From Pellico, L. H. (2012). *Focus on adult health.* Philadelphia, PA: Lippincott Williams & Wilkins.)

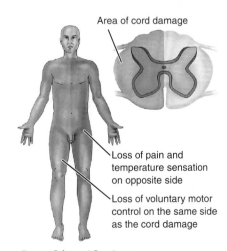

Figure 24.8 Cross section of the cord, illustrating the damage that results in Brown-Séquard syndrome. (From Pellico, L. H. (2012). *Focus on adult health.* Philadelphia, PA: Lippincott Williams & Wilkins.)

clinical signs of Brown-Séquard's syndrome generally include

Ipsilateral loss of motor function below the level of injury.

Ipsilateral reduction of deep touch and proprioceptive awareness. (There is a reduction rather than loss as many of these nerve fibers cross.)

Contralateral loss of pain, temperature, and touch.

Clinically, a major challenge presented by Brown-Séquard's syndrome is that the extremities with the greatest motor function have the poorest sensation.

■ Central Cervical Cord Syndrome

In this lesion, the neural fibers serving the upper extremities are more impaired than those of the lower extremities (Fig. 24.9). This occurs because the fibers that innervate the upper extremities travel more centrally in the cord and, as the name of the syndrome implies, the central structures are the ones that are damaged (Fig. 24.2). Injury to the central portion of the spinal cord is often seen, along with structural changes in the vertebrae. Most commonly, hyperextension of the neck, combined with a narrowing of the spinal canal, results in this type of injury. Because

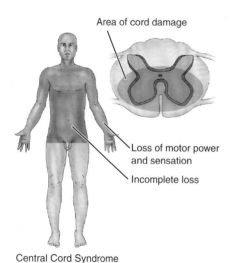

Central Cord Syndrome

Figure 24.9 Cross section of the cord, illustrating the damage resulting in central cervical cord syndrome. (From Pellico, L. H. (2012). *Focus on adult health.* Philadelphia, PA: Lippincott Williams & Wilkins.)

arthritic changes can lead to spinal canal narrowing, this syndrome is more prevalent in aging populations. The signs of central cord syndrome often include:

Motor and sensory functions in the lower extremities less involved than in the upper extremities.

Improvements in intrinsic hand function are generally evidenced last, if at all (Ackerman, Foy, & Tefertiller, 2013).

A potential for flaccid paralysis of the upper extremities, as the anterior horn cells in the cervical spinal cord may be damaged. Because these are synapse sites for the motor pathways, an LMN injury may result.

CAUDA EQUINA INJURIES

Cauda equina injuries do not involve damage to the spinal cord itself but rather to the spinal nerves that extend below the end of the spinal cord (Fig. 24.1). Injuries to the nerve roots and spinal nerves that constitute the cauda equina are generally incomplete. Because this type of injury actually involves structures of the peripheral nervous system (exiting spinal nerves), there is some chance for nerve regeneration and recovery of function if the roots are not too severely damaged or divided. These injuries are usually the result of direct trauma from fracture dislocations of the lower thoracic or upper lumbar vertebrae. Clinical signs of cauda equina injuries include

Loss of motor function and sensation below the level of injury.

Absence of a reflex arc, as the transmission of impulses through the spinal nerves to their synapse point is interrupted. Motor paralysis is of the LMN type, with flaccidity and muscle atrophy seen below the level of injury. Bowel and bladder function are also areflexic (American Spinal Injury Association, 2008).

CONUS MEDULLARIS INJURIES

Conus medullaris injuries are similar to cauda equina injuries. In many cases, it is very difficult to distinguish between these two types of injuries. They can both cause similar signs and symptoms such as local, referred, and radicular pain, loss of sphincter control, and gluteal and lower extremity sensation and weakness (Byrne, Benzel, & Waxman, 2000). Clinical signs of conus medullaris injuries include the following:

Loss of motor function and sensation below the level of injury, although typically not severe.

Absence of a reflex arc, as the transmission of impulses through the spinal nerves to their synapse point is interrupted. Motor paralysis is of the LMN type, with flaccidity and muscle atrophy seen below the level of injury. Bowel and bladder incontinence and sexual dysfunction are typically more severe than cauda equina injuries (Byrne et al., 2000).

COMPLETE VERSUS INCOMPLETE INJURIES

In both complete and incomplete injuries, the terms quadriplegia, tetraplegia, and paraplegia may be used to further describe the impact of the injury. Quadriplegia refers to lost or limited function of all extremities as a result of damage to cervical cord segments. The American Spinal Injury Association (ASIA) advocates the term tetraplegia over quadriplegia. Tetraplegia refers to impairment or loss of motor or sensory function in the cervical segments of the spinal cord that is the result of damage of neural elements within the spinal canal. Tetraplegia causes impairment of function in the arms as well as in the trunk, legs, and pelvic organs. It does not include brachial plexus lesions or injury to peripheral nerves outside the neural canal (American Spinal Injury Association/International Medical Society of Paraplegia, 2013). Paraplegia, which refers to lost or limited function in the lower extremities and trunk depending on the level of injury, occurs after lesions to thoracic, lumbar, or sacral cord segments. Spinal cord injuries are frequently classified further, based on the ASIA Impairment Scale (American Spinal Injury Association/International Spinal Cord Society, 2013), which contains the following levels:

Level A Complete; no motor or sensory function is preserved in the sacral segments S4 through S5.

Level B Sensory incomplete; sensory but not motor function is preserved below the neurological level and extends through the sacral segments S4 through S5.

Level C Motor incomplete; motor function is preserved below the neurological level, and the majority of key muscles below the neurological level have a muscle grade <3.

Level D Motor incomplete; motor function is preserved below the neurological level, and the majority of key muscles below the neurological level have a muscle grade of ≥3.

Level E Normal; motor and sensory function is normal.

A manual muscle test is performed to assess the strength of muscles and aid in the determination of the extent and nature of injury. Usually, strength is graded using the following scale (Moroz, 2015):

0 Total paralysis
1 Palpable or visible contraction
2 Active movement, full range of motion (ROM) with gravity eliminated
3 Active movement, full ROM against gravity
4 Active movement, full ROM against moderate resistance
5 Normal active movement, full ROM against full resistance
NT Not testable

COURSE AND PROGNOSIS

A prognosis implies that one can forecast or predict the outcome and chances for recovery from a particular disease or traumatic injury. That is somewhat challenging for SCIs. Although some aspects of SCI are highly predictable (e.g., specific muscle functions impaired with a complete lesion at C5), other aspects are much more vague.

Part of the ambiguity lies in the definitions of the term "recovery." One definition is to get back, or regain, which tends to be the client's focus. Another definition for recovery stresses compensation, which is often the thrust of the health care professional working with SCI. While the physiological prognosis of SCI will be discussed here, the clinician should always be aware, and acknowledge the validity, of the client's perspective on recovery. To "regain" and to "compensate for" are dramatically different frames of reference. When discussing prognosis with a person who has survived an SCI, the clinician should always be truthful but must also be acutely aware of the impact of what the client is hearing. Perhaps the most crucial indicators of an individual's functional outcome are personal characteristics such as motivation, use of support systems, and coping mechanisms. The clinician must be skilled at fostering these strengths while at the same time providing accurate information.

POSTTRAUMATIC COMPLICATIONS

■ Spinal Shock

The period of altered reflex activity immediately after a traumatic SCI is known as **spinal shock**. As a result of injury, spinal cord segments below the level of the lesion are deprived of excitatory input from higher CNS centers. What is observed clinically during this phase is a flaccid paralysis of muscles below the level of injury and an absence of reflexes. The bladder is also flaccid, requiring **catheterization**, which is a procedure to enable flow of urine by way of insertion of a latex tube into the bladder by way of the urethra when there is no voluntary control of the bowel. Depending on the level of the injury, the person with an SCI may require a ventilator because of lost or temporarily interrupted innervation to the diaphragm, intercostals, and abdominal muscles.

Spinal shock generally lasts from 1 week to 3 months after injury. Once spinal shock subsides, the areas of the spinal cord above the level of the lesion operate as they did premorbidly. Below the level of the lesion, reflexes will resume if the reflex arc is intact. This is an important concept to understand. Unlike a plant, which may die entirely if its stem is cut in half, the spinal cord is still alive and functional above and below the level of injury. The problem is one of communication; the brain cannot receive sensory information beyond the lesion site and cannot volitionally control motor function below that point.

After spinal shock subsides, there is often an increase in spasticity, especially in the flexor muscle groups. The reflex arc "fires," and the brain is unable to interfere. After this phase, there may be a period of 6 to 12 months after injury when an increase in the spasticity of the extensor groups is common. Usually, after 1 year postinjury, the wide fluctuations in tone will cease. An array of complications can greatly affect the prognosis of a person who has sustained an SCI. Some of the more common medical complications are addressed in the next section.

■ Respiratory Complications

People with spinal cord injuries at or below the level of T12 generally have a normal respiratory status. Injuries above that level, however, compromise the respiratory system to some degree. The abdominal musculature is innervated by segments T7 through T12, the intercostal muscles are served by segments T1 through T12, and the diaphragm is innervated by C4. People with complete injuries above C4 usually need a respirator. Some may be candidates for a phrenic nerve stimulator if the nerve shows the ability to conduct an impulse. Generally, people with complete injuries at C4 and below do not use respirators, but respiratory complications may persist. Breathing may be shallow, and the ability to cough productively may be compromised. Various deep-breathing and assisted-coughing techniques may be taught, along with other procedures to keep the lungs clear. Prevention and early management of respiratory complications are crucial. Currently, respiratory complications are the most common cause of death following SCI (Brown, DiMarco, Hoit, & Garshick, 2006).

■ Autonomic Dysreflexia (Hyperreflexia)

As implied by its name, **autonomic dysreflexia**, or hyperreflexia, involves an exaggerated response of the autonomic nervous system (ANS). A function of the ANS is the integration of body functions in the "fight-or-flight" response—heart rate, blood vessel constriction/dilation, regulation of glands, and smooth muscle. Autonomic dysreflexia usually occurs in people with spinal cord injuries above the T6 level. Signs to look for include a sudden, pounding headache, diaphoresis, flushing, goose bumps, and tachycardia followed by bradycardia. These signs are caused by an irritation of nerves below the level of injury. Common sources of irritation include an overfull bladder or bowel, urinary tract infections (UTIs), or decubitus ulcers. Even irritations such as ingrown toenails can trigger the response. These irritations would be bothersome to a person with an intact spinal cord—he or she would feel uncomfortable and act to remedy the situation. But the person with an SCI lacks this feeling, and autonomic dysreflexia is the body's way of warning that something is wrong below the level of the injury.

The most important aspect of managing autonomic dysreflexia is to find the cause and alleviate it. This may require emptying the bladder, checking for obstructions in external urinary drainage tubing, assessing for bowel impaction, or evaluating for other factors. It helps to decrease blood pressure if the person assumes an upright position. Most people with tetraplegia will experience an episode of autonomic dysreflexia at least once, but if the signs of autonomic dysreflexia appear frequently, medication may be indicated. Autonomic dysreflexia may appear suddenly and must be managed promptly. Because the blood pressure may elevate dramatically, there is risk of stroke or death if the situation is ignored or mismanaged. Although autonomic dysreflexia may be more prevalent in the initial months following injury, it has the potential of being an ongoing complication, and people with SCI must be educated about symptoms and management (Russo-McCourt, 2009).

Postural Hypotension

In contrast to autonomic dysreflexia, blood pressure decreases in postural hypotension. This condition, often seen in people who have sustained cervical or thoracic SCIs, also may be referred to as orthostatic hypotension (Krassioukov, Warburton, Teasell, & Eng, 2009). Blood tends to pool distally in the lower extremities as a result of reduced muscle tone in the trunk and legs. The symptoms of postural hypotension frequently occur when a person attempts to sit up after prolonged periods of bed rest. Symptoms include light-headedness, dizziness, pallor, sudden weakness, and unresponsiveness. Preventive measures include the use of antiembolism hosiery and abdominal binders, which externally assist circulation. Also, assuming an upright position slowly can help avoid these symptoms. If symptoms do occur, a semireclined or reclined position should be maintained until the symptoms subside.

Deep Vein Thrombosis

Deep vein thrombosis (DVT) can be a serious complication in many types of medical conditions. It is a potential complication in SCI for three main reasons: reduced circulation caused by decreased tone, frequency of direct trauma to legs causing vascular damage (e.g., repeated trauma during transfer or bed mobility activities), and prolonged bed rest. Edema is often seen in SCI for the same reasons. Clinical signs of DVT may include swelling in the lower extremities, localized redness, and a low-grade fever. However, a DVT may be relatively asymptomatic on bedside evaluation. Vigilant medical screenings for DVT should be performed in all cases of SCI. An undetected and unmanaged DVT may result in an embolism and death. In people with SCI, it appears the greatest risk of DVT is seen within the initial 2 weeks postinjury (American Spinal Injury Association, 2008; Consortium for Spinal Cord Medicine, 2006).

Thermal Regulation

It has already been seen that damage to the spinal cord can disrupt the ANS, possibly resulting in autonomic dysreflexia. Thermal regulation is another function of the ANS that can be disturbed after SCI. Maintaining the appropriate body temperature is often a problem for people whose injuries are above T6. During the first year after injury, the body tends to assume the temperature of the external environment. This condition is called poikilothermia (Wood, Binks, & Grundy, 2002). In time, some adjustment usually occurs. Cold weather often causes discomfort, as blood vessels below the level of injury do not constrict sufficiently to conserve the body's heat. Conversely, excessive sweating may occur above the level of injury in warmer weather but not below, which hampers the body's efforts to prevent hyperthermia. Because of this, extreme temperatures should be avoided, and attention should be given to the extent and type of clothing worn in all conditions.

Musculoskeletal

Spasticity

In people who have UMN lesions, increased tone appears in muscles below the level of injury after spinal shock subsides. Virtually all individuals with cervical cord injuries experience spasms, and the percentage of those experiencing spasms gradually decreases as the level of the lesion descends along the spinal cord column—with flexors and extensors experiencing the majority of spasms (Christopher & Dana Reeve Foundation, 2015b). An increase in spasticity can be triggered by a variety of factors including infections, positioning, pressure sores, UTIs, and heightened emotional states. Spasms are not necessarily disadvantageous. The ability to trigger spasms can help some individuals maintain muscle bulk, circulation, bowel and bladder management, transfers, and other activities of daily living (ADL). Excessive spasticity, however, may result in contractures, pain, and a reduced ability to participate in activities. At this point, pharmacological or surgical options may be recommended.

Heterotopic Ossification (Ectopic Bone)

Heterotopic ossification (HO) refers to the abnormal formation of bone deposits on muscles, joints, and tendons. It occurs most often in the hip and knee and less frequently in the shoulder and elbow. It has been estimated that 20% of all people with SCI have some degree of ectopic bone growth (Cipriano, Pill, & Keenan, 2009). Clinical signs of HO may include heat, pain, swelling, and a decrease in active or passive ROM. These signs should always alert the clinician, as they may also indicate other serious complications such as a DVT. Many facilities that specialize in the care of people with SCI routinely provide prophylactic medications that have shown promise in halting this abnormal calcification. In extreme cases in which HO permanently and severely limits ROM, surgery may be indicated.

■ Genitourinary Complications

UTIs are a common and dangerous complication of SCI. Prior to modern medical management, many people with SCI who survived the initial trauma died within a few years after injury, with one of the most common causes being kidney failure as a result of chronic UTI. For several reasons, individuals with SCI are prone to UTI or bladder infections. The bladder is composed of smooth muscle, innervated by sacral segments of the spinal cord. As such, it is affected by a loss of sensory and motor function, as are other parts of the body, depending on the level and extent of injury. The nature of bladder function will depend on whether the injury caused LMN or UMN deficits (Fig. 24.10). An injury affecting the UMN bladder is also referred to as a reflex or spastic bladder. In this case, the bladder can contract and void reflexively. Although this action is involuntary, some people with SCI can trigger the reflex through various stimuli, much as the knee-jerk reflex being triggered by tapping with a reflex hammer. This is because impulses can still enter the cord below the level of injury, synapse, and exit.

People with a UMN bladder may use various types of catheters and additional techniques to ensure that the bladder does not become distended or retain urine. They generally cannot rely on sensation to alert them that the bladder has exceeded its normal capacity; rather, they must rely on an established voiding schedule.

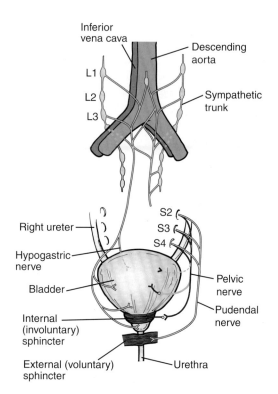

Figure 24.10 Bladder and corresponding spinal segment innervations. (From Rhoades, R. A., & Bell, D. R. (2012). *Medical physiology* (4th ed.). Philadelphia, PA: Lippincott Williams & Wilkins.)

An LMN bladder may also be referred to as a nonreflex or flaccid bladder. This type of bladder function is usually seen during the spinal shock phase and may remain if the injury has affected the cauda equina area. With an LMN bladder injury (Fig. 24.10), a reflexive emptying of the bladder cannot occur, as the reflex arc is destroyed. Because the bladder is flaccid and does not spontaneously empty, urine will accumulate continuously. People with an LMN bladder must catheterize according to a schedule or must apply external pressure to force urine from the bladder. The application of external pressure on the abdomen with their fists, starting at the umbilicus and pressing downward, is called **Credé's maneuver**. Another technique for generating force is called the Valsalva maneuver, which involves closing the glottis and contracting the abdominal muscles, as if resisting a forceful exhalation (Somers, 2010). Chronic use of Credé's maneuver may lead to multiple complications, including inguinal hernias, hemorrhoids, and vesicoureteral reflux (Chang, Hou, Dong,

& Zhang, 2000; Consortium for Spinal Cord Medicine, 2006; Somers, 2010).

With either type of bladder (UMN or LMN), voiding must occur routinely and completely. Chronic overstretching of the bladder will reduce its ability to empty adequately. Residual urine is a breeding ground for infections that can spread to all structures in the urinary system, including the ureters and kidneys. Chronic infections can lead to renal calculi (kidney stones), kidney failure, and, potentially, death. Warning signs of a UTI include urine that appears cloudy or has excessive particles, dark or foul-smelling urine, an elevated fever, chills, or an increase in spasticity. The best treatment of UTI is prevention—adhering to an effective voiding schedule, using clean or sterile techniques, maintaining a proper diet and adequate fluid intake, and prompt attention to warning signs.

■ Complications Associated with the Bowel

Normally, elimination occurs when stool is present in the rectum. Nerves in the rectal musculature are stimulated, triggering a reflexive **peristalsis**, which is a process of muscle contractions resulting in the movement of food through the digestive track and a relaxation of the rectal sphincters. A bowel movement may be prevented at this step of the process if the brain overrides this reflex, sending down an impulse to tighten the sphincter muscles until an appropriate time. We have all experienced the sensation of urgency caused by a full rectum, but perhaps we have not fully appreciated our brain's ability to allow us to forestall the process until a socially acceptable time.

Unfortunately, an SCI can interfere with bowel function in much the same way as it impedes the bladder. The bowel can become spastic or flaccid (Fig. 24.11). In this case, stool can be eliminated reflexively if nerves located in the rectum are stimulated. This stimulation may be done manually through digital stimulation or in conjunction with the use of suppositories. Establishing and following a regular schedule for bowel management can reduce occurrences of incontinence.

The bowel is usually flaccid during the phase of spinal shock and may remain in that state if the injury involves the areas illustrated at points B and C (Fig. 24.10). As with the flaccid bladder, the flaccid bowel cannot be stimulated to empty reflexively. Stool often remains in the rectum after attempts at evacuation, and it may be necessary to remove it manually to prevent impaction.

Constipation or impaction may result if elimination does not occur regularly. In addition to the general discomfort associated with this, autonomic dysreflexia may be triggered in people with lesions above the T6 level. Diarrhea is another complication that can be particularly frustrating for the person with an SCI who is trying to establish a set schedule for bowel management. This condition is always frustrating, but the majority of the general population have the benefit of intact sensation to provide a warning. The best strategies to prevent diarrhea for people with an SCI include making sure to use (not overuse) laxatives if they are prescribed, eating a proper diet, maintaining adequate hydration, and following a scheduled bowel program that reduces the chance of impaction, which can result in diarrhea.

■ Dermal Complications

The skin is the largest organ of the body, and it performs essential functions in maintaining health. Skin assists in thermal regulation, providing insulation in cold weather and sweating to prevent hyperthermia during hot conditions. Aside from literally keeping the body together, skin acts as a barrier to the external environment. At the cellular level, skin provides the site for O_2/CO_2 exchange through the capillary system. Keeping skin intact is essential and requires conscious effort by a person with an SCI, as sensations that would normally provide warning of potential skin damage, such as pain and extremes in temperature, are not perceived below the level of injury.

The story of our own modern-day Superman, Christopher Reeve, bears witness to the importance of skin integrity. What eventually took his life were not the leading causes of death for people with SCI such as renal failure, pneumonia, pulmonary emboli, or sepsis (NSCISC, 2009). What took the life of Superman was a pressure ulcer that became infected—ultimately resulting in organ failure.

Damage to the skin as a result of pressure sores, or **decubitus ulcers**, is a major reason for hospital admissions in SCI populations. The mechanism of injury is continued pressure due to lack of movement. Circulation is impaired because of the pressure, and capillary exchange is impeded. This can result rapidly in tissue

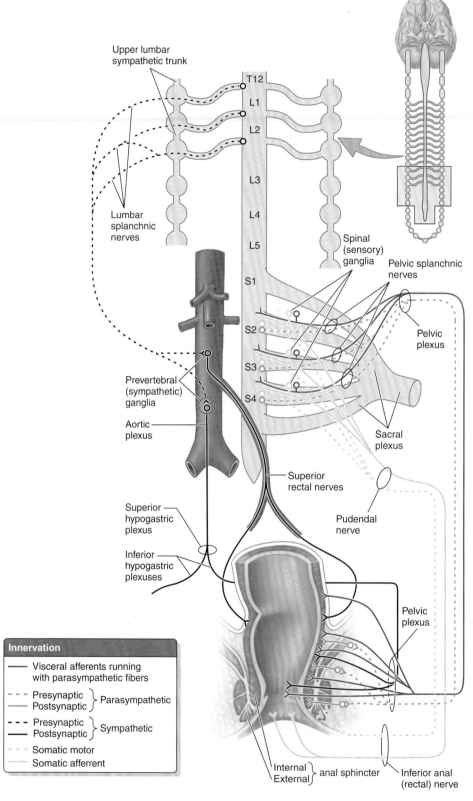

Figure 24.11 The bowel and corresponding spinal segment innervations. (From Moore, K. L., Agur, A. M., & Dalley, A. F. (2014). *Essential clinical anatomy* (5th ed.). Philadelphia, PA: Lippincott Williams & Wilkins.)

necrosis. The severity of pressure sores can be classified in four stages:

Stage I. Clinical signs are reddened or darkened skin. Damage is limited to more superficial (epidermal and dermal) layers. At this stage, merely removing pressure until the skin returns to its normal color can halt tissue breakdown.

Stage II. The skin now appears reddened and open. A blister or scab is present. The scab is not a sign of healing; rather, the tissue beneath it is necrotic. This involves the epidermal and dermal layers, as well as deeper adipose tissue. Wound dressings may be involved at this stage, and it is imperative that pressure be kept off the site.

Stage III. The skin breakdown is deeper, and the wound is now draining. Muscle may be visible through the open wound. An ulcer is developing in the necrotic tissue. In addition to wound dressings, surgical intervention may be indicated if more conservative treatment is unsuccessful.

Stage IV. All structures, from the superficial levels to the bone, are destroyed. Infection and bone decay occur. Surgical intervention is likely, and the person with a decubitus ulcer at this stage often must spend weeks after a skin graft with pressure totally removed from the involved site (Kroshinsky & Strazzula, 2015).

Pressure sores are preventable with diligent attention and preventative strategies. A person with SCI can use, or instruct another person to assist with, a variety of pressure relief methods. Also, visual skin inspections should be performed at least twice daily, taking particular note of areas most prone to breakdown. These would include areas where bony prominences (e.g., the sacrum, ischium, calcaneus, and scapula) can add to pressure. Proper nutrition also should be heeded, as healthy skin is less apt to break down and is more responsive to healing in early stages of pressure sore development.

Other dermal complications, such as burns or frostbite, are prevented by attentiveness and common sense. Even commonly encountered things, such as space heaters or exposed plumbing under a sink, can cause severe burns to people with an SCI without their immediate knowledge. It is important to be aware of the environment and to rely on other, intact senses to avoid injury.

■ Mental Health Challenges

Prevalent throughout the SCI literature is the high rate of depression in this population (Bombardier, Richards, Krause, Tulsky, & Tate, 2004), which, unaddressed, was found to be associated with greater incidence of pressure ulcers as well as decreased occupational performance (Fann et al., 2011). Depression significantly complicates daily living and is characterized by disinterest and feelings of worthlessness, fatigue, weight and appetite changes, and suicidal ideations (Kalpakjan, Bombardier, Schomer, Brown, & Johnson, 2009). The *Diagnostic and Statistical Manual of Mental Disorders, Fifth Edition* (DSM-5) is used to evaluate symptoms in regard to intensity and duration (APA, 2013). It is critical for occupational therapists to immediately refer patients with suspected depression to appropriate health care professionals and notify the treatment team accordingly.

MEDICAL/SURGICAL MANAGEMENT

Medical management of an SCI should begin immediately at the onset of injury. As typically injuries occur outside a hospital setting (roadways, lakes, sporting events), often first responders are not medical personnel. Any person with a suspected SCI should be immobilized with a backboard and neck brace before transport (Cooper, 2006). Diagnostic evaluation of the vertebral column and spinal cord must be completed to determine the next steps of intervention. Injuries may require surgical or nonsurgical intervention to decompress, realign, and stabilize the spine (Russo-McCourt, 2009). Surgical procedures such as laminectomies may be performed to remove the cause of pressure on the cord (such as a bony fragment or bullet) (Grundy et al., 2002). Spinal fusion may also be required to achieve stability. External alignment devices may be used following spinal surgery or may be sufficient substitutes for surgery (Wood et al., 2002). In thoracic injuries, a TLSO (thoracolumbosacral orthosis) or "clamshell" brace is often used. This device is a "total contact" molded 2-piece brace, applied to the anterior and posterior of an individual to limit trunk movement (University of California, San Francisco, 2015). Multiple devices also exist for external stabilization of cervical injuries. These orthoses typically restrict the chin and the posterior aspect of the skull, restricting cervical motion (Somers, 2010). Among the most restrictive cervical devices is the "halo" orthosis. This is composed of a metal ring affixed directly to the skull with screws (called "pins") at occipital and temporal points and steel bars mounted to a body vest (Somers, 2010). The determination of the need and/or type of orthosis required demands careful assessment of vertebral stability and the nature of movement the device is able to restrict.

Concurrent with spinal decompression, realignment, and stabilization, prompt pharmacologic management is vital (Russo-McCourt, 2009). In the most acute stages following injury, recent research headlines have reported that the use of steroids—specifically, methylprednisolone—may improve neurological outcomes of patients with SCI if administered within the first 8 hours after injury (Bracken, 2009). Additionally, select experimental drugs administered soon after injury, such as GM-1 ganglioside (Sygen) and 4AP, were hoped to aid in the preservation of damaged nerves and insulating them from the toxic level of chemicals the body releases during trauma and possibly reduce cell death (http://www.spinalcord.org/news). Study outcomes to date relating to the benefit of these drugs are mixed, and some concerns have been raised about potential adverse effects versus limited functional gains with some of these protocols. Another very recent acute experimental intervention that has been tried to mitigate spinal cord damage and hopefully improve outcomes is "therapeutic hypothermia." This process involves lowering the core body temperature to discourage spinal cord edema and reduce metabolic demands soon after injury occurs (Cappuccino, 2008). While this technique has been used historically for other diagnoses, its consideration in the management of SCI is relatively new. Perhaps the first introduction to this technique for many was during the 2007 National Football League season opening game, when millions watched live as Buffalo Bills' tight end Kevin Everett was involved in helmet-to-helmet contact that resulted in a cervical SCI. The team's orthopedic surgeon administered almost-immediate hypothermic intervention. The technique, which Everett has credited with his positive outcomes, was described for days in the media (Higgins, 2007). Certainly, significant additional research needs to be conducted in all aspects of the very acute management of SCI,

but improved initial treatments hold promise for better long-term outcomes.

On other fronts, while fetal stem cell research relating to spinal cord regeneration is prevalent in the news, meaningful functional outcomes have been limited. However, newer research related to stem cells found in a living donor's brain, spinal cord, or other structures may hold greater promise and potentially avoid problems of cell rejection found with fetal stem cells (NINDS, 2015). Headlines were made in the recent past regarding the treatment of spinal cord injuries with the use of stem cells from umbilical blood. This process reportedly resulted in a South Korean woman who had been paralyzed for 20 years being able to perform some level of ambulation with assistance (Gallagher, 2004.). Autologous (self-donated) bone marrow stem cell transplants have also been shown in select reported case studies to result in functional gains and quality of life improvements in spinal cord–injured recipients (Geffner, Santacruz, Izuretta, 2008). Additional research is being aimed at a variety of strategies, including pharmacologic and enzyme therapy, cloning of nerve cells, and the highly sophisticated altering of the cellular environment to encourage actual regeneration. As stated earlier, the spinal cord is typically intact above and below the level of injury; one goal of current research is to encourage functional reconnection of the disrupted pathways. A different picture is presented with cauda equina injuries or injuries involving the nerve root. These types of injuries carry the potential for regeneration if the nerve roots are not severely damaged or divided. The degree of regeneration that can be expected is very difficult to predict and should be addressed on an individual basis after extensive medical testing.

Aside from research on actual spinal cord cell replacement and regeneration, significant work is also being done with highly technical devices to compensate for paralysis. Retraining CNS circuits includes treatments such as epidural stimulation (ES), functional electric stimulation (FES), robotic-assisted therapy, and brain-computer interfaces (BCI) (NINDS, 2015). Epidural stimulation was used on a man with paralysis from an SCI along with intensive physical therapy. After 2 years of locomotor training, electrodes were surgically implanted over the paralyzed area thereby simulating the brain's signals to the spinal cord. Although locomotor training without ES is common practice in rehabilitation, inclusion of ES has the ability to relieve pain during training. This individuals' success provides hope for further investigations on how ES can help regain function in people with SCI paralysis (NINDS, 2015). People with UMN injuries have experienced increases in their functional abilities (improved ability to productively cough, upper extremity function, standing ability, ambulation) with the external application of electrodes that stimulate muscle contraction through FES. Although some may feel that the FES apparatus is cumbersome, unsightly, time consuming, and difficult to apply, refinements are ongoing. Many people with SCI feel that, although not ideal, the technology provides an appealing alternative to outcomes from traditional methods of rehabilitation. Another technological development is the use of neuro-prosthetic devices, which are surgically implanted FES systems. One device, the Freehand System, combines internal electrodes, stimulators, sensors, and transmission coils within an external control box. It allows a person with tetraplegia to achieve a degree of functional prehension, enhancing such ADL as eating, writing, and phone and computer use. Select studies have shown gains in the functional performance of individuals with C5 to C6 tetraplegia utilizing this system (Taylor, Esnouf, & Hobby, 2002). Research on robotic-assisted therapy is being used in various ways for people with incomplete SCI—to investigate assisted movement and enhanced sensation (AMES) technology by rotating the ankle and moving the leg, as well as through determining the effectiveness of body weight–supported treadmill training using a robotic gait trainer. Both areas of research are novel within the field of SCI recovery (NINDS, 2015). Finally, BCI technology has the ability to bypass damaged nerve circuits within the spinal cord, thereby providing a link from the brain to an assistive implanted device in order to restore paralyzed muscles with voluntary muscle control and coordination (NINDS, 2015). Electrodes are placed in the brain and through practice in directing their thoughts, patients can generate neural signals interpreted by the computer and translated into movement. This is currently being researched on people with UE paralysis as well as people with tetraplegia (NINDS, 2015). Overall, although actual regeneration of the cord may not be on the immediate scientific horizon, the advances in all phases of SCI management

are promising. Everyone has the right to hope for what is not yet reality, without being said to have unrealistic expectations. Assisting someone to be hopeful, while simultaneously working to maximize today's function, is to truly master the art of the therapeutic relationship.

IMPACT ON OCCUPATIONAL PERFORMANCE

Performance in areas of occupation relates to a person's ability to engage in or direct caregivers on activities that are essential and meaningful. Performance in areas of occupation includes ADL, instrumental activities of daily living (IADL), education, work, play, leisure, and social participation. Occupational performance for a person with an SCI can also include directing caregivers on how to assist with these fundamental aspects of their daily living (AOTA, 2014). Clearly, an SCI can have a catastrophic effect on a person's ability to function in these areas, because it can affect body function categories that support the ability to participate in these activities. Body function categories that may be impacted by an SCI include sensory functions and pain, voice and speech functions, functions of cardiovascular and respiratory systems, genitourinary and reproductive functions, neuromusculoskeletal and movement-related functions, functions of the skin and related structures, and select mental functions. The importance of understanding the theory of occupational performance cannot be overstated. We cannot begin to holistically treat a person with SCI until we can visualize the impact that this diagnosis has on the various aspects of that person's life. The following sections explore occupational performance areas and components to present a comprehensive view of the impact of SCI. Table 24.4 shows generally expected functional outcomes at various levels of complete injuries.

■ Instrumental Activities of Daily Living

Grooming, Oral Hygiene, Eating, Bathing, Dressing

For a person with tetraplegia, grooming, oral hygiene, and eating may be extremely laborious. The use of extensive adaptive devices or reliance on a caregiver may be necessary because

TABLE 24.4	Expected Functional Outcomes of Various Levels of Complete Injury (Noninclusive)
Last Spinal Cord Level Intact (Spared)	**Expected Functional Outcome**
C1–C3	Requires 24-h availability of caregiver
	Generally ventilator dependent; some individuals at C3 may be successfully weaned from a ventilator.
	Requires maximal assistance of another for pressure relief or requires an adapted switch and reclining chair
	May propel power chair independently with adapted switches (pneumatic, chin, head, mouthstick); requires maximal setup
	Maximal assistance needed for transfers, positioning, bed mobility, dressing, feeding, hygiene, grooming, and bowel/bladder care
	Dependent with driving
C4	Requires 24-h availability of caregiver
	Generally able to be weaned from ventilator; continued difficulty with productive coughing and deep breathing
	Pressure relief, wheelchair propulsion, transfers, bed mobility, dressing, hygiene, bowel/bladder care, and driving status comparable to C1–C3 level
	Adaptive feeding and grooming devices are available with set-up, although these tasks are very time-consuming and exhaustive for a person at this level and generally do not result in task independence
C5	May require 24-h availability of caregiver
	Decreased respiratory endurance, but not using ventilator
	A strong person with a C5 injury may be independent in pressure relief by leaning side to side; a weaker person may require maximal assistance.
	Independent on level surfaces with a power chair and occasionally wrist/forearm supports; a manual wheelchair with rim adaptations may be used by a strong person for short distances but is typically not a reasonable mobility strategy.
	Moderate to maximal assistance is required for all transfers, and generally, a sliding board or mechanical lift is used.
	Moderate assistance is required for bed mobility.
	A strong person with a C5 injury may assist with some dressing, hygiene, and grooming activities with the aid of adapted equipment. Feeding is generally possible with the use of adapted utensils and setup.
	Driving is feasible at this level (in the absence of additional complications such as extensive upper extremity tone/contractures); a person may be able to drive with specially adapted steering, braking, and acceleration hand controls and, due to transfer limitations, would drive directly from the wheelchair.

TABLE 24.4 *Continued*

Last Spinal Cord Level Intact (Spared)	Expected Functional Outcome
C6	Amount of assistance needed from another person varies from moderate to minimal with just a few specific activities.
	Some decreases in respiratory capacity and productive cough
	Has potential for independence in pressure relief
	Independently uses a manual wheelchair on level surfaces and gradual inclines; rim adaptations improve propulsion abilities. Generally requires a power wheelchair for long distances or rough terrain
	Ability to transfer varies. Some strong people with C6 injuries are able to transfer independently with the use of a sliding board to a car, chair, bed, commode, or tub seat.
	Has the potential for independent bed mobility and positioning with rails, power controls, and trapeze
	With some adapted devices, usually independent with hygiene, shaving, and grooming. Potential for independence in bathing and bowel/bladder care with equipment. Generally independent with upper extremity (UE) dressing, and potential for independence in lower extremity (LE) dressing with adaptive devices, although often, the latter is quite time consuming. Independent with feeding, although a wrist-hand orthosis (WHO) and setup may be required
	Generally able to drive independently using hand controls and adaptive devices; if transfers are challenging/inconsistent, driving directly from the wheelchair is indicated.
C7–C8	May be able to live independently without attendant care, although assistance required for high/low/heavy tasks
	Some decreased respiratory endurance
	Independent in pressure relief
	Independently uses manual wheelchair
	Generally able to transfer without a sliding board, depending on the surface characteristics
	Generally independent with positioning, bed mobility, hygiene, feeding, shaving, hair care, dressing, bathing, cooking, and light housekeeping. Generally independent with bowel/bladder care using adaptive equipment/techniques
	Drives independently with hand controls/steering adaptations
	Generally able to stand in parallel bars once assisted to upright position, with the use of a knee-ankle-foot orthosis (KAFO)
T1–T3	Can live independently, although assistance required for high/low/heavy tasks
	Respiratory capacity and coughing abilities significantly improved compared to previous levels
	All transfers generally independent unless other complicating factors (e.g., excessive tone challenges, contractures, shoulder dysfunction)

TABLE 24.4 *Continued*

Last Spinal Cord Level Intact (Spared)	Expected Functional Outcome
	Independent with all self-care
	Finger dexterity, strength, and coordination are functional.
	Drives independently with hand controls. Typically able to stow certain types of manual wheelchairs in a car but may be excessively time-consuming/energy-depleting/adversely impacting shoulders, and as such, a van may be indicated.
	Able to stand with minimal assistance, KAFO, and use of walker or parallel bars. Ambulation is generally not practical because of reduced trunk control/balance and high-energy expenditure.
T4–T8	Can live independently, although assistance required for high/low/heavy tasks
	Respiratory status stronger than T1–T3 level; only slightly decreased. Pressure relief, wheelchair use, positioning, bad mobility, and self-care all independent
	Driving: comparable to T1–T3 level
	May have potential to ambulate short distances with the use of a walker or Lofstrand crutches and KAFO on level surfaces only; however, even if able, high-energy output is required, and wheelchair use remains predominant form of mobility.
T9–T12	Respiration is functional.
	Pressure relief, wheelchair use, transfers, positioning, bad mobility, self-care, and homemaking (except heavy tasks) all independent
	Able to drive with hand controls
	Generally able to ambulate with KAFO and Lofstrand crutches as noted above, with somewhat less energy demands; wheelchair use remains predominant form of mobility.
L1–L3	Same as T9–T12 level with the addition of improved ambulation distances; a wheelchair is often required for long distances.
L4–L5	Same as above, with exceptions: Driving may be independent without adaptive devices; strength of ankle dorsiflexion and tone must be assessed. Generally able to ambulate with ankle-foot orthosis (AFO) and canes. Wheelchairs generally not needed for household ambulation but may be indicated for longer distances
S1–S2	A person with an S2-spared injury has the potential to ambulate without devices or orthoses.
	A wheelchair is generally not required. Hip extensors/abductors, knee flexors, and ankle plantar flexors are weak at the S1 level of injury. As with all other preceding levels, bowel and bladder functions are impaired but managed independently at the level through adapted devices/ techniques.

Developed with material from the Rehabilitation Institute of Michigan, 1996.

of deficits in sensory and neuromuscular performance components. People with paraplegia are generally independent in these tasks, but they must often think ahead, making sure that items are available and sufficient time is allocated. Bathing and dressing specifically present major challenges for people with quadriplegia. With higher-level injuries (C1 through C4), total assistance is required. At lower levels of injury, with varying amounts of adaptive equipment and assistance from others in some task components, the person with quadriplegia can be a more active participant. It is extremely important, however, for the person's own goals and contexts to be acknowledged. For example, if an individual with a complete C6 requires 60 minutes to dress with the use of adaptations, the question becomes, "Is this functional?" If a person is attempting reentry into the work force or return to school, is it "functional" to spend an entire hour, as well as all the physical energy, in just getting dressed? Or is it a sign of greater autonomy to delegate some tasks to a caregiver to allow participation in activities that are more meaningful?

Secondary conditions aside, individuals with paraplegia are usually independent in bathing and dressing. Some even have the strength to transfer to the bottom of a tub without assistive devices.

Toileting

Managing altered bowel and bladder function are challenges for virtually everyone with SCI. The two aspects to this challenge are the actual physiologic management and the various techniques and equipment used in the toileting process.

Medications may be required for physiologic management. Stool softeners are used, as well as suppositories, to assist in evacuation. A goal of effective bowel management is to eliminate or reduce reliance on medications. For people with injuries at C7 or below, independence in toileting can usually be achieved with an array of equipment that may include suppository inserters, digital stimulators (devices that trigger reflexes to relax the rectal sphincter in UMN injuries), catheterization devices, leg separators, mirrors, and adapted commode chairs that allow access to the perianal area for bowel-training procedures.

Aside from medications and equipment, additional strategies include maintaining a specific schedule for elimination, eating a healthy diet that promotes regularity, assuming positions

that facilitate elimination, and the use of Credé's method. If toileting appears to be tiring, then it has been portrayed correctly! But many people with SCI become adept at its management. It may be a very different picture, though, when a person attempts these procedures in a community environment (i.e., restrooms at work or school), due to accessibility, availability of equipment, and time limitations. In order to promote greater freedom and independence, some individuals opt to explore alternatives—such as undergoing surgical urinary diversion. Surgeries such as the Mitrofanoff procedure create a permanent stoma in the abdomen, which can allow an individual to catheterize through their navel. This presents benefits of easier anatomical access and significantly less adjustment of clothing versus traditional catheterizing. While not every individual is a candidate—and the procedure is certainly not without risk and potential long-term complication—studies have revealed that many who undertake it have been highly satisfied with the degree of freedom and independence it has allowed them (Merenda, Duffy, & Betz, 2007).

The person with a higher-level cervical injury faces greater challenges. Although the bowel and bladder management concepts are the same, neuromuscular deficits limit performance of the tasks, even with adaptive equipment. Generally, people with injuries above the C6 level require a caregiver to assist with or perform functions such as transfers to adaptive commode chairs, suppository insertion, digital stimulation, catheterization, and general perianal care. The person with an SCI must indicate who the caregiver will be, particularly for tasks that are socially sensitive. Even though family members may be willing to assist, it is perfectly justifiable for the person to request someone else as a caregiver. Some people may have no reservations about who assists them, whereas others may feel strongly that it would negatively affect established roles. Whatever the case, whenever feasible, the preferences of the person with an SCI should be the deciding factor in selecting caregivers for various tasks.

■ Personal Device Care

The extent of personal and adaptive devices required by an individual with an SCI can generally be predicted by the level of injury (Table 24.4). Additional complications, such as reduced ROM resulting from contractures, may require use of more extensive devices than are typically seen at a particular level. Usually, personal device care is performed by others for those with injuries at C4 and above. Those with injuries at the C5 level and below have progressively more ability to assist in personal device care and use, but this fluctuates greatly depending on the individual's endurance, motivation, resources, and priorities.

Health Maintenance

Fostering a healthy lifestyle is critical, but often challenging, after an SCI. Most people with an SCI are advised to follow lifelong exercise programs to preserve and enhance ROM and strength, as well as to promote good cardiovascular fitness and weight management. Many individuals report weight gains in the months after injury, as their energy demands are greatly altered in great part by use of a wheelchair for mobility. Attention also must be given to proper nutrition for weight management, impact on skin integrity, and bowel and bladder management. As mentioned earlier, routine attention to skin condition is crucial to avoiding dermal complications. A health maintenance routine may require the assistance of others, depending on the level of injury, for such activities as setting up weights and equipment, performing passive ROM, pressure relief, and aiding in skin inspection.

Socialization, Functional Communication, and Emergency Response

With a singular diagnosis of SCI, no cognitive deficits are inherent that would preclude a person from socializing in an appropriate contextual manner. What is challenging, though, are the variety of barriers that may inhibit socialization. Architectural, environmental, and transportation barriers; reduced endurance; and increased reliance on others may discourage or actually prevent someone from traveling to the places where they socialized before their injury. Psychological barriers also may prevent reintegration into a premorbid social support system, and these "barriers" are as real as physical ones.

In all but the highest of injuries, verbal communication is functional. People with injuries at C7 or below are generally independent with a variety of forms of communication (e.g., writing, keyboard use, phone use) without the use of adaptive equipment. Above this level, however, adaptive devices are progressively required.

The need to request assistance in emergencies is possible at virtually all levels of injury, depending on the environment and adaptive equipment available. For people with higher-level injuries, adaptive phone devices, emergency call systems, and environmental control units make contact with emergency agencies feasible. At the level of C4 and above, however, the availability of a caregiver 24 hours a day remains the most appropriate safety option. Individuals with injuries below this level may use a phone independently with possible adaptations but may be limited in other emergency responses, such as exiting a dwelling or attending to the physical needs of another injured person.

Functional Mobility

People with complete injuries at the thoracic levels of injury and above usually rely on wheelchairs for household and community mobility. Those with injuries at C6 or above may require additional assistance in manual wheelchair management; they may utilize a manual wheelchair with power-assist wheels, or a power wheelchair. Individuals with higher-level quadriplegia may use adapted orthotic devices to aid in controlling a power wheelchair, or alternative interfaces such as "puff and sip" or chin controls to maneuver the wheelchair in the absence of sufficient upper extremity function. Even at lower levels of injury, while an individual may be able to navigate a manual wheelchair under certain conditions, power wheelchairs may be considered due to community access needs (e.g., the need to navigate a large college campus routinely). A person with a lower level thoracic injury may be able to ambulate short distances with an ambulation device such as a walker or Lofstrand (forearm) crutch and lower extremity orthotic devices; however, the practicality of this in household and community settings must be evaluated. It is important to consider the need to avoid repetitive motion disorders in the upper extremities, which can become problematic if overused during ambulation activities. People with sacral injuries often can ambulate community distances without orthoses or devices.

Sometimes it is not so much the ability or inability of the person with an SCI but the inaccessibility of the environment that limits functional mobility. Whereas the home environment can be modified through creative thought, planning, and finances, the community environment is much harder to change. Although the Americans with Disabilities Act celebrated its 20th anniversary of enactment on July 26, 2010, most would agree that compliance with and enforcement of barrier-free environments are less than ideal. Many physically challenged people continue to fight discriminatory situations (e.g., inaccessible public transportation, restaurants, offices, classrooms). Ed Roberts, founder of the first Center for Independent Living, recalled a lighter side of the inaccessibility issue. He reminisced that early protestors in the disability rights movement were released from police custody because jail cells were inaccessible! (Price, 1990) In the vast majority of situations, however, an inaccessible environment is frustrating, demeaning, and personally violating. The health care team can do its part by helping physically, emotionally, or cognitively challenged people to be aware of their rights, as well as by providing them with information on advocacy groups.

Functional mobility includes driving as a consideration for many. A C5-injured person may be able to drive with specially adapted low-effort steering, braking, and acceleration hand controls. Usually, those with complete injuries above the C5 level cannot drive because of physical and respiratory limitations. People with C6 injuries and below may be able to drive independently using hand controls and adaptive steering devices. A van with a power lift or ramp may be recommended for someone who has difficulty transferring from his or her wheelchair or independently stowing the wheelchair in a vehicle. Often, finances more than need may dictate the type of transportation used, and clinicians can be invaluable in helping clients identify what financial and community resources may be available to help them meet their mobility needs.

■ Sexual Expression

As with bowel and bladder function, most people with SCI experience alterations in their ability to perform sexually as compared with their premorbid status. The nerves that innervate the genital area (both motor and sensory components) originate at the sacral spinal cord levels, so in the great majority of SCI cases, sexual function is affected.

For the most part, a person can participate in a variety of sexual activities despite SCI, although the level of sensation and motor response will vary, depending on the extent and level of injury. Specialists may recommend medications, surgical implants, and sexual enhancement devices, but this is highly individualized.

Advances in the field of fertility have improved the chances for a spinal cord–injured male to father a child. Although fertility rates for men with SCI are estimated at <10%, techniques such as electrostimulation to induce ejaculation in paraplegics have proven successful in many cases (Christopher & Dana Reeve Foundation, 2015a). Men may be well advised to delay a decision about surgical penile implants until at least 1 year after injury. This allows time to evaluate the full impact of the SCI on sexual function and to determine the extent, if any, of sensory or motor return in an incomplete injury. The reproductive capabilities of women are generally unaltered by an SCI, and women and their partners should be made aware that the potential for pregnancy exists (Spinal Outreach Team, 2014).

Addressing sexual function should be an integral part of each person's treatment plan, but a distinction should be made between purely physiological sexual performance—arousal, orgasm, and ejaculation—and sexuality, which is the totality of a person's attractiveness, personality, and self-perception as a sexual being. Sexuality does not have to rely on physiology. Whereas performance may be hampered as a result of an SCI, one's sexuality can be quite healthy and intact. The health care provider must make accurate information available and identify sources of more detailed information or expertise. It is entirely at the discretion of the person with an SCI to explore, or not explore, options available to them.

■ Home Maintenance

Tasks such as household maintenance, meal preparation, shopping, cleaning, clothing care, and safety procedures are included within the general category of home maintenance. Usually, people with a C6-level injury or above require assistance with all of these activities and need some personal attendant care. People with injuries at C7 or lower can often live independently (without attendant care) as they are able to perform their basic ADL tasks in accessible environments. However, they typically require assistance with heavier home maintenance tasks or activities requiring access to high or low areas.

■ Care of Others

An SCI can certainly make caring for others difficult, particularly if the injured person had been the primary caregiver for a child, spouse, or parent. Although a major goal of those with SCI is mastering personal self-care, a concurrent goal may be the introduction of activities (e.g., diapering, bathing a child) that can allow them to assume some premorbid roles. Often, many of these previous responsibilities must be delegated to others. In these cases, it is ideal if the person with SCI retains the responsibility for the verbal direction of care.

■ Education

People with SCI can generally resume educational activities, even while still inpatients in rehabilitation facilities. Many specialty hospitals retain the services of teachers from local school districts—or encourage the involvement of a student's premorbid teachers—and educational instruction is often scheduled along with other therapies for elementary, secondary, and high school students, encouraging smoother reintegration after discharge. The length of hospital admission following an SCI has decreased dramatically in the nearly three decades since more reliable statistics have been available; currently, the average length of combined acute/inpatient rehabilitation hospitalization following an SCI is 49 days (http://fscip.org//facts.htm). Certainly, a variety of factors can impact the length of hospitalization (e.g., level of injury, secondary diagnoses, complications, availability of specialty hospital resources), but the overall trend toward reduced inpatient hospitalization allows for individuals to reintegrate back into their premorbid roles and support systems much more rapidly than in the past. There are certainly advantages—but some inherent concerns—for children and adolescents returning more quickly to their previous school environments after the significant life changes brought on by an SCI. The ongoing support of the health care team can be critical in promoting successful reintegration.

College students would most likely be able to resume their studies following an SCI. Depending on their level of injury, however, people may reevaluate their course of study to prepare for a more feasible career.

Adaptive writing devices, page turners, recording devices, and computers have made returning to the classroom less intimidating. Laws have also improved the accessibility of public buildings. It is challenging, though, for a student with an SCI to manage bowel and bladder schedules, adjustment of clothing, eating devices, and so forth, but with planning and the assistance of others if needed, many individuals have successfully returned to the classroom.

■ Vocational

It is appropriate for a person with any level of SCI to begin to formulate vocational options, even as an inpatient, with the members of the health care team. Individual situations are so variable—premorbid occupation, level of injury, educational level, other vocational interests, family support, cognitive abilities, motivation, financial resources—making it impossible to say whether a person with a certain level of SCI can or cannot be gainfully employed. However, legislation mandates that work sites be accessible within reason. Also, many employers recognize the importance of a trained employee and will make additional accommodations to return a valued person to the workplace.

As we move from an industrial to an information society, the job market will continue to change, with positions requiring less physical labor than in the past. Job requirements will increasingly demand analytical thought, problem solving, and creativity, all of which are certainly intact after an SCI!

■ Leisure Activities

For most people, leisure pursuits are an integral part of a meaningful life. Although an SCI can alter the way in which one participates in leisure activities, it does not have to change the intensity of participation.

Sports, both individual and team, are excellent leisure pursuits that are growing in popularity for people with SCI. Virtually any sport can be undertaken, from basketball to tennis to archery. Adaptive equipment and modified regulations help make some sports more feasible for people with an SCI, and these modifications should not be viewed as detracting from the competitiveness of the sport. Consider that athletes in the general population use "adaptive" equipment all the time. How long would a catcher last in a baseball game without a mitt or a mask? Adaptive equipment need not detract from the legitimacy of the contest. It is heartening to see that, even internationally, the wheelchair athlete is recognized for excellence, with designated events in the Olympic games. People with an SCI who want to participate have numerous avenues open to them.

Aside from sports, opportunities for social activities from square dancing to traveling abound. Travel agencies and tour groups have recognized the market created by the wheelchair traveler and have responded. Most hospitals with specialized SCI rehabilitation units have well-established programs that help people get involved with special interest groups. Often, during the acute phase of SCI, people

cannot envision themselves participating again in the things they enjoy. The health care professional must be available for these individuals to encourage renewed interest in favorite leisure activities.

Several resources related to leisure activities, as well as other issues, have been discussed in this chapter. The reader is encouraged to consult the references and suggested readings at the end of this chapter for more information. Additionally, Table 24.4 gives an overview of specific expected outcomes for each level of SCI.

CASE STUDY

M.L. is a 24-year-old woman who sustained an SCI during a motor vehicle accident while on her honeymoon. Her husband was thrown from the vehicle but received only minor injuries. M.L. was transported by emergency medical services (EMS) to the local emergency department. She was diagnosed with a C5 through C6 vertebral subluxation and a C6 crush injury, resulting in a complete (ASIA-A) C6 SCI. She also sustained a left clavicular fracture. She received nasal O_2 for respiratory support. Once stabilized, she was transferred to the specialized trauma center near her home. A halo vest was applied, which stabilized her cervical spine. No operative procedures were indicated at that time. After 22 days, her endurance improved so that she could tolerate sitting upright in a chair for up to 1 hour. She was transferred to the nearby rehabilitation facility's SCI unit. During her 12 weeks there, the only complications she experienced were two episodes of autonomic hyperreflexia (apparently secondary to hard stool in the lower rectum) and a mild UTI. Spasticity developed in her wrists, elbows, and lower extremities.

Before her injury, M.L. was a recently graduated college student with a liberal arts degree. She and her new husband had recently signed a 1-year lease on an upstairs apartment close to the university, as she was anticipating pursuing graduate studies. She had been totally independent in all of her ADL and home management activities. Her leisure pursuits included recreational team sports (particularly softball) and more sedentary activities like reading and gourmet cooking. She was also involved with her family, particularly two sisters and her parents, who live close by.

Many body functions are significantly affected by M.L.'s injury. Her sensorimotor deficits are

consistent with those anticipated for a C6 complete quadriplegia. M.L. is challenged by the psychosocial/psychological issues facing her as a result of her SCI. She feels that her role has changed significantly, especially in her relationship with her husband. He has been willing to assist her in those activities in which she is physically limited; however, his assistance in some activities—particularly bowel management—has been difficult for her to accept. This has been a source of frustration for her, and she has discussed with him the possibility of hiring an attendant on a limited basis to assist with specific activities. He resists this idea, stating that it is his desire and duty to care for her. He took a temporary leave of absence from the family-owned landscaping company where he is employed when she was discharged 2 weeks ago. There is no definite timetable for his return. M.L. also is concerned about her ability to express herself sexually, as well as her potential to have children in the future. She attended classroom sessions on these topics in the rehabilitation facility, but she did not seek any individual counseling. M.L. states that she probably wasn't ready to hear anything specific then, but she now wishes she had someone to whom she could ask questions.

M.L. has not begun to consider her work activities or return to school. Even before her accident, she had been undecided about a career path. She has expressed interest, however, in exploring possible alternatives.

M.L. has stated that eventually, she might like to get involved in team sports again. In the 2 weeks since her discharge, though, her main leisure pursuits have been reading and watching television.

H. B. is a 6-year-old boy who sustained an incomplete (Brown-Séquard's) SCI, as the result of being struck by a stray bullet during a drive-by shooting in early August. He did not lose consciousness during transport to the emergency department. It was determined radiologically that the bullet, which entered from the right near the base of his neck/upper back, was lodged in the C7/C8 cervical spinal canal, and surgery was performed to remove the bullet soon after admission. H.B. is now 2 weeks postinjury and exhibits a loss of voluntary movement, reduced touch, and proprioceptive sensation on the right below the level of C7. He exhibits reduced pain, thermal, and some reduction in touch awareness on the left below the level of C7. The levels of C7 and above appear intact for both motor and sensory function. H.B. has had an uncomplicated hospital admission at this time. It is anticipated that he will remain in the acute children's specialty hospital for at least another 2 weeks and then transfer to the inpatient pediatric rehabilitation unit.

At the time of his injury, H.B. was living with his maternal grandmother, who is also his legal guardian. H.B. had been cocaine positive at birth, and his biological mother had relinquished her parental rights shortly after he was born. H.B.'s biological father is unknown. H.B.'s grandmother is also caring for another of H.B.'s siblings, an 8-year-old sister. H.B.'s grandmother reports that prior to his injury, he did not appear to have any overt behavioral/cognitive challenges and had successfully completed kindergarten. She related that he was a "normal, active boy" and enjoyed playing any type of outdoor games, as well as watching television. She states he did not have much exposure to computers or video games, as the family did not own these items. She states he had been looking forward to starting first grade, which is scheduled to begin in his district next week.

H.B. has been very cooperative with all of the health care providers working with him; he appears to enjoy the attention he is receiving from the staff, as well as the visitors from the neighborhood, his grandmother's church, and police department. His grandmother has expressed many concerns to the health care professionals working with H.B. Her overriding concern is fear that she will be unable to provide sufficient care—both from a physical and financial perspective—for H.B. following his inpatient rehabilitation stay. She related that the family residence is an older, rented duplex, with seven steps leading up to the front porch. She stated the interior of the residence is not conducive to any type of mobility devices, as the hallways and doorways are narrow, and all the bedrooms are on the second story of the unit. She also states concern about how he will be treated when he eventually starts school; although his older sister is in the same elementary school, H.B.'s grandmother states she has had very limited contact with teachers/administrators at the school and has no idea what resources are available to help him. She expressed frustration that H.B.'s shooter has not been apprehended and shared feelings of hopelessness and helplessness in her ability to protect H.B. and his sister from harm in the future.

RECOMMENDED LEARNING RESOURCES

Readings

Americans with Disabilities Act. Retrieved from http://www.ada.gov

Blackwell, T. L. (2001). *Spinal cord injury desk reference: Guidelines for life care planning and case management.* New York, NY: Demos Medical Pub.

Fehlings, M. G., Vaccaro, A. R., Boakye, M., Rossignol, S., Ditunno, J. F., & Burns, A. S. (2013).

Essentials of spinal cord injury: Basic research to clinical practice. New York, NY: Thieme Medical Publishers.

Field-Fote, E. C. (2009). *Spinal cord injury rehabilitation.* Philadelphia, PA: F.A. Davis Co.

Hall, M. (2012). *Across the street from hell: My spinal cord injury recovery.* Mark Anthony Hall.

Kirshblum, S., & Waring, W., III. (2014). Updates for the international standards for neurological classification of spinal cord injury. *Physical Medicine & Rehabilitation Clinics of North America*, *25*(3), 505–517, vii. doi: 10.1016/j.pmr.2014.04.001

Mayo Clinic. (2009). *Mayo clinic guide to living with a spinal cord injury*. New York, NY: Demos Health.

National Institute of Neurological Disorders and Stroke. Retrieved from http://www.ninds.nih.gov/

Ngonyani, J. B. (2008). *Living with spinal cord injury disability*. Dar es Salaam, Tanzania: Peramiho Printing Press.

Ozer, M. N. (1988). *The management of people with spinal cord injury*. New York, NY: Demos Publications.

Palmer, S., Kriegsman, K. H., & Palmer, J. B. (2008). *A guide for living: Spinal cord injury* (2nd ed.). Baltimore, MD: The Johns Hopkins University Press.

Pennsylvania Bar Institute. (2015). *The catastrophic injury case: Quadriplegia, paraplegia & spinal injury cases*. Mechanicsburg, PA: Pennsylvania Bar Institute.

Selzer, M. E., & Dobkin, B. H. (2008). *Spinal cord injury*. New York, NY: Demos Medical Pub.; AAN Press, American Academy of Neurology.

Senelick, R. C., & Dougherty, K. (1998). *The spinal cord injury handbook for patients and their families*. Birmingham, AL: HealthSouth Press.

Simonds, A. K. (2007). *Non-invasive respiratory support: a practical handbook* (3rd ed.). London, UK: Hodder Arnold.

Somers, M. F. (2010). *Spinal cord injury: Functional rehabilitation* (3rd ed.). Upper Saddle River, NJ: Pearson.

Sutton, A. L. (2011). *Disabilities sourcebook: Basic consumer health information about disabilities that affect the body, mind, and senses* (2nd ed.). Detroit, MI: Omnigraphics.

Tabak, H. (2005). *No whining. Craig hospital spinal injury rehab: Reaching new heights*. Lincoln, NE: iUniverse Inc.

Patient/Family Resources

Alpert, M. J., & Wisnia, S. (2008). *Spinal cord injury and the family: A new guide*. Cambridge, MA: Harvard University Press; Christopher & Dana Reeve Foundation. Retrieved from http://www.christopherreeve.org/site/c.ddJFKRNoFiG/b.4048063/k.67BA/The_Christopher_amp_Dana_Reeve_Foundation__Paralysis_amp_Spinal_Cord_Injury.htm

Jefferson University Hospitals. (2009). *Spinal cord injury: Patient family teaching manual*. Retrieved from http://www.spinalcordcenter.org/consumer/manual.html

Neville, J. B. (2012). *How I roll: Life, work, and love after a spinal cord injury*. Pennsylvania, PA: Winans Kuenstler Publishing, LLC.

Spinal Cord Injury Information Network. Retrieved from http://www.uab.edu/medicine/sci/

The Miami Project to Cure Paralysis. University of Miami School of Medicine. P.O. Box 016960, Mail Locator R-48, Miami, FL 33101. Retrieved from www.miamiproject.miami.edu

General Neuroanatomy Reviews

Gertz, S. D., & Tadmor, R. (2007). *Liebman's neuroanatomy made easy and understandable* (7th ed.). Austin, TX: PRO-ED.

Kiernan, J. A., & Barr, M. L. (2009). *Barr's the human nervous system: An anatomical viewpoint* (9th ed.). Philadelphia, PA: Wolters Kluwer Health/Lippincott Williams & Wilkins.

REFERENCES

Ackerman, P. M., Foy, T. A., & Tefertiller, C. (2013). *Traumatic spinal cord injury. Umphred's neurological rehabilitation* (6th ed., pp. 459–520). St. Louis, MO: Elsevier.

American Occupational Therapy Association (AOTA). (2014). Occupational therapy practice framework: Domain and process (3rd ed.). *American Journal of Occupational Therapy*, *68*(Suppl. 1), S1–S48. Retrieved from http://dx.doi.org/10.5014/ajot.2014.682006

American Psychiatric Association (APA). (2013). *Diagnostic and statistical manual of mental disorders* (5th ed.). Washington, DC: American Psychiatric Association.

American Spinal Injury Association. (2008). *American spinal injury association international standards for neurological classification of spinal cord injury*. Atlanta, GA: American Spinal Injury Association.

American Spinal Injury Association/ International Spinal Society. (2013). *International standards for neurological classification of spinal cord injury*. Retrieved from http://www.asia-spinalinjury.org/elearning/ASIA_ISCOS_high.pdf

Bombardier, C. H., Richards, J. S., Krause, J. S., Tulsky, D., & Tate, D. G. (2004). Symptoms of major depression in people with spinal cord injury: Implications for screening. *Archives of Physical Medicine Rehabilitation*, *85*(11), 1749–1756.

Bracken, M. B. (2009). Steroids for acute spinal cord injury. *Cochrane Database of Systematic Reviews*,

2002(2), 1–45. Retrieved from http://www.escriber.com/userfiles/ccoch/file/CD001046.pdf

Brown, R., DiMarco, A. F., Hoit, J. D., & Garshick, E. (2006). Respiratory dysfunction and management in spinal cord injury. *Respiratory Care*, *51*(8), 853–870.

Byrne, T. N., Benzel, E. C., & Waxman, S. G. (2000). *Diseases of the spine and spinal cord*. New York, NY: Oxford University Press.

Cappuccino, A. (2008). Moderate hypothermia as treatment for spinal cord injury. *Orthopedics*, *31*(3), 243–246.

Chang, S. M., Hou, C. L., Dong, D. Q., & Zhang, H. (2000). Urologic status of 74 spinal cord injury patients from the 1976 Tangshan earthquake, and managed for over 20 years using the Credé Maneuver. *Spinal Cord*, *38*(9), 552–554.

Christopher & Dana Reeve Foundation. (2015). *Sexual health for men*. Retrieved from http://www.christopherreeve.org/site/c.mtKZKgMWKwG/b.4453431/k.552C/Sexual_Health_for_Men.htm

Christopher & Dana Reeve Foundation. (2015). *Spasticity*. Retrieved from http://www.christopher-reeve.org/atf/cf/%7B173bca02-3665-49ab-9378-be009c58a5d3%7D/SPASTICITY6-13.PDF

Cipriano, C. A., Pill, S. G., & Keenan, M. A. (2009). Heterotopic ossification following traumatic brain injury and spinal cord injury. *Journal of American Academy of Orthopedic Surgeons*, *17*, 689–697.

Consortium for Spinal Cord Medicine. (2006). *Bladder management for adults with spinal cord injury: A clinical practice guideline for health-care providers*. Washington, DC: Paralyzed Veterans of America.

Cooper, G. (2006). *Essential physical medicine and rehabilitation*. Totowa, NJ: Humana Press.

Fann, J. R., Bombardier, C. H., Richards, S., Tate, D. G., Wilson, C. S., & Temkin, N. (2011). Depression after spinal cord injury: Comorbidities, mental health service use, and adequacy of treatment. *Archives of Physical Medicine*, *92*, 352–360.

Gallagher, M. V. (November 29, 2004). *Paralyzed South Korean woman walks thanks to adult stem cell research*. *Lifenews.com*. Retrieved from http://archive.lifenews.com/bio582.html

Geffner, L. F., Santacruz, P., & Izurieta, M. (2008). Administration of autologous bone marrow stem cells into spinal cord injury patients via multiple routes is safe and improves their quality of life: Comprehensive case studies. *Cell Transplantation*, *17*, 1277–1293.

Grundy, D., Tromans, A., & Jamil, F. (2002). Later management and complications-I. In D. Grundy & A. Swain (Eds.), *ABC of spinal cord injury* (4th ed., pp. 65–69). London, UK: BMJ Books.

Guttmann, L. (1976). *Spinal cord injuries*. Oxford, UK: Blackwell Scientific.

Hayes, K. C., Hsieh, J. T., Wolfe, D. L., Potter, P. J. & Delaney, G. A. (2000). Classifying incomplete spinal cord injury syndromes: Algorithms based on the international standards for neurological and functional classification of spinal cord injury patients. *Archives of Physical Medicine and Rehabilitation*, *81*, 644–652.

Higgins, M. (September 12, 2007). Doctor's say Bills' Everett will walk again. *The New York Times*. Retrieved from http://www.nytimes.com/2007/09/12/sports/football/12everett.html?_r=1

Kalpakjan, C. Z., Bombardier, C. H., Schomer, K., Brown, P. A., & Johnson, K. L. (2009). Measuring depression in people with spinal cord injury: A systematic review. *Journal of Spinal Cord Medicine*, *32*(1), 6–24. Retrieved from http://www.ncbi.nlm.nih.gov/pmc/articles/PMC2647502/#i1079-0268-32-1-6-b02

Krassioukov, A., Warburton, D. E. R., Teasell, R., & Eng, J. J. (2009). A systematic review of the management of autonomic dysreflexia following spinal cord injury. *Archives of Physical Medicine and Rehabilitation*, *90*(4), 682–695.

Kroshinsky, D., & Strazzula, L. (2015). *Pressure sores: Bedsores, decubitus ulcers, pressure ulcers*. *Merck Manual*. Retrieved from http://www.merck-manuals.com/home/skin-disorders/pressure-sores/pressure-sores

Russo-McCourt, T. A. (2009). Spinal cord injuries. In K. A. McQuillan, M. B. F. Makic, & E. Whalen (Eds.), *Trauma nursing: From resuscitation through rehabilitation* (4th ed., pp. 565–613). St. Louis, MO: Saunders.

Mayo Clinic. (2011). *Spinal cord injury causes*. Retrieved from http://www.mayoclinic.com/health/spinal-cord-injury/DS00460/DSECTION=causes

Merenda, L., Duffy, T., & Betz, R. (2007). Outcomes of urinary diversion in children with SCI. *Journal of Spinal Cord Medicine*, *30*(Suppl. 1), 41–47.

DiZazzo-Miller, R. (2015). Spinal cord injury induced by gun shot wounds: Implications for occupational therapy. *The Open Journal of Occupational Therapy*, *3*(1), Article 7. doi:10.15453/2168-6408.1127

Moroz, A. (2015). *Physical therapy (PT): Grades of muscle strength*. Merck Manual Professional Version. Retrieved from http://www.merck-manuals.com/professional/special-subjects/rehabilitation/physical-therapy-pt

National Institute of Neurological Disorders and Stroke (NINDS). (2013). Spinal cord injury: Hope through research. Retrieved from https://www.ninds.nih.gov/disorders/sci/detail_sci.htm

National Institute of Neurological Disorders and Stroke (NINDS). (2015). *Spinal cord injury: Hope through research*. Retrieved from https://www.ninds.nih.gov/disorders/sci/detail_sci.htm

National Spinal Cord Injury Statistical Center (NSCISC). (2014). *2014 Annual Statistical Report.* Birmingham, AL: University of Alabama at Birmingham. Retrieved from https://www.nscisc. uab.edu/PublicDocuments/reports/pdf/2014%20 NSCISC%20Annual%20Statistical%20Report%20 Complete%20Public%20Version.pdf

National Spinal Cord Injury Statistical Center (NSCISC). (2013). *Spinal cord injury facts and figures at a glance.* Birmingham, AL: University of Alabama at Birmingham. Retrieved from https:// www.nscisc.uab.edu/PublicDocuments/fact_ figures_docs/Facts%202013.pdf

National Spinal Cord Injury Statistical Center (NSCISC). (2009). Spinal cord injury statistics. *Foundation for spinal cord injury prevention, care & cure.* Retrieved from http://www.fscip.org/ facts.htm

Price, D. (March 18, 1990). Building lives with no barriers (pp. 17–33A). *The Detroit News Washington Bureau.*

Somers, M. F. (2010). *Spinal cord injury functional rehabilitation* (3rd ed.). Upper Saddle River, NJ: Pearson.

Spinal Outreach Team. (2014). *The impact of spinal cord injury on pregnancy, labour and delivery: What you need to know.* Brisbane, Australia: Queensland Health. Retrieved from https://www.health.qld.gov. au/qscis/documents/pregnancy-sci.pdf

Taylor, P., Esnouf, J., & Hobby, J. (2002). The functional impact of the freehand system on tetraplegic hand function: clinical results. *Spinal Cord, 40,* 560–566.

University of California, San Francisco Orthopaedic Institute. (2015). *Orthotics and prosthetics: Thoraco-lumbo-sacral orthosis.* Retrieved from http://orthosurg.ucsf.edu/oi/patient-care/divisions/ orthotics-and-prosthetics/services/spinal-orthotics/ thoraco-lumbo-sacral-orthosis-tlso/

Wood, C., Binks, E., & Grundy, D. (2002). Nursing. In D. Grundy & A. Swain (Eds.), *ABC of spinal cord injury* (4th ed., pp. 41–48). London, UK: BMJ Books.

25 Orthopedics

Nancy Hock, Heather Javaherian-Dysinger
and Sharon L. Pavlovich

KEY TERMS

Arthroplasty
Closed fracture
Comminuted fracture
Complex regional pain
 syndrome (CRPS)
Compound fracture
Delayed union
Ecchymosis
Greenstick fracture
Heterotopic ossification
Malunion
Nonunion
Open fracture
Open reduction internal
 fixation (ORIF)
Osteoarthritis
Osteopenia
Osteoporosis
Pathologic fracture
Remodeling
Rheumatoid arthritis
Volkmann's deformity

M ary is a 68-year-old widow who lives alone in a small two-story home. Though obese and managing diabetes, she is very active. She volunteers at her church and the community hospital. She loves to garden, walk, play cards with her friends, and do crossword puzzles. At home, she cooks simple meals and does light housework as the pain in her hip and hands makes it too difficult to carry out the activities that she did in the past. Mary was an avid square dancer, but with the hip pain and loss of her husband, she gave up dancing, a valued occupation.

After much encouragement from her friends and children, Mary finally went to the doctor and told him about the severity of her pain. After a few tests, he diagnosed her with arthritis. She started anti-inflammatory medication to manage her pain and discomfort. Over the past year, however, her right hip became more and more painful. She had difficulty getting out of bed in the morning and had to ask her children to help with the housework and gardening. She cried on the phone as she told her daughter, "I can't do anything anymore." She missed being out in her garden and tending to the plants as it gave her peace and helped her feel connected to the memories of her husband. She also missed socializing, walking, and playing cards with her friends. When they came over to check on her, they encouraged her to talk to her doctor again.

After seeing her doctor, who confirmed that she had severe arthritis in her hip and degeneration, Mary chose to have an elective total hip replacement (THR). Plain radiographs obtained from the right hip revealed severe arthritic changes. Her physician thoroughly discussed the benefits and risks of the surgery with her. She was seen for preassessment training, which involved meeting with several members of the orthopedic total joint team. During this time, she met with both an occupational and physical therapist. The occupational therapist asked her several questions about her postoperative goals, the design of her home, her family support, and the activities in which she liked to engage. The occupational therapist explained that she would receive occupational therapy after the surgery to help her regain independence in daily activities while safely following her hip precautions. The occupational therapist told her that it would take about 6 weeks to recover and that she should be walking with her friends, meeting them for card night, working in the garden with possible modifications, and, most importantly, enjoying life again.

DESCRIPTION AND DEFINITION

Orthopedic conditions involve injury and disease of bones, joints, and their related structures, which include ligaments, tendons, and muscles. The severity of the injury determines the extent of involvement of those supporting structures. Orthopedic conditions may be caused through a variety of circumstances and disease including traumatic injury, motor vehicular accident (MVA), or arthritis. Injuries during sports such as snowboarding, leisure activities including hiking, and unexpected falls that happen while going about one's day contribute to many of the conditions we see in occupational therapy. Orthopedic conditions may also be caused by rheumatic diseases such as **osteoarthritis** and **rheumatoid arthritis** as well as **osteoporosis**. Osteoarthritis is a result of wear and tear causing joint damage, whereas rheumatoid arthritis is an autoimmune disorder. Osteoporosis is caused by a decrease or loss in bone density. As a result of these diseases, people may need a joint replacement or **arthroplasty** to promote participation in daily activities and to help improve their quality of life with severe arthritis.

One of most common orthopedic conditions is a fracture, which is a break in the continuity of the bone. When one considers the forces involved in an injury such as the impact to the wrist as an older woman tries to protect herself from falling, or from the force of a door crushing against a finger, it is easy to understand that the ligaments and tendons surrounding the involved joint or bone are often injured as well. Though this is common in orthopedic conditions, the focus of this chapter is on conditions related directly to bones and joints.

ETIOLOGY

■ Fractures

Fractures are caused by a trauma or disease of the bone or joint. There are two critical factors involved in the determination of a fracture: (1)

the amount of force applied to the bone and (2) the strength of the bone (Kunkler, 2002). Forces can be high energy such as those experienced in a motor vehicle accident (MVA) or low energy such as those experienced in a fall or through chronic stress as seen in long-distance running. Consequently, these are called stress fractures. The second determining factor is bone strength, which may be normal or weakened from pathological conditions such as tumors or osteoarthritis and osteoporosis. In addition, the age of a person and the size of the bone further influence the bones' ability to withstand a force. These factors negatively affect bone density, elasticity, and supportive structures, thus making the bone more vulnerable to fracture. For example, an older adult who has decreased bone density from osteoporosis has a weak bone that may be unable to sustain normal forces experienced during daily activities. Thus, the bone may fracture while the person simply bends over or gets out of bed. This type of fracture is called a **pathologic fracture** as the fracture was caused by weakening of the bone from another disease. Osteoarthritis and osteoporosis are common conditions that contribute to a pathologic fracture.

■ Osteoarthritis

Osteoarthritis, also referred to as degenerative joint disease, is a noninflammatory joint disease that results in deterioration of articular cartilage and the formation of new bone or osteophytes on the joint surface. These changes often result in pain, joint edema, and impaired participation in life activities. Osteoarthritis is the most common joint disease in the upper extremity. Osteoarthritis of the knee tends to cause the most disability as it impacts one's ability to walk, go up and downstairs, and engage in leisure and work activities. As a result of osteoarthritis, many individuals seek elective surgery for hip and knee replacements to return to a more active and pain-free lifestyle. In the United States, approximately 719,000 total hip and 332,000 knee replacements are performed annually (CDC, 2015b). This number is expected to increase with the aging of the population (National Institute of Arthritis and Musculoskeletal and Skin Diseases, 2009). The technology of joint replacements continues to evolve making them essential in promoting participation in daily activities and improving quality of life in people with severe arthritis.

■ Other Orthopedic Conditions

Osteoporosis is a disease characterized by low bone density and deterioration of bone. It is common in postmenopausal women due to the cessation of estrogen production. The National Osteoporosis Foundation (2010) estimates that over 10 million people in the United States have osteoporosis. A person with osteoporosis may fracture a bone through normal movement such as turning to reach an item of clothing when getting dressed in the morning. The most common sites for these fractures according to data gathered in 2005 are the vertebrae, the wrist, the hip, and the pelvis with approximately 547,000 vertebral fractures, 397,000 wrist fractures, and approximately 297,000 hip fractures (National Osteoporosis Foundation, 2010). It is estimated that half of all women and as many as one out of four men aged 50 and older will experience a fracture related to osteoporosis (US Dept. of Health and Human Services, 2004).

Osteopenia is a reversible weakening of the bone. It is estimated that nearly 34 million people have low bone mass (National Osteoporosis Foundation, 2010). As osteopenia is a reversible condition, it is important to take advantage of bone density screenings offered at health fairs and follow up with your physician. Measures to help decrease the risk of osteopenia and halt further progression into osteoporosis include a balanced diet, supplements, weight-bearing exercise, and bone density screenings.

Heterotopic ossification (HO) is an orthopedic condition resulting in abnormal bone formation in extraskeletal soft tissues (Moore & Cho, 2010). This condition is often associated with traumatic injuries including severe burns, spinal cord injuries, and head injuries as well as other bone-forming diseases such as ankylosing spondylitis (Moore & Cho, 2010). The exact cause and pathophysiology of HO is still unclear. The massive trauma sustained by the body creates a whole-body response, and in some instances, fibroblasts inappropriately start forming bone. This results in excessive bone growth near joints causing stiffening and loss of movement. This painful and debilitating condition is still not clearly understood, but it can have a significant impact on a person's functional abilities.

INCIDENCE AND PREVALENCE

■ Fractures

In 2007, the National Center for Injury Prevention (NCIP) reported unintentional falls as the leading cause of nonfatal injuries in the United States across all age groups. The most common fractures that result from falls are those of the spine, hip, forearm, leg, ankle, pelvis, upper arm, and hand (Scheffer, Schuurmans, VanDijk, & VanDerHoof, 2008). Chung and Spilson (2001), following review of nearly 1.5 million fractures, determined that 44% of all fractures involve the distal radius. Falls are the leading cause of fractures among older adults (Bell, Talbot-Stern, & Hennessy, 2000). In 2001, more than 1.6 million older adults were treated for fall-related injuries, which included fractures and other conditions. The 2000 census reported that there are 360,000 to 480,000 fall-related fractures in older adults per year involving the hip, wrist, humerus, vertebrae, and pelvis, with the most serious being a hip fracture (National Center for Injury Prevention and Control, 2004). Older adult women sustain approximately 80% of all hip fractures (Stevens & Olson, 2000). Population studies project, with the rising number of older adults, a significant increase in rates of hip fractures, which are expected to reach 289,000 annually by 2030. This is an increase of 12%. Fortunately, the hip fracture rate declined significantly from 1996 to 2010 (CDC, 2015a). Hip fractures, however, continue to be a significant condition contributing to long-term functional impairment as well as increased nursing home admissions (CDC, 2015a).

Hip fractures are one of the primary causes of disability and mortality in the older adult. Statistics suggest that one in five patients dies within the first year of sustaining a hip fracture (Farahmand, Michaelsson, Ahlbom, Ljunghall, & Baron, 2005). Some people will not return to their premorbid functional level and may rely on adaptive equipment or modifications to their daily activities (Crottty et al., 2010). A randomized trial by Hagsten, Svensson, and Gardulf (2004), however, found that occupational therapy intervention increased a patient's ability to perform activities of daily living (ADL) sooner than those who did not receive occupational therapy. Thus, patients receiving occupational therapy were more likely to return to an independent living situation and require less postoperative care. This charges occupational therapy practitioners with the role of promoting life participation and well-being among individuals who are recovering from fractures as well as other orthopedic conditions.

■ Osteoarthritis

Arthritis is one of the leading causes of disability impeding people's capacity to engage in meaningful and necessary daily occupations due to pain, weakness, and loss of range of motion (ROM) (Healthy People 2010, 2010). According to the Centers for Disease Control and Prevention (2013), 52.5 million people have arthritis worldwide. In the United States alone, it is estimated that 27 million people age 25 and older have osteoarthritis (Lawrence et al., 2008). Arthritis was also found to result in estimated $128 billion in medical care costs and lost earning in the United States in 2003 (CDC, 2013). Osteoarthritis typically affects the knee, distal interphalangeal joints, proximal interphalangeal joints, and the first carpal metacarpal joint.

■ Other Orthopedic Conditions

According to the National Osteoporosis Foundation, 10 million people have osteoporosis, of which 80% are women (National Osteoporosis Foundation, 2010). Early signs of osteoporosis are seen in younger women in the form of osteopenia. This trend emphasizes the importance of prevention and lifestyle management as once the disease progresses beyond osteopenia to osteoporosis, bone regeneration is no longer reversible. Nguyen, Eisman, Center, and Nguyen (2007) identified that postural instability, quadriceps weakness, and a history of a fall or previous fracture are shown to be significant predictors of future osteoporotic fractures.

HO is a common complication after traumas such as fractures, arthroplasties, traumatic amputations, spinal cord injuries, head injuries, and burns with the incidence varying depending on the injury (Wheeless, 2015b). Though it is a common complication, only 10% to 20% of people who develop HO will have significant functional limitations (Bruno-Petrina, 2008). Most people will be asymptomatic and most likely diagnosed when it is seen on an x-ray. HO usually occurs 1 to 4 months after the traumatic injury (Wheeless, 2015b). HO may occur after a fracture especially in those who have an open reduction internal fixation (Bruno-Petrina, 2008). In injuries and fractures to the elbow, the incidence may be as high as 90% (Bruno-Petrina, 2008). The incidence of HO in hip arthroplasties is generally 50%, although only one-third of the people experience clinically significant symptoms such as limited ROM and pain (Kocic, Lazovic, Mitkovic, & Djokic, 2010). Revisions to hip and knee replacements increase the risk of developing HO (Moore & Cho, 2010). With the increase in combat-related injuries over the last several years, we have seen more soldiers with traumatic amputations. The incidence of HO in these amputations was found to be 63%, which is much higher than previously expected (Potter, Burns, Lacap, Granville, & Gajewski, 2007). Fortunately, the majority of the cases are successfully managed or the soldiers are asymptomatic. HO occurs in 40% to 50% of people who have a spinal cord injury, with it primarily affecting the knee, pelvis, and hip (Moore & Cho, 2010). Research suggests it also occurs in 20% of people who have a traumatic brain injury (Bruno-Petrina, 2008). The incidence of HO appears to be much higher in fractures and neurological injuries involving spasticity than it does in burns. Factors that can impact occurrence of HO in burns are found to be the percentage and location of the burn, the amount of forceful manipulation, and the time period of immobilization and time for wound closure (Klein, Logsetty, & Costa, 2007).

SIGNS AND SYMPTOMS

■ Fractures

The general symptoms of a break are localized pain at the fracture site, deformity, edema, and **ecchymosis**, which is often seen after 24 to 48 hours of onset (Altizer, 2002). Ecchymosis is described as a discoloration of the skin that is caused by bleeding. There are several types of fractures. A **closed fracture** refers to a fracture that has not broken through the skin, whereas in an **open fracture**, the bone breaks through the skin surface. Open fractures, also known as **compound fractures**, have an increased chance for infection. The term **comminuted** is applied to fractures that have two or more fragments. A displaced fracture involves segments that have become separated or shifted from the bone (Altizer, 2002). **Greenstick fractures** are often seen in children whose bones are still soft and growing. Rather than snapping into two, the bone breaks on one side and bends on the other. It is similar to how a young twig or tree limb breaks, thus the name greenstick fracture.

Fractures are further described by the type of fracture line. A complete fracture involves a break in the full continuity of the bone. An incomplete fracture involves a partial disruption in the continuity of the bone. Such breaks are often called cracks or hairline fractures (Altizer, 2002). A transverse fracture occurs when the fracture line is at a right angle to the longitudinal axis of the bone. An oblique fracture involves a fracture line that is diagonal or slanted. Torsional stress applied to bone causes a twisting fracture line, which is called a spiral fracture.

Distal Radial Fractures

Distal radial fractures may cause loss of sensation, strength, movement, and limited functional use of the hand and possibly the arm. As most of these injuries are caused by a fall on an outstretched arm, the entire upper extremity should be examined for injury. Several different classification systems have been used to describe distal radius fractures. These systems are used to identify fracture fragment patterns and lead the surgeon's management decisions (Michlovitz & Festa, 2011). Physicians evaluate distal radius fractures based on volar or dorsal displacement, comminution of the fracture, whether there is articular involvement or involvement of the ulna, or whether there are additional soft tissue injuries associated with the fracture (Chen, Huang, Trumble, & Jupiter, 2010).

Hip Fractures

A hip fracture generally refers to a fracture of the proximal femur. It may be intracapsular or extracapsular. Intracapsular fractures involve the femoral neck such as a subcapital or transcervical fracture (Fig. 25.1). Extracapsular fractures involve the trochanters such as a subtrochanteric or intertrochanteric fracture. An individual with a hip fracture may experience referred pain to the knee, be unable to bear weight on the involved

lower extremity, and will often have a leg-length discrepancy.

Humeral Fractures

The incidence of humeral fractures in the United States has increased as a result of the aging of our population, increased participation in sports, and the rise of osteoporosis (Gill, 2002). A humeral fracture may present with humeral displacement and malposition of the distal limb. Radial nerve injury is found in approximately 18% of humeral shaft fractures (Wheeless, 2015a). A spiral fracture may lacerate the radial nerve, or it may be damaged by displaced bony segments. Clinical signs of radial nerve involvement include loss of wrist extension and impaired sensation on the dorsal aspect of the wrist. Seventy-five to ninety percent of individuals who have closed humeral fractures have recovery of the radial nerve in 3 to 4 months (Wheeless, 2015a).

Fractures that occur at the distal end of the humerus just above the medial and lateral condyles are referred to as supracondylar fractures. These fractures are commonly known as elbow fractures. The medial and lateral condyles serve as an origin site for many muscles of the forearm and have bony connections to the radius and ulna of the forearm. Nerves and arteries pass along this area; therefore, a supracondylar fracture can also result in injury to muscles, nerves, and tissue that further affect the function of the entire arm. Understandably, it is associated with a high risk for complications such as **malunion** and **Volkmann's deformity**. Volkmann's deformity is a condition that results from severe damage to tissues and muscles caused by increased pressure in the forearm compartments (Kare, 2008). Increased compartmental pressures may be caused by several factors such as ischemia, compartmental bleeding, and excessively tight bandages (Kare, 2008). Signs of ischemia include pale or bluish skin, absence of radial pulse, decreased sensation, and severe pain. Suspected cases of increased compartmental pressure should be immediately reported to the physician as it can result in nerve damage and necrosis.

Scaphoid Fractures

The position of the scaphoid in the proximal row of the carpal bones makes it particularly vulnerable to injury. It is the most commonly fractured bone in the wrist with an incidence of 35,000 to

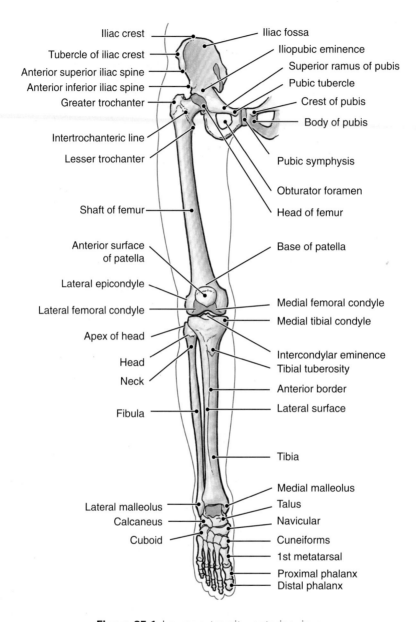

Figure 25.1 Lower extremity, anterior view.

50,000 fractures annually (Dell, Dell, & Griggs, 2011). Scaphoid fractures are commonly seen in young males with a sports injury resulting in wrist hyperextension >90 degrees with radial deviation. Fractures of the middle and proximal poles of the scaphoid are susceptible to avascular necrosis because of its poor blood supply (Dell et al., 2011). Plain radiographs are commonly used to classify the scaphoid fracture; however, other radiographic procedures may be necessary to evaluate its healing.

Arthritis

There are other conditions in addition to fractures that affect the integrity of the bone, such as rheumatic diseases. Rheumatic diseases include an array of progressive conditions leading to impairments in joints and soft tissue. Examples include osteoarthritis and rheumatoid arthritis. Rheumatic diseases are closely associated with the term arthritis, which means joint inflammation. Arthritis is a general term used to describe a host of conditions characterized by joint pain, redness, swelling, and stiffness (Deshaies, 2006).

Osteoarthritis symptoms build up gradually and often begin with notable aches with movement especially after inactivity. Osteoarthritis is often characterized by joint pain, inflammation, stiffness, tenderness, limited ROM, and crepitus, which is an audible or palpable crunching or popping in the joint caused by the irregularity of opposing cartilage surfaces (Hochberg as cited in Deshaies, 2006).

Other Orthopedic Conditions

Osteoporosis is gradual and somewhat silent as it emerges. In the early stages of osteoporosis, symptoms are not usually present. Over time, however, advanced symptoms present themselves through pain, height loss, and kyphosis. The primary clinical signs include skeletal fractures and recurring pathological fractures (Dal Bello-Haas, 2009). Osteopenia is a predecessor to osteoporosis. Even more silent, there are no clinical signs or presentation for osteopenia.

HO usually begins with pain, joint warmth, swelling, and decreased ROM approximately 1 to 4 months after an injury (Adler, 2006). There may be a palpable mass, which becomes harder as the bone forms.

COURSE AND PROGNOSIS

The prognosis and functional outcomes for orthopedic conditions vary depending on the condition itself and the health of the person. The general course and prognosis of fractures are dependent upon several factors: age, type of fracture, fracture location, severity of the fracture, and the patient's intrinsic motivation and premorbid health status. It is important to note, however, that considering all of the orthopedic conditions, hip fractures are a leading cause of morbidity and mortality in older adults (Stevens & Olson, 2000). Therefore, occupational therapy practitioners should work closely with the referring physician for the appropriate protocol and precautions. This statistic also emphasizes the importance of addressing fall prevention and community wellness programs for older adults.

The way in which the bone heals influences the patient's course and prognosis. There are two types of tissues that form bone: cancellous

and cortical. Cancellous bone or spongy bone is the inner layer that houses the bone's vascular supply. It is essential for nutrients to help form strong healthy bones. Cortical bone is the hard outer layer of the bone that provides support and protection. The periosteum is a dense fibrous membrane consisting of connective tissues, elastic fibers, and nerve fibers, which line the outer surface of most bones (Gray, 2004). Depending on the location, a fractured bone normally takes 6 to 12 weeks to heal (Kunkler, 2002).

To achieve optimal healing, it is important that the fracture site receive immediate vascular circulation and appropriate immobilization. The healing process involves five stages (Kunkler, 2002). First, a hematoma forms and seals the damaged blood vessels, and then osteoclasts reabsorb the damaged bone and tissue. The second stage is the formation of a granular or fibrocartilage tissue, which increases the stability of the bone fragments. The third stage involves the formation of a callus. This takes place between 2 and 6 weeks. The formation of the callus has a significant influence on the outcome of the fracture. The fourth stage is ossification and the formation of a bony union. The fifth or final stage is often referred to as consolidation and **remodeling** occurring between 6 weeks and 1 year. To reiterate, the amount of healing time depends on the severity of the fracture and any premorbid health conditions. During remodeling, the bone is ideally reshaped to its original form to enable it to resume its intended function as best as possible.

In some instances, the bone heals abnormally. Abnormal healing can be caused by several factors including an open fracture, severe soft tissue damage, infection, poor vascularization, nerve damage, phlebitis, or compartment syndrome. Such complications can result in **delayed union**, **malunion**, and **nonunion**. A delayed union is when the bone takes more time to heal than is expected; it heals slowly. It may be suspected when pain and tenderness persist at the fracture site 3 months to 1 year after the injury (Kunkler, 2002). Delayed unions may be caused by several factors including infection, poor vascularization, or inadequate immobilization. Once the causing factor is identified and corrected, the bone will typically heal. In a malunion fracture, the fracture heals in an abnormal or deformed position. Contributing factors include muscle imbalance and inadequate protection and positioning of the fracture (Altizer, 2002). A malunion fracture has significant functional implications as the person will often experience limited ROM, strength, and coordination. Nonunion fractures refer to a fracture in which the bone is not healing. A non-union fracture may be caused by several factors such as vascular and tissue damage, poor alignment, stress to the fracture site, and infection (Altizer, 2002). The scaphoid bone has a high risk for nonunion due to its limited blood supply.

■ Arthritis

The course and prognosis of arthritis vary. Idiopathic osteoarthritis, which is the most common, may show itself by osteophytes or "bone spurs" on the proximal interphalangeal joints (Bouchard's nodes) and distal interphalangeal joints (Heberden's nodes). These may become painful and inflamed, limiting functional use. In cases where there is significant pain and joint degeneration, an arthroplasty may be warranted. This is most common in the carpometacarpal joint of the thumb (Cooper, 2014).

■ Other Orthopedic Conditions

Osteopenia may progress to osteoporosis if untreated through lifestyle changes including calcium supplements, a calcium-enriched diet, and added weight-bearing exercise. As mentioned before, this condition is silent and will transform into osteoporosis without any signs. Osteoporosis is irreversible. In regard to prognosis, a person can live a productive and active life but will need to take extra caution in joint protection and fall prevention to avoid a resulting fracture due to the weakened bone.

In the case of HO, 10% to 20% of patients will have permanent functional loss (Bruno-Petrina, 2008; Wheeless, 2015b). The severity of the functional limitations will depend on the joints involved. For instance, there may be more functional implications for a person who has had a burn and develops HO in the dominant upper extremity versus if it develops in the hip joint of someone who has paraplegia. The course of the condition, however, can be complicated if there is additional nerve compression due to the ossification and lymphedema. Medical management, which will be covered in the next section, is important in maintaining ROM and decreasing functional limitations and pain.

DIAGNOSIS

Following an injury with suspected fracture, a physician first performs a clinical evaluation obtaining information on the signs and symptoms and the circumstances surrounding the fracture. The physician usually refers the person to radiology to confirm and determine the degree and classification of the fracture. The radiologist also evaluates for other associated findings such as a pathological fracture (bone weakened by a tumor), stress fracture, or other preexisting conditions that may have affected the integrity of the bone. The diagnosis is commonly confirmed through plain films or x-ray, though other studies may be ordered depending on the physician, suspected injury, and location of the suspected injury.

Fractures of the distal radius are also diagnosed through x-ray. To evaluate the wrist for fracture, the standard views are posteroanterior, lateral, and oblique. Scaphoid fractures can be more challenging to diagnose and, therefore, may require what is known as a scaphoid view. Scaphoid fractures may also present with dorsal wrist pain and tenderness with palpation to the anatomic snuffbox at clinical examination. Given that this fracture is difficult to diagnose, a CT scan or bone scan may be necessary (Sendher & Ladd, 2013).

Osteoarthritis can occur at any joint. Diagnosis begins with clinical exam as patients complain of pain, stiffness, and swelling. The severity of osteoarthritis is diagnosed by x-ray or radiographs. This demonstrates the amount of joint damage that has occurred.

Osteoporosis is typically identified through a bone mineral density scan. Osteopenia is often evident in bone scans, which may be used to confirm the diagnosis (Li, Smith, Tuohy, Smith, & Koman, 2010). It may be initially diagnosed in health screenings or when an adult has several risk factors such as being female, smoking, consuming excessive alcohol, having a low body weight (US Department of Health & Human Services, 2005), and a parent who has had a hip fracture due to osteoporosis (Ahlborg et al., 2010; Khosla & Melton, 2007; National Osteoporosis Foundation, 2010).

HO can sometimes be difficult to diagnose as it may be misdiagnosed as a scarring or joint contracture. Patients with HO may present with a "locking sign." This presents at the end range of either flexion or extension of the joint. X-ray is the most economical method to confirm the diagnosis of HO; if suspected from clinical evaluation (Chen, Yang, Chuang, Huang, & Yang, 2009), HO can also be diagnosed by a radiologist through bone scan, ultrasonography, or CT scan (Moore & Cho, 2010).

MEDICAL AND SURGICAL MANAGEMENT

The medical management of orthopedic conditions varies depending on the specific condition. Some require conservative treatment consisting of over-the-counter medications, splinting, and home exercise programs, while others may require surgery. Below, we have provided a brief summary of the medical management of the more common conditions that we have discussed in this chapter.

■ Fractures

Hip Fractures

Most hip fractures require surgical intervention. The type of procedure depends on several factors such as the severity of the fracture, prefracture functional level of the patient, age of the patient, the presence or absence of comorbid conditions, and the preference of the surgeon (Beloosesky et al., 2002; Lowe, Crist, Bhandari, & Ferguson, 2010). Patients who are more active prior to their fracture often have fewer complications and more positive results after surgery thus emphasizing the importance of a healthy lifestyle (Beloosesky et al., 2002). There is still mixed evidence on the morbidity and mortality rates and surgical approach for the very elderly (Lowe et al., 2010). Therefore, physicians will carefully consider these factors and make necessary preoperative referrals to medically stabilize the patient while keeping in mind complications and further discomfort that might arise with a delay in surgery (Holt, Smith, Duncan, & McKeown, 2010).

The goal of surgical intervention for a hip fracture is to align and immobilize the fracture site to allow for normal healing. Hip fractures are treated with closed reduction and immobilization or open reduction and internal fixation (ORIF). Closed reduction involves realigning the fracture fragments through manual manipulation or traction, which may be done under general or local anesthesia (Kunkler, 2002). Immobilization can be accomplished through casts, traction, splints, or braces. Open reduction on the other hand involves surgically opening and reducing the fracture site. Internal fixation is commonly done after an open reduction to secure the fracture. Internal fixation involves securing the fracture site with pins, rods, plates, and screws. This promotes healing and allows for early mobilization, which can reduce complications often associated with immobility. Some hip fractures, such as an intracapsular femoral neck fracture, may be treated with hemiarthroplasty or a THR (Brunner & Eshilian-Oates, 2003). A hemiarthroplasty is a partial joint replacement in which the femoral head and neck are replaced by a metal prosthesis. A total arthroplasty or THR may be indicated depending on the patient's age and whether the femur and acetabulum were damaged from the injury or a preexisting disease.

Distal Radial Fractures and Humeral Fractures

Management of distal radius fractures has changed over the last 10 years secondary to changes in fixation (Michlovitz & Festa, 2011). Distal radial and humeral fractures may be reduced or realigned manually or with surgery. Closed fractures may be reduced manually and immobilized with a cast. Fractures that are unstable or cannot be manually reduced require surgery. This procedure is called an **open reduction and internal fixation** (ORIF), which secures the fracture site with screws, pins, plates, and rods. Open and comminuted fractures often require ORIF. Figure 25.2 is a radiograph of an ORIF in which two plates and screws were used to surgically stabilize displaced fractures of the radius and ulna of a woman who had been in an MVA. As described earlier, all distal radius fractures are not equal and, therefore, must be managed individually. Typically, the immobilization phase following a distal radius fracture can last 1 to 6 weeks (Michlovitz & Festa, 2011). During this phase, it is important to control edema and pain while also addressing ROM in the shoulder and digits if allowed. Complications such as nerve compression, tendon rupture, stiffness, **complex regional pain syndrome** (CRPS), and pain may also impact progression and outcome (Michlovitz & Festa, 2011). CRPS presents as

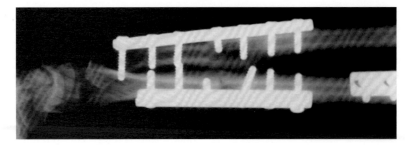

Figure 25.2 Open reduction internal fixation.

chronic pain with autonomic dysfunction. The most common precursor to this complication is fracture (Li et al., 2010).

Scaphoid Fractures

A nondisplaced scaphoid fracture is typically immobilized with a thumb spica cast for approximately 8 to 10 weeks (Dell et al., 2011) (see Fig. 25.3). Proximal scaphoid fractures may require a long-arm thumb spica cast followed by the use of a short-arm thumb spica cast to promote healing for as long as 6 weeks to 6 months. Displaced or unstable scaphoid fractures require an ORIF with a compression screw (Dell et al., 2011). Following the ORIF, a wrist orthosis should be used for 2 to 4 weeks for soft tissue healing. A percutaneous fixation technique using a Herbert

screw is a common and effective approach used in the treatment of acute scaphoid fractures. This technique has been found to be associated with a more rapid return of hand function, higher client satisfaction, and minimal complications (Jeon, Oh, Park, Ihn, & Kim, 2003). The physician and therapist should closely monitor the fracture to ensure proper vascularization.

■ Arthritis

Arthritis may be controlled with various medications, and patients should be followed closely by a rheumatologist. Arthroplasty may be indicated in joints that have severe pain and joint deterioration that significantly limits participation in daily activities. Arthroplasties or joint replacements may be done in the hands, shoulder, and other

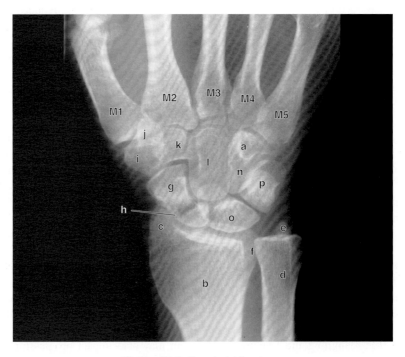

Figure 25.3 Scaphoid fracture.

joints though it is most common in the hip and knee as they are our weight-bearing joints.

Arthritis of the Hip

THRs are typically indicated for those who have severe arthritis causing pain and stiffness that significantly limits the person's participation in daily activities or, as mentioned above, when there is damage to the acetabulum or femur during a fall. This is a common condition seen by occupational therapy practitioners working in acute care and inpatient rehabilitation. THRs are often seen in individuals 55 years and older. The procedure involves replacement of the acetabulum and ball of the femur with artificial implants. These may be secured by bone cement or a cementless prosthesis, which allows for bone growth. Hip replacements or arthroplasties generally last for 10 to 25 years (Roberts, 2002), though researchers continue to evaluate implant wear.

Following a THR, there are several precautions that a patient must follow for 6 to 8 weeks after the surgery (Maher, 2014; Rasul & Wright, 2010). These precautions include no hip adduction and rotation of the operated leg, and no hip flexion beyond 90 degrees of the operated leg (Table 25.1). If the surgeon uses an anterior approach, the patient must also avoid hip extension. Oftentimes, therapists will encourage their clients to avoid hip rotation in general to ensure that the surgical hip is protected. These precautions are currently the standard of care; however, recent research suggests that an anterolateral surgical approach rather than strict adherence to traditional hip precautions was more likely to be associated with a low rate of dislocation (Peak et al., 2005). Depending on the severity of the condition, the surgical approach and procedure, and the orthopedic surgeon, there may be weight-bearing precautions for patients who undergo a THRs and ORIFs. Common weight-bearing statuses include non–weight bearing, touchdown or toe-touch weight bearing, partial weight bearing, weight bearing as tolerated, and full weight bearing (Table 25.2).

Hip precautions have functional implications for the person in a variety of daily activities. Occupational therapy practitioners must educate clients on the hip precautions and teach them adaptations for sitting, dressing, bathing, reaching for items, and driving among others. In regard to driving, patients are to avoid driving for 4 to 6 weeks following surgery (Ganz, Levin, Peterson, & Ranawat, 2003). At this time, most patients have reached their preoperative driving reaction time and continue to show improvements in reaction time for up to 1 year.

Arthritis of the Knee

The first line of management of arthritis of the knee is conservative treatment, which often begins with over the counter anti-inflammatory medications and heat and ice. If pain and functional limitations progress, the patient's primary physician or rheumatologist may prescribe medications to effectively control the arthritis. When conservative treatment does not work, the patient may be a candidate for a partial or total knee replacement (TKR). This is also referred to as a knee arthroplasty. A TKR involves resurfacing the entire knee joint with metal and plastic prosthetic components. The procedure typically involves a femoral component, tibial plate, and a patellar button (Roberts, 2002) and may be done unilaterally or bilaterally.

After surgery, it is important to begin the rehabilitation process (Bade, Kohrt, & Stevens-Lapsley, 2010; Rasul & Wright, 2010). Treatment involves pain medication and early mobilization to strengthen the quadriceps and prevent loss of ROM. A continuous passive motion machine may be prescribed while in the hospital or at home to help improve circulation and movement at the knee joint depending on the patient's postoperative health and functional abilities. Mizner, Petterson, and Snyder-Mackler (2005), identified

TABLE 25.1 Total Hip Precautions

1. Avoid hip flexion beyond 90 degrees.
2. Avoid hip rotation of operated leg.
3. Avoid hip adduction of operated leg (avoid crossing legs).

TABLE 25.2 Weight-Bearing Status	
Weight-Bearing Status	**Percentage and Description**
Non–weight bearing	0%. No WB on the operated leg, it should not touch the floor.
Touchdown or toe-touch weight bearing	10%–15%. Foot of operated leg may rest on floor.
Partial weight bearing	30%–50%. May put 30%–50% of weight through the operated leg.
Weight bearing as tolerated	Patient may put as much weight through operated leg as tolerated without unnecessary pain or discomfort.
Full weight bearing	75%–100%. Patient bears full weight on the operated leg.

Modified from Goldstein, T. S. (1999). *Geriatric orthopedics: Rehabilitative management of common problems* (2nd ed.). Gaithersburg, MD: Aspen.

quadriceps weakness as a primary impairment following TKR and found a high correlation between quadriceps strength and functional performance over knee ROM or pain.

To maximize the results of the surgery and functional outcomes, the patient needs education on several precautions such as avoiding putting a pillow under the knee while in bed, resting both feet on the floor when sitting to increase knee ROM, and wearing an immobilizer as instructed by the physician to protect the knee joint until the muscle is strong enough to support it (Rasul & Wright, 2010). The immobilizer may be required when walking, while in bed, or at all times. Kneeling should be avoided. Other considerations include not driving, running, and jumping until cleared by the physician. Generally, patients are able to return to most of their normal daily activities after 3 to 6 weeks though high-impact activities may need to be modified. Driving may be resumed around 4 to 6 weeks as long as the patient is able to bend his or her knee enough to get in and out of the car and have appropriate muscle strength and control to operate the pedals. Patients need to follow up with their physician to monitor for complications and ensure continued progress.

IMPACT ON OCCUPATIONAL PERFORMANCE

Occupational therapy practitioners use a holistic approach to examine specific client factors residing within the person to understand their impact on occupational performance (AOTA, 2014). Systems of values, beliefs and spirituality, body functions, and body structures are client factors that are often affected by illness or disability (AOTA, 2014). Client factors are an important consideration when working with a person who has an orthopedic condition to help them engage in daily occupations such as dressing, working, managing the home, and leisure pursuits. We will discuss client factors that are commonly affected by an orthopedic condition.

During the initial evaluation, it is important to carefully assess the nature and circumstances surrounding the onset of the orthopedic condition. For example, children and adults are likely to sustain fractures during play and sports activities, whereas older adults may experience a fracture as a result of a fall or osteoporosis. In some circumstances, however, a fracture may also be a result of child abuse or domestic violence. The nature of the circumstance surrounding the injury or condition may impact secondary injuries and psychosocial involvement. It is important therefore to conduct a thorough history of the fall and a radiologic analysis of the fracture (American Academy of Pediatrics, 2000) and, for children, to ascertain their developmental level.

Orthopedic conditions may compromise participation in several areas of occupation including ADLs, instrumental activities of daily living (IADL), sleep, education, work, play, leisure, and social participation (AOTA, 2014). The degree of impairment depends upon the severity of the injury, location of the injury, and the client's premorbid health status. Several client factors

TABLE 25.3	Client Factors Commonly Involved in Orthopedic Conditions (AOTA, 2014)

1. Values, beliefs, and spirituality
2. Body functions
   - Mental functions
   - Sensory functions and pain
     - Vestibular function (balance)
     - Pain
     - Protective functions of the skin
   - Neuromusculoskeletal and movement-related functions
     - Joint mobility
     - Joint stability
     - Muscle power
     - Muscle tone
     - Muscle endurance
   - Skin and related structure functions
     - Repair function of the skin
3. Body structures
   - Structures related to movement
   - Skin and related structures

may be compromised by orthopedic conditions (Table 25.3). The main client factors that will affect one's participation in occupation are neuromusculoskeletal and movement-related functions and structures and sensory and pain functions and structures. Joint mobility, stability, and alignment are directly affected by a fracture or a condition such as osteoarthritis. Therefore, in the case of fractures, it is necessary to reduce or realign them in a timely manner. Limited joint mobility may affect an individual's ability to participate in daily activities such as dressing, cooking, and cleaning. This in turn can affect one's role performance. For example, a woman with a distal radius fracture may initially have difficulty fulfilling her mothering role with an infant. Until the pain and swelling are reduced and the fracture is stabilized, she may be unable to lift her baby and have difficulty doing things such as changing diapers.

Muscle strength and endurance are often affected by orthopedic conditions as a result of immobilization of a joint during recovery. These limitations may also be caused and worsened by disuse of the involved extremity. A person will often hold their involved extremity in a dependent or guarded position and refrain from using it. This further compounds the patient's symptoms and often leads to loss of ROM, strength, and pain in other joints and musculature that were initially uninvolved. Limitations in muscle strength and

endurance directly impact one's performance and participation in daily activities. A person recovering from a humeral fracture may find it difficult to golf or may find that his or her arm tires easily when painting or doing household chores.

Orthopedic conditions may affect sensation function and pain in the areas of balance, sensation, and pain. When recovering from a THR or hip fracture, an individual may struggle with balance as he or she tries to walk, move around in the bathroom, and get dressed while following weight bearing precautions. As a result, the individual may need to modify how he or she does certain activities in order to prevent a fall. Sensation may be affected if there is nerve involvement at the fracture site. Depending on the degree of sensory involvement, an individual may have difficulty picking things up. Pain, as noted earlier in the discussion, is a common sign of an injury. Pain will vary depending on the person, severity of the injury, and complications. Sharp or continuous pain may affect an individual's ability to complete daily tasks. The pain experienced by people who develop CRPS can be so overwhelming that it affects their ability to work and carry out their life roles.

Joint pain, inflammation, and limited ROM from osteoarthritis often affect participation in daily life activities as the integrity of the bone is compromised. As such, an individual may require the use of adaptive equipment to help with tasks such a dressing and grooming. Fluctuations in movement-related functions can vary from day to day secondary to medications, pain, and efforts put forth in energy conservation and work simplification techniques.

In addition, functions of the skin and related structures and mental functions may be impacted by orthopedic conditions. Compound fractures that break through the skin will result in a wound at risk for infection. This type of fracture will involve more medical management and may consequently limit an individual's ability to participate in a variety of daily occupations due to pain, wound care procedures, and type of fixation.

Mental functions such as one's self-concept, motivation, and interests may be impacted by an orthopedic condition. A distal radius fracture, for example, may present with skin changes, edema, and severely limited movement in the fingers. As a result, the individual may have difficulty doing many tasks such as dressing, grooming, and writing. The inability to perform these daily tasks that we often take for granted may impair one's self-concept and thus affect a person's motivation such as when one withdraws from activities that he or she is normally interested in. This emphasizes the importance for the occupational therapy practitioner to continually assess and address the person's values, beliefs, and spirituality as these factors will impact the person's coping strategies and mental well-being throughout the healing process.

CASE STUDY 1

Josh is a 16-year-old boy who enjoys participating in several sports during the winter months. On a recent snowboarding venture, Josh was taken to a local emergency room after he fell on his right arm while performing an air stunt. The on-call physician evaluated Josh and ordered x-rays to confirm a distal radial fracture. After confirmation of a closed fracture, the physician manually reduced the fracture and immobilized Josh with a cast. After 5 weeks, the cast was removed and occupational therapy was ordered to address ADL.

The occupational therapy evaluation found Josh to have impaired strength and limited ROM in his forearm. Josh reported having difficulty turning his forearm to dress and shares that his arm does not feel strong enough to hold all of his school books.

Questions

1. What are three possible signs and symptoms of a distal radial fracture?
2. Approximately how long should a cast be worn for Josh's type of fracture?
3. What additional difficulties do you anticipate Josh may experience?
4. What client factors do you feel should be addressed first?
5. What tips can you give Josh regarding energy conservation and work simplification?

CASE STUDY 2

Ana is a 57-year-old woman who fractured her humerus in an MVA. She was taken to the emergency room (ER) where the physician conducted a clinical assessment and ordered x-rays to confirm the suspected fracture. The radiologist report confirmed that there was a closed transverse fracture of the middle third of the right humeral shaft. The physician was able to reduce the fracture without surgery. He immobilized the arm in a sling. Four weeks later, Ana still had significant pain and tenderness in her upper arm. Radiological tests revealed that the bone was forming a malunion. The physician determined that it was necessary to surgically reduce the fracture and stabilize it with internal fixation. Radiologic studies showed signs of healing 6 weeks after the second reduction as well as signs of osteopenia. The physician wrote a prescription for occupational therapy.

The occupational therapist evaluated Ana. He noted that she held her arm in a dependent position and was very hesitant to move it or let him examine it. She reported significant pain and had atrophy of her upper arm and forearm muscles. Her skin appeared shiny in comparison to her left arm. Ana had limited movement and reported that her husband had to help her with everything. She had been unable to return to work as an office manager because the pain was just too great.

RECOMMENDED READINGS AND RESOURCES

Books

Bonder, B. R., & Dal Bello-Haas, V. (2009). *Functional performance in older adults* (3rd ed.). Philadelphia, PA: F.A. Davis.

Skirven, T. M., Osterman, A. L., Fedorczyk, J. M., & Amadio, P. C. (2011). *Rehabilitation of the hand and upper extremity* (6th ed.). St. Louis, MO: Mosby.

Radomski, M. V., & Trombly-Latham, C. A. (2014). *Occupational therapy for physical dysfunction* (7th ed.). Philadelphia, PA: Lippincott Williams & Wilkins.

Journals

American Journal of Occupational Therapy
www.aota.org

American Journal of Orthopedics
http://www.amjorthopedics.com/

Journal of American Geriatrics Society
http://www.wiley.com/bw/journal.asp?ref=0002-8614&site=1

Orthopaedic Nursing
http://journals.lww.com/orthopaedicnursing/pages/default.aspx

Websites

American Occupational Therapy Association. Evidence-Based Practice & Research
http://www.aota.org/Educate/Research.aspx

Centers for Disease Control and Prevention
http://www.cdc.gov

Healthy People 2020
http://www.healthypeople.gov/hp2020/

Lewis, W. H. (Ed). *Gray's anatomy* (12th ed.). New York: Bartleby.com. Retrieved from http://www.bartleby.com/107

United States Department of Health & Human Services
http://www.hhs.gov/

Wheeless, C. R. (2015). *Wheeless' textbook of orthpaedics*. http://www.wheelessonline.com

REFERENCES

Adler, C. (2006). Spinal cord injury. In M. B. Early (Ed.), *Physical dysfunction practice skills for the occupational therapy assistant* (2nd ed., pp. 528–550). St. Louis, MO: Mosby.

Ahlborg, H., Rosengren, B., Jarvinen, T., Rogmark, C., Nilsson, J., Sernbo, I., & Karlsson, M. (2010). Prevalence of osteoporosis and incidence of hip fracture in women—Secular trends over 30 years. *BMC Musculoskeletal Disorders*, *11*(1), 48. doi:10.1186/1471-2474-11-48

Altizer, L. (2002). Fractures. *Orthopaedic Nursing*, *21*, 51–59.

American Academy of Pediatrics. (2000). Diagnostic imaging of child abuse. *Pediatrics*, *105*, 1345–1348. doi: 10.1542/peds.2009-0558

American Occupational Therapy Association. (2014). Occupational therapy practice framework: Domain and process (3rd ed). *American Journal of Occupational Therapy*, *68*(Suppl. 1), S1–S48. doi: 10.5014/ajot.2014.682006

Bade, M. J., Kohrt, W. M., & Stevens-Lapsley, J. E. (2010). Outcomes before and after total knee arthroplasty in health adults. *Journal of Orthopaedic & Sports Physical Therapy*, *40*(9), 559–567. http://www.jospt.org/. doi: 10.2519/jospt.2010.3317

Bell, A. J., Talbot-Stern J. K., & Hennessy A. (2000). Characteristics and outcomes of older patients presenting to the emergency department after a fall: A retrospective analysis. *eMedical Journal of Australia*,

173, 179–182. Retrieved from www.mja.com.au. *The Journal of Bone and Joint Surgery (American)*. 2007;89:476–486. doi:10.2106/JBJS.F.00412

Beloosesky, Y., Grinblat, J., Rivka, B., Epelboym, B., Weizz, A., Grosmann, B., & Hendell, D. (2002). Functional gain of hip fracture patients in different cognitive and functional groups. *Clinical Rehabilitation, 16*(3), 321–328. doi: 10.1191/0269215502cr497oa

Brunner, L. C., & Eshilian-Oates, L. (2003). Hip fractures in adults. *American Family Physician, 67*, 537–542.

Bruno-Petrina, A. (2008). Posttraumatic heterotopic ossification. *Emedicine*. Retrieved from http://emedicine.medscape.com/article/326242-overview

Centers for Disease Control and Prevention (CDC). (2013). *Arthritis: Morbidity and Mortality Weekly Report: Prevalence of doctor-diagnosed arthritis and arthritis-attributable activity limitations—United States, 2010–2012*. doi: 10.2337/dc12-0046. Retrieved from http://www.cdc.gov/mmwr/preveiw/mmwrhtml/mm6244al.html, August 28, 2015.

Centers for Disease Control and Prevention (CDC). (2015a). *Injury prevention and control: Home and recreational safety: Hip fractures among older adults*. Retrieved from http://www.cdc.gov/HomeandRecreationalSafety/Falls/adulthipfx.html, August 28, 2015.

Centers for Disease Control and Prevention (CDC). (2015b). *National hospital discharge survey. Inpatient surgery, 2010*. Retrieved from http://www.cdc.gov/nchs/fastats/inpatient-surgery.htm, August 28, 2015.

Chen, N. C., Huang, J. I., Trumble, T. E., & Jupiter, J. B. (2010). Fractures and malunions of the distal radius. In T. E. Trumble, G. M. Rayan, J. E. Budoff, & M. E. Baratz (Eds.), *Principles of hand surgery and therapy* (2nd ed., pp. 135–153). Philadelphia, PA: Saunders.

Chen, H. C., Yang, J. Y., Chuang, S. S., Huang, C. Y., & Yang, S. Y. (2009). Heterotopic ossification in burns: Our experience and literature reviews. *Burns, 35*(6), 857–862. doi: 10.1016/j.burns.2008.03.002

Chung, K. C., & Spilson, S. V. (2001). The frequency and epidemiology of hand and forearm fracture in the United States. *Journal of Hand Surgery, 26*(5), 908–915. http://dx.doi.org/10.1053/jhsu.2001.26322

Cooper, C. (2014). Hand impairments. In M. V. Radomski & C. A. Trombly Latham (Eds.), *Occupational therapy for physical dysfunction* (7th ed., pp. 1129–1160). Philadelphia, PA: Lippincott Williams & Wilkins.

Crottty, M., Unroe, K., Cameron, I. D., Miller, M., Ramirez, G., & Couzner, L. (2010). Rehabilitation interventions for improving physical and psychosocial functioning after hip fracture in older people. *Cochrane Database of Systematic Reviews, 1*, CD007624. doi: 10.1002/14651858

Dal Bello-Haas, V. (2009). Neuromusculoskeletal and movement function. In B. R. Bonder & V. Dal Bello-Haas (Eds.), *Functional performance in older adults* (pp. 130–176). Philadelphia, PA: F.A. Davis.

Dell, P. C., Dell, R. B. & Griggs, R. (2011). Management of carpal fractures and dislocations. In T. M. Skirven, L. Osterman, J. M. Fedorxzyk, & P. C. Amadio (Eds.), *Rehabilitation of the hand and upper extremity* (6th ed., pp. 988–1001). St. Louis, MO: Mosby.

Deshaies, L. (2006). Arthritis. In H. M. Pendleton & W.S. Krohn (Eds.), *Occupational therapy practice skills for physical dysfunction* (pp. 950–982). St. Louis, MO: Mosby.

Farahmand, B. Y., Michaelsson, K., Ahlbom, A., Ljunghall, S., & Baron, J. A. (2005). Swedish Hip Fracture Study Group. Survival after hip fracture. *Osteoporosis International, 16*(12), 1583–1590. doi: 10.1007/s00198-005-2024-z

Ganz, S. B., Levin, A., Peterson, M. G., & Ranawat, C. S. (2003). Improvement in driving reaction time after total hip arthroplasty. *Clinical Orthopaedics, 413*, 192–200. doi: 10.1097/01.blo.0000072468.32680.ff

Gill, M. (2002). Managing distal and humeral shaft fractures. *Journal of the National Association of Orthopedic Technologists, 4*, 1–4.

Gray, H. (2004). Bone. In W. H. Lewis (Ed). *Gray's anatomy* (12th ed). New York: Bartleby.com. Retrieved from http://www.bartleby.com/107

Hagsten, B., Svensson, O., & Gardulf, A. (2004). Early individualized postoperative occupational therapy training in 100 patients improves ADL after hip fracture. *Acta Orthopaedica, 75*, 177–183. http://dx.doi.org/10.1080/00016470412331294435

Healthy People 2010. (2010). *Arthritis, osteoporosis, and chronic back conditions*. Retrieved from www.healthypeople.gov/document/html/volume1/02arthritis.htm, July 26, 2010.

Holt, G., Smith, R., Duncan, K., & McKeown, D. W. (2010). Does delay to theatre for medical reasons affect the peri-operative mortality in patients with a fracture of the hip? *Journal of Bone and Joint Surgery (British), 92*(6), 835–841. doi: 10.1302/0301-620X.92B6.24463

Jeon, I., Oh, C., Park, B, Ihn, J., & Kim, P. (2003). Minimal invasive percutaneous Herbert screw fixation in acute unstable scaphoid fracture. *Hand Surgery, 8*, 213–218. doi: 10.1142/S0218810403001807

Kare, J. A. (2008). Volkmann contracture. *Emedicine*. Retrieved from http://www.emedicine.com/orthoped/topic578.htm

Khosla, S., & Melton, J. (2007). Osteopenia. *The New England Journal of Medicine, 356*(22), 2293–2300. doi: 10.1056/NEJMcp070341

Klein, M., Logsetty, S., & Costa, B. (2007). Extended time to wound closure is associated with increased risk of heterotopic ossification of the elbow. *Journal of Burn Care & Research, 28,* 447–450. doi: 10.1097/BCR.0B013E318053D378

Kocic, M., Lazovic, M., Mitkovic, M., & Djokic, B. (2010). Clinical significance of the heterotopic ossification after total hip arthroplasty. *Orthopedics, 33,* 16. doi: 10.3928/01477447-20091124-13

Kunkler, C. E. (2002). Fractures. In A. B. Maher, S. W. Salmond, & T. A. Pellino (Eds.), *Orthopedic nursing.* Philadelphia, PA: Saunders.

Lawrence, R. C., Felson, D. T., Helmick, C. G., Arnold, L. M., Choi, H., Deyo, R. A., ... Wolfe, F. (2008). Estimates of the prevalence of arthritis and other rheumatic conditions in the United States: Part II. *Arthritis and Rheumatism, 58*(1), 26–35. doi: 10.1002/art.23176

Li, Z., Smith, B. P., Tuohy, C., Smith, T. L., & Koman, L. A. (2010). Complex regional pain syndrome after hand surgery. *Hand Clinics, 26*(2), 281–289. doi: 10.1016/j.hcl.2009.11.001

Lowe, J. A., Crist, B. D., Bhandari, M., & Ferguson, T. A. (2010). Optimal treatment of femoral neck fractures according to patient's physiologic age: An evidence-based review. *Orthopedic Clinics of North America, 41*(2), 157–166. doi: 10.1016/j.ocl.2010.01.001

Maher, C. (2014). Orthopaedic conditions. In M. V. Radomski & C. A. Trombly Latham (Eds.), *Occupational therapy for physical dysfunction* (7th ed.). Philadelphia, PA: Lippincott Williams & Wilkins.

Michlovitz, S., Festa, L., (2011). Therapist's management of distal radius fractures. In T. M. Skirven, L. Osterman, J. M. Fedorczyk, & P. C. Amadio (Eds.). *Rehabilitation of the hand and upper extremity* (6th ed., pp. 949–962). St. Louis, MO: Mosby.

Mizner, R. L., Petterson, S. C., & Snyder-Mackler, L. (2005). Quadriceps strength and the time course of functional recovery after total knee arthroplasty. *Journal of Orthopaedic & Sports Physical Therapy, 35*(7), 424–436. doi: 10.2519/jospt.2005.35.7.424

Moore, D. S., & Cho, G. (2010). Heterotopic ossification. *eMedicine.* Retrieved from http://emedicine.medscape.com/article/390416-overview

National Center for Injury Prevention and Control. (2004). *Falls and hip fractures among older adults.* Retrieved from http://www.cdc.gov/NCIPC/factsheets/falls

National Institute of Arthritis and Musculoskeletal and Skin Diseases. (2009, April). *Arthritis.* NIH Publication No. 09–5149. Retrieved from http://www.cdc.gov/nchs/fastats/inpatient-surgery.htm

National Osteoporosis Foundation. (2010). *Fast facts on osteoporosis.* Retrieved from http://www.nof.org/osteoporosis/diseasefacts.htm, August 16, 2010.

Nguyen, N. D., Eisman, J. A., Center, J. R., & Nguyen, T. V. (2007). Risk factors for fracture in nonosteoporotic men and women. *The Journal of Clinical Endocrinology & Metabolism, 92*(3), 955–962. doi: 10.2519/jospt.2005.35.7.424

Peak, E., Parvizi, J., Ciminiello, M., Purtill, J. J., Sharkey, P. F., Hozack, W. J., & Rothman, R. H. (2005). The role of patient restrictions in reducing the prevalence of early dislocation following total hip arthroplasty. A randomized, prospective study. *Journal of Bone and Joint Surgery (American Volume), 87*(2), 247–253. doi: 10.2106/JBJS.C.01513

Potter, B., Burns, T., Lacap, A., Granville, R., & Gajewski, D. (2007). Heterotopic ossification following traumatic and combat-related amputations prevalence, risk factors, and preliminary results of excision. *Journal of Bone and Joint Surgery (American), 89,* 476–486. doi: 10.2106/JBJS.F.00412

Rasul, A. T., & Wright, J. (2010). Total joint replacement rehabilitation. *eMedicine.* Retrieved from http://emedicine.medscape.com/article/320061-overview, September 17, 2010.

Roberts, D. (2002). Degenerative disorders. In A. B. Maher, S. W. Salmond, & T. A. Pellino (Eds.), *Orthopedic nursing.* Philadelphia, PA: Saunders.

Scheffer A. C., Schuurmans, M. J., VanDijk, N., & VanDerHoof, T. (2008). Fear of falling: Measurement strategy, prevalence, risk factors and consequences among older persons. *Age and Ageing, 37,* 19–24. doi: 10.1093/ageing/afm169

Sendher, R., & Ladd, A. L. (2013). The scaphoid. *Orthopedic Clinics of North America, 44*(1), 107–120. doi: 10.1016/j.od2012.09.003

Stevens, J. A., & Olson, S. (2000). *Reducing falls and resulting hip fractures among older women.* National Center for Injury Prevention and Control. Retrieved from http://www.cdc.gov/mmwr/preview/mmwrhtml/rr4902a2.htm

United States Department of Health & Human Services. (2004). *Public Health Service, Office of the Surgeon General. Bone health and osteoporosis: A report of the surgeon general* (p. 436). Rockville, MD: US GPO. Retrieved from http://www.ncbi.nlm.nih.gov/books/NBK45513?pdf?TOC.pdf

United States Department of Health & Human Services. (2005). *Osteonecrosis, osteoporosis, and osteopenia.* Retrieved from http://www.aidsinfo.nih.gov/ContentFiles/OsteonecrosisOsteoporosisOsteopenia_FS_en.pdf, September 16, 2010.

Wheeless, C. R. (2015a). Fractures of the humerus. *Wheeless' textbook of orthpaedics.* Retrieved from http://www.wheelessonline.com

Wheeless, C. R. (2015b). Heterotropic ossification. *Wheeless' textbook of orthopaedics.* Retrieved from http://www.wheelessonline.com

26 Low Vision Disorders

Diane Powers Dirette

KEY TERMS

Age-related macular
  degeneration
Angle-closure glaucoma
Aqueous humor
Cataracts
Central scotomas
Central vision
Contrast sensitivity
Glare sensitivity
Intraocular pressure
Neovascular glaucoma
Macula
Metamorphopsia
Myopia
Opacifications
Open-angle glaucoma
Peripheral vision
Retina
Trabecular meshwork

George was leading a leisurely retirement and enjoying the time he had to kick back and do all the things he couldn't do while he was working. He was finally able to spend time fishing at his cottage and taking care of his grandkids when his daughter needed his help. George knew his vision wasn't what it used to be, but he started using reading glasses and felt like he was getting by. One day while driving home from the store, he stopped at a four-way intersection and then drove straight into the side of a car that had stopped before him. Luckily no one was hurt, but after that, his daughter insisted that he see an ophthalmologist who diagnosed him with a low vision disorder called age-related macular degeneration. George was devastated. He feared he would become blind and lose his ability to live alone.

Low vision disorders are progressive diseases that lead to chronic loss of sight and limit everyday function. Low vision disorders are one of the most common causes of disability in United States of America with an estimated 3 million people 40 years and older affected (Rosenberg & Sperazza, 2008). It is estimated that 80% of the population of people with low vision is over age 65 years (Massof, 2002). Because of the aging of the population, the number of people with low vision disorders is expected to continue to increase with projected estimations of 5.5 million people in the United States by the year 2020 (Rosenberg & Sperazza, 2008).

In the United States, the three most common causes of low vision for people who are over 40 years old are macular degeneration, glaucoma, and cataracts (Rosenberg & Sperazza, 2008). Because of the prevalence of these diagnoses, most occupational therapists (OTs) will work with people who have one of these conditions as either a primary or a secondary diagnosis. Diabetic retinopathy is also a common low vision disorder, but that condition will be covered in the Diabetes chapter in this textbook.

Low vision is the third most common cause of impaired function in people who are older than 70 years (Rosenberg & Sperazza, 2008). Low vision disorders not only limit a person's ability to function independently but also increase the risk of depression, social isolation, fall injuries, and a general decline in overall health (Rosenberg & Sperazza, 2008). There is also a fear of blindness among people with low vision. Blindness is one of the most feared diseases in the United States (Burack-Weiss, 1992).

Macular Degeneration

■ Description and Definitions

Age-related macular degeneration (AMD) is a low vision disorder that results from loss of function of the **macula**, the center of the **retina** (Bressler & Gills, 2000; Lim, Mitchell, Seddon, Holz, & Wong, 2012). There are two types of AMD including dry AMD (atrophic/geographic atrophy) and wet AMD (neovascular/exudative) (Lim et al.). Dry AMD is progressive atrophy of the retinal pigment epithelium, choriocapillaris,

and photoreceptors in the macula. Wet AMD is an ingrowth of new blood vessels that break through the neural retina and leak fluid, lipids, and blood into the subretinal space leading to fibrous scarring (Chong et al., 2008; Hirami et al., 2009) (see Fig. 26.1).

AMD is also classified as either early or late. Early AMD is the beginning signs that the disease is developing and late AMD is when the disease has progressed to the macula (Chong et al., 2009). In early AMD, the retina is unhealthy and predisposed to visually threatening complications or late AMD (see Fig. 26.2).

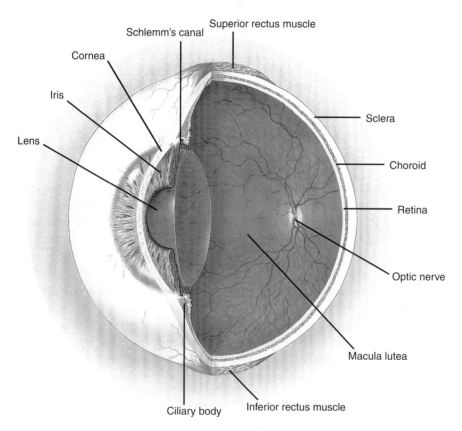

Figure 26.1 Anatomy of the eye. (From Anatomical Chart Co.)

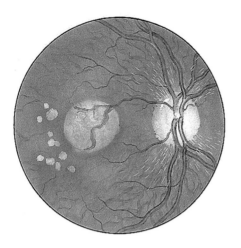

Figure 26.2 Macular degeneration. (From Anatomical Chart Co.)

Etiology

Research indicates that the cause of AMD is probably a combination of genetic and environmental factors (Chong et al., 2009; Wang et al., 2008). The complement factor H gene and gene variants BF and C2 have been associated with higher rates of AMD (Wang et al., 2008). Several other genes may also be involved including vascular endothelial growth factor (Lim et al., 2012). Genetic susceptibility, however, can be modified by altering environmental influences that are linked to the development of AMD.

Many environmental factors including smoking; obesity; dietary intake low in vitamins A, D, E, zinc, lutein, and omega-3 fatty acids; and ultraviolet light exposure are linked to the development of AMD (Goodman, Parmet, Lynm, & Livingston, 2012; Lim et al., 2012). Cigarette smoking has been found to trigger or promote the development of AMD or contribute significantly to higher risks for AMD (Wang et al., 2008). Diets high in red meat consumption are associated with early AMD (Chong et al., 2009), and diets high in fish consumption are associated with decreased risk for late AMD (Montgomery et al., 2010; Wang et al., 2008). An unhealthy lifestyle that results in cardiovascular problems, such as hypertension, is also associated with AMD. Long-term, regular use of aspirin is significantly associated with an increased risk of wet AMD (Klein et al., 2012). Ocular risk factors include darker iris pigmentation, cataract surgery, and hyperopic refraction (Lim et al.).

Incidence and Prevalence

AMD is the leading cause of severe vision loss for people older than 50 years in the United States and other developed countries (Friedman et al., 2004) and is the leading cause of vision loss worldwide (Lim et al., 2012). The prevalence of AMD increases with age with 2% prevalence among people 40 years of age and as many as 25% of people by age 80 years (Ambati & Fowler, 2012). Current studies find that AMD is more prevalent in Caucasian and Asian populations. Because the population is continuing to age, the incidence of AMD is increasing with an expected increase to 3 million cases of late AMD in the United States by the year 2020. Dry AMD accounts for 80% of AMD cases in Western countries, whereas other parts of the world have higher incidence of wet AMD (e.g., Japan) (Hirami et al., 2009).

Signs and Symptoms

The primary symptom of wet AMD is acute loss of **central vision** that becomes permanent as the retina atrophies and is replaced by fibrous tissue. Wet AMD usually results in rapid loss of central vision. Dry AMD can also result in the loss of central vision, but the progression is much slower taking years to develop. Initially, a person with AMD may be asymptomatic (Lim et al., 2012). Over time, loss of visual acuity for discrimination of details, **metamorphopsia** (distortion of objects), **central scotomas** (dark patches), increased **glare sensitivity**, decreased **contrast sensitivity,** and decreased color vision can develop (Rosenberg & Sperazza, 2008).

Although the loss of vision can be profound and greatly impair function, people with AMD frequently do not notice the symptoms in the early stages. The visual loss does not result in black or white spots but is spotty loss that is filled in by the surrounding vision that is still intact (Table 26.1).

Course and Prognosis

The course of AMD varies from person to person. Dry AMD does not always advance into wet AMD, but wet AMD always is preceded by dry AMD and therefore, dry AMD is considered a risk factor for wet AMD (Ambati & Fowler, 2012). The timeline for the progression of dry or wet AMD is variable. Some people have dry AMD for years before it develops into wet AMD and others develop wet AMD right away (Mogk & Mogk, 2003).

TABLE 26.1 Signs and Symptoms of Low Vision Disorders

Macular Degeneration	Glaucoma	Cataracts
Acute loss of central vision	Slow loss of peripheral vision	Decreased visual acuity
Loss of visual acuity	Decreased ability to see in dim light	Cloudy, blurry, or foggy vision
Metamorphopsia (distortion of objects)	Decreased contrast sensitivity	Decreased contrast sensitivity
Central scotomas	Poor adaptation to changes in lighting	Increased glare sensitivity
Increased glare sensitivity	Increased glare sensitivity	Nearsightedness (myopia)
Decreased contrast sensitivity	Blurred vision	Decreased color perception especially to blue hues
Decreased color vision	Decreased depth perception	
	Ocular pain	
	Eventual loss of central vision	

Overall, 1% of people with early AMD will progress to late AMD each year (Lim et al., 2012). So, in 5 years, 5% of people with early AMD will progress to late AMD and in 15 years, 15% of those people will progress from early AMD to late AMD.

The prognosis for loss of central vision due to AMD also varies. For some people, loss of central vision will proceed rapidly and others will have AMD for years and still maintain a functional level of central vision (Mogk & Mogk, 2003). Wet AMD progresses much more rapidly than does dry AMD (Ambati & Fowler, 2012). Regardless of the speed of progression, AMD does not cause total blindness. AMD results in loss of central vision, but it does not affect **peripheral vision**. Therefore, the person will retain peripheral vision even if he or she has late AMD.

Diagnosis

An Amsler grid test may be used initially by an eye doctor to screen for signs of AMD, but diagnosis relies on more invasive tests (Goodman et al., 2012). The diagnosis of AMD is made through examination by an ophthalmoscope. In early AMD, the formation of drusen, small yellow deposits in the center of the retina, can be seen when the pupil is dilated (Bressler & Gills, 2000; Lim et al., 2012). In dry AMD, the pigmented layer of the retina slowly atrophies.

In wet AMD, abnormal new blood vessels in the choroidal layer of the eye that nourishes the outer retina grow and proliferate with fibrous tissue within the drusen material are detected through fundus fluorescein angiography, an examination of the vascular system of the eye using an intravenous injection of yellow dye. The bleeding accumulates within and beneath the retina, and the retina atrophies or becomes replaced with fibrous tissue.

Medical/Surgical Management

There is no medical treatment for early dry AMD. There are two medications that have been developed in the last several years, however, that aid in the prevention of vision loss due to wet AMD and even lead to the improvement of vision in some cases (Lim et al., 2012). Those medications are ranibizumab and bevacizumab. Both medications work to suppress the vascular endothelial growth factor and are delivered through intravitreal injections usually on a monthly basis (Lim et al., Martin, et al., 2011). In countries where these medications are used routinely, there has been a significant reduction in legal blindness due to AMD (Cheung & Wong, 2013). Bevacizumab (Avastin, Genentech), although developed for the treatment of colon cancer, is also used as it is related to the medication ranibizumab. Aflibercept was also recently approved for the treatment of wet AMD, but it has not been widely adopted (Cheung & Wong, 2013). In addition, high-dose regimens of zinc and antioxidants (vitamin C, vitamin E, and beta-carotene) are recommended (Rosenberg & Sperazza, 2008). Lipid-lowering drugs such as statins have been tested as a treatment for AMD but have not been found to be effective in the treatment or prevention of AMD (Chuo, Wiens, Etminan, & Maberley, 2007).

Laser treatments are used for wet AMD to burn the area of the retina with neovascularization and photodynamic therapy, which uses the drug verteporfin with the laser treatment to selectively destroy lesions (Bressler & Gills, 2000; Goodman et al., 2012). This treatment is usually repeated every 3 or 4 months to prevent growth of blood vessels.

In addition to medical treatments, people with AMD are assessed for impairments in mobility and activities of daily living with a referral to physical therapy or occupational therapy if necessary. They may also benefit from psychological evaluation for anxiety or depression as persons with AMD have been found to have significant emotional distress and profoundly reduced quality of life (Rosenberg & Sperazza, 2008; Williams, Brody, Thomas, Kaplan, & Brown, 1998).

GLAUCOMA

◾ Description and Definitions

Glaucoma is a group of conditions with differing causes that result in damage to the optic nerve head (King, Azuara-Blanco, & Tuulonen, 2013). This low vision disorder is characterized by progressive loss of the ganglion cell layer of the retina usually caused by increased **intraocular pressure** (IOP) (Rosenberg & Sperazza, 2008; Wittstrom et al., 2010). Recent findings, however, reveal that 20% to 52% of people with glaucoma have IOP that measures within the normal range (King et al.).

Three types of glaucoma include **open-angle glaucoma**, **angle-closure glaucoma**, and **neovascular glaucoma**. Angle-closure glaucoma is the obstruction by the iris to the outflow pathway of **aqueous humor** through the trabecular network at the angle between the peripheral cornea and the iris (King et al., 2013; Subak-Sharpe, Low, Nolan, & Foster, 2009). In **open-angle glaucoma**, there is not an obstruction of the aqueous humor, but the damage to the retina is caused by increased IOP. **Neovascular glaucoma** is a secondary disorder that results from other diseases, such as diabetes mellitus or tumors, which cause new blood vessels to grow and obstruct the outflow of aqueous humor (Shazly & Latina, 2009). See Figure 26.3.

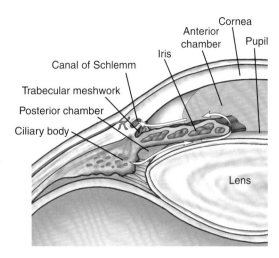

Figure 26.3 Path of aqueous flow. (From Porth, C. (2014). *Essentials of pathophysiology* (4th ed.). Philadelphia, PA: Lippincott Williams & Wilkins.)

◾ Etiology

As with AMD, glaucoma is thought to be caused by a combination of genetic and environmental factors. A family history of glaucoma increases a person's chances of developing the disease (Hollands et al., 2013). Although several genes have been identified in relation to glaucoma, they account for only a small portion of cases (Leske, 2007). Other factors that may contribute to glaucoma include abnormal blood pressure, diabetes, cataracts, myopia, and hypothyroidism (King et al., 2013; McDaniel & Besada, 1996; Subak-Sharpe et al., 2009).

Several pharmacological interventions have also been linked to angle-closure glaucoma (Subak-Sharpe et al., 2009). Bronchodilators, antidepressants, anticholinergics (used for overactive bladder), antihistamines, botulinum toxin, and sildenafil (Viagra) are all pharmaceuticals that have been linked to angle-closure glaucoma. Also, recreational drug use of cocaine and ecstasy has been shown to cause angle-closure glaucoma.

◾ Incidence and Prevalence

Glaucoma is the second most common cause of blindness worldwide accounting for 4.5 million people or 12% of cases, but it is the leading cause of blindness among people of African descent accounting for 32% of cases (Hollands et al., 2013; Leske, 2007; Lin & Yang, 2009). As of 2010, glaucoma accounted for 2% of cases of visual impairment and 8% of cases of blindness globally (King et al., 2013). It is uncommon in people under the age of 20 years with fewer than 3 per 100,000 in the United States for all forms of glaucoma (Quigley, 2011).

Open-angle glaucoma is the most common form of glaucoma in Western cultures, but angle-closure glaucoma accounts for 50% of blindness worldwide and is more common in Asian populations (Leske, 2007; Subak-Sharpe et al., 2009). Although variation is noted, most studies report higher incidence and prevalence of glaucoma in men than in women (Leske, 2007) and higher incidence and prevalence in people of African descent (Rosenberg & Sperazza, 2008).

There is a marked increase in the prevalence of glaucoma among people older than 40 years with an overall prevalence of 0.3%. Prevalence increases to 3.3% in people older than 70 years. Because of aging populations, the incidence of glaucoma is expected to rise (King et al., 2013). Variations in the prevalence of open-angle glaucoma among people older than 40 years can be seen throughout the world with estimates of 1% to 5% in the United States, 1% to 3% in Europe, 1% to 4% in Asia, 1% to 8% in Africa, and 2% to 3% in Australia (Leske, 2007). The highest prevalence is in the Caribbean with 7% to 9%. Most people in the Caribbean have ancestry linked to West Africa where open-angle glaucoma is very common.

Signs and Symptoms

Open-angle glaucoma begins with a slow loss of peripheral vision that can eventually lead to loss of central vision (King et al., 2013; Rosenberg & Sperazza, 2008). Other symptoms include decreased ability to see in dim light, decreased contrast sensitivity, poor adaptation to changes in lighting, sensitivity to glare, blurred vision, and decreased depth perception (Lin & Yang, 2009). In the early stages, however, many of these symptoms may not occur or may develop so gradually that people are not aware of their condition (Beleforte et al., 2010; Quigley, 2011). By the time visual loss appears, there is usually already significant and permanent damage.

The symptoms of closed-angle and neovascular glaucoma, however, may have a more rapid onset. The symptoms include significant ocular pain, headache, nausea, vomiting, and loss of or blurred vision. As many as 75% of people with closed-angle glaucoma may not have an acute attack but remain asymptomatic or have such gradual loss of peripheral vision that the symptoms are unnoticed until the disease has progressed significantly (Quigley, 2011).

Course and Prognosis

Angle-closure glaucoma has three stages. The first stage is marked by contact between the peripheral iris and the **trabecular meshwork**. This progresses to the formation of adhesions, which cause increased IOP. If not treated, this may progress to cause glaucomatous optic neuropathy, which causes significant functional impairment of the vision (Subak-Sharpe et al., 2009). Open-angle glaucoma tends to progress at a slower rate and the patient may not notice that he or she has lost vision until the disease has progressed significantly (King et al., 2013). Neovascular glaucoma begins when a fibrovascular membrane initially obstructs aqueous outflow in an open-angle fashion and later contracts to produce secondary angle-closure glaucoma (Shazly & Latina, 2009).

If left untreated, glaucoma will lead to blindness. If treated, however, people with glaucoma usually retain some level of functional vision for their whole life (Ang & Eke, 2007). In developed countries, 3% to 12% of people with glaucoma are blind in one or both eyes (King et al., 2013).

Diagnosis

Early diagnosis and treatment are important to prevent vision loss. Diagnosis of open-angle glaucoma is based on visual field defects, disc defects, and abnormally increased IOP (Hollands et al., 2013; King et al., 2013; Sonnsjo & Krakau, 1993). There is some debate about the use of IOP in the diagnosis of glaucoma because this increase is not always seen (Heijl, 2015; Hollands et al.; Leske, 2007; Quigley, 2011). When increase IOP is detected, however, it is used to aid in the diagnosis. Angle-closure glaucoma is diagnosed using gonioscopy or other screening techniques to examine the anterior chamber angle for contacts or adhesions (Subak-Sharpe et al., 2009). Neovascular glaucoma is diagnosed through the detection of new blood vessels in the iris, a closed anterior chamber angle, and high IOP (Shazly & Latina, 2009).

Medical/Surgical Management

Glaucoma is treated with topical ocular medications, such as eye drops, oral medications, laser therapy, and surgery. The first line of treatment is usually glaucoma drop monotherapy with different types of drops added to the regime as needed to control IOP.

A trabeculectomy, the removal of part of the trabecular meshwork, is the most common surgical procedure used to reduce IOP. Glaucoma filtration surgery may also be used to decrease IOP pressure in open-angle glaucoma (Wittstrom et al., 2010). Laser surgery, such as a goniopuncture, may be used to perforate the trabecular meshwork to increase aqueous flow (King et al., 2013).

For angle-closure glaucoma, surgical procedures may include an iridotomy or an iridoplasty (King et al., 2013; Subak-Sharpe et al., 2009). An iridotomy is a procedure in which a laser is used to create a hole in the iris to allow for drainage of the aqueous humor and an iridoplasty is a procedure in which a laser is applied to the peripheral iris to remove adhesions to the trabecular meshwork and open the angle. Cataract surgery to allow the iris to move away from the drainage pathway may also be used (King et al.). Topical ocular medications may be given to constrict the pupil and thus pull the peripheral iris away from the trabecular meshwork. Oral medications may also be given to reduce IOP for all types of glaucoma.

Future treatments that are currently being explored are intraocular implants to deliver medication, therapeutic treatments that provide neuroprotection for the retinal ganglion cells, stem cells or gene transfer to improve trabecular meshwork outflow and reduce IOP, and stem cell transplants for retinal ganglion cell regeneration (King et al., 2013; Quigley, 2011).

Cataracts

■ Description and Definitions

Cataracts are **opacifications** of the crystalline lens of the eye, which result in a decreased amount of light reaching the retina. Cataracts are made up of broken proteins that stick together and form sheathlike obstructions in the lens (Armitage, 2015). The incoming light is scattered, and visual acuity is decreased. While there are some variant cataract conditions such as congenital cataracts due to rubella, the focus of this chapter will be on the most common type, age-related cataracts (see Fig. 26.4).

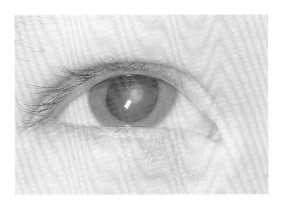

Figure 26.4 Cataract. (From Dudek, R. W. (2013). *High-yield embryology*. Philadelphia, PA: Lippincott Williams & Wilkins.)

■ Etiology

As with other low vision disorders, the cause of cataracts is a combination of factors. Risk factors for the development of cataracts include aging, cigarette smoking, ocular UVB and radiation exposure, drug use, systemic diseases (e.g., diabetes), and dietary nutritional intake with increasing age being the strongest risk factor by far (Rosenberg & Sperazza, 2008). Some of the drugs associated with increased cataract risk are corticosteroids, antipsychotics, chemotherapy agents, cholesterol-lowering medications, and tranquilizers. Heavy alcohol consumption has been labeled a risk factor for the development of cataracts, but recent meta-analyses refute that claim (Wang & Zhang, 2014). The use of statins has been disputed as either increasing or decreasing the risk of cataracts, but recent research has not found any evidence of statins being effective for reducing the risk of cataracts and may actually contribute to the problem (Hoster, 2013). Those studies, however, are confounded by high levels of bad cholesterol from a poor diet, and researchers continue to recommend increased consumption of fruits and vegetables to reduce risks.

Meat consumption when compared to the vegetarian or vegan diets is associated with increased risk for cataracts (Appleby, Allen, & Key, 2011). Lutein (found in dark green leafy vegetables and eggs), vitamin C, and vitamin E intake have shown some associations with reduced risks for the development of cataracts (Lyle, Mares-Perlman, Klein, Klein, & Greger, 1999). Iodine deficiency and injuries to the lens are also risk factors for cataracts.

Incidence and Prevalence

Cataracts are the third leading cause of blindness in the United States, accounting for about 9% of all cases (Sperduto, 1994), and are a leading cause of blindness worldwide (Wang & Zhang, 2014). Nearly 17.2% of Americans over age 40 years are diagnosed with cataracts (Armitage, 2015). They are more prevalent among females than males and are more prevalent among people of African descent (Rosenberg & Sperazza, 2008; Sperduto, 1994). Cataracts also vary in prevalence among different age groups with approximately 4% of people aged 52 to 64 years, 28% of people aged 65 to 74 years, and 46% of people aged 75 to 85 years.

As the population ages, the number of people worldwide who will be blind due to cataracts is expected to increase dramatically over the next few decades (Sperduto, 1994). The number of people who are blind due to cataracts could reach close to 40 million by the year 2025. As the ozone layer is depleted, there is an increase in ultraviolet radiation and this is expected to also increase the incidence of cataracts worldwide.

Signs and Symptoms

Decreased visual acuity, decreased contrast sensitivity, glare disability, nearsightedness (**myopia**), and decreased color perception especially to blue hues are all common symptoms of cataracts (Rosenberg & Sperazza, 2008). Complaints of cloudy, blurry, or foggy vision are often noted. The vision of people with cataracts is sometimes described as viewing the world through a steamy glass (Armitage, 2015). Some people may experience temporary improvement in near acuity as the shape of the lens is changed by the cataract.

Course and Prognosis

When a person is young, the lens is transparent and incoming light has no difficulty reaching the retina. Over time, however, the lens becomes less transparent as a cloudy, opaque cataract develops in the lens. One eye is usually affected earlier than the other, but eventually, both eyes are usually involved. If left untreated, cataracts may lead to blindness or develop into other eye diseases such as AMD or glaucoma (Rosenberg & Sperazza, 2008).

Diagnosis

A diagnosis of cataracts is done using pupil dilation, acuity charts, and tonometry. Tonometry is done to examine ocular fluid pressure inside the eye. Some cataracts can be detected with a visual examination that reveals a cloudy lens, but pupil dilation is done to further examine the back of the eye.

Medical/Surgical Management

Initially, the cataracts may be managed by prescription lenses, tobacco cessation, and UV protection, but the only medical treatment for cataracts is the surgical removal of the lens by either laser or scalpel (Armitage, 2015). When the cataract has advanced to a stage that it interferes with a person's ability to function, surgery is performed to remove the molecular grout that builds up in the eye (Armitage, 2015; Sperduto, 1994). Sometimes the lens is replaced. Research is currently being conducted that aims to develop a steroid-based eye drop that could dissolve cataracts (Armitage, 2015).

IMPACT OF CONDITIONS ON OCCUPATIONAL PERFORMANCE

Visual function is the client factor that is impaired in low vision disorders. The extent of the impact on occupational performance depends on the type of low vision disorder, the stage of progression of that disorder, and the treatment that has been received. Loss of central vision is the main concern for people with AMD and cataracts, and loss of peripheral vision is the main concern for people with glaucoma. For most people, cataracts will be surgically removed when they interfere with the person's ability to function. There are standardized assessments, such as the Impact of Vision Impairment Scale and the Visual Function Questionnaire, that may be useful to help therapists ascertain the impact of a person's visual loss on occupational performance (Lamoureux et al., 2008; Magacho et al., 2004).

Activities of Daily Living

Because of the loss of central vision, the self-care skills that require visual acuity are most affected by AMD and cataracts (Lim et al., 2012). These include skills such as make-up application, dental care, nail care, and shaving. Reading and inability to recognize faces are common problems (Bennion, Shaw, & Gibson, 2012). Management of medications may be difficult due to difficulty reading labels and identifying various medications. Eating may also be visually challenging in advanced stages of the disorders.

Safety during functional mobility is a concern for all low vision disorders. The loss of central vision in AMD and cataracts and the loss of peripheral vision in glaucoma can impact a person's ability to safely navigate both within and outside the home (Wu et al., 2010). Within the home, entryways and stairs are especially difficult particularly at night. Adaptations, such as increased lighting, railings, and visual contrasts, may need to be made to increase safety. Outside the home, unfamiliar places may pose challenges for both locating points of interest and negotiating varying surfaces.

Instrumental Activities of Daily Living

Driving is impacted by all low vision disorders (King et al., 2013). Because driving represents independence for most people, it can also be the most difficult occupation to address. In addition, driving is necessary for most other instrumental activities of daily living (IADLs) such as shopping, going to the post office, and making appointments (Bennion et al., 2012).

Home management including cleaning, doing laundry, making home repairs, and maintaining a yard can all be impacted by low vision disorders. Being able to perform meal preparation accurately and safely is also a concern as loss of visual acuity will interfere with seeing food items, utensils (e.g., knives, measuring spoons, measuring cups), appliance settings, and recipes.

Money management for reading bills, paying bills, keeping records, and identifying and handling money can all be impacted by a loss of central vision. Large-print electronic systems may be useful for assisting with money management.

Education

Because all of these low vision disorders are likely to be age related, most people with these disorders will have completed their formal education. If participation in education is still essential, functional mobility and reading may interfere with successful completion of education-related occupations.

Work

The age of retirement has progressively increased, and therefore, the person may still be involved in work occupations when low vision disorders progress to the point that they interfere with function. Depending on the area of work in which the person participates, visual deficits in central and peripheral vision can impact the person's ability to successfully complete work tasks. Work-related activities such as reading, working on the computer, using the telephone, working on an assembly line, and driving can all be impaired by visual deficits.

Play and Leisure

Many leisure activities can be affected by low vision disorders. Many people with low vision disorders are retired and fill their time with leisure activities. In addition, these leisure activities may be part of the person's identity providing life purpose and satisfaction. Painting, knitting, sewing, gardening, playing games, completing puzzles, watching television, reading, and participating in sports are just some of the many leisure activities that may be difficult for a person with a low vision disorder.

Social Participation

Low vision disorders can impact social function in many ways. People with AMD frequently complain about difficulty recognizing faces, which may lead to feelings of humiliation and embarrassment in social situations. People with low vision disorders may also have difficulty negotiating crowded places such as concerts, restaurants, and ceremonies. In restaurants, they may have difficulty reading the menu in addition to navigating the physical layout. They may become distressed if they collide with people or objects. All of these factors may lead the person into a life with more isolation. The combination of the loss of independence and anxiety about the ability to function in social situations can often lead to depression (Bennion et al., 2012). When people become depressed, they are less likely to pursue social contact and a cycle of isolation and depression can be worsened.

CASE STUDY 1

Maria is a 72-year-old woman who has been referred to occupational therapy due to vision loss. Maria was diagnosed with wet age-related macular degeneration 2 years ago and is having difficulty functioning in her home. The recent death of her husband, who was able to help her in the home, has left her trying to find ways to manage on her own. She has two children. Her daughter lives about 1 hour away with her three children, and her son lives about 2 hours away in a large urban area. Her children are reportedly concerned that she is no longer safe to live independently.

Maria worked for many years as a legal assistant until she retired at age 62. Since then, she has been enjoying traveling with her husband, spending time with her grandchildren, and participating in various leisure activities, such as knitting, reading, gardening, and playing mahjong. She was once an avid tennis player but had to stop playing due to her vision loss.

Maria now lives alone in a four-bedroom, split-level home and would like to remain there for as long as possible. She is having difficulty accepting the fact that driving is dangerous for her and she tries to get by using a GPS. She also gets embarrassed when she doesn't recognize people, so she has started to avoid social situations where she is expected to interact with people who don't know about her vision loss.

Maria has been getting monthly injections of ranibizumab since she was diagnosed, but because they don't improve her vision, she has difficulty understanding why she needs more treatments. She is also taking high doses of zinc, vitamin C, vitamin E, and beta-carotene, but she states that sometimes she is not sure if she has taken the right pills. She has been referred to occupational therapy for evaluation and treatment. Her primary goal is to maintain her current lifestyle as long as possible.

CASE STUDY 2

Bob is known among his friends as Bob the Builder. He retired from his job as a site manager 10 years ago but has been busier than ever helping his friends with home improvement projects. Bob's wife says he is so busy helping their friends that he never has time to get to their own home improvement needs. Bob and his wife, Sharon, live in a four-bedroom century-old farmhouse that they have been fixing up since they moved in 10 years ago. Their home is on a 40-acre lot, but they rent out the land to a local farmer.

Bob and Sharon have been married for 15 years. They don't have children of their own, but both have children from previous marriages. All of their four children live within an hour of them and they have seven grandchildren between them.

Last year, Bob went to his eye doctor for a routine checkup. It had been about 5 years since his last checkup. His kids were teasing him about his outdated glasses and he decided to get a new style. Bob hadn't noticed any significant changes in his vision. He knew he was having some difficulty seeing when it was dim lighting, but he thought this was just due to his eyes getting older. He was very surprised when the eye doctor told him that he suspected that he had glaucoma.

The eye doctor referred him to a specialist who confirmed the diagnosis. The ophthalmologist explained that he had what is called open-angle glaucoma and showed him diagrams of how much peripheral vision he had already lost. Bob and his family were surprised. Bob felt healthy and never really noticed the significant loss of vision. His mother had glaucoma, but he didn't connect that to the possibility that he would one day develop it as well.

Bob uses eye drops and recently underwent surgery to reduce the pressure in his eye. He has been referred to occupational therapy to see if adaptations can be made to his environment and lifestyle to help him maintain as much function as possible in the coming years.

CASE STUDY 3

Elizabeth, who is known as Beth to her family and friends, has been dealing with increasingly limited vision due to cataracts. Beth is 68 years old and has lived with her partner, Sue, for the last 26 years in a high-rise condo in an urban area. Beth has a daughter from a previous relationship and she lives within walking distance to her mother's home. Beth is retired from her career as an architect, but Sue still works as a teacher and has an hour commute to and from work.

Since her retirement, Beth spends most of her time participating in leisure activities. She loves to paint, swim, and work out in the building's gym facilities. She is also an avid reader but has been frustrated with her visual deficits when trying to read. Her daughter owns and operates a local coffee shop, so she frequently stops by there to hang out or help out her daughter as needed.

Beth has been very aware of her increasingly limited vision over the past several years. She describes her vision as cloudy, blurry, and sensitive to "bad lighting." She started wearing glasses a few years ago, but now, her vision loss is starting to interfere with her ability to function around the home and within her community.

Beth's eye doctor discussed routine eye surgery to remove the cataracts from both eyes. Once the eye doctor discovered that Beth had scarring on her retina in the right eye due to an old injury, however, she decided that the surgery would only benefit the left eye. Beth, therefore, will continue to have a significant loss of vision in her right eye even after the surgery is done.

Beth was referred to occupational therapy for an evaluation and intervention to assist her in making any adaptations necessary to increase her ability to function independently in her home and her community.

RECOMMENDED LEARNING RESOURCES

American Academy of Ophthalmology
http://www.aao.org
American Council of the Blind
http://www.acb.org

American Foundation for the Blind
http://www.afb.org

MACULAR DEGENERATION

MedlinePlus
www.nlm.nih.gov/medlineplus/maculardegeneration.html

MayoClinic.com
www.mayoclinic.com/health/macular-degeneration
Macular Degeneration Foundation
www.eyesight.org/

GLAUCOMA

Glaucoma Research Foundation
www.glaucoma.org/
Mayo Clinic
www.mayoclinic.com/health/glaucoma

National Eye Institute
www.nei.nih.gov

CATARACTS

MedlinePlus
www.nlm.nih.gov/medlineplus/cataract.html
National Eye Institute
www.nei.nih.gov

Mayo Clinic
www.mayoclinic.com/health/cataracts

REFERENCES

Ambati, J., & Fowler, B. J. (2012). Mechanisms of age-related macular degeneration. *Neuron*, *75*(1), 26–39. http://dx.doi.org/10.1016/j.neuron.2012.06.018

Ang, G. S., & Eke, T. (2007). Lifetime visual prognosis for patients with open-angle glaucoma. *Eye*, *21*, 604–608.

Appleby, P. N., Allen, N. E., & Key, T. J. (2011). Meat consumption linked to cataracts? *American Journal of Clinical Nutrition*, *93*(5), 128–135.

Armitage, H. (2015). *Eye drops could dissolve cataracts. The American Association for the Advancement of Science.* http://dx.doi.org/10.1126/science.aac8893

Beleforte, N. A., Moreno, M. C., de Zavalia, N., Sande, P. H., Chianelli, M. S., Keller Sarmiento, M. I., & Rosenstein, R. E. (2010). Melatonin: A novel neuroprotectant for the treatment of glaucoma. *Journal of Pineal Research*, *48*, 353–364. http://dx.doi.org/10.1111/j.1600-079X.2010.00762.x

Bennion, A. E., Shaw, R. L., & Gibson, J. M. (2012). What do we know about the experience of age related macular degeneration? A systematic review and meta-synthesis of qualitative research. *Social Science & Medicine*, *75*(6), 976–985. http://dx.doi.org/10.1016/j.socscimed.2012.04.023

Bressler, N. M., & Gills, J. P. (2000). Age related macular degeneration: New hope for a common problem comes from photodynamic therapy. *BMJ*, *321*, 1425–1427. http://dx.doi.org/10.1136/bmj.321.7274.1425

Burack-Weiss, A. (1992). Psychological aspects of aging and vision loss. In: E. Faye & C. S. Stuen (Eds.). *The Aging eye and low vision: A study guide for physicians* (pp. 29–34). New York: Lighthouse.

Cheung, C. M. G., & Wong, T. Y. (2013). Treatment of age-related macular degeneration. *The Lancet*, *382*(9900), 1230–1232. http://dx.doi.org/10.1016/S0140-6736(13)61580-9

Chong, E. W.-T., Simpson, J. A., Robman, L. D., Hodge, A. M., Aung, K. Z., English, D. R., … Guymer, R. H. (2009). Red meat and chicken consumption and its association with age-related macular degeneration. *American Journal of*

Epidemiology, *169*(7), 867–876. http://dx.doi.org/10.1093/aje/kwn393

Chuo, J. Y., Wiens, M., Etminan, M., & Maberley, D. A. L. (2007). Use of lipid-lowering agents for the prevention of age-related macular degeneration: A meta-analysis of observational studies. *Ophthalmic Epidemiology*, *14*(6), 367–374. http://dx.doi.org/10.1080/09286580701421684

Friedman, D. S., O'Colmain, B. J., Munoz, B., Tomany, S. C., McCarty, C., de Jong, P. T., … Kempen, J. (2004). Prevalence of age-related macular degeneration in the United States. *Archives of Ophthalmology*, *122*(4), 564–572. http://dx.doi.org/10.1001/archopht.122.4.564

Goodman, D. M., Parmet, S., Lynm, C., & Livingston, E. H. (2012). Age-related macular degeneration. *Journal of the American Medical Association*, *308*(16), 1702. http://dx.doi.org/10.1001/jama.2012.4091

Heijl, A. (2015). Glaucoma treatment: By the highest level of evidence. *The Lancet*, *385*(9975), 1264–1266. http://dx.doi.org/10.1016/S0140-6736(14)62347-3

Hirami, Y., Mandai, M., Takahashi, M., Teramukai, S., Tada, H., & Yoshimura, N. (2009). Association of clinical characteristics with disease subtypes, initial visual acuity, and visual prognosis in neovascular age-related macular degeneration. *Japanese Journal of Ophthalmology*, *53*, 396–407. http://dx.doi.org/10.1007/s10384-009-0669-4

Hollands, H., Johnson, D., Hollands, S., Simel, D. L., Jinapriya, D., & Sharma, S. (2013). Do findings on routine examination identify patients at risk for primary open-angle glaucoma? *Journal of the American Medical Association*, *309*(19), 2035–2042.

Hoster, M. (2013). Do statins cause or prevent cataracts? *Review of Optometry*, *150*(10), 4. Retrieved from http://www.reviewofoptometry.com/content/d/news_review/c/44383/

King, A., Azuara-Blanco, A., & Tuulonen, A. (2013). Glaucoma. *British Medical Journal*, *346*, f3518. http://dx.doi.org/10.1136/bmj.f3518

Klein, B. E. K., Howard, K. P., Gangnon, R. E., Dreyer, J. O., Lee, K. E., & Klein, R. (2012). Long-term use of aspirin and age-related macular degeneration. *Journal of the American Medical*

Association, 308(23), 2469–2478. http://dx.doi. org/10.1001/jama.2012.65406

Lamoureux, E. L., Pallant, J. F., Pesudova, K., Tennant, A., Rees, G., O'Connor, P. M., & Keeffe, J. E. (2008). Assessing participation in daily living and the effectiveness of rehabilitation in age related macular degeneration patients using the impact of vision impairment scale. *Ophthalmic Epidemiology, 15*, 105–113. http://dx.doi. org/10.1080/09286580701840354

Leske, M. C. (2007). Open-angle glaucoma—an epidemiological overview. *Ophthalmic Epidemiology, 14*, 166–172. http://dx.doi. org/10.1080/09286580701501931

Lim, L. S., Mitchell, P., Seddon, J. M., Holz, F. G., & Wong, T. Y. (2012). Age-related macular degeneration. *The Lancet, 379*(9827), 1728–1738. http:// dx.doi.org/10.1016/S0140-6736(12)60282-7

Lin, J., & Yang, M. (2009). Correlation of visual function with health-related quality of life in glaucoma patients. *Journal of Evaluation in Clinical Practice, 16*, 134–140. http://dx.doi. org/10.1111/j.1365-2753.2009.01135.x

Lyle, B. J., Mares-Perlman, J. A., Klein, B. E. K. Klein, R., & Greger, J. L. (1999). Antioxidant intake and rick of incident age-related nuclear cataracts in the Beaver Dam eye study. *American Journal of Epidemiology, 149*(9), 801–809. http:// dx.doi.org/10.1093/oxfordjournals.aje.a009895

Magacho, L., Lima, F. E., Nery, A. C. S., Sagawa, A., Magacho, B., & Avila, M. P. (2004). Quality of life in glaucoma patients: Regression analysis and correlation with possible modifiers. *Ophthalmic Epidemiology, 11*(4), 263–270. http://dx.doi. org/10.1080/09286580490515251

Martin, D. F., Maguire, M. G., Ying, G.-S., Grunwald, J. E., Fine, S. L., & Jaffe, G. J. (2011). Ranibizumab and bevacizumab for neovascular age-related macular degeneration. *The New England Journal of Medicine, 364*(20), 1897–1908. http://dx.doi.org/10.1056/NEJMoa1102673

Massof, R. W. (2002). A model of the prevalence and incidence of low vision and blindness among adults in the U.S. *Optometry and Vision Science, 79*, 31–38. http://dx.doi. org/10.1097/00006324-200201000-00010

McDaniel, D., & Besada, E. (1996). Hypothyroidism—A possible etiology of open-angle glaucoma. *Journal of the American Association, 67*(2), 109–114.

Mogk, L. G., & Mogk, M. (2003). *Macular degeneration: The complete guide to saving and maximizing your sight.* New York: Random House.

Montgomery, M. P., Kamel, F., Pericak-Vance, M. A., Haines, J. L., Postel, E. A., Agarwal, A., … Schmidt, S. (2010). Overall diet quality and

age-related macular degeneration. *Ophthalmic Epidemiology, 17*(1), 58–65. http://dx.doi. org/10.3109/09286580903450353

Quigley, H. A. (2011). Glaucoma. *The Lancet, 377*(9774), 1367–1377. http://dx.doi.org/10.1016/ S0140-6736(10)61423-7

Rosenberg, E. A., & Sperazza, L. C. (2008). The visually impaired patient. *American Family Physician, 77*(10), 1431–1438.

Shazly, T. A., & Latina, M. A. (2009). Neovascular glaucoma: Etiology, diagnosis and prognosis. *Seminars in Ophthalmology, 24*, 113–121. http:// dx.doi.org/10.1080/08820530902800801

Sonnsjo, B., & Krakau, C. E. T. (1993). Arguments for vascular glaucoma etiology. *Acta Ophthalmologica, 71*, 433–444. http://dx.doi. org/10.1111/j.1755-3768.1993.tb04615.x

Sperduto, R. D. (1994). Age-related cataracts: Scope of problem and prospects for prevention. *Preventive Medicine, 23*, 735–739. http://dx.doi. org/10.1006/pmed.1994.1126

Subak-Sharpe, I., Low, S., Nolan, W., & Foster, P. J. (2009). Pharmacological and environmental factors in primary angle-closure glaucoma. *British Medical Bulletin, 93*, 125–143. http://dx.doi. org/10.1093/bmb/ldp042

Wang, W., & Zhang, X. (2014). Alcohol intake and the risk of age-related cataracts: A meta-analysis of prospective cohort studies. *PLoS One, 9*(9), e107820. http://dx.doi.org/10.1371/journal. pone.0107820

Wang, J. J., Rochtchina, E., Smith, W., Klein, R., Klein, B. E. K., Joshi, T., … Mitchell, P. (2008). Combined effects of complement factor H genotypes, fish consumption, and inflammatory markers on long-term risk for age-related macular degeneration in a cohort. *American Journal of Epidemiology, 169*(5), 633–641. http://dx.doi. org/10.1093/aje/kwn358

Williams, R. A., Brody, B. L., Thomas, R. G., Kaplan, R. M., & Brown, S. I. (1998). The psychosocial impact of macular degeneration. *Archives of Ophthalmology, 116*, 514–520. http://dx.doi. org/10.1001/archopht.116.4.514

Wittstrom, E., Schatz, P., Lovestram-Adrian, M., Ponjavic, V., Bergstrom, A., & Andreasson, S. (2010). Improved retinal function after trabeculectomy in glaucoma patients. *Graefe's Archive for Clinical and Experimental Ophthalmology, 248*, 485–495. http://dx.doi.org/10.1007/ s00417-009-1220-5

Wu, P., Guo, W., Xia, H., Lu, H., & Xi, S. (2010). Patients' experience of living with glaucoma: A phenomenological study. *Journal of Advanced Nursing, 67*(4), 800–810. http://dx.doi. org/10.1111/j.1365-2648.2010.05541.x

Cancer

Suzänne Fleming Taylor

Mark, a 49-year-old male, could not get rid of his nagging cough. As a construction worker, he was used to the changing weather, and he had not had trouble before. Over the next few weeks, Mark noticed he was fairly tired throughout the day and tended to become short of breath carrying items that previously caused him no trouble. After his roommate commented on the noticeable weight loss, Mark decided to make an appointment with his primary care physician. Upon learning the recent symptoms, the physician ordered an x-ray of his lungs. The results showed an abnormal mass in the left upper lobe, prompting the physician to recommend consultation with an oncologist. Mark was told to expect to undergo a tissue biopsy as his physician suspected lung cancer.

DEFINITION AND DESCRIPTION

In 2014, there were nearly 14.5 million people living with cancer in the United States, and in 2015, an estimated 1,658,370 new cases will be diagnosed, bringing the total to nearly 16.2 million cancer survivors in the United States (National Institutes of Health: Surveillance, Epidemiology, and End Results Program, 2015). As cancer survivors are living longer after diagnosis, the challenge becomes one of ensuring quality of life and optimal functional and cognitive abilities.

The focus of this chapter is to provide an overview of cancer including definitions, etiology, signs and symptoms, medical and surgical management including common side effects, and the impact of cancer on occupational performance. Readers are encouraged to utilize the resources listed to further enhance their understanding of this complex and chronic disease.

Cancer refers to a collection of related diseases in which some of the body's cells divide without control and are able to invade other tissues. This occurs when the normal process of cell division, growth, and death is not properly regulated, allowing old or damaged cells to

513

continue to survive, and new cells are unnecessarily formed, leading to an abnormal growth, or neoplasm. Cancer can start almost anywhere in the body and is typically named for the organ or cell where it originates. For example, lung cancer originates in the lungs, breast cancer originates in the breast, and so forth.

The basic tumor cell types are classified as benign, in situ, or malignant. The cells in a **benign** tumor remain differentiated, or genetically similar to the original cell, and therefore are unable to spread to other tissues, structures, or organs. Since benign tumors are not able to spread, they are not considered cancerous. **In situ** translates to "in position" or "in place." This is an early stage of cancer in which the cancerous, or **neoplastic**, cells remain in the original site from which they arose. While these cells have not spread, unlike benign tumors, they have a very high likelihood of progression to becoming undifferentiated and spreading to surrounding tissues, structures, and/or organs. In situ may also be referred to as pre-malignant. A **malignant** tumor invades surrounding tissues and is usually capable of spreading to distant tissues, or metastasizing. Malignant tumors are typically capable of recurring after removal and may recur as **metastatic disease**, which means the cancer from one organ or part of the body has spread to another organ or part of the body not directly connected. For example, an individual may have a history of breast cancer, status post mastectomy with chemotherapy and radiation, now in remission, and years later have recurrence as metastatic bone disease.

Cancers are generally referred to as either a "solid tumor" or "liquid tumor." **Solid tumors** begin in a solid structure such as bone, muscle, or organ and include carcinoma and sarcoma. **Liquid tumors** are also known as blood cancers or hematological tumors. They arise from and affect the blood, bone marrow, and lymphatic system and include leukemia, lymphoma, and myeloma.

■ Classification of Solid Tumor

There are hundreds of different cancers and several methods of classification. The various methods include by site of origin, by histological (tissue) type, and by stage and grade. Classification by site of origin simply names the primary, specific type such as lung cancer, prostate cancer, and

liver cancer. The International Classification of Diseases for Oncology, Third Edition (ICD-O-3) groups cancer into six categories based on histological type: carcinoma, sarcoma, myeloma, leukemia, lymphoma, and mixed types. **Carcinomas** are cancerous tumors that arise in epithelial tissues of skin, blood vessels, and lining of the cavities and organs. Carcinomas account for 80% to 90% of all cancers. **Sarcomas** are cancerous tumors that arise in supportive and connective tissues including bones, tendons, cartilage, muscle, and fat. **Myeloma** is a malignant tumor that originates in the plasma cells of bone marrow. **Leukemia**, which means "white blood" in Greek, is a cancer that begins when the blood-forming cells of the bone marrow and other blood-forming organs create an excess of abnormal white blood cells (WBC). **Lymphoma** is a cancer that develops in the glands or nodes of the lymphatic system causing abnormal cellular reproduction of WBC called lymphocytes, which are a vital part of the immune system. **Mixed-type cancer** is cancer that has different tissue types or components from more than one type of cancer.

■ Staging of Solid Tumor

Solid tumors are staged to describe the severity of the cancer based on the size of the primary tumor and whether or not it has spread in the body. The TNM classification of malignant tumors (TNM) is the most widely used cancer staging system (Table 27.1). This system was developed, and is maintained, by the American Joint Committee on Cancer (AJCC). "TNM" is the abbreviation for: the size of the tumor (T), the involvement of nearby lymph nodes (N), and the presence of metastasis (M). This provides a quick and standardized method for understanding the involvement of the cancer. Healthcare providers use cancer staging to assess prognosis and determine treatment(s). Cancer staging is used in research to determine efficacy of treatments, compare treatment centers, and as a means of cancer surveillance and control.

After the values for TNM have been determined, the cancer is assigned an overall stage. Staging groups use roman numerals and range from I through IV (plus 0). Certain cancers are further defined using the letters A and B. The higher cancer stages (III and IV) are associated

TABLE 27.1 TNM Classification

Tumor size—describes the size of the primary tumor

Tx	Cannot be evaluated
Tis	Carcinoma in situ
T0	No signs of tumor
T1	Size/extent of primary tumor
T2	Size/extent of primary tumor > than T1
T3	Locally advanced
T4	Spread to distant

Lymph Node—degree of spread to regional lymph nodes

Nx	Cannot be evaluated
N0	No involvement
N1	Present in regional lymph node
N2	Presence beyond regional lymph nodes
N3	Presence in distant lymph nodes

Metastasis—presence of distance metastasis

M0	No metastasis
M1	Metastasis beyond regional lymph nodes

with more advanced cancer and poorer prognosis compared to the lower cancer stages (I and II).

Stage 0: carcinoma in situ; early in development, not all cancers have stage 0

Stage I: localized cancer; often has a good prognosis

Stage II and III: locally advanced; criteria for II and III dependent on type of cancer

Stage IV: metastasized; cells have become undifferentiated

It is important to note that cancers are staged when they are first diagnosed and the stage does not change over time, even if the cancer shrinks, progresses, becomes metastatic, or recurs after remission. This information is simply added to the diagnosis. For example, a 76-year-old male with stage II prostate cancer has progression of disease despite treatment. An example of an updated diagnosis would be "Stage II prostate cancer with metastatic disease to the pelvis." This is to facilitate an improved understanding of treatments by stage and associated survival rates. On a rare occasion, the cancer might be restaged to determine the response to treatment. If this is done and the new stage is used, a lower care "r" will appear in front of the new stage.

■ Classification and Staging of Liquid Tumor

Liquid tumors, also referred to as blood cancers, include leukemia, lymphoma, and myeloma. Liquid tumors arise from and affect the bone marrow, blood cells, and the lymphatic system. **Myeloblasts** and **lymphoblasts** are immature blood cells in the bone marrow. Myeloblasts develop into granulocytes and lymphoblasts develop into either B or T lymphocytes. When there is malfunctioning or errors within these processes, immature blood cells may be released into and accumulate in the peripheral blood. Myeloblasts in the peripheral blood leads to myleoblastic leukemia, and lymphoblasts in the peripheral blood leads to lymphocytic leukemia. The term "**blasts**" is often used as a shortened version, indicating immature blood cells found in the peripheral blood, and reported in percentages.

There are a variety of classification systems and staging criteria for liquid tumors, each of which is dependent upon the disease type and often includes subtypes. The following section provides an overview of classification and staging for liquid cancers.

Leukemia may be either acute or chronic. Acute leukemia is often classified using a cellular or cytologic level. The classification system that is most widely used is the French-American-British (FAB) system. This system divides acute leukemia into eight subtypes of acute myelogenous leukemia (AML) and three subtypes of acute lymphocytic leukemia (ALL). The World Health Organization (WHO) classification uses chromosome translocations and evidence of dysplasia. Other factors included in the staging are number of myeloblasts (immature WBC) found in the blood or bone marrow.

Chronic lymphocytic leukemia (CLL) is frequently staged in the United States using the Rai staging system, while the Binet system is widely used in Europe. The Rai system divides CLL into five stages based upon absence or enlargement of the lymph nodes, spleen, or liver as well as the counts of red blood cells (RBC) and platelets. All stages have lymphocytosis or an increase in the number of lymphocytes in the blood. The five Rai stages are as follows:

Stage 0: low risk
Stage I: intermediate risk
Stage II: intermediate risk
Stage III: high risk
Stage IV: high risk

Chronic myelogenous leukemia (CML) typically develops and progresses slowly, over months or years, even without treatment. CML is divided into three phases dependent upon clinical manifestation, laboratory values, and the percentage of blood and bone marrow blasts. The chronic phase typically lasts four to five years although some people have remained in the chronic phrase for more than 20 years. Many people do not experience any symptoms and the diagnosis is often by chance during blood testing for an unrelated reason, reveling blasts of less than 10%. Treatment during this phase is through the use of tyrosine kinase inhibitor (TKI) which targets the oncogene BCR-ABL. This gene is not found in normal cells and it causes the growth of CML. Over several years, CML progresses to an accelerated phase during which the disease process speeds, leukemia cells accumulate more quickly, and the blood and bone marrow have 10-19% blasts. This phase typically lasts from 6-24 months before progression. Treatment depends upon treatments received thus far. An allogeneic stem cell transplant may be the best option for those eligible. The final phase of CML is the blast crisis, which often behaves as an acute leukemia. The blood and bone marrow contain 20% or more blasts and symptoms are more severe. People in blast crisis often have fevers, an enlarged spleen, weight loss, and report a general feeling of being unwell. Treatment includes chemotherapy, however success is difficult at this stage with fewer people reaching remission, and remissions lasting shorter periods of time. Many times people in the blast crisis of CML cannot be cured therefore, palliative treatments may be used to alleviate bothersome symptoms including radiation to reduce pain from areas of bone damage and to shrink an enlarged spleen. Approximately 85% of patients are diagnosed in the chronic phase (Tefferi, 2006).

Lymphoma, the most common blood cancer, occurs when a subset of WBC called lymphocytes grow abnormally. Lymphocytes are a vital part of the immune system and are divided into B and T cells. Dependent upon the specific lymphocyte involved, lymphoma is classified as either Hodgkin lymphoma (HL) or non-Hodgkin lymphoma (NHL). Although the growth rate and prognostic factors are not taken into account, the Ann Arbor staging is commonly used for staging lymphoma. There are four stages as follows:

Stage I: one nodal group or lymphoid region
Stage II: two or more nodal groups, same side of the diaphragm
Stage III: nodal groups on both sides of the diaphragm
Stage IV: spread beyond the lymph nodes, most often to the liver, bone marrow, or lungs

Many oncologists consider NHL stages III and IV as one category as treatment and prognosis do not differ.

Myeloma begins in the bone marrow and is a cancer of a different type of WBC, the plasma cells, or plasma B cells. There are four types of myeloma:

Multiple myeloma: the most common, constituting approximately 90% of all myeloma
Plasmacytoma: only one site of myeloma cells evident
Localized myeloma: found in one site with extension into surrounding tissue
Extramedullary myeloma: involves tissue other than the bone marrow such as skin

Myeloma may be considered asymptomatic (smoldering) or symptomatic. Asymptomatic myeloma progresses slowly and there are no symptoms, while symptomatic myeloma progresses quicker and has related symptoms including anemia and kidney damage.

ETIOLOGY

By definition, cancer is a disease of the genes. A gene is a distinct portion of deoxyribonucleic acid (DNA) that encodes, or instructs, the production of proteins and ribonucleic acid (RNA), which in turn form the basis for how our body grows and functions. Cells in our body continually grow, divide, and replace themselves, which may lead to potential errors in coding or damage to the DNA. Likewise, factors from the environment may damage DNA. The DNA repair process allows the cell to identify and correct such damages. If the damage is not repaired, the gene becomes mutated, which means the change is permanent, and this may cause the production of faulty proteins. As the abnormal cell continues to divide uncontrollably, it forms a neoplasm or tumor. These gene mutations and damage to DNA that cause cancer are attributable to factors within three general categories: genetic inheritance, environmental carcinogens, and lifestyle choices. It is important to remember that research in the field of oncology continues to add evidence to our understanding of the etiology, the risk factors, and the best interventions for cancer. The following information represents the most current understanding in the field of oncology at the time of this writing.

■ Genetics

The National Institutes of Health (NIH), National Cancer Institute (NCI), reports that inherited mutations in a person's chromosomes, genes, or proteins play a role in only 5% to 10% of cancers, while the majority of cancers (90% to 95%) are attributable to environmental carcinogens and/or lifestyle choices. There are some types of cancers that tend to recur in some family generations such as breast, colon, ovarian, and uterine. Current research suggests that it is possible to inherit certain genes that increase an individual's susceptibility to certain cancers such as early-onset breast cancer (National Cancer Institute, 2015d).

■ Environmental Carcinogens

The International Agency for Research on Cancer (IARC), a part of the WHO, the United States National Toxicology Program (NTP), and the United States Environmental Protection Agency (EPA) have ongoing efforts to identify and educate on carcinogens. While all three of these agencies have methods of classification of agents, the most widely used system is from the IARC:

Group 1: Carcinogenic to humans
Group 2A: Probably carcinogenic to humans
Groups 2B: Possibly carcinogenic to humans
Group 3: Unclassifiable as to carcinogenicity in humans
Group 4: Probably not carcinogenic to humans

The IARC has evaluated over 900 agents and placed them in one of the above groups. Most are listed within Groups 2A, 2B, and 3 due to the difficulty in testing. There are over 100 agents placed in group 1, known to be carcinogenic to humans. It is important to note that carcinogens do not cause cancer at all times, under all circumstances. Sometimes the agent is only carcinogenic when exposed in a certain manner such as touching versus ingesting. Others may only cause cancer in the setting of specific genetics. Sometimes, an agent is carcinogenic after brief exposure, while others take repeated exposure. For specific details, readers are encouraged to visit the IARC, NTP, and EPA Web sites directly.

Radiation

There are several different types of radiation, some of which increase the risk of cancer. The electromagnetic spectrum of radiation ranges from low frequency to high frequency. The lower frequencies, or radiofrequency (RF), are nonionizing. This means there is enough energy to move atoms in a molecule enough to vibrate, but not enough to ionize. Microwaves, radio waves, full-body scanners, cell phones, and cell phone towers are all forms of low-frequency, nonionizing radiation. As such, they do not have enough energy to cause cancer by directly damaging cellular DNA. The higher frequencies, with higher energy, are ionizing radiation. Radiation on this end of the electromagnetic spectrum has enough energy to change an atom or molecule by removing an electron. This level of energy is able to damage the DNA inside the cells, thus increasing the risk of cancer. Gamma rays, x-rays, and ultraviolet (UV) waves from sunlight are examples of ionizing radiation.

Ultraviolet Radiation

The sunlight that reaches the surface of Earth is made of two types of rays, both of which are harmful: long-wave ultraviolet A (UVA) and short-wave ultraviolet B (UVB). These rays cause premature aging of the skin, damage to the eyes leading to low vision and cataracts, and they cause skin cancer. This damage occurs because of the changes to the cellular DNA and resulting mutations. The WHO lists UV radiation as a proven human carcinogen, as well as the leading cause of basal cell carcinoma (BCC), squamous cell carcinoma (SCC), and nonmelanoma skin cancers (NMSC) (Lucas, McMichael, Smith, & Armstrong, 2006). Artificial UV-emitting devices, such as tanning beds and sun lamps, are also known to be a human carcinogen. Studies have shown the dose of UVA emitted from tanning beds to be as high as 12 times of that of the sun. People who use tanning beds are 2.5 times more likely to develop SCC and 1.5 times more likely to develop BSC (Lucas et al., 2006).

Air Pollution

Air pollution occurs as a result of introducing contaminants into the atmosphere. The most common cause of air pollution is exhaust from transportation and factories. While air pollution had previously been recognized as a factor that increases respiratory and heart diseases, data from the WHO's Global Burden of Disease Project showed 223,000 deaths from lung cancer associated with air pollution worldwide. Following these findings, in 2013, the IARC classified outdoor air pollution as a carcinogen (Simon, 2013). The following highlights five common air pollutions that are carcinogenic.

Secondhand Tobacco Smoke

Secondhand tobacco smoke, or passive smoking, includes both the smoke given off by the burning tobacco product and the exhaled smoke from the smoker and is classified as a known human carcinogen. There have been more than 7,000 chemicals identified in tobacco smoke, including more than 250 harmful substances. The known carcinogens in tobacco smoke include arsenic, benzene, beryllium, carbon monoxide, ethylene oxide, hydrogen cyanide, and polonium-210. The known carcinogens in tobacco smoke are directly linked to cancer of the lung, esophagus, larynx, mouth, throat, kidney, bladder, liver, pancreas, stomach, cervix, colon, rectum, and acute myeloid leukemia. It may also play a role of increasing the risk of other cancers including breast cancer and skin cancer (National Cancer Institute, 2015g).

Benzene

Benzene is widely used as a starting chemical for the production of plastics, rubbers, dyes, drugs, and pesticides. It is present in motor vehicle exhaust and in cigarette smoke. Benzene is known to cause blood cancers, in particular leukemia, through damaging the DNA in marrow cells (Leukemia & Lymphoma Society, 2015).

Diesel Engine Exhaust

Diesel engine exhaust is now classified as a known human carcinogen. Research has shown an increase in the lifetime risk of lung cancer and has linked diesel engine exhaust to an estimated 6% of lung cancer deaths annually (Vermeulen et al., 2014). The two parts of diesel engine exhaust are gas and soot in which the substances include carbon dioxide, carbon monoxide, nitric oxide, nitrogen dioxide, and polycyclic aromatic hydrocarbons (PAHs) (American Cancer Society, 2015d).

Asbestos

Asbestos, a naturally occurring group of minerals, has been widely used in the United States since the late 1800s. Uses have included building materials, ceiling and floor tiles, paint, plastics, vermiculite-containing garden products, and insulation. When the tiny fibers of asbestos are disturbed and released into the air, they can easily be breathed, allowing the fibers to accumulate in the lungs. Regular exposure to asbestos greatly increases the risks of both lung cancer and mesothelioma, a cancer in the membranes lining the chest and abdomen (National Cancer Institute, 2015a). The EPA banned all new use of asbestos in 1989.

Radon

Radon is a naturally occurring radioactive gas with no color, no odor, and no taste. As radon gas in the air breaks down, it creates radioactive elements called radon progeny. Breathing these elements allows them to become lodged in the lining of the lungs where they can give off radiation. While cigarette smoking is the leading cause of lung cancer in the United States, radon is the second leading cause (United States Environmental Protection Agency, 2015).

■ Lifestyle

Research has shown that a significant number of cancers may be prevented with improved lifestyle choices (Anand et al., 2008). The lifestyle choices that contribute to cancer include use of tobacco, excessive alcohol, increased weight, physical inactivity, poor diet, and contracting infectious agents.

Tobacco Use

Tobacco, whether it is smoked or smokeless, is a carcinogen. Of the estimated 589,430 cancer deaths in the United States in 2015, smoking tobacco caused approximately 171,000. This includes those smoking cigarettes and cigars and those exposed to passive or secondhand smoke (National Cancer Institute, 2015g). Of all lung cancers, 80% to 90% occur in smokers. Researchers have shown that smoking also contributes to cancers in the upper respiratory tract, the esophagus, and the larynx along with the bladder and pancreas. Liver, stomach, and kidney cancers have also been linked to smoking (Centers for Disease Control and Prevention, 2015).

Excessive Alcohol

While there is evidence that alcohol in small amounts may have health benefits, such as reduction of the risk of heart disease, excessive or heavy use of alcohol negates these benefits and increases the risks of cancers (American Cancer Society, 2015a; National Institutes of Health: NIAAA, 2000; Vincenzo, Blangiardo, LaVecchi, & Corrao, 2015). The generally accepted definition of moderate alcohol use is up to one drink per day for women and up to two drinks per day for men. Excessive, or heavy, alcohol use is defined as five or more drinks on a single occasion, and 5 or more days in the past 30 days. A meta-analysis of over 200 studies showed consistent evidence that heavy alcohol use significantly increased risks of cancer involving the mouth, pharynx, larynx, and esophagus (Bagnardi, Blangiardo, La Vecchia, & Corraro, 2001). Heavy use of alcohol also increases the risk of cancer involving the stomach, colon, rectum, liver, breast, and ovaries (American Cancer Society, 2015a). The component that increases the risk of cancer is the alcohol itself, chemically known as ethanol or ethyl alcohol, not the other ingredients. The structural formula for ethanol is CH_3CH_2OH and is abbreviated as EtOH. Different types of beverages have different levels of ethanol within them; however, as far as the body is concerned, all alcohol is the same at the unit level. As the risks of cancer are attributable to the ethanol, the greater amounts of ethanol have higher associated risks (Bagnardi et al., 2001). Along with alcoholic beverages, ethanol is also used as an additive for gasoline, as a solvent in the manufacturing of varnishes and perfumes, and as a disinfectant. Ethanol is a neurotoxic psychoactive drug that has direct effects on the nerve cell. Additionally, once ingested, ethanol in the liver metabolizes into acetaldehyde, a toxic chemical. Acetaldehyde encourages liver cells to grow faster, increasing the risk of errors that could lead to mutations in DNA. When alcohol is used in combination with tobacco, the risk significantly increases for cancers involving the mouth, pharynx, larynx, and esophagus, well above the risk levels associated with either tobacco or alcohol alone (Bagnardi et al., 2001; National Institutes of Health: NIAAA, 2000). This stems from tobacco and ethanol working in tandem. For example, ethanol increases the absorption of tobacco into the linings of the mouth and esophagus, increasing the exposure of those areas to the harmful effects of tobacco.

Increased Weight

Each year, close to 500,000 new cancer cases worldwide are associated with obesity (Arnold et al., 2015; International Agency for Research on Cancer, 2002). Obesity is associated with cancers involving the breast, ovaries, uterus, pancreas, gallbladder, prostate, colon, and rectum (Key et al., 2004). Obesity is defined by a body mass index (BMI) of 30 or higher. Researchers have proposed several possible mechanisms to explain the link between obesity and cancer (National Cancer Institute, 2015f):

Obesity causes a chronic low-level inflammation, which is associated with increased risk of cancer.

Obesity leads to increased levels of insulin and insulin-like growth factor in the blood, which may contribute to the growth of certain tumors.

Fat cells produce hormones that may stimulate or inhibit cell growth.

Fat tissue produces excess amounts of estrogen, and high levels of estrogen are linked with breast and endometrial cancers.

Physical Inactivity

The NCI reports that people who exercise on a regular basis have a 40% to 50% lower risk of colon cancer and a 30% to 40% lower risk of breast cancer compared to people who do not exercise on a regular basis. The WHO reports that sedentary lifestyles increase all causes of mortality including the risk of colon cancer and the risk of obesity. Physical inactivity leads to slower bowel function, increasing the length of time the colon is exposed to potential carcinogens. When coupled with tobacco use and poor diet, physical inactivity is contributing to the rise of complications and mortalities with chronic diseases including cancer (World Health Organization, 2002). Research also supports regular exercise leading to a lower risk of lung cancer and prostate cancer.

Poor Diet

Approximately 35% of all cancers are directly related to dietary causes (Stadler, 2009) and include cancers of the breast, ovaries, uterus, gallbladder, pancreas, colon, rectum, and prostate (World Health Organization, 2011). Poor diet choices, which increase the risk of cancers, include foods containing high fat and oxidized fats. The chemicals produced by certain meat preparation methods including charcoaling, smoking, and grilling may also increase the risk of cancer. Chemicals called PAHs are emitted from combustion of charcoal, gas, and wood. Research has shown that lab animals exposed to PAHs had higher risks of developing cancer in the skin, liver, and stomach (Gehle, 2009). More recently, researchers at Oregon State University discovered compounds that are produced by certain chemical reactions that are hundreds of times more mutagenic than the parent compounds of PAHs (Mishamandani, 2014). When meat is exposed to high heat, a chemical reaction occurs involving the released meat nitrates and the PAHs, forming nitrated PAHs (NPAHs). This research showed the mutagenic abilities of NPAHs to be as much as 432-fold increase over PAHs. Processed meat products contain sodium nitrite as a preservative and colorant. When sodium nitrite is exposed to high temperatures, it combines with proteins called amines and forms nitrosamines, most of which are carcinogenic (International Agency for Research on Cancer, 2015). Nitrosamines are also found in pickled and salted foods. Recent studies have linked smoked meats to an increased risk of colorectal, pancreatic, and prostate cancer (National Cancer Institute, 2015b). Current research continues to study the risk of cancer and the role of PAHs, NPAHs, sodium nitrites, nitrosamines, and other chemicals associated with the processing of food.

■ Infectious Agents

Research over the past decades has shown that approximately 15% of cancers are attributable to viruses (Liao, 2006; National Cancer Institute, 2015e) including human papillomavirus (HPV), hepatitis B virus (HBV), hepatitis C virus (HCV), and human immunodeficiency virus (HIV) (Table 27.2).

■ Aging and Cancer

One of the greatest risk factors for cancer is aging (Hurria et al., 2010). Research currently speculates that increased risk of cancer from aging

TABLE 27.2 Infectious Agents

Virus	Associated Cancer(s)
Human papillomavirus (HPV)	Cervical cancers
Hepatitis B virus (HBV)	Hepatocellular carcinoma (liver cancer)
Hepatitis C virus (HCV)	Hepatocellular carcinoma (liver cancer)
Human immunodeficiency virus (HIV)	Lymphoma, Kaposi's sarcoma
Epstein-Barr virus (EBV)	Lymphoma, Hodgkin's, leiomyosarcoma, nasopharyngeal carcinoma
Human herpesvirus 8 (HHV-8)	Kaposi's sarcoma

may be a result of having a greater length of time for exposure to factors that damage DNA, and it may be also the aged tissues' potential decreased ability to adequately complete the DNA repair process, thus creating a cellular environment that has increased susceptibility to mutations within an immune system that is less capable of responding (Hurria et al., 2010; Ukraintseva & Yashin, 2003).

INCIDENCE AND PREVALENCE

Survivorship, a common term referring to individuals who have been diagnosed with cancer, begins at the time of diagnosis and continues through the person's end of life. In 2015, there were approximately 14.5 million cancer survivors in the United States (National Institutes of Health: Surveillance, Epidemiology, and End Results Program, 2015). The average lifetime risk of developing cancer in the United States is one in two men and one in three women. It is expected that 1,658,370 new cases of cancer will be diagnosed in 2015, and this does not include carcinoma in situ. The most common types of cancer are prostate, breast, and lung (American Cancer Society, 2015b) (Table 27.3).

■ Adolescent and Young Adult Cancer (Ages 0 to 14 Years)

Approximately 10,380 new cases of childhood cancer were diagnosed in 2015 in the United States, representing <1% of all new cancer diagnosis. An estimated 1,250 deaths in 2015,

childhood cancer is the second leading cause of death behind accidents (American Cancer Society, 2015c). Leukemia represents approximately 25% of all childhood cancers, while brain and other central nervous system tumors represent 24% (Kupfer, 2015).

■ Older Adult Oncology (Ages 65 Years and Older)

In 2010, approximately 40 million people living in the United States were aged 65 years or older, representing 13% of the general population (Agency for Healthcare Research and Quality, 2015). The growth of the population of older adults is projected to continue increasing such that by 2030 approximately 72 million or 20% to 25% of the general population (Agency for Healthcare Research and Quality, 2015). As the incidence of cancer increases with age, the majority of cancers are diagnosed in persons aged 65 years and older (Tariman, 2009; Ukraintseva & Yashin, 2003; National Institute on Aging, 2015). Rates of cancer for aged 65 and older are as follows: males 4× greater and females 2× greater than those aged 45 to 64 years (Baranovsky & Myers, 1986; National Institute on Aging, 2015). As aging is complex and each person ages at a different rate, successful cancer treatment for older adults requires an understanding of how the natural aging process, physiological age, comorbidities, level of function, and the expectations for treatment all play a role. For example, age-associated decline in kidney function leads to a decrease in the body's ability to clear medications (Weinstein & Anderson,

TABLE **27.3** Leading Sites of New Diagnoses—2015 Estimates	
Cancer Site	**Estimated New Cases in 2015**
Breast	234,190
Lung and bronchus	221,200
Prostate	220,800
Urinary system	138,710
Colon and rectum	132,700
Lymphoma	80,900
Thyroid	62,450
Leukemia	54,270

Source: American Cancer Society, 2015 Fact Sheet.

2010). This increases chemotherapy toxicity limits, which causes dosing to be lowered compared to similar diagnoses in a younger population (Hurria et al., 2010). As a result, the overall effectiveness of treatment is lowered. Likewise, cardiac, lung, and neurological comorbidities increase the risk of adverse effects of chemotherapy and radiation. Additionally, older adults tend to have rapid progression of disease, a poorer tolerance to neutropenia, shorter remissions, and a higher likelihood of complications (Hurria et al., 2010). However, older adults who are healthy, active, and have fewer comorbidities have equal benefit with equal treatments (Berger et al., 2006; Warburton, Nicol, & Bredin, 2006).

SIGNS AND SYMPTOMS

The signs and symptoms of cancer will depend upon the location and the size of the cancer, as well as whether the cancer is affecting nearby tissues or organs. General signs and symptoms of cancer include an unexplained weight loss, lingering fatigue, coughing blood, persistent headaches, chronic pain, persistent low-grade fever, skin changes, and repeated infections. The American Cancer Society uses the acronym "CAUTION" as a reminder of the general symptoms of cancer. It is important to remember that there are many other diseases that could cause these symptoms; therefore, it is advisable to seek medical advice to determine the underlying problem.

Change in bowel or bladder habits
A sore that does not heal
Unusual bleeding or discharge (blood in urine or stools)
Thickening or lump in the breast, testicles, or elsewhere
Indigestion or difficulty swallowing
Obvious change in the size, color, shape, or thickness of a wart, mole, or mouth sore
Nagging cough or hoarseness

COURSE AND PROGNOSIS

The NIH considers cancer a chronic disease model and places emphasis on recognizing not only the effects of cancer itself but also the short- and long-term effects of the treatments, all of which impact quality of life. The course and prognosis of cancer depends upon the type of cancer, the location and stage of the cancer, the age of the individual and his or her premorbid health, and how well the individual responds to treatment. Statistics are used to predict the future course and outcome of cancer, as well as the likelihood of recovery. Five-year survival rates are commonly used measures. This refers to the proportion of the people expected to be alive, 5 years after the initial diagnosis, compared with a demographically similar population that is without cancer. While the survival rates for many cancers have continued to improve, cancer overall remains the second leading cause of death following heart diseases (Table 27.4).

DIAGNOSIS

The process of diagnosing cancer involves several steps. These steps may begin following a routine screening that produces abnormal results or if an individual presents with lingering

TABLE 27.4 Risk of Mortality 2013

Rank and Cause of Death	No. of Deaths	% of Deaths
1. Heart diseases	611,105	38.1
2. Cancer	**584,881**	**36.4**
3. Chronic lower respiratory diseases	149,205	9.4
4. Accidents (unintentional injuries)	130,557	8.1
5. Cerebrovascular disease	128,978	8.0

Source: US Mortality Data 2013, National Center for Health Statistics, Centers for Disease Control and Prevention, 2015.

complaints. After gathering a recent medical history, the physician conducts a full examination to look for abnormalities in color, texture, lumps, swelling, tenderness, or thickening of tissue. Laboratory tests of blood, urine, and/or other body fluids are frequently ordered. For concerns of solid tumor, initial imaging may be conducted using computed tomography (CT) scans, magnetic resonance imaging (MRI), or ultrasound. Nuclear medicine scans such as positron emission tomography (PET) scans and bone scans are used to diagnose, stage, and monitor cancer. PET scans focus on the organs of the body, while bone scans are specific to detecting bone involvement. The process of having a nuclear medicine scan begins with a small amount of radioactive substance, typically injected into a vein, that is absorbed by organs and tissues throughout the body. Cancer cells tend to use more energy than healthy cells and thus absorb more of the radioactive substance. The nuclear scan image shows those areas of high radioactive tracer uptake (Fig. 27.1). A tissue biopsy may be conducted by removing a small portion of tissue from the area in question. Experts then review the samples under a microscope to determine if cellular changes are suggestive of cancer. At times, the physician may recommend genetic testing for known genetic mutations linked to particular cancers. For example, three abnormal genes, BRCA1, BRCA2, and PALB2, are inheritable genes with a mutation that significantly increases the risk of breast cancer in women (National Cancer Institute, 2015c).

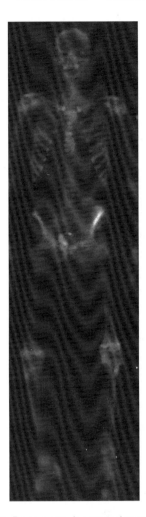

Figure 27.1 Bone scan. Increased uptake is seen at the left iliac crest in the setting of osteosarcoma.

MEDICAL MANAGEMENT

The primary goals of cancer treatment are to remove all or as much as possible of the tumor and prevent recurrence or spread of the primary tumor. The recommended course of treatment(s) is determined on an individual basis and with consideration for balancing the likelihood of curing the cancer with the anticipated side effects of the treatment, as well as the patient's preference. There are situations when the cancer is identified at a late stage and is widely metastatic or when the primary cancer is aggressive and cure is not possible, at which point the focus becomes relieving symptoms and controlling the cancer.

■ Surgery

Surgery is used to diagnose, stage, treat, and/or palliate solid tumors and is the most commonly used cancer treatment for solid tumors. There are several types of surgeries:

Preventive: to keep cancer from occurring. Examples of preventive surgery are removal of precancerous polyps or a mastectomy for a high-risk person.

Diagnostic (biopsy): removing some, or all, of the tumor for examination. This can be done through a fine needle aspiration (FNA), incisional, or excisional biopsy.

Staging: to determine the extent of the cancer. This is sometimes completed through endoscopic or laparoscopic procedures.

Curative: the removal of cancerous tumor. This is most effective on localized cancer and is often followed by radiation and/or chemotherapy.

Supportive: to help with other cancer treatments. An example of supportive surgery is placing of a port or an Ommaya reservoir for chemotherapy treatment.

Palliative: is not meant to cure or prevent. The purpose of a palliative surgery is to ease pain or disability and improve quality of life. Tumor debulking to alleviate symptoms in gastrointestinal cancer is an example of a palliative surgery.

Surgical interventions may damage nerve and muscle tissue, potentially leading to weakness and sensory changes. There may also be lingering complaints of pain. While these changes are typically localized to the surgical area(s), if left untreated, over time the individual may self-restrict his or her daily routines and/or roles, leading to a decline in function and in overall quality of life.

■ Radiation Treatment

Radiation treatment (XRT) may be used as curative, adjuvant (in addition to the primary treatment to maximize effectiveness), neoadjuvant (given before the primary treatment to reduce the size or extent of cancer), or palliative (to relieve symptom burden). There are two methods of receiving radiation: internally and externally. Internal radiation, known as brachytherapy, involves the placement of a radioactive substance in a pellet or liquid into or at the cancerous site. External radiation involves aiming the beam at the tumor from outside the body. This is a multistep process including imaging to accurately locate the targeted area, a simulation session to accurately mark the body and detail positions for the machine, and the radiation treatments. The ionizing radiation damages the cellular DNA of the cancerous cells, leading to cell death. The radiation beams are strategically placed in order to focus the larger absorbed dose on the tumor. The surrounding healthy tissue is exposed to radiation as well, but in much lower doses. Radiation side effects are classified as early adverse effects and late adverse effects. Early adverse effects are proportional to the dosing of radiation and include changes to radiosensitive tissues such as oral mucosa, stomach, small bowel, colon, vagina, and lymph nodes. Fatigue is a common complaint

that worsens as treatments progress. Erythema, a reddening of the skin, is common across the radiation site(s). Late adverse effects can take months to years to develop and include changes and tissue fibrosis to the radiated areas and changes to the lymph vessels increasing the risk of lymphedema. Secondary cancers are also possible. It is very important for individuals who received radiation across their abdominal region to remain mindful of maintaining regular bowel movements and using stool softeners, especially with any constipating medications such as opioids. Constipation and passing hard stool through tissues weakened by effects of radiation may lead to a fistula. A **fistula** is an abnormal connection or pathway between structures caused by disease, injury, or surgery. In this example, the bowel becomes weakened by radiation and cannot retain structural integrity, forming a fistula. A common treatment for a fistula involving the bowel is a colostomy, which may become permanent. Although developing a fistula is not always preventable, care should be taken to decrease the risk.

■ Chemotherapy

Chemotherapy is a medicine that may be taken orally, topically, or by injection intra-arterial (IA), intravenous (IV), or intraperitoneal (IP). There are over 100 chemotherapy agents, often used in combination. Induction chemotherapy, used to induce a remission, is commonly used to treat acute leukemia and is typically given while admitted to the hospital. Chemotherapy may also be administered on an outpatient basis. Chemotherapy works on cells that grow and divide quickly. As cancer cells divide more frequently than normal cells, they are more affected by the chemotherapy. However, other cells that grow and divide quickly are also affected including those that line the mouth and intestines and those that cause hair to grow. This leads to many side effects, of which fatigue is the most common. Other side effects may include nausea, vomiting, constipation, diarrhea, taste changes, appetite changes, cognitive dysfunction, bleeding problems, anemia, hair loss, sun sensitivity, and an increased risk of infection. **Chemotherapy-induced peripheral neuropathy** (CPIN), a side effect of chemotherapy that causes altered sensations of tingling, numbness, and weakness impacting primarily the hands and/or feet, occurs as chemotherapy spreads throughout the body, damaging the distal portions of the nerves. These symptoms may occur immediately following chemotherapy or weeks to months later and typically begin distally, progress proximally, and are bilateral. Symptoms often get worse as treatments progress. Chemotherapy is a cardiotoxic agent leading to long-term cardiac changes including heart failure, arrhythmias, and hypertension. Individuals who have undergone chemotherapy treatment are generally advised to have annual cardiac examinations.

■ Hormone Therapy

Hormone therapy, often used as an adjuvant therapy, is used for those types of cancers that are hormone dependent and grow faster in the presence of particular hormones. This includes prostate, breast, and uterine cancers. By blocking the production or action of the hormone, the tumor growth is slowed and survival may be extended for several months or years. Side effects of hormone therapy are dependent upon the specific hormone; however, general side effects include tiredness, memory problems, mood changes, thinning hair, and headaches. There might be complaints of joint pain initially, and some hormones may cause thinning of the bones.

■ New Approaches to Treatment

One new focus in cancer treatment is the use of targeted cancer therapy: drugs or substances that target specific molecules or proteins to block the growth and spread of cancerous cells. Targeted therapies are different from chemotherapy in that they work on specific targets associated within the cancerous cell rather than on rapidly dividing cells. This helps avoid healthy cells from cellular death, thus decreasing the risk of side effects. Another difference is that targeted therapies are cytostatic (block cell division) and chemotherapy is cytotoxic (kill the cell). Immunotherapy, or biologic therapy, uses the body's own immune system to destroy cancer cells. This type of treatment is being studied in clinical trials and is not yet widely available.

■ Bone Marrow Transplantation

Bone marrow transplant (BMT) is a procedure in which the damaged or destroyed stem cells are replaced with healthy stem cells. Stem cells are primarily found in bone marrow but may also be harvested from peripheral blood or umbilical cord blood from newborns. For purposes of clarification, stem cell transplant (SCT) refers to a transplantation using peripheral blood stem cells; the procedure itself is still referred to as BMT. **Bone marrow**, the spongy center of certain bones, forms three types of blood cells: RBC, WBC, and platelets. RBC, also called erythrocytes, carry oxygen throughout the body and bring carbon dioxide back to the lungs. WBC, also called leukocytes, help fight infection. Platelets, also called thrombocytes, assist in the clotting factor of blood. Lymphocytes, also formed in the bone marrow, work with the lymphatic system to help fight infections. Cancer occurs when stem cells become damaged and start producing abnormal cells or too few blood cells. The first BMT occurred in 1956 between identical twins. Twelve years later in 1968, after improved understanding of the role of human leukocyte antigens (HLA) and the importance of matching, the first BMT was performed between siblings. Then in 1973, the first unrelated BMT was performed. There are three types of BMT: autologous BMT, allogeneic BMT, and umbilical cord blood transplant. In an **autologous bone marrow transplant**, stem cells are removed from the individual while in remission from cancer and are kept frozen. After the individual undergoes high-dose chemotherapy or radiation, those stem cells are replaced to begin making new blood cells. Advantages of autologous BMTs include the following: there is no need to locate a donor; the individual receives his or her own stem cells and is not at risk of receiving an infection from the donor, nor is there a risk of the graft attacking the body (graft vs. host). A disadvantage is the increased rate of relapse or recurrence of the original cancer. In an **allogeneic bone marrow transplant** the individual undergoes high-dose chemotherapy or radiation and then receives stem cells from a HLA-matched donor. Umbilical cord transplants are a form of allogeneic in that the stem cells are from another individual (donor), in this case a newborn baby's umbilical cord. In an allogeneic BMT, the stem cells make their own immune cells, which could help destroy any remaining cancerous cells. This is called graft versus cancer, a preferable outcome. **Graft versus host disease** (GVHD) is a significant disadvantage in allogeneic transplants and occurs when the newly formed immune system views the recipient's body as foreign and attacks systems and/or organs. The most common GVHDs involve the gastrointestinal system, the skin, and the liver (National Cancer Institute, 2015h). GVHD is considered acute if it begins within the first 100 days posttransplant, chronic if it begins after. This complication requires hospitalization with close monitoring, and the treatment often includes immune-suppressing medications, steroids, and, if the gastrointestinal system is involved, artificial nutrition. As a result, the survivor is at high risk of an overall decline in physical and cognitive abilities as well as from a psychosocial standpoint.

ONCOLOGIC EMERGENCIES

Oncologic emergencies are defined as an acute and potentially life-threatening event caused by cancer or the associated treatments. These emergencies require immediate intervention to prevent loss of life or quality of life (Lewis, Hendrickson, & Moynihan, 2011; McCurdy & Shanholtz, 2012).

■ Tumor Lysis Syndrome

Tumor lysis syndrome (TLS) refers to a group of metabolic disorders that are potentially life threatening and includes the rapid development of hyperuricemia (high blood uric acid), hypocalcemia (low blood calcium), and hyperphosphatemia (high blood phosphorus); symptoms include severe muscle weakness or paralysis, sudden mental incapacity, extrapyramidal movement disorders, and myopathy. TLS is common in acute leukemia although it may occur in other cancers including lymphoma. Higher numbers of blasts, or abnormal immature WBC, increase the risk of TLS once the person begins chemotherapy. As the malignant cells go through lysis, breaking down of a cell membrane, the intracellular contents are released into the systemic circulation and may exceed the abilities of the kidneys leading to this metabolic emergency.

■ Hyperleukocytosis and Leukostasis

Hyperleukocytosis is a high leukocyte (WBC) count, and this condition can cause **leukostasis**, which is a clumping or sludging of the microcirculation that tends toward clotting. This oncologic emergency occurs more frequently in AML. Impairment in vascular flow and local hypoxemia is common in the pulmonary and cerebral vascular systems. The coronary circulation may also be affected. Early pulmonary involvement presents as mild dyspnea and

respiratory alkalosis, which is excessive alkaline, causing weakness and cramps. Cerebral involvement can range from confusion to somnolence to frank intracerebral bleeding and coma.

■ Disseminated Intravascular Coagulopathy

Disseminated intravascular coagulopathy (DIC) is an oncologic emergency encompassing both excessive bleeding and thromboembolic events and is common in leukemia, in particular acute promyelocytic leukemia (APL). The characteristic trait is excess thrombin generation. This is an enzyme in blood plasma that causes clotting by changing fibrinogen to fibrin. The typical presentation is episodes of thrombosis rather than bleeding; however, there is a high risk of bleeding from injury. While signs and symptoms of DIC vary as the clots can occur throughout the body, bleeding is often the first sign of acute DIC and includes bruising more frequently or more severe than expected, red spots on the skin, nosebleeds or epistaxis, bleeding from the gums, coughing up blood or hemoptysis, and dark, tarry stools.

■ Superior Vena Cava Syndrome

Superior vena cava syndrome (SVCS) is an oncologic emergency resulting in diminished blood return to the heart, causing symptoms of facial edema, edema of the neck and upper extremities, dyspnea, cough, and shortness of breath or orthopnea and is most commonly caused by lung cancer. The initial temporary measure is to elevate the head and apply supplemental oxygen.

■ Fever and Neutropenia

When the cancer involves the immune system, or immunosuppressive chemotherapy as a treatment, patients often have a period of **neutropenia**, which is defined as an absolute neutrophil count lower than $500/mm^3$. Neutrophils are the most abundant type of WBC, formed from stem cells in the bone marrow, and are an essential part of the immune system. During neutropenic states, the immune system becomes very susceptible to infections, particularly from gram-negative organisms, staphylococci, and fungi.

■ Metastatic Spinal Cord Compression

Metastatic spinal cord compression (MSCC) occurs when cancer grows on or near the spine, causing compression on the dural sac and the contents, in particular the spinal cord. There are approximately 12,700 new cases of MSCC per year (Quinn, 2000). Compression of spinal cord may be due to growth of a mass around the vertebrae, growth within the spinal column, or collapse of bone. The thoracic region is the most common at 70%, lumbar-sacral at 20%, and cervical at 10% (Dubey & Koul, 2009). Aggressive lymphomas such as Burkitt, multiple myeloma, and solid tumors with high risk for bone metastases (lung, breast, and prostate cancers) may lead to spinal cord compression(s). Back pain is the most common symptom present; neurological changes may or may not be present. Immediate interventions, no longer than 48 hours following symptoms, are required to alleviate pressure on the spinal cord with the goal of preventing permanent neurological changes (George et al., 2008). Interventions include stabilizing and decompressing surgeries, procedures such as kyphoplasty (surgically filling the collapsed vertebrae), local radiation, and/or high-dose steroids. Temporary measures include restricting activity pending stabilization and/or support of the compromised region(s).

■ Increased Intracranial Pressure

Mass lesions or obstructions of flow of cerebrospinal fluid by tumor tissue may cause increased intracranial pressure. Increased intracranial pressure requires immediate medical intervention; when left untreated, herniation and mortality may result. The symptoms include complaints of headache, cranial nerve symptoms, nausea and vomiting, and the onset of seizures. The initial temporary measure is to elevate the head to 30 degrees higher than the level of the heart.

■ Altered Mental Status

Altered mental status, always an emergency, may occur as a result from the primary cancer or from metastatic brain disease. It may also occur from metabolic changes, infections, or organ failure. The symptoms range from confusion and decreased attention through delirium and coma.

■ Neurological Changes

Changes in neurological status may warrant immediate medical attention. Signs and symptoms include disorientation, complaints of dizziness or light-headedness, complaints of blurred vision, changes in sensation, and ataxia or change in motor planning.

IMPACT ON CLIENT FACTORS AND OCCUPATIONAL PERFORMANCE

Both cancer and the associated treatments have significant implications across all client factors and areas of occupational performance (American Occupational Therapy Association, 2015a, c). Along with optimizing physical, cognitive, and psychosocial functioning, it is imperative for occupational therapy practitioners to work with survivors and their family and/or caregivers to help them understand the changing trajectory and how to live within these changes. Effective occupational therapy interventions will make a positive impact on the quality of life through facilitating posttreatment recovery including increasing functional and cognitive independence, reducing or eliminating pain, instructing on management of changes to sleep, addressing impacts on sexual abilities and intimacy, addressing social and psychosocial impacts, assisting with return to work, and redefining occupational roles (Penfold, 1996; Pergolotti, Cutchin, Weinberger, & Meyer, 2014; Silver, Baima, & Mayer, 2013; Silver & Balma, 2013; Silver & Gilchrist, 2011). Additionally, patients must maintain the best level of function possible as a loss of function, increased need for sedentary time, or increased time in bed may preclude further treatment. The Eastern Cooperative Oncology Group (ECOG), is one of the common scales used by oncologists to determine if further cancer treatment is appropriate (Oken, 1983) (Table 27.5).

■ Common Effects of Cancer and Treatments

Pain

A systematic meta-analysis review of 40 years of studies showed that across all cancers, at all stages, >50% of patients experience pain and more than one-third rated their pain as moderate or severe (Everdingen et al., 2007). The causes of cancer pain include spinal cord compression, metastatic bone involvement, surgical pain, side effects of chemotherapy and radiation, psychological responses to the diagnosis and treatments, and cancer itself such as an expanding mass pressing on organs. Cancer-related pain syndromes include peripheral neuropathies, axillary

TABLE 27.5 Karnofsky Performance Status

Able to care on normal activity and to work; no special care needed	100	Normal with no complaints; no evidence of disease
	90	Able to carry on normal activity; minor signs or symptoms of disease
	80	Normal activity with effort; some signs and symptoms of disease
Unable to work; able to live at home and care for most personal needs; varying amount of assistane needed	70	Cares for self; unable to carry on normal activity or do active work
	60	Requires occasional assistance, but able to care for most of his/her personal needs
	50	Requires considerable assistance and frequent medical care
Unable to care for self; requires equivalent of institutional or hospital care; disease may be progressing rapidly	40	Disabled; requires special care and assistance
	30	Severely disabled; hospital admission is indicated although death is not imminent
	20	Very sick; hospital admission necessary; active supportive treatment necessary
	10	Moribund; fatal processes progressing rapidly
	0	Dead

web syndrome (cording), and radiation fibrosis. Pain can lead to a loss of function in routines and roles due to guarding movements, self-restriction of activities, and generalized weakness associated with inactivity, leading to a low quality of life. Occupational therapy plays a vital role as a part of a multidisciplinary approach to pain management. Interventions include patient education, training in proactive pain management, safe body mechanics, neuromuscular re-education, muscle tension reduction training, and pacing activities (American Occupational Therapy Association, 2015b). Pain must be assessed during every occupational therapy session using objective measures such as patient-reported pain ratings, adult nonverbal pain scale, and Wong-Baker FACES pain rating scale. Documentation must also include the location, any patient-reported description of the pain such as stabbing or burning, and if movement leads to an increase or decrease in the complaint(s) of pain. Types of pain include visceral, somatic, neuropathic, and mixed type. Visceral pain arises from internal organs and is described as dull, often difficult to pinpoint. Somatic pain arises from the skin and deep tissues and is generally described as a musculoskeletal pain with a more precise location. Neuropathic pain arises from nerve damage and may result in localized complaints of numbness or hypersensitivity. Accurately understanding the patient's complaints of pain is necessary for the development of an appropriate intervention, as the occupational therapy intervention will vary according to the root cause of the pain. For example, a patient may have complaints of pain in the general hip and gluteal region. This may stem from soft tissue tumor burden, spinal cord compression, or metastatic bone disease. Further questioning and assessment of the pain, coupled with the known diagnosis, will dictate if it is appropriate to attempt standing (to don clothing or complete toileting) or if recommendations should be made for further imaging due to concern for unstable bone. When uncertain, err on the side of caution.

Compromised Bone

Compromised bone due to metastatic disease or primary bone cancer can lead to pathological fractures. Almost all cancers can spread to bone, but certain cancers commonly spread to bone including breast, lung, prostate, thyroid, and kidney. The liquid cancer multiple myeloma arises from plasma cells in the bone marrow and frequently causes weakening of bones. Along with facilitating overgrowth of plasma cells that crowd the normal blood-forming cells, multiple myeloma interferes with the cells that maintain bone integrity:

osteoblasts, which form new bone, and osteoclasts, which lyse or dissolve bone. Typically, new bone is being formed while old bone is being dissolved. Multiple myeloma speeds the process of osteoclasts, thus leading to weaker bones as the bones are broken down without forming new ones. As cancer spreads to the bone, it causes bone lesions. **Osteoblastic lesions**, or blastic lesions, result when cancer increases the activity of osteoblasts, causing that area of the bone to be harder. Although harder, the structure is abnormal and these areas break more easily than normal bone. Prostate cancer typically causes osteoblastic lesions. **Osteolytic lesions**, or lytic lesions, occur when greater numbers of osteoclasts are lysing the bone. This causes areas so weak that the bone can break even under its own weight. Breast, lung, and multiple myeloma cancers typically cause osteolytic lesions. Bones that break other than by trauma are considered a **pathological fracture**. Pathological fractures are managed differently than traumatic fractures, as healing is poor due to abnormal bone structure. Internal stabilization is the most common intervention. If there is a reason that the individual is not able to have surgical intervention, the occupational therapy plan must include protection for the unstable area(s), instruction of proper body mechanics to avoid weight-bearing across the unstable area(s), instruction on the impact to the individual's daily routine, and issuance of adaptive equipment and durable medical equipment as needed. Occupational therapy practitioners may be hesitant to mobilize patients with known metastatic bone disease, but without mobilization, the overall functional abilities including participation in their daily routine declines due to the negative impact of inactivity. Bunting and Shea (2001) published a study reviewing pathological fractures in 54 patients with metastatic bone disease who were undergoing rehabilitation. Results showed a total of 16 fractures in 12 patients. Only one occurred during rehabilitation, nine were silent fractures, and six occurred during rest. The **Mirel's scoring** system is a tool used to guide the management of bones with cancer in order to help prevent a pathological fracture (Table 27.6). Remember, all pathological fractures were once not fractured, and intervention including internal stabilization is considerably easier when impending pathological fractures are identified (Figs. 27.2 and 27.3). This is done through understanding the primary diagnosis and proper pain assessment.

Although continued mobilization is vital to maintain maximum levels of activity and engagement with their routine and roles, there may be times when mobilization is no longer safe due to the location of the unstable bone. At this point, it may be most appropriate to modify the individual's routine and roles to a bed level. This requires significant involvement from occupational therapy in order to successfully educate the caregivers on proper care and proper positioning and to assist the individual in adjustment of his or her life to a bed level.

TABLE 27.6 Mirel's Scoring

Mirel's Score	Scores		
	1	2	3
Site	Upper limb	Lower limb	Peritrochanter
Pain	Mild	Moderate	Severe
Lesion	Blastic	Mixed	Lytic
Size	<1/3	1/3–2/3	>2/3

Score	Clinical Recommendations
≤7	Radiotherapy and observation
8	Use clinical judgment
≥9	Prophylactic fixation

Score each: site, pain, lesion, and size from 1 to 3. Total the score for clinical recommendations.
"Size" is the size/diameter of the lesion in relationship to the size of the bone; look at imaging.

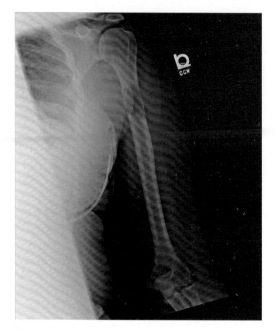

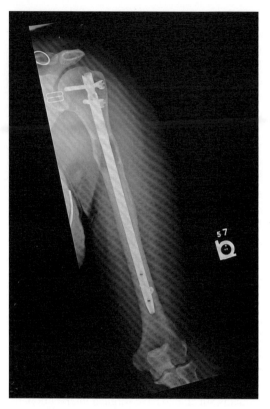

Figure 27.2 Impending pathological fracture. Example wording of an imaging report: Cortical thinning is present in the proximal humeral metaphysis. There is no definite associated fracture or soft tissue mass. A second lucent lesion may also be present in the left posterior lateral fifth rib. Shoulder and elbow joints are anatomically aligned. Bone mineralization is otherwise normal. Visualized left lung is clear. Impression: Lytic lesions in the left proximal humerus and left posterior fifth rib compatible with patient's known metastatic renal cell carcinoma.

Figure 27.3 Postoperative intramedullary (IM) rod to prevent pathological fracture. Example wording of an imaging report: The patient is status post ORIF with placement of a long intramedullary rod and interlocking screws crossing a 4-cm lytic lesion in the proximal humeral shaft. When compared with the prior exam, the overall size of the lesion does not appear to have changed. The lesion shows slight interval thickening of the remaining cortex. No other lesions are identified in the left humerus. Impression: Multiple lytic lesions as described above. No increase in size of the above lesions and some increased margination and perhaps increased new bone formation around the lesions suggest the possibility of some interval healing or positive response to treatment.

Cancer-Related Fatigue

Cancer-related fatigue (CRF) is a common side effect of cancer and the associated treatments. CRF impacts anywhere from 40% to 100% of people with cancer (American Cancer Society, 2015a). CRF is not the same as a regular or general fatigue as CRF does not get better with rest. Often described as feeling weak and drained, minimal activity can cause exhaustion such as walking from the bed to the bathroom or even just getting out of the bed to eat. The level of fatigue can vary from day to day and throughout each day. CRF can last for months and years after treatment ends (American Cancer Society, 2015a). The hazard with CRF is the tendency for survivors to decrease daily activity, restrict roles, and become inactive, directly and negatively impacting the overall quality of life. Additionally, decreased functional status may preclude the survivor from receiving continued cancer treatments such as chemotherapy. CRF is currently understood to be a combination of cancer and the treatments. Other factors that may contribute include low levels of certain blood cells, stress, pain, poor sleep, lack of exercise, and poor nutrition. The National Comprehensive Cancer Network (NCCN) provides clinical guidelines for management of CRF and recommends assessment of fatigue at diagnosis and management of symptoms and treatable contributing factors including pain, emotional distress, sleep disturbance, and decreased functional status (2015). Occupational therapy's role in CRF includes instruction in energy conservation balanced with continued daily activity and engagement in routines and roles; intervention to improve strength, balance, and physical abilities to complete daily activities; and educating on good sleep hygiene.

Cancer-Related Cognitive Dysfunction

Previously referred to as "chemo brain," **cancer-related cognitive dysfunction** (CRCD) refers to various cognitive weaknesses an individual may experience following chemotherapy treatments (Porter, 2013; Staat & Segatore, 2005). These cognitive changes are common following chemotherapy treatments (Raffa et al., 2006), with current research showing that 75% cancer patients experience mental impairments and upward of 35% persist for months or years (Janelsins et al., 2011). CRCD includes difficulty with attention, concentration, memory, and processing speed, areas that directly impact executive functioning (Evens & Eschiti, 2009; Janelsins et al., 2011; Raffa, 2010, 2013).

Potential causes of CRCD include primary brain disease, metastatic brain disease, hypoxia, fluid or electrolyte abnormalities, psychological impact of the diagnosis, stress, impaired sleep, chemotherapy treatment, brain radiation, and treatment duration. Occupational therapists should use standardized cognitive assessments in order to objectively measure and track cognitive abilities. This is particularly important at the time of diagnosis, prior to the introduction of treatments that potentially impact cognition such as chemotherapy. This allows both an understanding of (near) baseline cognitive abilities and the ability to identify subtle changes that may not be recognized during general conversations. Engaging in mentally stimulating and cognitive exercising tasks has been shown to positively impact cognitive functioning (Evens & Eschiti, 2009; Porter, 2013; Staat & Segatore, 2005). The role of occupational therapy for individuals with CRCD includes education of the individual, the family/caregivers, and the treatment team on the noted areas of impairment and the anticipated impact on the daily routine, along with facilitating treatment plans to include

cognitive retraining. For example, a mild cognitive impairment in the area of attention and mental flexibility places the individual at risk of error in medication management and household finances. During the time of impairment, it is advisable to have assistance with these tasks as errors could be detrimental to the individual's overall well-being. Meanwhile, the occupational therapy plan of care includes interventions to facilitate improvement in these areas and standardized testing to track progress.

Immobility

A variety of reasons may cause an individual to become immobile including cancer and treatment-related fatigue, weakness, pain, depression, fear of movement, and hospitalization(s). Regardless of the underlying reason for immobility, the immobility itself leads to a further decline in function beginning at a physiological level. Research has demonstrated that immobility leads to orthostasis and thrombus formation (Olsen & Thompson, 1967) as well as an increase in accumulation of secretions (Olsen & McCarthy, 1967). This places the individual at an increased risk of complications including orthostatic hypotension, which further limits tolerance for out-of-bed activity, and may preclude the individual from receiving further chemotherapy treatments. Additionally, prolonged immobility may lead to critical illness polyneuropathy (CIP), a multilevel weakness with high rates of mortality (Latronico & Bolton, 2011). Immobility also leads to decreased strength, decreased joint integrity, and an overall decrease in physical functioning (Bryant, Grigsby, Swenso, Scarbro, & Baxter, 2007; Bunting & Shea, 2001; Chambers, Moylan, & Reid, 2009). A landmark longitudinal study, the Dallas Bed Rest and Training study, demonstrated the significant changes to the cardiovascular system following immobility. In 1966, five 20-year-old men participated in the Dallas Bed Rest and Training study. It began with a series of tests on physiological capacity, followed by 3 weeks of bed rest. At the end of the 3 weeks, the men were retested, underwent 8 weeks of heavy endurance training, and were retested again. The results showed a significant decline in their cardiovascular system. Thirty years later, the same five men were evaluated and the results were profound. A greater deterioration in cardiovascular performance, specifically maximal oxygen uptake (VO_{2max}), was found after 3 weeks of bed rest than in 30 years of natural aging (McGuire et al., 2001). A final follow-up to this study was published in 2009 (McGavock et al., 2009). The same five men, 40 years after the original assessments, were evaluated. The net proportional decline in maximal oxygen uptake for a period of 40 years of life was comparable with that experienced after 3 weeks of strict bed rest as a 20-year-old. Reflect for a moment: this study was conducted on five *healthy* 20-year-olds. How much greater is impact of bed rest for an older individual, or in someone with comorbidities, or in someone who has cancer? The role of occupational therapy is to facilitate participation with daily routines and roles, to provide therapy interventions to improve function, to modify tasks and/or routines as needed, and to provide recommendations for adaptive equipment or durable medical equipment.

Lymphedema

The lymphatic system, composed of groups of lymph nodes and a network of lymphatic vessels throughout the body, drains excess fluids from the body's tissues. It also helps defend the body against disease through lymphocytes, a type of WBC. When there is disruption to the lymphatic system following surgery or radiation in the area of the lymph nodes, rather than circulating through the lymphatic system, the lymph fluid builds in the fatty tissue just under the skin, resulting in lymphedema. **Lymphedema** is a condition resulting from the disrupted flow of the lymph system and is a lifelong side effect that cannot be cured but must be managed. As examples, lymphedema may occur in the arm following axillary lymph node dissection for breast cancer or in the leg following inguinal lymph node dissection for a soft tissue sarcoma or cervical cancer. Lymphedema may also occur in the genitals, the trunk, or the head and neck region, dependent upon the surgical or radiation area. Factors that increase the risk of lymphedema include extensive surgery or radiation, an infection in the affected limb, trauma to the affected limb, inadequate muscle contraction, obesity, hypertension, and chronic venous insufficiency. Lymphedema goals include decreasing the volume in the affected area and developing the best system to maintain the lowest volume. Patients and caregivers are educated on risk reduction, early detection, and treatment, as well as the risk for infection and guidelines for proper skin care. Lymphedema treatments consist of manual lymph drainage, use of elastic sleeves and short-stretch bandaging systems to continue decreasing volume, and ordering custom-fit compression garments. Occupational therapists may become certified lymphedema therapists (CLT) after participating in a training and certification program.

Psychosocial Disruption

A certain amount of anxiety, despair, and fear is normal following a diagnosis of cancer as the individual has concerns about potential changes in daily routine and life plans, has changes in the body (loss of hair, postoperative changes, skin changes following radiation), has a fear of death, or has legal or financial concerns (American Cancer Society, 2013a). However, clinical anxiety and depression may co-occur with cancer to a greater rate than the general population without cancer and may impact the overall medical management and outcomes (Hewitt, Greenfield, & Stovall, 2006). Research has shown the prevalence of clinical anxiety ranging from 19% to 24%, clinical depression from 6% to 13%, and mixed anxiety/depression from 9% to as high as 30% (Boyes et al., 2013; Brintzenhofe-Szoc, Levin, Li, Kissane, Zabora, 2009; Linden, Vodermaier, MacKenzie, & Greig, 2012). The percentages are higher when subclinical symptoms are included. The Diagnostic and Statistic Manual of Mental Disorders, 5th edition (DSM-5) provides diagnoses for both anxiety disorder and depressive disorder "due to another medical condition" and includes parameters for clinical diagnosis. The role of occupational therapy is to recognize when these changes in mood are impacting the individual's ability to complete his or her daily routine and to share this information with the individual, family, and treatment team. Through examination of the individual's routines and roles, the occupational therapy practitioner can recommend modifications and instruct on balance both of tasks and roles, thus encouraging continued daily engagement in activity.

■ Special Considerations

As cancer and the treatments impact areas across all client factors, occupational therapy practitioners must have special considerations for the following areas in order to effectively and safely guide treatment sessions.

Cardiovascular Considerations

Research has shown that chemotherapy treatments and radiation across the chest increase the risk of cardiac problems including heart failure, myocardial ischemia, arrhythmias, hypertension, and thromboembolism (Bovelli, Plataniotis, & Roila, 2010). Regular monitoring for cardiac signs and symptoms is important for early detection and intervention including the following:

> Complaints of chest pain.
> Resting pulse is >100 beats per minute or lower than 50 beats per minute.
> Resting blood pressure is >145/95 or systolic is lower than 85 mm Hg.
> Swelling is noted at bilateral ankles.
> If the patient is on any medication(s) that controls the heart rate, the target heart rate during exercise will not be attainable; do not overexert, and watch for clinical signs and symptoms such as increased breathing and diaphoresis (sweating) or increased complaints of fatigue.
> If the patient has lymphedema or is at risk for lymphedema, compression garments should be worn on the affected limb during exercise.
> If the patient has a known premorbid risk of cardiac disease, then it is medically recommend to be supervised during exercise testing and training.

Potential Contraindications

The following list of potential contraindications is defined as *potential* because patients undergoing cancer treatments may very well fall below these parameters; however, the risk of inactivity may outweigh the risk of mobility with these potential contraindications: deep vein thrombosis (DVT) or pulmonary embolism (PE), oxygen saturation below 90%, orthostasis, unstable bone, platelets below 20,000 (20k), and hemoglobin (Hgb) below 8.0. Clinical judgment and close attention to clinical signs and symptoms associated with these values are important during occupational therapy sessions.

Cancer and Nutrition

Consideration must be given to the patient's nutritional status as cancer and the treatments may lead to poor oral intake or poor metabolism of intake. At times, patients may have complaints of decreased appetite, decreased sense of taste, nausea, or vomiting. If the patient has been vomiting or had diarrhea within the last 24 to 36 hours, dehydration must also be considered. When not adequately addressed, these issues may lead to failure to thrive and/or **cancer cachexia**, an often irreversible syndrome leading to substantial weight loss including skeletal muscle and body fat (Acreman, 2009). At times, artificial nutrition may be used; options include total parenteral nutrition (TPN) infused intravenously, a percutaneous endoscopic gastrostomy (PEG) tube, and a nasogastric (NG) tube. The amount of energy (calories) expended during occupational therapy sessions and throughout the day should not exceed the number of calories the body is processing, especially in the setting of cancer cachexia.

Cancer and Sexuality and Intimacy

The changes in sexuality and intimacy following a cancer diagnosis and the associated treatments have been shown to negatively impact both the cancer survivor and his or her partner and lead to a decreased quality of life. Multiple factors have been identified including physical changes following surgeries and cancer treatments, decreased libido, CRF, mood disturbances including anxiety and depression, changes in body image, emotional distancing, and role changes from intimate partners to patient-caregiver (Beck, Robinson, & Carlson, 2012; Hawkins et al., 2009; Loaring, Larkin, Shaw, & Flowers, 2015; Low et al., 2009; Rolland, 1994; Ussher, Perz., & Gilbert, 2012). Changes in sexuality and intimacy have been reported in as many as 76% of individuals with cancer and 84% of partners caring for individuals with cancer (Hawkins et al., 2009). Occupational therapy practitioners should address the roles of sexuality and intimacy in order to effectively optimize the overall quality of life.

CASE STUDY 1

Janice, a 62-year-old female, had difficulty with a persistently infected wound that had been nonhealing for several months. Further medical workup revealed acute myeloid leukemia with 63% circulating blasts. Janice was immediately admitted to the hospital for induction chemotherapy. As the 14-day bone marrow biopsy showed residual disease, she underwent a reinduction, which was successful in helping her achieve remission. Overall, the hospital course proceeded without medical complications. Her function declined slightly and she had generalized weakness, as expected, but she remained independent with her basic daily routine. Cognitive testing during occupational therapy sessions showed a mild cognitive impairment in executive functioning, specifically with cognitive flexibility and working memory. She has been completing cognitive self-exercises. Now medically stable, and after 47 days of hospitalization, Janice is ready to return home with her husband. Due to the lengthy medical course for acute leukemia, she had to stop working as a real-estate assistant; therefore, she plans on spending most of her time at home. While she enjoys socializing with her friends and is typically active in her church, she verbalized a good understanding of the need to balance her routine within her tolerance, as well as the importance of avoiding close contact with individuals who may be contagious. She expressed both excitement and apprehension regarding the medical plan for a BMT. An HLA-matched donor has been located, and the process is scheduled for approximately 6 weeks from now.

CASE STUDY 2

Sonya is a 43-year-old female with stage IIa breast cancer. Unfortunately, the disease has been refractory to multiple rounds of chemotherapy and has continued to progress. She now has metastatic disease to the liver, spleen, and bones. Sonya resides with her husband and two sons aged 10 and 13 years old in a single-level home. Previously an elementary school teacher, Sonya stopped working approximately 6 months earlier due to disease progression and became a stay-at-home mother. While this transition was emotionally difficult for her, she took pride in keeping the home "ready for when everyone gets home each day." Three months ago during a hospital admission, her occupational therapist instructed her that she could no longer bend, could no longer lift more than 5 lb, and needed to avoid twisting her back. This change in her routine was made due to the findings of multiple bony lesions including at T8, which required medical intervention to stabilize, and at L3 and L5. She was encouraged to complete her own self-care, to remain active each day within her precautions, and to "teach her sons" when they arrived home from school to complete portions of tasks such as lifting laundry, placing casseroles in the oven, and vacuuming. Sonya is now admitted to the hospital following complaints of progressive bilateral leg weakness to the point of being unable to move and increasing neck pain. Imaging shows a new lesion at C5 with cord edema, and there is a concern for metastatic disease involving the CNS with differential diagnoses including metastatic dural disease versus leptomeningeal disease. Her mother and father are willing to have her live with them so they can take care of her while her husband continues to work full-time to maintain finances. Although in tremendous pain, Sonya wishes to be able to use the bedside commode instead of a bedpan.

RECOMMENDED LEARNING RESOURCES

Academy of Nutrition and Dietetics: Oncology Nutrition
http://www.oncologynutrition.org

American Cancer Society
http://www.cancer.org

American Lung Association
http://www.lung.org

American Society for Blood and Marrow Transplantation
http://www.asbmt.org

International Agency for Research on Cancer
http://www.iarc.fr

Leukemia and Lymphoma Society
http://www.lls.org

National Cancer Institute: SEER Training Modules
http://www.training.seer.cancer.gov

National Cancer Institute: Comprehensive Cancer Information
http://www.cancer.gov

National Comprehensive Cancer Network
http://www.nccn.org/

National Lymphedema Network
http://www.lymphnet.org

National Hospice and Palliative Care Organization
http://www.nhpco.org

Occupational Therapy in Oncology
http://www.otoncology.org

Palliative Care Video
http://www.palliativecarevideo.com

World Health Organization: Cancer
http://www.sho.init/cancer/en/

RECOMMENDED READING

The Immortal Life of Henrietta Lacks by Rebecca Skloot; New York: Crown Publishers, 2010.

The Emperor of All Maladies by Siddhartha Mukherjee; New York: Scribner, 2010.

REFERENCES

Acreman, S. (2009). Nutrition in palliative care. *British Journal of Community Nursing*, *14*(10), 427–431.

Agency for Healthcare Research and Quality. (2015). *AgingStats: Federal interagency forum on aging-related statistics*. Retrieved from www.againstats.gov

American Cancer Society. (2013). *Anxiety, fear, and depression*. Publication. Retrieved from www.cancer.org/acs/groups/cid/documents/webcontent/002816-pdf.pdf

American Cancer Society. (2015a). *Cancer Facts & Figures 2015*. Publication. Atlanta. Retrieved from http://www.cancer.org/research/cancerfactsstatistics/cancerfactsfigures2015/

American Cancer Society. (2015b). *Cancer in children*. Retrieved from http://www.cancer.org/cancer/cancerinchildren/index

American Cancer Society. (2015c). *Learn about cancer*. Retrieved from http://www.cancer.org/Cancer/index

American Cancer Society (2015d). *Diesel exhaust and cancer*. Retrieved from www.cancer.org/cancer/cancercauses/othercarcinogens/pollition/diesel-exhaust-and-cancer

American Occupational Therapy Association. (2015a). *Cancer care and oncology*. Retrieved from http://www.aota.org/Practice/Rehabilitation-Disability/Emerging-Niche/Cancer.aspx

American Occupational Therapy Association. (2015b). *Occupational therapy and pain rehabilitation*. Retrieved from http://www.aota.org/-/media/Corporate/Files/AboutOT/Professionals/WhatIsOT/HW/Facts/Pain %Rehabilitation fact sheet.pdf

American Occupational Therapy Association. (2015c). *Role of occupational therapy in oncology*. Retrieved from http://www.aota.org/-/media/Corporate/Files/AboutOT/Professionals/WhatIsOT/RDP/Facts/Oncology fact sheet.pdf

Anand, P., Kunnumakara, A. B., Sundaram, C., Harikumar, K. B., Tharakan, S. T., Lai, O. S., … Aggarwai, B. B. (2008). Cancer is a preventable disease that requires major lifestyle changes. *Journal of Pharmacy Research*, *25*(9), 2097–2116.

Arnold, M., Pandeya, N., Brynes, G., Reneham, A. G., Stevens, G. A., Ezzati, M., ...Soerjomataram, I. (2015). Global burden of cancer attributable to high body-mass index in 2012: A population-based study. *The Lancet Oncology*, *16*(1), 36–46.

Bagnardi, V., Blangiardo, M., La Vecchia, C., & Corraro, G. (2001). Alcohol consumption and the risk of cancer: A meta-analysis. *Alcohol Research & Health*, *25*(4), 263–270.

Baranovsky, A., & Myers, M. H. (1986). Cancer incidence and survival in patients 65 years of age and older. *CA: A Cancer Journal for Clinicians*, *36*(1), 27–41.

Beck, A. M., Robinson, J. W., & Carlson, L. E. (2012). Sexual values as the key to maintaining satisfying sex after prostate cancer treatment: The physical pleasure-relational intimacy model of sexual motivation. *Archives Sexual Behavior*, *42*, 1637–1647. doi: 10.1007/s10508-013-0168-z

Berger, N. A., Savvides, P., & Miller, R. H. (2006). Cancer in the elderly. *Transactions of the American Clinical and Climatological Association*, *117*, 147–156.

Bovelli, D., Plataniotis, G., & Roila, F. (2010). Cardiotoxicity of chemotherapy agents and radio-therapy-related heart disease: ESMO clinical practice guidelines. *Annuals of Oncology*, *21*(Suppl. 5), v277–v282. doi: 10.1093/annonc/mdq200

Boyes, A. W., Girgis, A., D'Este, C. A., Zucca, A. C., Lecathelinais, C., & Carey, M. L. (2013). Prevalence and predictors of the short-term trajectory of anxiety and depression in the first year after a cancer diagnosis: A population-based longitudinal study. *Journal of Clinical Oncology*, *31*(21), 2724–2729.

Brintzenhofe-Szoc, K. M., Levin, T. T., Li, Y., Kissane, D. W., & Zabora, J. (2009). Mixed anxiety/depression symptoms in a large cancer cohort: Prevalence by cancer type. *Psychosomatics*, *50*(4), 383–391.

Bunting, R. W., & Shea, B. (2001). Bone metastasis and rehabilitation. *Cancer*, *92*(Suppl. 4), 1020–1028.

Bryant, L. L., Grigsby, J., Swenso, C., Scarbro, S., & Baxter, J. (2007). Chronic pain increases the risk of decreasing physical performance in older adults: The San Luis Valley Health and Aging Study. *The Journals of Gerontology Series A: Biological Sciences and Medical Sciences*, *62*(9), 989–996.

Centers for Disease Control and Prevention. (2015). *Smoking and cancer*. Retrieved from www.cdc. gov/tobacco/campaign/tips/diseases/cancer.html

Chambers, M. A., Moylan, J. S., & Reid, M. B. (2009). Physical inactivity and muscle weakness in the critically ill. *Critical Care Medicine*, *37*(10), S337–S346.

Dubey, A., & Koul, R. (2009). Malignant spinal cord compression: An overview. *The Internet Journal of Oncology*, *7*(2). ISPUB.com/IJO/7/2/3125

Evens, K., & Eschiti, V. S. (2009). Cognitive effects of cancer treatment: "Chemo brain" explained. *Clinical Journal of Oncology Nursing*, *13*(6), 661–666.

Everdingen, M. H., Riijke, J. M., Kessels, A. G., Schouten, H. C., Kleef, M., & Patijn, J. (2007). Prevalence of pain in patients with cancer: A systematic review of the past 40 years. *Annuals of Oncology*, *18*, 1437–1449.

Gehle, K. (2009). Toxicity of polycyclic aromatic hydrocarbons (PAHs). *Agency for Toxic Substances and Disease Registry (ATSDR)*. Retrieved from www.atsdr.cdc.gov/csem/pah/docs/pah.pdf

George, R., Jeba, J., Ramkumar, G., Chacko, A. G., Leng, M., & Tharyan, P. (2008). Interventions for the treatment of metastatic extradural spinal cord compression in adults. *Cochrane Database System Review*, *8*, CD006716.

Hawkins, Y., Ussher, J., Gilbert, E., Perz, J., Sandoval, M., & Sundquist, K. (2009). Changes in sexuality and intimacy after the diagnosis and treatment of cancer. *Cancer Nursing*, *32*(4), 271–280.

Hewitt, M, Greenfield, S., & Stovall, E. (Eds.). (2006). *From cancer patient to cancer survivor: Lost in translation*. Washington, DC: The National Academies Press.

Hurria, A., Browner, I. S., Cohen, H. J., Denlinger, C. S., deShazo, M., Extermann, M., ... Wildes, T. (2010). Senior adult oncology: Clinical practice guidelines in oncology. *Journal of National Comprehensive Cancer Network*, *10*, 162–209.

International Agency for Research on Cancer. (2002). *IRAC handbooks of cancer prevention. Weight control and physical activity*. Lyon, France: IRAC.

International Agency for Research on Cancer, 2010. Ingested nitrate and nitrite, and cyanobacterial peptide toxins. *IARC Monographs on the evaluation of carcinogenic risks to humans, 94*: Lyon, France

Janelsins, M. C., Kohli, S., Mohile, S. G., Usuki, K., Ahles, T. A., & Morrow, G. R. (2011). An update on cancer- and chemotherapy-related cognitive dysfunction: Current status. *Seminars in Oncology*, *38*(3), 431–438. doi: 10.1053/j. semioncol.2011.03.014

Key, T. J., Schatzkin, A., Willett, W. C., Allen, N. E., Spencer, E. A., & Travis, R. C. (2004). Diet, nutrition, and the prevention of cancer. *Public Health Nutrition*, *71*(1A), 187–200. doi: 10.1079/ PHN2003588

Kupfer, G. M. (2015). *Childhood cancer epidemiology*. Retrieved from http://www.emedicine.med-scape.com/article/989841-overview-a3

Latronico, N., & Bolton, C. F. (2011). Critical illness polyneuropathy and myopathy: A major cause of muscle weakness and paralysis. *Lancet Neurology*, *10*(10), 931–941. doi: 10.1016/ S1474-4422(11)70178-8

Leukemia & Lymphoma Society. (2015). *Acute myeloid leukemia*. Retrieved from https://www.lls.org/leukemia/acute-myeloid-leukemia

Lewis, M. A., Hendrickson, A. W., & Moynihan, T. J. (2011). Oncologic emergencies: Pathophysiology, presentation, diagnosis, and treatment. *Cancer Journal for Clinicians, 61*(5), 287–314. doi: 10.3322/caac.20124

Liao, J. B. (2006). Viruses and human cancer. *The Yale Journal of Biology and Medicine, 79*(3–4), 115–122.

Linden, W., Vodermaier, A., MacKenzie, R., & Greig, D. (2012). Anxiety and depression after cancer diagnosis: Prevalence rates by caner type, gender, and age. *Journal of Affective Disorders, 141*, 343–351.

Loaring, J. M., Larkin, M., Shaw, R., & Flowers, P. (2015). Renegotiating sexual intimacy in the context of altered embodiment: The experiences of women with breast cancer and their male partners following mastectomy and reconstruction. *Health Psychology, 34*(4), 426–436. doi: 10.1037/hea0000195

Low, C., Fullarto, M., Parkinson, E., O'Brien, K., Jackson, S., Lowe, D., & Rogers, S. (2009). Issues of intimacy and sexual dysfunction following major head and neck cancer treatment. *Oral Oncology, 45*(10), 898–903. doi: 10.1016/j.oraloncology.2009.03.014

Lucas, R., McMichael, T., Smith, W., & Armstrong, B. (2006). *Solar ultraviolet radiation: Global burden of disease from solar ultraviolet radiation. Environmental Burden of Disease Series, No. 13.* Geneva, Switzerland: World Health Organization, Public Health and the Environment.

McCurdy, M. T., & Shanholtz, C. B. (2012). Oncologic emergencies. *Critical Care Medicine, 40*(7), 2212–2222. doi: 10.1097/CCM.0b013e31824e1865

McGavock, J. M., Hastings, J. L., Snell, P. G., McGuire, D. K., Pacini, E. L., Levine, B. D., & Mitchell, J. H. (2009). A forty-year follow-up of the Dallas bed rest and training study: The effect of age on the cardiovascular response to exercise in men. *Journals of Gerontology Series A: Biological Sciences & Medical Sciences, 64A*(2), 293–299.

McGuire, D. K., Levine, B. D., Williamson, J. W., Snell, P. G., Blomqvist, C. G., Saltin, B., & Mitchell, J. H. (2001). A 30-year follow up of the Dallas bed rest and training study II: Effect of age on cardiovascular adaption to exercise training. *Circulation, 104*(12), 1358.

Mishamandani, S. (2014). Study identifies novel compounds more mutagenic than parent PAHs. *NIH: National Institute of Environmental Health Sciences*. Retrieved from http://www.niehs.nih.gov/news/newsletter/2014/2/science-NPAHs/

National Cancer Institute. (2015a). *Asbestos exposure and cancer risk*. Retrieved from http://www.cancer.gov/about-cancer/causes-prevention/risk/substances/asbestoes/asbestos-fact-sheet

National Cancer Institute. (2015b). *Chemicals in meat cooked at high temperatures and cancer risk*. Retrieved from http://www.cancer.gov/about-cancer/causes-prevention/risk/diet/cooked-meats-fact-sheet

National Cancer Institute. (2015c). *Genetics of breast and gynecologic cancers for health professionals*. Retrieved from http://www.cancer.gov/types/breast/hp/breast-ovarian-genetics-pdq-section/_88

National Cancer Institute. (2015d). *Genetic testing for hereditary cancer syndromes*. Retrieved from http://www.cancer.gov/about-cancer/causes-prevention/genetics/genetic-testing-fact-sheet

National Cancer Institute. (2015e). *Infectious agents*. Retrieved from http://www.cancer.gov/about-cancer/causes-prevention/risk/infectious-agents

National Cancer Institute. (2015f). *Obesity and cancer risk*. Retrieved from http://www.cancer.gov/about-cancer/causes-prevention/risk/obesity/obesity-fact-sheet

National Cancer Institute. (2015g). *Secondhand smoke and cancer*. Retrieved from http://www.cancer.gov/about-cancer/causes-prevention/risk/tobacco/second-hand-smoke-fact-sheet-q3

National Cancer Institute. (2015h). *Stem cell transplant side effects*. Retrieved from http://www.cancer.org/treatment/treatmentsandsideeffects/treatmenttypes/bonemarrowandpheralbloodstemcelltransplant/stem-cell-transplant-long-term-problems-after-transplant

National Comprehensive Cancer Network. (2015). *Cancer-related fatigue: Version 1.2014*. Retrieved from https://www.pfizerpro.com/resources/minisites/oncology/docs/NCCNFatigueGuidelines.pdf

National Institute on Aging. (2015). *Health and aging: Cancer Facts for People over 50*. Retrieved from https://www.nia.hih.gov/health/publication/cancer-facts-people-over-50

National Institutes of Health: National Institute on Alcohol Abuse and Alcoholism. (2000). *10th Special Report to the U.S. Congress on Alcohol and Health: Highlights from current research*. Retrieved from http://www.pubs.niaaa.nih.gov/publications/10Report/10thSpecialReport.pdf

National Institutes of Health: Surveillance, Epidemiology, and End Results Program. (2015). *Cancer Statistics*. Retrieved from http://www.seer.cancer.gov/statfacts/html/all.html

Oken, M. M., Creech, R. H., & Tormey, D. C. (1983). Toxicity and response criteria of the Eastern Cooperative Oncology Group. *American Journal of Clinical Oncology, 5*(6), 649–655.

Olsen, E. V., & Thompson, L. F. (1967). Immobility: Effects on cardiovascular function. *American Journal of Nursing, 67*(4), 781–782.

Olsen, E. V., & McCarthy, J. A. (1967). Immobility: Effects on respiratory function. *American Journal of Nursing, 67*(4), 783–784.

Penfold, S. (1996). The role of the occupational therapist in oncology. *Cancer Treatment Reviews, 22*, 75–81.

Pergolotti, M., Cutchin, M. P., Weinberger, M., & Meyer, A. M. (2014). Occupational therapy use by older adults with cancer. *American Journal of Occupational Therapy, 68*, 597–607. Retrieved from http://dx.doi.org/10.5014/ajot.2014.011791

Porter, K. E. (2013). "Chemo brain"—Is cancer survivorship related to later-life cognition?: Findings from the health and retirement study. *Journal of Aging and Health, 25*, 960. doi: 10.1177/0898264313498417

Quinn, D. (2000). Neurological emergencies in the cancer patient. *Seminars in Oncology, 27*(3), 311–321.

Raffa, R. B. (2010). Is a picture worth a thousand (forgotten) words?: Neuroimaging evidence for the cognitive deficits in 'chemo-fog'/'chemo-brain.' *Journal of Clinical Pharmacy and Therapeutics, 35*, 1–9. doi: 10.1111/j.1365-2710.2009.01044.x

Raffa, R. B. (2013). Cancer 'survivor-care': II. Disruption of prefrontal brain activation top-down control of working memory capacity as possible mechanism for chemo-fog/brain (chemotherapy-associated cognitive impairment). *Journal of Clinical Pharmacy and Therapeutics, 38*, 265–268. doi: 10.1111/jcpt.12071

Raffa, R. B., Duong, P. V., Finney, J., Garber, D. A., Lam, L. M., Mathew, S. S., … Jen Weng, H. F. (2006). Is 'chemo-fog'/'chemo-brain' caused by cancer chemotherapy? *Journal of Clinical Pharmacy and Therapeutics, 31*, 129–138.

Rolland, J. S. (1994). In sickness and in health: the impact of illness on couples' relationships. *Journal of Marital Family Therapy, 20*(4), 327–335.

Silver, J. K., Baima, J., & Mayer, R. S. (2013). Impairment-driven cancer rehabilitation: an essential component of quality care and survivorship. *Cancer Journal for Clinicians, 63*(5), 295–317.

Silver, J. K., & Balma, J. (2013). Cancer prehabilitation: An opportunity to decrease treatment-related morbidity, increase cancer treatment options, and improve physical and psychological health outcomes. *American Journal of Physical Medicine and Rehabilitation, 92*(8), 715–727. doi: 10.1097/PHM.0b013e31829b4afe

Silver, J. K., & Gilchrist, L. S. (2011). Cancer rehabilitation with a focus on evidence-based outpatient physical and occupational therapy interventions. *American Journal of Physical Medicine and Rehabilitation, 90*(5 Suppl. 1), S5–S15. doi: 10.1097/PHM.0b013e31820be4ae

Simon, S. (2013). *World Health Organization: Outdoor air pollution causes cancer.* Retrieved from http://www.cancer.org/cancer/news/world-health-organization-outdoor-air-pollution-causes-cancer

Staat, K., & Segatore, M. (2005). The phenomenon of chemo brain. *Clinical Journal of Oncology Nursing, 9*(6), 713–720.

Stadler, K. M. (2009). *The Diet and Cancer Connection.* Virginia: Cooperative Extension Publications and Educational Resources. Blacksburg, Virginia. Retrieved from pubs.ext.vtedu/348/348-141/348-141.html

Tariman, J. D. (contributing editor). (2009). Half of patients with cancer are older than 65: Do you know how to care for older adults? *Oncology Nursing Society Connect, 24*(12), 8–11.

Tefferi, A. (2006). Classification, diagnosis and management of myeloproliferative disorders in the JAK2V617F era. *Hematology/the Education Program of the American Society of Hematology*, 240–245. doi: 10.1182/asheducation-2006.1.240 PMID 17124067

Ukraintseva, S. V., & Yashin, A. I. (2003). Individual aging and cancer risk: How are they related? *Demographic Research 9*(8), 163–196. doi: 10.4054/DemRes.2003.9.8

United States Environmental Protection Agency. (2015). *Radon health risks.* Retrieved from https://www2.epa.gov

Ussher, J. M., Perz, J., & Gilbert, E. (2012). Changes to sexual well-being and intimacy after breast cancer. *Cancer Nursing, 35*(6), 456–465. doi: 10.1097/NCC.0b013e3182395401

Vermeulen, R., Silverman, D. T., Garshick, E., Vlaanderen, J., Portengen, L., & Steenland, K. (2014). Exposure-response estimates for diesel engine exhaust and lung cancer mortality based on data from three occupational cohorts. *Environmental Health Perspectives, 122*, 2. doi: 10.1289/ehp.1306880

Vincenzo, B., Blangiardo, M., LaVecchi, C., & Corrao, G. (2015). *Alcohol consumption and the risk of cancer: A meta-analysis. NIH: National Institute on Alcohol Abuse and Alcoholism.* Retrieved from http://pubs.niaaa.nih.gov/publications/arh25-4/263-270.htm

Warburton, D. E. R., Nicol, C. W., & Bredin, S. S. D. (2006). Health benefits of physical activity: The evidence. *Canadian Medical Association Journal,* *174*(6), 801–809.

Weinstein, J. R., & Anderson, S. (2010). The aging kidney: Physiological changes. *Advanced Chronic Kidney Disorder, 17*(4), 302–302. doi: 10.1053/j. ackd.2010.05.002

World Health Organization. (2002). *Physical inactivity a leading cause of disease and* *disability, warns WHO.* Retrieved from http://www.who.int/mediacentre/news/releases/release23/en/

World Health Organization. (2011). *Cancer linked with poor nutrition.* Retrieved from http://www.euro.who.int/en/health-topics/noncommunicable-diseases/cancer/news/news/2011/02/cancer-linked-with-poor-nutrition

28 Obesity

Shirley Blanchard

Carl is a 56-year-old man who is a part-time assistant pastor of a small church congregation in the rural South. With a height of 6'3", his weight had been stable at 240 lb until he had a sudden onset of a rare neurological condition, Parsonage-Turner Syndrome. He was unable to return to work as a furniture machinist secondary to the inability to perform shoulder and arm motions, perceive arm position, and lift and carry objects. Since the diagnosis, he has gained 230 lb and has adopted a sedentary lifestyle. He and his wife cook traditional Southern meals such as biscuits, gravy, and fried foods. His current weight of 470 lb makes it difficult to tolerate activity, perform functional mobility, find suitable clothing for church, participate in home maintenance, and get in and out of the car. He was recently hospitalized for hypertension, lower extremity cellulitis, and edema. He is edentulous due to persistent gingivitis and periodontal disease that resulted in complete teeth extraction. His physician prescribed antibiotics for systemic inflammation and recommended weight loss and consultation with a dietician. When asked about his eating habits he states, "I have to have some enjoyment." The client's mental health status was not assessed.

DESCRIPTION AND DEFINITIONS

Obesity is a public health concern and a complex social problem. The University of Rochester Minnesota Department of Senior Health Research (URMCR) reports that of the top ten most common health issues, being overweight and obesity ranked second to physical inactivity and nutrition (URMCR, 2015). A constellation of factors contribute to obesity including health behaviors, diet, physical inactivity, and genetics. Health disparities such as environment, socioeconomic status, health literacy, and access to health education may also impact obesity.

Obesity is a modifiable risk factor associated with type II diabetes, cardiovascular disease, heart disease, gallbladder and liver disease, sleep apnea, gynecological problems (fibroid disease), neurological (such as atherosclerosis, hypertension, and peripheral vascular disease), and musculoskeletal changes such as osteoarthritis (OA). **Metabolic syndrome** and **diabesity** refer to the presence of a combination of risk factors including obesity, diabetes, hypertension, high cholesterol, elevated fasting blood sugar, high triglycerides, systemic inflammation, and a tendency to form blood clots (Blanchard, 2012; Kresser, 2015).

The relationship of obesity to cancer has received less attention; however, existing evidence suggests that increased adipose tissue may increase the risk of breast, prostrate, and colon cancer. Additionally, increased body weight increases circulating insulin, which affects multiple types of cancer cells (Calle & Thung, 2004). Recent research examined a possible link between obesity and Alzheimer's disease. Chuang et al. (2015) studied 142 elders with an average age of 83 when diagnosed with Alzheimer's. Findings imply that those who were overweight by age 50 tended to develop a decline in memory earlier. Higher BMI at age 50 was related to early onset of the disease and at autopsy demonstrated increased brain tangles. The Centers for Disease Control and Prevention (CDC, 2015a) advise that obesity is associated with poorer mental health outcomes and reduced quality of life. Figure 28.1 represents a summary of associated complications and the impact of obesity on client factors and body structure.

The terms overweight, **obesity**, and morbid (or extremity obesity) refer to excess body weight (Foti, 2005). Currently, the CDC, World Health Organization ([WHO], 2015), and the American College of Sports Medicine ([ACSM], 2012) define obesity by using the **body mass index** (BMI) measure. The BMI was developed by the Nutrition/Metabolism Laboratory, Cancer Research Institute in Boston (Blackburn & Kanders, 1987). The BMI is an international standard used to determine degree of obesity relative to height and is calculated by multiplying weight in (pounds) × 703 and then dividing by the height in inches squared. A BMI < 24.9 kg/m^2 is considered normal, while a BMI in excess of 25 is considered overweight with increased risk for disease (ASCM 2000, 2014). BMI may also be calculated electronically using the National Heart Lung and Blood Institute (NHLBI) Guidelines (NIH Web site or with smart phone apps; graphs are available for tracking BMI (NHLBI, 2015).

Along with **waist circumference**, BMI is used to describe the degree of obesity and predict the level of disease risk. Waist size indicates

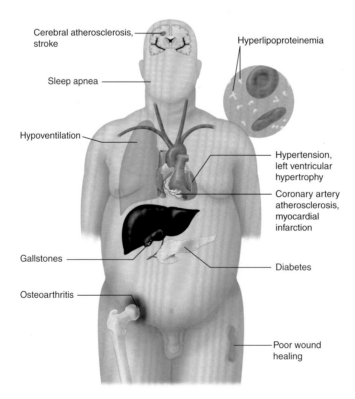

Figure 28.1 Complications of obesity. (From Braun, C. A., & Anderson, C M. 2011. *Pathophysiology: A clinical approach*. Philadelphia, PA: Wolters Kluwer.)

the amount of fat distribution in the abdominal area. An accumulation of body fat in this area results in an apple shape body and is associated with increased risk of heart disease and diabetes (ACSM, 2014). Specifically, a waist size > 35 in. or 88 cm for women and 40 in. for men is associated with higher risk for high blood pressure, high cholesterol, and heart disease (ACSM, 2014; CDC, 2015a). More recently, the CDC suggest that a waist size > 35 for women and 37 for men is associated with increased for disease (CDC, 2015b). Jacobs (2010) found that a waist size of 47 in. or larger for men and 42 in. for women increased risk for death compared to those with a waist size of 35 and 30 respectively. An adult with a BMI between 25 and 29.9 kg/m^2 is considered overweight, and an adult with a BMI higher than 30 kg/m^2 is considered obese (Table 28.1). A BMI between 39 and 40 is considered morbidly obese with extremely high risk for disease. BMI > 50 may be classified as super obesity or super morbid obesity (Dallas Center for Obesity Surgery, 2013). The term morbid obesity refers to patients who are 50% to 100% or 100 lb above their ideal body weight (Kolata, 2015).

The term **bariatrics** is often associated with persons who are morbidly obese. Current literature defines this condition as the medical study of the causes, evaluation, and intervention for individuals who are obese (Foti, 2005; Purnell, 2011; Stedman's Medical Dictionary, 2006). Medical and surgical management of bariatrics will be discussed later in the chapter.

■ Childhood Obesity

Obesity among children and adolescents continues to be a health concern. Obesity is defined in children and adolescents aged 2 to 19 years of age as a BMI at or above the 95th percentile according to gender, age, and growth chart (CDC, 2011). The lack of a diagnosis of obesity and an immediate plan for intervention during annual medical examinations exposes children to the same health conditions and comorbidities experienced by adults. Children may develop hypertension, systemic inflammation, dyslipidemia, type II diabetes, sleep apnea, and increased rate of obesity. Shah et al. (2015) examined adolescent and young adults with obesity and found increased cardiovascular risk factors (e.g. C-reactive protein, increased blood pressure, type 2 diabetes, and arterial wall thickness). Bout-Tabaku et al. (2015) assessed musculoskeletal pain among 233 teens average age 17 with a median BMI of 50.4. Seventy-six percent of the teens reported musculoskeletal pain, low back pain (63%), hip pain (31%), knee pain (49%), and ankle and foot pain (53%). Results suggest that adolescents with morbid obesity experience musculoskeletal pain that limits physical function and quality of life.

The American Academy of Pediatrics (APA) recommends annual monitoring of BMI to prevent childhood and adolescent obesity (Flower, Perrin, Viadro, & Ammerman, 2007).

Flower et al. (2007) interviewed pediatricians and parents and found lack of assessment,

---

TABLE **28.1** Body Mass Index, Waist Size, and Disease Risk

Weight	BMI, kg/m²	88 cm = waist size 35 in.[a]	
		Women ≤ 88 cm Men ≤ 102 cm	Women ≥ 88 cm Men > 102 cm
Underweight	<18.5		
Normal	18.5–24.9		
Overweight	25.0–29.9	Increased	High
Obesity Class I	30.0–34.9	High	Very high
Obesity Class II	35.0–39.9	Very high	Very high
Obesity Class III	≥40	Extremely high	Extremely high

[a]Classification of disease risk based on waist circumference: <88 to >88 cm.
Adapted from American College of Sports Medicine. (2014). Classification of disease risk based on BMI and waist circumference. *ACSM's resources for the personal trainer* (4th ed., p. 311). China: Lippincott Williams & Wilkins.

identification, reporting, and discussion about children's obesity. Themes from focus groups also suggest that there are several barriers to using BMI screening with children, including lack of access to accurate BMI charts and accurate height and weight measurements, outdated growth charts, and lack of time to calculate BMI. BMI results may also stigmatize children as being obese and cause issues with self-esteem. This creates added psychosocial stress and pressure to be thin (Schvey, et al., 2015), which may be further perpetuated by the media, peers, friends, and family members. Dissatisfaction with body image, depression, and failed attempts to achieve weight loss through dieting may result in weight gain, altered metabolic function (insulin sensitivity), and secretion of cortisol. Combined stressors, obesity, and psychosocial challenges may lower school performance and reduce quality of life (Tonetti, Fabri, Filardi, Martoni, & Natale, 2015). Today, the requirement of electronic medical records automatically calculates BMI, tracks risk factors, and compares measurements over time (Flower et al., 2007). BMI results may be used to raise parent and child awareness and discuss and set goals for lifestyle change and weight management.

Elder Obesity

Obesity among elders may result from a decline in physical activity and a change in independent living (Blanchard & Mosley, 2010). As elders transition from independent living to long-term care facilities and a more sedentary lifestyle, they are often positioned in and confined to wheelchairs. Weight gain may be associated with chronic conditions, immobility, and altered eating habits. This immobility limits range of motion and strength and hinders energy expenditure necessary to maintain a healthy weight. Elders who were active and lived independently are now exposed to an increase in social eating, which also increases BMI. Limited participation in occupations, deconditioning, and loss of muscle mass (sarcopenia) influences physical function and metabolic rate. Obesity among elders can negatively impact pulmonary, cardiovascular, cognitive status (vascular dementia), cholesterol, and joint pain associated with OA (Sperling, Laviolette, O'Keefe, et al., 2009). Long-term care facilities are now monitoring elder BMI through the Minimum Data Set (MDS). This Centers for Medicare and Medicaid (CMS) resident assessment tool requires a reassessment of BMI every 30 days. Section K of the MDS monitors BMI (CMS, 2010).

Obesity as Disease

Recently, the American Medical Association (AMA) approved the classification of obesity as a disease. The organization defines disease as: "(1) an impairment of the normal functioning of some aspect of the body; (2) characteristic signs and symptoms; and (3) causes harm or morbidity" (Sales-Martinez, 2013, paragraph 2, p. 1). The AMA and Jones (2015) of the Rudd Center for Health Policy and Obesity further propose advantages and disadvantages to classifying obesity as disease. Classifying obesity as a disease raises awareness, increases insurance coverage and reimbursement for treatment, and expands federal and private funding for research, which may lead to new public policies regarding obesity intervention and prevention (Smith, 2013).

Proponents of the new classification support early diagnosis through primary screening and argue that chronic obesity may be prevented through follow-up care, weight loss, and reducing associated stigma. Obesity may also be viewed as an addiction. The new classification suggests that persons will take the initiative to seek intervention. However, motivation for compliance with diet, increased physical activity, or other lifestyle changes is uncertain (Sales-Martinez, 2013).

Opponents of the AMA decision argue that obesity is a risk factor for other chronic diseases, that BMI does not measure fat mass, and that patients diagnosed as overweight or obese may still be healthy. Padro, Gonzales, Heymsfield, et al. (2015) agree that BMI does not differentiate between the contributions of lean body mass opposed to adipose tissue. This lack of well-defined overall body composition confounds the documented health consequences for morbidity and mortality associated with obesity across populations (Sales-Martinez, 2013). Therefore, it is felt that the disease classification is not warranted. Perceived lack of control over weight results in taking less responsibility for weight management. For example, individuals may seek a "quick fix" through pharmacological intervention or surgery (Sales-Martinez, 2013). Classification of obesity as a disease has the potential to reduce stereotypes and place the responsibility on the individual; however, the classification still must consider environmental, social, cultural, and psychological issues that may impact this complex health issue (Sales-Martinez, 2013; Smith, 2013).

■ Obesity and Stigma

Existing evidence supports that persons who are obese may be shunned by others. Stunkard and Sorensen (1993) refers to "obesity as the last socially acceptable form of prejudice" (p. 1037). Stigma associated with obesity is seen across population groups, among health care professionals, and across the lifespan. Persons who are obese may experience verbal abuse and verbal and physical bullying and be more vulnerable to depression, reduced self-esteem, and poor self-concept (Puhl & Latner, 2007). Unfortunately, health care professionals such as nurses, physicians and students perpetuate negative attitudes towards persons who are obese. Many fear the doctor's response that is often stated as "I can't help you if you don't lose weight" (Bailey, 2016, p. 8).

As the BMI increases, health providers are less tolerant and attentive, do not address health concerns in a timely manner, and view the person with obesity as a "waste of time," which results in negative psychosocial health and quality of life (Teachman & Brownell, 2001; Wang, Brownell, &Wadden, 2004). Blodorn, Major, Hunger, and Miller (2015) found that over time, constant rejection associated with higher BMI threatened social identity and increased the expectation of a negative response. Allison and Lee (2015) compared attitudes toward 185 overweight female university students. Results from participants read one of six vignettes to describe a female student with varying weights indicated that overweight targets were viewed more negatively than average weight or underweight targets.

Persons who are obese may be perceived as dishonest, sloppy, lacking self-control, lazy, unattractive, intellectually impaired, gluttonous, and socially impaired (Crandall, 1994; Flint, 2015). Persons who are obese report discrimination in the workplace, doctor's office, school, or other social or public settings. Rejection, stereotyping, and disrespect results in social isolation, overeating, and an increased potential for self-harm (Bailey, 2016; Faith, Matz, & Jorge, 2002; Puhl & Brownell, 2006). Choice of terms such as overweight or unhealthy weight is preferred to thick, chubby, or morbidly obese (Dutton, Tan, Perri, et al., 2010; Tailor & Ogden, 2009). Children who are obese may experience similar adult comorbidities and stigmatizations that perpetuate health disparities across the lifespan (Flint, 2015).

■ Obesity and Depression

Obesity is considered to be a medical but not a mental health diagnosis. The relationship between emotional state, behavior, excessive food intake, and low energy expenditure may reflect a significant mental health or psychosocial issue. The Diagnostic and Statistical Manual of Mental Disease Version-5 (DSM-5) does not include overeating but focuses on binge eating (Grever, 2013; Walsh, 2010). The American Psychiatric Association included bulimia (purging syndrome) and night eating syndrome in the most recent edition of the DSM-5, but failed to include obesity secondary to lack of acceptance of the diagnosis as a mental health disorder (Devlin, 2007; Grever, 2013; Walsh, 2010). Depression is one of the most prevalent psychiatric disorders and a major contributor to the United States (US) burden of disease. Bailey (2016) suggests that up to 80% of persons who are obese have some level of depression. Onset of depression and obesity may be related to geographical location and seasonal affective disorder (SAD) (Atkinson, 2005). Faith et al.'s (2002) meta-analysis implies an association between obesity and depression in childhood, during midlife, and among elders.

The relationship between obesity and depression may also differ by gender and race. Several studies support a biological and psychological basis for overeating and weight gain. Xiang and Ruopeng (2014) correlated the BMI of 6,514 adults born between 1931 and 1941 with the Center for Epidemiology Studies Depression Scale (CESDS). The CESDS defines symptoms of clinical depression over a 2-week period. Results indicated that unhealthy body weight was associated with future onset of depression. Blanchard (2009) examined the relationship of BMI and Depression among 378 African American women. Eighty-six percent of the sample had an average BMI of 32.78 with a high risk for disease. CESDS scores ranged from some to severe symptoms of depression with 73 (23.5%) reporting mild symptoms of depression, 79 (25.4%) moderate, and 29 (9.4%) severe symptoms. Women also reported overeating when stressed. Dixon, Dixon, and Obrien (2003) reported that weight loss following bariatric surgery was associated with a decline in depression scores 1 to 4 years postsurgery. Other researchers report that psychological well-being following bariatric surgery depends on presurgery eating patterns, social support, self-esteem, body image, coping strategies, and the amount of weight loss after surgery (Ortega, Fernandez-Canet, Alvarez-Valseita, Cassinello, & Baguena-Puigcerver, 2012).

Biological contributions to obesity include an increase in the stress hormone **cortisol**, which is a steroid hormone that is activated in response to stress and hypoglycemia and is believed to trigger depressive symptoms. In addition, medications used to treat depression may result in weight gain.

■ Obesity and Stress

Stress and anxiety may also interfere with one's ability to lose and manage weight. Various types of stress may contribute to obesity including emotional stress. Stress results in the secretion of cortisol, which has been shown to increase central adipose tissue and secondary risk factors for disease such as metabolic syndrome. Women may be more predisposed to stress than men due to increased central fat. Studies are beginning to focus on secretion of cortisol in women. Epel et al. (2015) exposed 59 women (30 with high hip to waist ratio, and 29 with a low hip to waist ratio) to three stressful sessions and one rest session. Women with the high hip to waist ratio secreted significantly more cortisol and reported greater challenges when stressed than did the low hip to ratio group. Another study examined the relationship between chronic stress, food cravings, and BMI for a community-based sample of adults ($N = 619$). Chronic stress had a significant effect on food cravings, and food cravings had a significant effect on BMI. Findings are consistent with research that chronic stress is related to motivation for reward-seeking behaviors and indicate that high food cravings may contribute to stress-related weight gain (Chaol, Grilo, White, & Sinha, 2015). Repeated stress associated with altered sleep habits and routines such as rotating work shifts are examples of environmental factors that may also increase weight.

■ Obesity and Vitamin D Deficiency

Vitamin D deficiency is common among children, adults, and elders. Research findings support that most tissues and cells of the body have a vitamin D receptor. Current research aims to discern the role of vitamin D in the prevention of chronic diseases such as cancer, cardiovascular, depression, and obesity (Holick, 2007). Vitamin D deficiency is defined as a 25-hydroxy vitamin D level of <20 ng/mL; 30 is considered sufficient, and toxicity may occur at 150 ng/mL. Wortsman, Matsuoka, Chen, Lu, and Holick (2000) found low levels of vitamin D in a sample of persons who were obese and that oral vitamin D corrected the deficiency. They further postulate that because of low physical activity levels, persons who are obese spend less time exposed to the sun and thus have lower vitamin D levels. Solar radiation is required for synthesis of vitamin D. It is also thought that vitamin D deficiency is linked to osteoporosis and muscle weakness that may be associated with observed immobility in persons who are obese (Holic, 2007). Seppa (2013) reported that persons with low Vitamin D levels were not prone to obesity and that losing weight could reverse vitamin D deficiency. Vitamin D supplements may not be effective as a weight loss regime. While vitamin D is stored in fat tissue, the mechanism for the role of vitamin D in weight loss requires additional research.

ETIOLOGY

A variety of factors influence obesity. The consequence of physical inactivity and its relationship to obesity is well documented in the public health literature. An imbalance between calories consumed and energy expenditure during occupational performance create a positive energy balance resulting in weight gain and obesity. Even a modest energy imbalance over a sustained period of time may increase BMI. Research has shown that losing 5% to 10% of excess weight may prevent disease (Diabetes Care, 2011). Location of grocery stores, food choices, and availability account for some obesity. Previously, lack of available food resulted in storing fat to prevent starvation. Now the type of food (such as fast, convenient, or refined) and high availability result in increased stored fat and the prevalence of obesity (Mance, Veach, & Veach, 2013).

■ Genetic Factors

Genetic factors combined with lifestyle choices increase the risk or predisposition for familial obesity. Patterns of childhood obesity are similar in appearance to adult obesity. Family, and adoption studies attribute obesity to a phenotype or observed characteristics of a group (e.g., family members who resemble each other in appearance) (MOSBY's Medical Dictionary, 1994, p. 1208). Studies examining the relationship of genetics to obesity report that 40% to 70% of the variance in body mass is related to social environment (type of food consumed, factors related to heredity, and physical inactivity). Clement, Boutin, and Froguel (2002) used genome scans to identify the location of 68 obesity genes on several chromosomes that aid in the regulation of appetite and satiety. A more recent study of genetics and obesity in 249,796 European participants identified 32 loci or markers associated with BMI. These markers, however, explained only 1.5% of the variance in BMI (Volkow, Wang, & Baler, 2011). Available research on genotyping and obesity has yielded small, uncertain, and limited explanation of the contribution of genetic markers to obesity. Inconsistent effects make it difficult to generalize results across populations.

■ Obesity Hypothalamus and Hypothyroidism

The inability of the hypothalamus to recognize satiety along with thyroid dysfunction may also result in obesity. The thyroid gland secretes the hormone thyroxin into the blood stream that is essential to the regulation of normal body growth and metabolism (processing food into energy). Thyroid cells absorb and use iodine. The pituitary gland and hypothalamus both control the thyroid. When thyroid hormone levels drop too low, the hypothalamus secretes TSH releasing hormone (TRH), which alerts the pituitary to produce thyroid stimulating hormone (TSH) (Sargis, 2015). **Hypothyroidism** occurs when cells of the thyroid gland are damaged by inflammation resulting from an associated autoimmune response or secondary medical interventions. The most common cause of thyroid gland failure is called autoimmune thyroiditis (Hashimoto's thyroiditis), a form of thyroid inflammation caused by the patient's own immune system (Sargis, 2015).

An endocrinologist may diagnose hypothyroidism with a medical and family history, risk factors, and physical examination. A definitive diagnosis may be achieved with a blood test called a TSH; additional laboratory analyses such as thyroxine or T4, and triiodothyronine or T3 also support the

diagnosis. Normally, the thyroid gland produces 80% T4 and 20% T3; T3 is the stronger of the two hormones (Sargis, 2015). Combined, T3 and T4 increase the rate of metabolism, affect body temperature, and regulate protein, fat, and carbohydrate catabolism (conversion of nutrients into energy) in the cells of the body. Without intervention, fatigue, weakness, weight gain, or increased difficulty losing weight increases. The inability to burn fat normally is often referred to as having a "fast" or "slow" metabolism (Mosby's Medical Dictionary, 1994, p. 1555). It is believed that weight loss may lead to decreased systemic inflammation that may restore thyroid function (Longhi & Radetti, 2013). Pharmacologic interventions such as synthetic hormones (Synthroid, levothyroxine sodium, liothyronine sodium) may be used to regulate hormone function (Sargis, 2015). Care must be taken to avoid a rapid increase in dosage to avoid symptoms of hyperthyroidism such as nervousness, tremor, tachycardia, arrhythmia, or menstrual irregularity (Carl, Gallo, & Johnson, 2014).

Hunger is associated with increased blood flow to the hypothalamus, thalamus, and frontal and temporal lobes. Destruction or trauma to the ventromedial hypothalamus, which regulates appetite and feeding behavior, may increase food intake and reduce metabolic rate resulting in obesity. **Leptin** is a hormone that is present in adipose tissue and signals receptors in the brain of satiety, or when one is full. Diminished leptin in the brain results in impaired signaling of satiety, thus promoting overeating. Females tend to have a higher percent of body fat or adipose tissue than do males; thus, with low levels of leptin they experience weight gain, increased hunger, and reduced metabolic rate (Atkinson, 2005; Couillard et al., 2002; Meyers, Leibel, Seeley, & Schwartz, 2010). For elders, low leptin levels, increased fat tissue, and loss of muscle mass are referred to as **sarcopenia**.

Gorden and Gavrilova (2003) report that leptin replacement leads to reduced food intake, weight loss, and reduced percent body fat. Satiety has also been achieved in both human and mouse models, but an increased resting metabolic rate only occurred in mice, suggesting that a loss of fat mass may impact resting metabolic rate.

■ Obesity and Neuroscience

Available research indicates that there is inconclusive but plausible evidence linking the neurobehavioral effects of overeating, obesity, and addiction (Ziauddeen, Farooq, & Fletcher, 2012). Neuroscientists are aware of neural structures that contribute to obesity; addiction research infers that addiction to food is similar to addiction to drugs both in behavioral and neurological response (Ziauddeen et al., 2012). Food addiction literature reports that foods high in fat, salt, and sugar are enjoyed by those who are obese. Processed foods may be more addictive than foods in their natural state such as fruits and vegetables (Benton, 2010). The addiction model supports the premise that obesity is related to food addiction and binge eating. Binge eating is characterized by uncontrolled, rapid consumption of large amounts of food in isolation and in the absence of hunger despite the negative impact on health, social or financial limitations. Multiple failed attempts to alter behavior results in feelings of guilt, remorse, distress, and failure (Smith & Robbins, 2013). The Yale Food Addiction Scale (YFAS) used DSM-5 addiction criteria to format questions that identify those who may exhibit signs of addiction toward certain foods (such as high fat, salt, and sugar). Knowledge of which foods trigger overeating and food addiction has the potential to impact food marketing strategies across the lifespan and may impact public policy (Gearhardt, Corbin, & Brownell, 2008).

Several neural structures are thought to contribute to addictive behavior and obesity. The hypothalamus regulates **satiety** or the feeling of fullness. The prefrontal cortex is associated with habitual and compulsive overeating; the dorsal striatum is responsible for loss of executive control over the behavior. Impulsive eating or initiating behavior without considering the consequences may be related to lower levels of dopamine. Insufficient dopamine may increase seeking of the feelings of reward and result in overeating (Volkow et al., 2002, 2011).

The more food that is consumed, the more one loses control and awareness of the amount of food consumed. Results of positron emission tomography studies show that striatal dopamine receptors are reduced in persons who are obese compared to leaner counterparts and that they tend to overeat to compensate for reduced striatal sensitivity (Mahapatra, 2010). Thus, long-term overeating of pleasurable foods alters the chemical response in the brain and sensitizes the brain to "crave certain foods"; thus the motivation and drive to eat and consume certain food increases

with environmental cues (Volkow & Wang, 2005; Volkow et al., 2011). Researchers are focusing on food addiction rather than diet and the possibility of prescribing pharmacological agents to artificially alter dopamine as an intervention for obesity. Proposed medications may be addictive and only recommended for those with morbid obesity and urgent health risks (Devlin, 2015).

PREVALENCE AND INCIDENCE

The global public health epidemic of obesity is often referred to as "**globesity**." Nationally obesity has doubled since 1980. The CDC, National Center for Health Statistics (NCHS) Data Brief (2015b) reports that the prevalence of obesity from 2011 to 2014 was 36% for adults and 17% for youth; for adults aged 20 to 39 and 40 to 59, the prevalence of obesity was higher among women than men; more than one-third of adults and youth in the United States were obese. If people who are classified as overweight are included, the estimate increases to 69% or two-thirds of the population (Mance et al., 2013). Harvard medical school researchers estimate that overweight, obesity, and physical inactivity were responsible for 1 in 10 deaths in the U.S. (Mance et al., 2013).

Regarding race, higher rates were noted with women who are African American at 56.9%, women who are Hispanic at 45.7%, men who are Hispanic at 39.9%, and 37.5% for men who are African American. People who are Asian tended to have lower rates of obesity at 11.9%. The average weight for men in the U.S. in 2011 was 88.3 kg (about 195 lb), and for women it was 74.7 kg (or 165 lb). Depending on BMI, this represents a significant increase (Mance et al., 2013). Recent findings by Ogden, Carroll, Kit, and Flegal (2014) reveal no significant reduction in obesity, and prevalence remains high.

Table 28.2 summarizes the prevalence of obesity across the lifespan.

Certain states and areas of the country have a high incidence of obesity No state had a prevalence of obesity <20%; 5 states and the District of Columbia had a prevalence of obesity between 20% and <25%; 23 states, Guam, and Puerto Rico had a prevalence of obesity between 25% and <30%; 19 states had a prevalence of obesity between 30% and <35%; 3 states (Arkansas, Mississippi, and West Virginia) had a prevalence

TABLE 28.2 Obesity Prevalence

Lifespan	Age	Prevalence of Obesity
Preschool	2–5	8.9%
School children	6–11	17.5%
Adolescents	12–19	20.5%
Young adults	20–39	32.3%
Middle adults	40–59	40.2%
Older adults	60 or >	37%

Adapted from the Center for Disease Control and Prevention National Center for Health Statistics Data Brief. (2015). *Prevalence of obesity among adults and youth: United States, 2011–2014.* Retrieved from http://www.cdc.gov.nchs/data/databriefs/db219.htm

of obesity of 35% or greater; and the Midwest had the highest prevalence of obesity (30.7%), followed by the South (30.6%), the Northeast (27.3%), and the West (25.7%) (CDC, 2014).

SIGNS AND SYMPTOMS

Classic signs and symptoms of obesity include pannus and abdominal fat, lymphedema, and OA. Obesity may also be described by the location and distribution of adipose or fat tissue, or **pannus** and its characteristic anthropometric shape. Dionne (2006) identified six body types: **apple ascites**, **apple pannus**, **pear abducted**, **pear adducted**, **gluteal shelf**, and **posterior adipose**. Each body type may be predisposed to challenges with activities of daily living, functional mobility, gait, and activity tolerance. These body types are described in Table 28.3.

■ Obesity and Lymphedema

Persons with obesity may experience compromised skin integrity secondary to skin on skin contact and impaired lymph drainage. Diabetes may further complicate wound healing and increase the risk of infection. For clients who are immobile, the **Braden Scale** may be used to predict risks for pressure sores (15 to 16 = low risk, 13 to 14 = moderate risk, 12 or less = high risk) (Braden, 2014).

A BMI > 50 often results in bilateral lower extremity edema associated with lymphatic dysfunction. Adipose tissue is composed of adipocytes or fat cells that produce hormones referred to as adipokines. These hormones cause a chemical reaction that impedes the function of the lymph system causing lymphatic leakage or **lymphedema** (swelling) (Greene, 2015). Obesity combined with decreased muscle pumping action further limits lymphatic function. The number of

TABLE 28.3 Body Type & Pannus Distribution

Body Type	Description
Apple Ascites	Weight centered around the abdomen
Apple Pannus	Increased hip width and weight around the pelvis
Pear Abducted	Weight located on the hips and upper thighs
Pear Adducted	Pannus located on the thighs
Gluteal Shelf	Pannus protrudes posteriorly
Posterior Adipose	Pannus distributed on the posterior trunk

Adapted with permission from Dionne's (2006) Six Body Types Images and Lisle E. Veach, PTcourses.com, 2013.

patent lymphatic vessels cannot keep up with the demand of new and proliferative adipose tissue; thus, the extra weight increases resistance to the distal and proximal flow of lymph (Bertsch, 2015; Greene, 2015). Impaired lymph node regeneration and abnormal swelling associated with cycles of weight loss and gain is known as primary lymphedema and may develop early in infancy, childhood, or adolescence and continue into adulthood (Greene, 2015). A diagnosis of lymphedema is made using lymphoscintigraphy, which verifies backflow or blocked lymphatics (Greene, 2015).

Abdominal obesity such as that observed in the apple ascites or apple pannus body type may compress the lymphatics in the abdominal and groin area and add to lower extremity edema. Weight loss may improve lymphatic function but may not reverse the condition (Bertsch, 2015). Decongestive therapy, dietary intervention, and weight loss are recommended as primary interventions.

■ Obesity and Osteoarthritis

Osteoarthritis is also known as degenerative joint disease (DJD) or a "wear and tear" disease. Clients 75 and older with obesity report higher knee pain and are more likely to be disabled (Jordan et al., 1996). Oviatt (2009) reports that 65% of adults with DJD are overweight or obese; 44% of those with DJD report limited physical activity. Persons 85 years of age and older, who are obese, account for 57% of annual hip and knee replacements. CDC Behavioral Risk Surveillance System data from 2009 revealed that 53% of adults with DJD had no leisure time activity, limited access to a fitness center for appropriate exercise, and lack of fitness instructors who are knowledgeable about DJD (Morbidity and Mortality Weekly Report 2011). BMI levels of ≥ 30 kg/m^2 increases joint loading and causes misaligned joints and failure of weakened quadriceps to contract adequately and absorb forces needed to transition from sit to stand (Sowers & Karvonen-Gutierrez, 2010). Coggon et al. (2001) suggest that those with obesity were nearly three times more likely than were those of normal weight to develop severe knee pain over a 3-year period. Of those who are overweight and obese, a reduction of weight by 5 kg, and achieving a BMI within the recommended normal range, would result in an estimated 24% reduction in knee surgeries associated with OA. Strong support for public health initiatives aimed at reducing the burden of knee OA by controlling obesity is needed.

■ Obesity Hypoventilation Syndrome

Sleep apnea is referred to as **obesity hypoventilation syndrome** (OHS) or pickwickian syndrome. OHS results from excess weight compressing on the chest, preventing breathing, and increasing the amount of carbon dioxide in the blood; lack of oxygen contributes to poor sleep quality and hypoxia (Mance et al., 2013). As weight increases around the neck, trunk, and abdomen, temporary lapses in breathing compromise respiratory function. Clients with obesity may benefit from using a larger electric hospital bed with the head of the bed elevated between 45 degrees to 90 degrees known as the **Fowler position** or elevating the head of the bed to 90 degrees and placing the arms over a bed table in a **orthopneic position**. Continuous positive airway pressure (CPAP) may also be used to achieve positive flow of air into the nasal passages in order to keep the airway open.

COURSE AND PROGNOSIS

Failure to achieve a sustained healthy weight with nonsurgical procedures, pharmacological intervention, dietary changes, and some physical activity will lead to more invasive procedures such as bariatric surgery. Outcome data focus on the total amount of weight lost, reduction in chronic health conditions, and number of prescribed pharmacological interventions used to treat comorbidities. Following bariatric surgery a weight loss of 50% to 70% is expected (Health Grades, 2013). There is a significant decrease or reversal of chronic conditions including type II diabetes and high cholesterol; improvements in blood glucose levels may appear within days following bariatric surgery (Health Grades, 2013). For clients with a BMI of 35 or with comorbidities, bariatric surgery resolves migraines (57%), hypertension (52% to 92%), cardiovascular disease (82%), dyslipidemia (63%), metabolic syndrome (80%), type II diabetes (83%), obstructive sleep apnea (74%), fatty liver (90%), gastroesophageal reflux disease (72% to 98%), urinary stress incontinence (44%), gout (72%), DJD (41% to 76%), polycystic ovarian syndrome (79%), depression (55%), reduced quality of life (95%), and mortality (89%) (Brethauer, Chand, & Schauer, 2006). Long-term health benefits also include lower risk of cardiovascular and cerebrovascular events with improved quality of life (Health Grades, 2013).

Quality of life following bariatric surgery depends on type of surgery and procedure, residual intestinal and digestive problems, discomfort and pain, and presence of excess skin folds. Clients requiring body contouring to reduce loose skin a year following surgery reported improved quality of life (Lier, Aastrom, & Rortveit, 2015). Occupational therapy faculty and student researchers surveyed 11 clients post bariatric surgery using an activity and functional health and well-being assessment. Average weight loss was 105.1 with highest loss of 189 lb. Although this was a small sample size, several themes emerged from the study. Post–bariatric surgery participants reported a significant increase in participation in instrumental activities of daily living (IADLs) that require physical movement, leisure pursuits, social interaction, and health maintenance. Even though participants achieved weight loss, some clients transferred food addiction to alcohol or other drug use. Additionally, clients experienced relationship changes and divorce and often reverted to previous unhealthy eating patterns and habits (Mata, Mikkola, Loveland, & Hallowell, 2015). Ortega et al. (2012) surveyed 60 morbidly obese clients (46 women and 14 men) 1 year post–bariatric surgery. Findings indicate that negative preoperative body image improved after surgery but self-esteem did not change. Overall findings suggest that psychological intervention is needed to prepare clients for realistic expectations following surgery and to improve postsurgical outcomes.

MEDICAL AND SURGICAL MANAGEMENT

Diet and exercise may be recommended at various levels of intervention. Clients at risk for a diagnosis of obesity (BMI 25) may receive primary health screenings to increase awareness about the health risk factors associated with obesity. Secondary intervention aims to prevent the progression of obesity (BMI >25 to 30) from becoming a chronic health issue and tertiary intervention (BMI > 30) attempts to maintain quality of life with chronic obesity (Garvey, Mechanick, & Einhorn, 2014).

Following a comprehensive review of systems, modifiable risk factors, and laboratory evaluations of blood work, clients may be prescribed pharmacological intervention or psychiatric consultation. More often, immediate interventions for weight loss, such as pharmacological interventions, are used to increase motivation and promote weight loss. It is important to recognize that side effects of some medications increase hunger, promote overeating, and result in weight gain or obesity. Glucocorticoids produce an increase in truncal adipose tissue and insulin and oral hypoglycemic drugs increase fat in tissues of persons with diabetics. Antipsychotics such as phenothiazine and antidepressants (selective serotonin reuptake inhibitors) also produce weight gain. Adrenergic antagonists such as propranolol reduce sympathetic nervous system acidity and lead to weight gain (Atkinson, 2005). Some of the Food and Drug Administration (FDA)–approved medications for the treatment of obesity may cause serious side effects and must be monitored. Currently, orlistat (Xenical) is used to absorb fats, decrease side effects including oily and frequent bowel movements, and increase absorption of fat-soluble vitamins (A, D, E, and K), so a multivitamin may be prescribed. Alli is a similar, less potent over-the-counter (OTC) version of orlistat. Qsymia, previously known as Qnexa, reduces appetite, contributes to satiety, and alters the taste of food. Belviq alters serotonin levels in the brain and may lead to addiction (Mance et al., 2013). Cortisol blockers are not yet FDA approved for weight management but may be used in the future to reduce the formation of central adipose tissue (Zeratsky, 2015).

There are many diets that claim to result in various levels of weight loss. Popular diets used for weight loss include Atkins, Human chorionic growth hormone (HCG) South Beach, Weight Watchers, the Zone, and Body for Life. The Atkins diet is a low-carbohydrate, high-protein diet that burns fat for fuel. Side effects may include reduced brain glucose and increased blood lipid levels. HCG is extracted from the urine of pregnant women and injected, while prescribing a restriction of calories to 500 per day. There is minimal evidence to support the efficacy of HCG, and it is not FDA approved. The South Beach diet is supported by research; balances carbohydrates, protein, and fat; and does not limit fruits and vegetables, which is a disadvantage for maintaining a restricted pattern of eating. The Zone diet requires 30% each of fats, protein, and carbohydrates and focuses on healthy grains and fiber. Body for Life program encourages six small meals per day to maintain stable blood sugar. Weight Watchers is well researched and uses a point system, a balanced meal plan, and a support group or online participation. Although there are many diets from which to select, a 69% obesity rate continues in the U.S.

■ Bariatric Surgery

Bariatric surgery is often recommended for persons with super or morbid obesity or for a BMI ≥ 40; a BMI of 35 with accompanying metabolic syndrome or sleep apnea may also benefit from surgical intervention. The goal of bariatric surgery is to lose 50% of body weight or achieve a healthy target weight. An interprofessional bariatric health care team may include a bariatric physician or surgeon, nurse, psychiatrist, dietician or nutritionist, physical therapist, and occupational therapist.

Bariatric surgery produces a quick reduction in weight; when combined with a healthy diet and consistent physical activity, weight loss can be sustained over a period of time. There are two general surgical strategies: stapling and banding. Within these two categories, there are several surgical procedures available. Each may be associated with complications such as diarrhea, bleeding, infection, malabsorption and lower extremity blood clots (Table 28.4; Figure 28.2).

TABLE 28.4 Advantages and Disadvantages of Different Types of Bariatric Surgery		
Surgery Type	**Advantage**	**Disadvantage**
Gastric band • A band is placed around the upper stomach	• Restricts amount of food consumed • Food is absorbed • Band is adjustable • Slower weight loss • Surgery can be reversed	• Access port may leak • Band may erode stomach wall • Band may slip • Slower weight loss
Roux-en-Y • A pouch limits food intake • Y-shape bypasses the small intestine; reduces absorption	• Substantial weight loss • Reduced absorption of calories • Resolves metabolic syndrome	• Impedes absorption of nutrients, iron, and calcium • Increased bone deficiency • Procedure is permanent/nonreversible
Biliopancreatic diversion with duodenal switch • Creates a sleeve stomach • Duodenum: divided for pancreatic and bile drainage	• Resolves metabolic syndrome • Eat a larger meal	• Initial liquid bowel movements • Abdominal bloating • Foul-smelling stool or gas • Increased risk of gallstones • Intestinal irritation and ulcers
Orbera intragastric balloon • Inserted in stomach and filled with saline	• BMI > 30 and <40 kg/m^2 • Multiple failed weight loss attempts • Required 12-month lifestyle change • After 30–50 lb weight loss • Balloon is removed • 6 month follow-up	• Balloon may deflate • Weight loss will slow

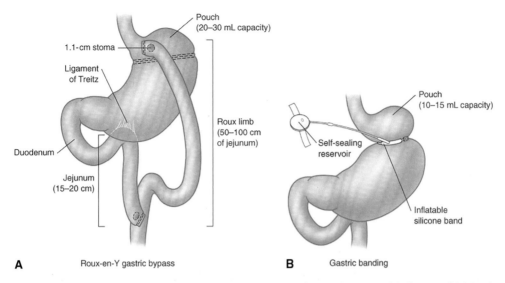

Figure 28.2 Two surgical procedures for morbid obesity. **A.** Gastric bypass with Roux-en-Y. A horizontal row of staples creates a pouch with a capacity of 50 mL or less. The proximal jejunum is transected and the distal end anastomosed to the new pouch. The proximal segment is anastomosed to the jejunum. **B.** Laparoscopic gastric banding. The silicone adjustable band component of the lap band is placed around the upper part of the stomach, forming a small gastric pouch (15 mL) to limit intake and slow gastric emptying. Size is adjusted by injection of saline into a subcutaneous reservoir that is connected to the lap band. (From Farrell, M., & Dempsey, J. (2010). *Smeltzer and Bare's textbook of medical–surgical nursing* (2nd ed.). Philadelphia, PA: Wolters Kluwer.)

IMPACT ON OCCUPATIONAL PERFORMANCE

Obesity is a modifiable risk factor that impacts multiple client factors and performance skills, patterns, and occupational engagement. Persons with obesity may experience changes in mental functions (mood) associated with altered levels of serotonin. Medications used to treat depression may result in weight gain but aid in appetite control. Excess weight aggravates symptoms of OA resulting in loss of joint structures, destruction of cartilage, and spinal and peripheral nerve compression. Joint pain, malalignment, reduced range of motion, and disuse atrophy limit mobility and activity tolerance.

Diminished skin integrity is another challenge for persons with obesity. Loose skin may cause friction and reduced skin integrity between the thighs during ambulation. Excess skin may need to be camouflaged by wearing larger rather than fitted clothing. Because of multiple skin folds associated with pannus under the breasts, around the abdomen, and perineal area, it is difficult to maintain hygiene following urination or bowel movement. Clients may become embarrassed to have a family member or caregiver perform this task. Skin may have poor vascularization secondary to atherosclerosis and lymphedema. Prolonged sitting in one position or changing position may result in skin shearing, abrasions, or other pressure sores. Clients may be dependent for pressure relief including lateral weight shifts and raises.

Performance of occupations (such as activities of daily living) that are usually performed in the bathroom (bathing and toileting) and self-feeding a meal in the kitchen or dining room are now performed in the same location, which is often in bed. These clients may experience shame and loss of self-esteem and prefer social isolation. Loss of intimacy and lack of human touch may also hinder self-concept. Lack of mobility and tolerance to supine and prone positions in bed may interfere with breathing. Positioning in a wheelchair or chair may be ill tolerated secondary to neuropathy, peripheral vascular disease, or pressure sores related to type II diabetes. Clients may perform at a slower pace and require a wheelchair or other mobility aide to access the community. The increased cost for larger assistive technology such as a wheelchair and accessible van may not be reimbursed by the insurance provider. The inability to fit into a standard-size chair, car seat, or restaurant booth restricts driving, social participation, educational pursuits and work.

The lack of awareness of clearly defined occupations that promote planned energy expenditure versus energy conservation may impede progressive and graded physical activity needed to achieve a steady reduction in weight over time. Altered roles, habits and previously performed routines must be modified to achieve maximum participation in occupations.

CASE STUDY 1

Candice is a 10-year-old female who is 5′4″ and weighs 234 lb. She has three brothers who are active in a variety of sports and are of normal weight. Both parents are slightly overweight and believe Candice will grow out of her obesity. Candice snacks throughout the day and prefers cookies, candy, and fried chicken fingers for lunch. She consumes 3 to 4 cans of sugared soda daily. During the last physician's visit, a thyroid panel consisting of a T4 and T3 was ordered along with a screening for depression. The thyroid panel was negative, but Candice demonstrated signs and symptoms of depression. She informed her mother that she has been feeling stressed at school because she is being bullied and teased about her weight. Her brothers usually hang out with their friends and were not aware of the teasing and bullying. Candice has asked her parents if she can get bariatric surgery to help lose weight so that she may be treated like other girls. Her parents are slow to agree with the surgery because the bullying may not change after the surgery. Candice's parents have asked her if she would like to transfer to another school.

CASE STUDY 2

Mildred is an 85-year-old woman who is a resident of a long-term care facility. She has lived at the facility for 10 years, and her BMI has increased from 30 (260 lb) to 40 (380 lb). She has difficulty sleeping in a flat position in bed. Her roommate informed the nurse that Mildred's snoring and breathing keeps her awake at night. Mildred complains of knee pain associated with OA and increasing difficulty with standing and ambulation; a wheelchair is used for long distances. The nursing staff noticed that her participation in transfers to bed, toilet, and shower chair are becoming more difficult. Over the last 3 months, the facility replaced two commodes that cracked when the client sat down. The occupational therapist is recommending a commode with a load capacity of 500 to 1,000 lb. The certified nursing assistant (CNA) reported that Mildred's feet continue to swell and she has developed a rash between breast, abdominal, and perineal skin folds. The facility administrator and director of nursing is concerned about the safety and well-being of the client and staff and adherence to state nursing home regulations. Mildred has expressed a desire to remain at this facility because the staff treats her like family. She realizes she does not have the willpower to lose weight and has requested to be moved to a room that has a larger bed, commode, and mechanical lift that can handle her weight. Patient rights indicate that the client has the right to eat and gain weight.

LEARNING RESOURCES

Center for Disease and Prevention Adolescent Growth Charts

http://www.cdc.gov/healthyweight/assessing/bmi/childrens_bmi/about_childrens_bmi.html

Center for Disease Control and Prevention BMI Calculation for BMI Percentile Calculator for Child and Teen English Version

https://nccd.cdc.gov/dnpabmi/calculator.aspx

BARIATRIC SURGERY RESOURCES

- http://obesityreporter.com/bariatric-weight-loss-surgery-statistics-updated-2015/
- https://asmbs.org/patients/bariatric-surgery-misconceptions
- http://www.bariatric-surgery-source.com/obesity-united-states-statistics.html
- http://www.medpagetoday.com/Surgery/GeneralSurgery/39629
- https://asmbs.org/resources/estimate-of-bariatric-surgery-numbers

- http://www.pharmacytimes.com/publications/issue/2014/July2014/Complications-of-Bariatric-Surgery-Dumping-Syndrome-and-Drug-Disposition
- http://www.ncbi.nlm.nih.gov/pubmed/20622654
- http://www.sciencedirect.com/science/article/pii/S1550728909005309

REFERENCES

Allison, M., & Lee, C. (2015). Too fat, too thin: Understanding bias against overweight and underweight in an Australian female university student sample. *Psychology and Health*, *30*(2), 189–202. doi: 10.1080/08870446.2014.954575

American College of Sports Medicine (2000). *Guidelines for exercise testing and prescription* (6th ed., p. 64). Philadelphia, PA: Lippincott Williams & Wilkins.

American College of Sports Medicine. (2012). *Measuring and evaluating body composition*. Retrieved from http://www.acsm.org/public-information/articles/2012/01/12/measure

American College of Sports Medicine. (2014). Classification of disease risk based on BMI and waist circumference. *ACSM's resources for the personal trainer* (4th ed., p. 311). China: Lippincott Williams & Wilkins.

Atkinson, R. L. (2005). Etiologies of obesity. In D. J. Goldstein (ed.), *The management of eating disorders and obesity* (2nd ed., pp. 107–109). Totowa, NJ: Humana Press. Retrieved from http://www.iub.edu/~k536/articles/etiology/etiology%20atkinson%202005.pdf

Bailey, M. (2016). Understanding obesity and depression. *Healthy Living*, *5*(1), 19.

Benton, D. (2010). The plausibility of sugar addiction and its role in obesity and eating disorders.

Clinical Nutrition, *29*(3), 288–303. doi: 10.1016/j.clnu.2009.12.001

Bertsch, T. (2015). Obesity related lymphedema. *Lymph Link*, *28*(3), 1–2. Retrieved from http://www.lymphnet.org/pdfDocs/Vol_28-N3_PP_Obesity-related_LE.pdf

Blackburn, G. L., & Kanders, B. S. (1987). Medical evaluation and treatment of the obese patient with cardiovascular disease. *American Journal of Cardiology*, *60*(21), 55G–58G.

Blanchard, S. (2009). Variables impacting obesity among African American women in Omaha. *American Journal of Occupational Therapy*, *63*(1), 58–68.

Blanchard, S. (2012). Societal statement on obesity. *Journal of American Occupational Therapy*, *66*(6), S81–S82.

Blanchard, S., & Mosley, L.J. (2010). Geriatric obesity. *American Occupational Therapy Association Gerontology Special Interest Section Quarterly*, *3*(2), 1–4.

Blodorn, A., Major, B., Hunger, J., & Miller, C. (2015). Unpacking the psychological weight of weight stigma: A rejection-expectation pathway. *Journal of Experimental Social Psychology*, *63*, (20116), 69–76. doi: 10.1016/j.jesp.2015.12.003

Bout-Tabaku, S., Michalsky, M. P., Jenkins, T. M., Baughcum, A., Zeller, M. H., Brandt, M. L., ...

Inge, T. H. (2015). Musculoskeletal pain, self-reported physical function, and quality of life in the teen—Longitudinal assessment of bariatric surgery (teen-labs) cohort. *Journal of the American Medical Association Pediatrics, 169*(6), 552–559. doi: 10.1001/jamapediatrics.2015.0378

Braden, B. (2014). *Braden scale score.* Retrieved from http://www.phca.org/education/docs/webinars/webinar-20140805.pdf

Brethauer, S. A., Chand, B., & Schauer, P. R. (2006). Risks and benefits of bariatric surgery: Current evidence. *Cleveland Clinic Journal of Medicine, 73,* 1–15. Retrieved from https://my.clevelandclinic.org/ccf/media/files/Bariatric_Surgery/schauerbest.pdf

Calle, E. E., & Thung, M. J. (2004). Obesity and cancer. *Oncogene, 23,* 6365–6378. doi: 10.1038/sj.onc.1207751

Carl, L. L., Gallo, J. A., & Johnson, P. R. (2014). Medications used to treat thyroid disease, parathyroid disease, and osteoporosis. In L. L. Carl, J. A. Gallo, & P. R. Johnson (Eds.), *Practical pharmacology in rehabilitation* (pp. 502–524). Champaign, IL: Human Kinetics.

Center for Disease Control and Prevention. (2011). *Childhood obesity facts: Prevalence of childhood obesity in the United States, 2011–2012.* Retrieved from http://www.cdc.gov/obesity/data/childhood.html

Center for Disease Control and Prevention. (2014). *Obesity prevalence maps.* Retrieved from http://www.cdc.gov/obesity/data/prevalence-maps.html

Center for Disease Control and Prevention. (2015a). *Defining overweight and obesity.* Retrieved from http://www.cdc.gov/obesity/adult/defining.html

Center for Disease Control and Prevention National Center for Health Statistics Data Brief. (2015b). *Prevalence of obesity among adults and youth: United States, 2011–2014.* Retrieved from http://www.cdc.gov/nchs/data/databriefs/db219.htm

Centers for Medicare and Medicaid. (2014). *MDS3.0 information.* Retrieved from http://www.ahcancal.org/facility_operations/Documents/RAI_3.0/MDS%203%200%20Chapter%203%20Section%20K%20V1.02%20May%2028,%202010.pdf

Chaol, A., Grilo, C. M., White, M. A., & Sinha, R. (2015). Food cravings mediate the relationship between chronic stress and body mass index. *Journal of Health Psychology, 20,* 721–729.

Chuang, Y. F., An, Y., Bilgel, M., Wong, D. F., Troncoso, J. C., O'Brien, R. J., ... Thambisetty, M. (2015). Midlife adiposity predicts earlier onset of Alzheimer's dementia, neuropathology and presymptomatic cerebral amyloid accumulation. *Molecular Psychiatry.* doi: 10.1038/mp.2015.129

Clement, K., Boutin, P., & Froguel, P. (2002). Genetics of obesity. *American Journal of Pharmacogenomics, 2*(3), 177–187. doi: 10.2165/00129785-200202030-00003

Coggon, D., Reading, I., Croft, P., McLaren, M., Barrett, D., & Cooper, C. (2001). Knee osteoarthritis and obesity. *International Journal of Obesity and Related Metabolic Disorders, 25*(5), 622–627. doi: 10.1038/sj.ijo.0801585

Couillard, C., Mauriege, P., Prud Homme, D., Nadeau, A., Trerrblay, A., Bouchard, C., et al. (2002). Plasma leptin response to an epinephrine infusion in lean and obese women. *Obesity Research, 10*(1), 6–13.

Crandall, C. S. (1994). Prejudice against fat people: Ideology and self-interest. *Journal of Personality and Social Psychology, 66,* 882–894.

Dallas Center for Obesity Surgery. (2013). *BMI classifications.* Retrieved from http://www.obesitysurgerydallas.com/bmi.html

Devlin, M. J. (2007) Is there a place for obesity in DSM-V? *International Journal of Eating Disorders, 40,* S83–S88. doi: 10.1002/eat.

Devlin, F. (2015). *The real cause of obesity: Addicted to food.* Retrieved from www.youramazingbrain.org.uk/General_HC_Flora_Devlin.pdf

Diabetes Care. (2011, July), *34*(7), 1481–1486. doi: 10.233371/dc 10-2415. Epub 201 May 18, accessed May 24, 2013.

Dionne, M. (2006). *Among giants: Courageous stories of those who are obese and those who care for them* (pp. 70–95). LuLu Press. Retrieved from http://www.bariatricrehab.com

Dixon, J. B., Dixon, M. E., & Obrien, P. E. (2003). Depression in association with severe obesity changes with weight loss. *Archives of Internal Medicine, 163,* 2058–2065. Retrieved from http://dx.doi.org/10.1001/archinte.163.17.2058

Dutton, G. R., Tan, F., Perri, M. G. et al. (2010). What words should we use when discussing excess weight? *Journal of the American Board of Family Medicine, 23,* 606–613.

Epel, E. S., McEwen, B., Seeman, T., Matthews, K., Castellazzo, G., Brownell, K. D., ... Ickovics, J. R. (2015). Stress and body shape: Stress induced cortisol is consistently greater among women with central fat. *Psychosomatic Medicine, 62*(5), 623–632.

Faith, M. S., Matz, P. E., & Jorge, M. N. (2002). Obesity-depression associations in the population. *Journal of Psychosomatic Research, 53,* 935–942. Retrieved from http://dx.doi.org/10.1016(50022-3999)(02)00308-2

Flint, S. W. (2015). Obesity stigma: Prevalence and impact in healthcare. *British Journal of Obesity, 1*(1), 14–18.

Flower, K. B., Perrin, E. M., Viadro, C. I., & Ammerman, A. S. (2007). Using body mass index to identify overweight children: Barriers and facilitators in primary care. *Ambulatory Pediatrics, 7*(1), 38–44.

Foti, D. (2005, February 7). Caring for the person of size. *OT Practice,* 9–14.

Garvey, W. T., Mechanick, J. I., & Einhorn, D. (2014). *2014 advanced framework for a new diagnosis of obesity as a chronic disease.* The American Association of Clinical Endocrinologists and the American College of Endocrinology. Retrieved from https://www.aace.com/files/2014-advanced-framework-for-a-new-diagnosis-of-obesity-as-a-chronic-disease.pdf

Gearhardt, A. N., Corbin, W. R., & Brownell, K. D. (2008). Preliminary validation of the Yale food addiction scale. *Appetite, 52,* 430–436.

Gorden, P., & Gavrilova, O. (2003). The clinical uses of leptin. *Current Opinion in Pharmacology, 3,* 655–659. doi: 10.1016/j.com.2003.06.006

Greene, A. K. (2015) Obesity-induced lymphedema. In A. K. Green, S. A. Summer, & H. Brorson (Eds.), *Lymphedema presentation, diagnosis and treatment* (pp. 97–104). Retrieved from http://link.springer.com/chapter/10.1007/978-3-319-14493-1_9#page-1

Grever, J. (2013). *APA: Obesity rejected as psychiatric diagnosis in DSM 5.* Retrieved from www.medpagetoday.com/MeetingCoverage/APA/20381

Health Grades. (2013). *Health grades bariatric surgery report 2013.* Retrieved from https://d2dcgio-3q2u5fb.cloudfront.net/

Holic, M. (2007). Vitamin D deficiency. *The New England Journal of Medicine, 357,* 266–281.

Jacobs, E. (2010). Larger waist size increases health risk. *Archives of Internal Medicine.* Retrieved from http://www.cancer.org/Cancer/news/News/larger-waist-size-increases-health-risks

Jones, D. P. (2015, May 13). *Press release: Rudd Center study finds support for obesity designation as disease.* Retrieved from http://today.uconn.edu/2015/05/rudd-center-study-finds-support-for-obesity-designation-as-disease/

Jordan, J., Luta, G., Renner, J., Linder, F., Dragomir, A., Hochberg, M., & Fryer, J. (1996). Self-reported functional status in osteoarthritis of the knee in a rural southern community: The role of sociodemographics factors, obesity, and knee pain. *Arthritis Care and Research, 9*(4), 273–278.

Kolata, G. (2015, November 3). Morbid obesity. *New York times Health Information.* Retrieved from http://www.nytimes.com/health/guides/symptoms/morbid-obesity/

Kresser, C. (2015). *Let's take back your health-starting now.* Retrieved from http://chriskresser.com/diabesity/

Lier, H. O., Aastrom, S., & Rortveit, K. (2015). Patients' daily life experiences five years after gastric bypass surgery—A qualitative study. *Journal of Clinical Nursing, 25*(3–4), 322–331. doi: 10.1111/jocn.13049

Longhi, S., & Radetti, G. (2013). Thyroid function and obesity. *Journal of Clinical Research in Pediatric Endocrinology, 5*(Suppl. 1), 40–49. doi: 10.4274/Jcrpe.856

Mahapatra, A. (2010). Overeating, obesity, and dopamine receptors. *American Chemical Society Neuroscience, 1,* 346–347. doi: 10.1021/cn100044y

Mance, P., Veach, M., & Veach, L. E. (2013). *Mobilizing bariatric patients* (p. 13). Retrieved from info@OTcourses.com

Mata, H., Mikkola, A., Loveland, J., & Hallowell, P. T. (2015). Occupational therapy and bariatric surgery: Discovering occupation after weight-loss surgery. *OT Practice, 20*(1), 11–15.

Meyers, M. G., Leibel, R. L., Seeley, R. J., & Schwartz, M. W. (2010). Obesity and leptin resistance: Distinguishing cause form effect. *Trends in Endocrinology and Metabolism, 21*(11), 643–651. doi: 10.1016/j.tem.2010.08.002

Morbidity and Mortality Weekly Report (2011, December 9). State-specific prevalence of no leisure time physical activity among adults with and without doctor-diagnosed arthritis—United States, 2009. *Weekly, 60*(48), 1641–1645. Retrieved from http://www.cdc.gov/mmwr/preview/mmwrhtml/mm6048a1.htm

Mosby's Medical, Nursing, & Allied Health Dictionary. (1994). *Thyroid gland* (p. 1555). St. Louis, MO: Mosby.

National Heart Lung and Blood Institute. (2015). *Aim for a healthy weight. Calculate your BMI.* Retrieved from http://www.nhlbi.nih.gov/health/educational/lose_wt/BMI/bmicalc.htm

Ogden, C. L., Carroll, M. D., Kit, B. K., & Flegal, K. M. (2014). Prevalence of childhood and adult obesity in the United States, 2011–2012. *Journal of the American Medical Association, 311*(8), 806–814. doi: 10.1001/jama.2014.732

Ortega, J., Fernandez-Canet, R., Alvarez-Valseita, S., Cassinello, N., & Baguena-Puigcerver, M. J. (2012). Predictor of psychological symptoms in morbidly obese patients after gastric bypass surgery. *Surgery for Obesity and Related Diseases, 8*(2012), 770–776. doi: 10.1016/j.soard.2011.03.015

Oviatt, J. (2009). *Obese are three times as likely to need a hip or knee replacement.* Canadian Institute of Health Information. Retrieved from http://secure.cihi.ca/cihiweb/dispPage.jsp?cw_page=media_17aug2005_e

Padro, C. M., Gonzales, M. C., & Heymsfield, S. B. (2015). Body composition, phenotypes, and obesity paradox. *Current Opinion Clinical Nutrition, Metabolic Care, 18*(6), 535–551. doi: 10.10971MCO:0000000000000216

Puhl, R. M., & Brownell, K. D. (2006). Confronting and coping with weight stigma: An investigation of overweight and obese adults. *Obesity (Silver Spring), 14,* 1802–1815.

Puhl, R. M., & Latner, J. D. (2007). Stigma, obesity, and the health of the Nation's children.
Psychological Bulletin, 133, 557–580.

Purnell, J. Q. (2011). *Obesity.* Retrieved from http://online.
statref.com/Document.aspx?docAddress=y8WQZw
DPhnJaDA-oItwrwg%3d%3d&SessionId=2224496L
QUSTYXSK&Scroll=1&goBestMatch=true&
Index=1&searchContext=define+bariatrics|c0||10|1|0|
0|0|0||c0&minimalsize=1,doi:10.2310/7900.1051

Sales-Martinez, S. (2013). *AMA declares obesity a
disease: Should we like this decision?* Retrieved
from https://www.nutrition.org/asn-blog/2013/08/
ama-declares-obesity-a-disease

Sargis, R. M. (2015). *Thyroid gland overview.*
Retrieved from http://www.endorineweb.com/
endocrinology/overview-thyroid

Schvey, N. A., Shomaker, L. B., Kelly, N. R.,
Pickworth, C. K., Cassidy, O., Galescu, O., et al.
(2016). Pressure to be thin and insulin sensitivity among adolescents. *Journal of Adolescent
Health, 58,* 104–110. Retrieved from http://dx.doi.
org/10.1016/j.jadohealth.2015.09.010

Seppa, N. (2013). *Link between obesity and vitamin D
clarified.* Retrieved from https://www.sciencenews.
org/article/link-between-obesity-and-vitaminD

Shah, A. S., Dolan, L. M., Khoury, P. R., Gao, Z.,
Kimball, T. R., & Urbina, E. M. (2015). Severe
obesity in adolescents and young adults is associated with sub-clinical cardiac and vascular changes.
*Journal of Clinical Endocrinology & Metabolism,
100*(7), 2751–2757. doi: 10.1210/jc.2014-4562

Smith, L. (2013). *A name by any other? AMA
declares obesity as disease.* Retrieved from
http://www.nutrition.org/asn-blog/2013/08/
ama-declares-obesity-a-disease

Smith, D. G., & Robbins, T. W. (2013). The neurological underpinnings of obesity and binge eating: A
rationale for adopting the food addiction model.
Biological Psychiatry, 73, 804–810. Retrieved from
http://dx.doi.org/10.1016/j.biopsych.2012.08.026

Sowers, M., & Karvonen-Gutierrez, C. A. (2010).
The evolving role of obesity in knee osteoarthritis. *Current Opinion in Rheumatology, 22*(5),
533–537. doi: 10.1097/BOR.0b013e32833b4682

Sperling, R. A., Laviolette, P. S., O'Keefe, K., O'Brien,
J., Rentz, D. M., Pihlajamaki, M., et al. (2009). Early
warning: Key Alzheimer's brain changes observed in
unimpaired older humans. *Neuron, 63,* 178–188.

Stedman's Medical Dictionary. (2006). *Bariatrics.*
Wolters Kluwer Health, Lippincott Williams &
Wilkins. Retrieved from http://online.statref.com/
Splash.aspx?SessionID=2224496LQUSTYXSK

Stunkard, A. J., & Sorensen, T. I. A. (1993). Obesity
and socioeconomic status—A complex relation.
New England Journal of Medicine, 329, 1036–1037.

Tailor, A., & Ogden, J. (2009). Avoiding the term
"obesity": An experimental study of the impact

of doctor's language on patients' beliefs. *Patient
Education and Counseing, 76,* 260–264.

Teachman, B. A., & Brownell, K. D. (2001). Implicit
anti-fat bias among health professionals, is anyone
immune? *International Journal of Obesity and
Related Metabolic Disorders, 25,* 1525–1531.

Tonetti, L., Fabri, M., Filardi, M., Martoni, M., &
Natale, V. N. (2015). The association between
higher body mass index and poor school performance in high school students. *Pediatric Obesity.*
doi: 10.1111/ijpo.12075

University of Rochester Minnesota. (2015). *Top
10 most common health issues.* Retrieved from
https://www.urmc.rochester.edu/senior-health/
common-issues/top-tenaspx

Volkow, N. D., & Wang, R. A. (2005). How can drug
addiction help us understand obesity. *Lancet, 357,*
354–357.

Volkow, N. D., Wang, G. J., & Baler, R. D.; National
Institute of Health Public Access. (2011). Reward
dopamine and the control of food take: Implications
for obesity. *Trends in Cognitive Science, 15*(1),
37–46. doi: 10.1016/j.tics.2010.11.001

Volkow, N. D., Wang, G. J., Fowler, J. S., Logan,
J., Jayne, M., Franceschi, D., et al. (2002).
"Nonhedonic" food motivation in humans involves
dopamine in the dorsal striatum and methvlpheni-
date amplifies this effect. *Synapse, 44,* 175–180.

Walsh, B. (2010). *Approaches to the diagnosis and
classification of eating disorders in DSM-V* (p.
106). APA. Retrieved from http://www.medpageto-
day.com/MeetingCoverage/APA/20381

Wang, S. S., Brownell, K. D., & Wadden, T. A.
(2004). The influence of the stigma of obesity on
overweight individuals. *International Journal of
Obesity, 28,* 1333–1337.

World Health Organization. (2015). *Global health
observatory data: Mean body mass index (BMI).*
Retrieved from http://www.who.int/gho/ncd/
risk_factors/bmi_text/en/

Wortsman, J., Matsuoka, L. Y., Chen, T. C., Lu, Z., &
Holick, M. F. (2000). Decreased bioavailability of
vitamin D in obesity. *American Journal of Clinical
Nutrition, 72,* 690–693.

Xiang, X., & Ruopeng, A. (2014). Obesity and
onset of depression among middle-aged and
older adults. *Journal of Psychosomatic Research,
78*(2015), 242–248. Retrieved from http://dx.doi.
org/10.1016/j.jpsychores2014.12.0080022-3999

Zeratsky, K. (2015). *Can cortisol blockers such as
CortiSlim help me lose weight?* Retrieved from http://
www.mayoclinic.org/healthy-lifestyle/weight-loss/
expert-answers/cortisol-blockers/faq-20058132

Ziauddeen, H., Farooq, I. S., & Fletcher, P. C. (2012).
Obesity and the brain: How convincing is the
addiction model? *Nature Reviews Neuroscience,
13*(4), 279–286. doi: 10.1038/nrn3212

Index

Page numbers followed by *f* or *t* refer to illustrations or tables, respectively

O